AF293594

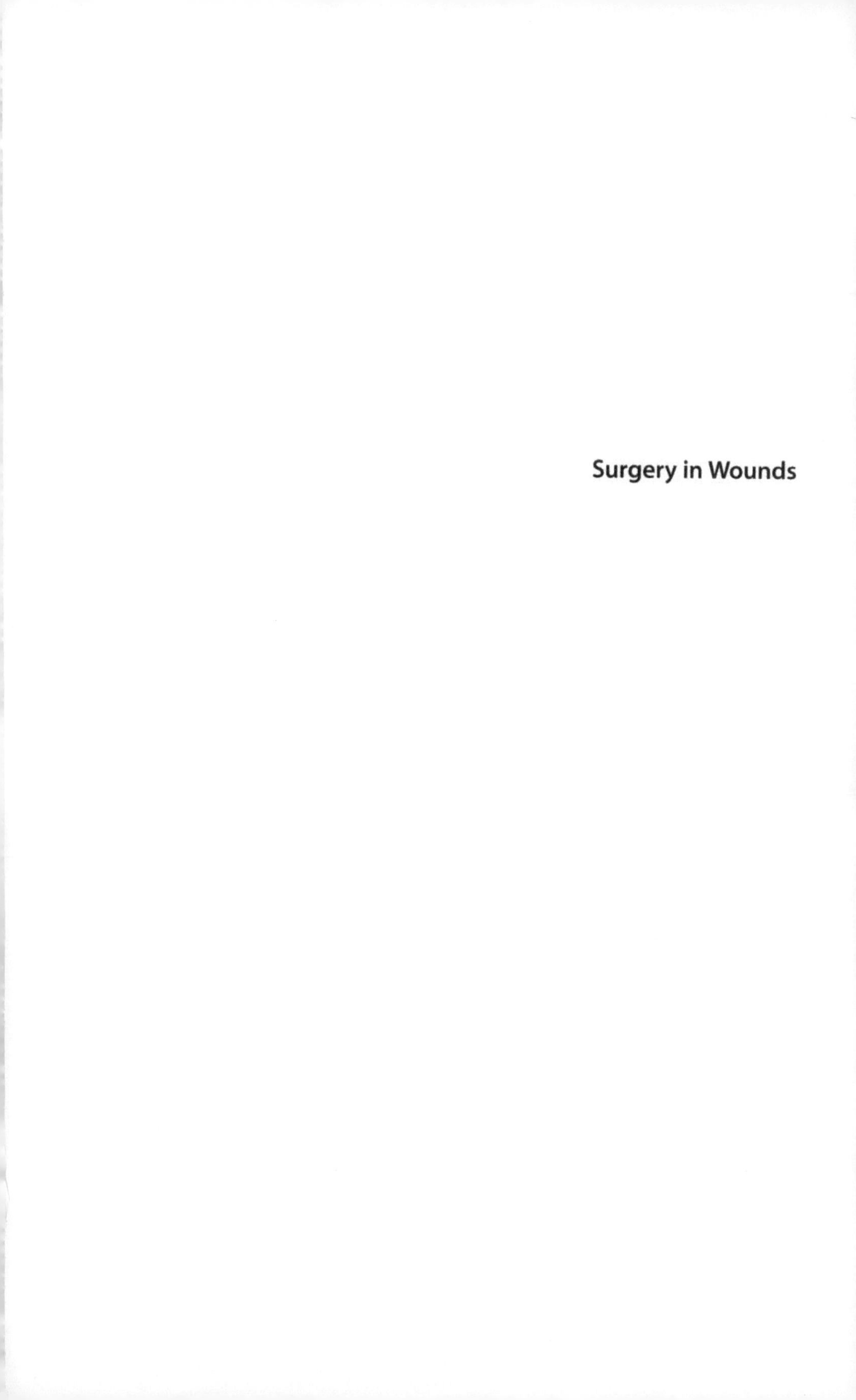

**Surgery in Wounds**

Springer

*Berlin*
*Heidelberg*
*New York*
*Hong Kong*
*London*
*Milan*
*Paris*
*Tokyo*

L. Téot · P.E. Banwell · U.E. Ziegler (Eds.)

# Surgery in Wounds

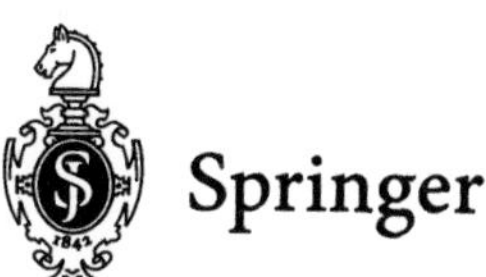

Springer

**Luc Téot**, Professor
Service des Brûles
Hôpital Lapeyronie
391 Avenue du Doyen Giraud
34255 Montpellier Cedex
France

**Ulrich E. Ziegler**, Dr. med.
Plastische Chirurgie und Handchirurgie
Chirurgische Universitätsklinik
Josef-Schneider-Str. 2
97080 Würzburg
Germany

**Paul E. Banwell**, BSc MB BS FrCS
Department of Plastic Surgery
Radcliffe Infirmary
Woodstock Road
Oxford
Oxon OX2 8HE
United Kingdom

ISBN-13: 978-3-642-63929-6     e-ISBN-13: 978-3-642-59307-9
DOI: 10.1007/978-3-642-59307-9

Cataloging-in-Publication Data applied for
A catalog record for this book is available from the Library of Congress.

Bibliographic information published by Die Deutsche Bibliothek
Die Deutsche Bibliothek lists this publication in the Deutsche Nationalbibliografie;
detailed bibliographic data is available in the Internet at http://dnb.ddb.de



Springer-Verlag  Berlin  Heidelberg  New York
a member of Springer Science+Business Media GmbH

http://www.springer.de/medizin



Cover Design: design & production GmbH, Heidelberg
Typesetting: Hilger VerlagsService, Heidelberg

Printed on acid-free paper          SPIN 11008019          5 4 3 2 1 0

# Foreword

Wounds have existed since the beginning of time, and records of their nature and treatment are found in the earliest documents. Interestingly, many of these treatments are now being rediscovered or re-used in modern-day clinical practice. In addition to the diverse nature of treatments that have been suggested as being beneficial for wounds, over many centuries there has been a range of clinicians who have cared for patients with wounds, and in many parts of the world today it is not doctors but other professional colleagues – e.g. nurses or podiatrists – who are the most knowledgeable persons on wounds and wound treatments. Finally, the nature of wounds seen in clinical practice is changing. Increasing destructive power is resulting in more severe injuries occurring in patients involved in conflict. Developments in surgical techniques have enabled new surgical procedures to be offered to patients, but novel and more severe complications can result from such technical advances. In addition, many societies around the world are having to deal with an increasing ageing population, and huge increases in the number of patients suffering from chronic wounds are being seen.

In summary, expanding treatment options, diverse groups of clinicians caring for patients and changes in the nature of wounds seen in clinical practice are real issues that have to be faced, and solutions have to be found if patients are to receive optional care for their wounds. This book, that addresses the role of surgery and wounds, is a timely reminder that surgical interventions can be beneficial for a large majority of patients suffering from wounds and wound-healing difficulties. The challenge remains of which patient, which treatment option and who is to provide such care for the patients.

The relatively recent expansion of knowledge relating to the underlying pathophysiology of the body's response to injury has provided a platform for recognising what needs to be done both to create healing and to minimise the problems of scarring in patients with wounds. The recognition that not all treatments or interventions are employed to produce closure of a wound in a single step is evidence of the maturing thought processes of individuals involved in this area. The new term wound-bed preparation is probably nothing more than good clinical care, but provides a framework for determining what is intended by the use of a particular intervention.

The explosion of dressings, devices, biological and physical therapies also produces an increasing range of therapeutic modalities and an added confusion for many clinicians who care for patients with wounds. The appropriate selection of these interventions also provides enormous challenges for the modern-day clinician.

In many hospitals, cities, countries and continents the role of surgery in wounds is not always given due consideration as part of a comprehensive and forward-looking means of treating patients with wounds – both acute and chronic. Many would say this is due to the lack of interest in surgeons performing surgical interventions on patients with wounds or their belief that other more interesting and challenging aspects of a surgical procedure are more important than considering healing of the tissues involved. This book dispels many of these myths and preconceptions. The biological basis for healing is addressed, as is the range of other interventions available to treat patients with wounds, and perhaps more importantly, the management of pain, post-operative complications, rehabilitation and prevention of further problems are all covered. It also provides an insight into the role of surgical interventions in patients with wounds and an international perspective as a consequence of the various chapter authors' country of work. Surgeons are definitely a key member of the multidisciplinary team needed to provide optimal care for patients with wounds, and surgical interventions are often not available or used only after all other therapeutic modalities have been considered. This situation is clearly inacceptable and this book will – I am sure – provide not only a source of reference for surgeons wanting to know more about wounds and wound healing but will also stimulate surgeons to become engaged with others in managing patients with wounds.

Much further work needs to be done to address the issues of the evidence base to support the use of all wound interventions – including surgery. The changing nature of wound types appearing across the world will unquestionably benefit from surgical approaches. The role of the surgeon or other professionals trained in offering surgical approaches for patients with wounds has to be refined, but the work presented in this book provides information, challenges and opportunities for all to consider surgery as a key component of comprehensive, professional and 21st-century clinical practice of wound healing.

K. Harding

# Preface

Covering wounds has always been a challenge for physicians. For 30 years, solutions have been essentially orientated towards surgical techniques, allowing to close the wound after surgical debridement, most of the time realised in the same stage. We participated to the flap development and could analyse the functional improvements provided by these techniques.

For less than a decade, alternative solutions have begun to develop, some of them revolutionising the field. These techniques propose a series of consecutive wound-management techniques and local cares, interacting with the natural stages of wound healing. Solutions for debridement, granulation-tissue formation, keratinisation and scar maturation appeared and demonstrated some evidence. A step-by-step-staging reconstruction can now reasonably be anticipated, issuing to a mature scar, at least equivalent aesthetically and functionally to the one obtained with flaps. This last point is crucial when attempting to prevent the recurrences. A well-matured scar has recovered suppleness, local humidity is maintained enough to make the scar mechanically resistant, hyperkeratosis is prevented.

One of the most important points concerns education of surgeons to the practices of new dressings and the use of the new techniques. Surgeons are not usually trained to use them and to prescribe them with the same precision they can choose the best flap for a specific loss of substance.

These techniques have drastically changed surgeon's behaviour in the management of acute limbs trauma and of post-operative infections in critically ill patients. The techniques, even if some of them were designed by non-surgeons, are considered as best practices in chronic wounds now. They can be transposed to many situations like burns, acute wounds, bites, necrotising fasciitis, war wounds, fistulas and other difficult wounds as well as in most of the wound situations. Some solutions, designed by surgeons, have on the contrary demonstrated their universality. The are used nowadays by every caregiver.

What changed in the mind of the pioneers was the progressive conviction of a better management of wound infection.

The tremendous changes in practicing reconstructive surgery, in finding new areas of performance for our specialities, is described in this book, with the pretention of being exhaustive at the moment, but keeping in mind that wound-healing solutions are changing very fast.

LUC TÉOT, ULRICH ZIEGLER, PAUL BANWELL

# Table of Contents

## VI Chronic Wound Problems



## VII Burns



## VIII Treatment of Scaring



## IX Future Perspectives in Wound Management



## X Conclusions



## XI Appendix

# Editors and Contributors

This book was coordinated by a group of three surgeons involved in wound healing for the past ten years, with the help of an International Panel of colleagues who kindly accepted to join their forces to produce this book, considered as the first issue of the World Union of Wound Healing Educational Program.

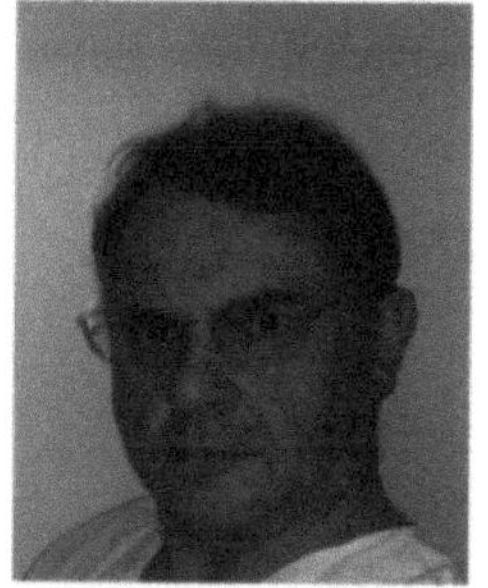

**Luc Téot** is Plastic Surgeon, working at the Montpellier University Hospital . He founded the French Wound Healing Society, one of the most prominent group in wound healing in the world with more than 3000 participants each year. He is becoming President of the European Tissue Repair Society. He organises the II. World Union of Wound Healing Societies in July 2004 in Paris, a group he becomes President the same year.

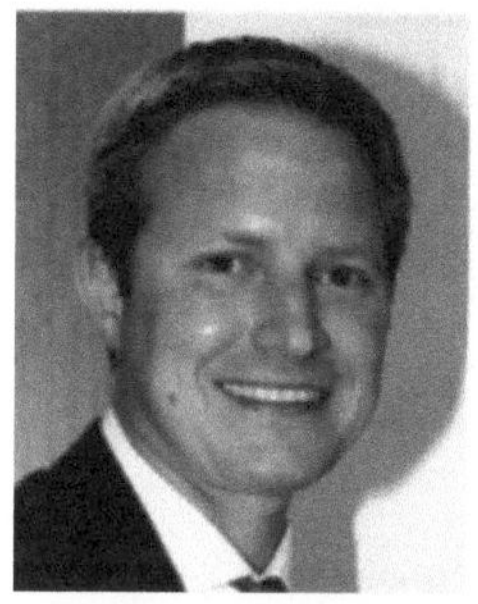

**Paul E. Banwell** is Plastic Surgeon, working at the Oxford University Hospital. Twice a year he organises important events in new surgery, from his negative-pressure-therapy experience. He develops new technologies in this field and has allowed the emergence and the federation of an international group of surgeons interested in reconstructive surgery.

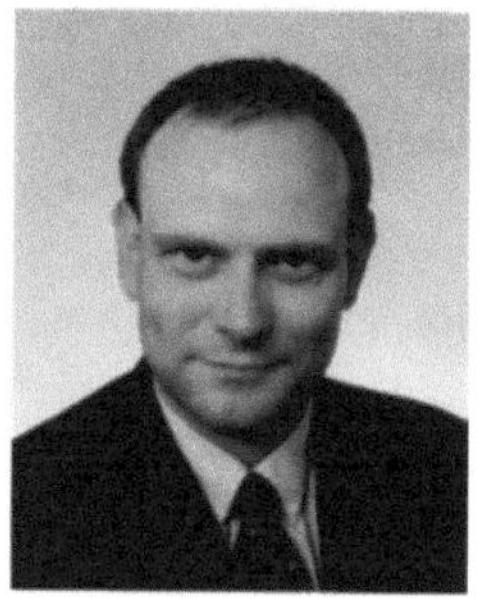

**Ulrich E. Ziegler** is Plastic Surgeon and General Surgeon working at the Wuerzburg University Hospital. Member of the German Wound Healing Society, organiser of several meetings in Germany and co-founder of the European Wound Institute. He is leading one of the most active Wound Healing Groups in Europe. He is recognised as an international referent for dermal substitutes applications, treatment of chronic/acute wounds and flaps in chronic wounds.

On the following pages the adresses of the first authors of all chapters are listed in alphabetical order.

**D.G. ARMSTRONG**, Professor of Surgery, Chair of Research and Assistant Dean, Dr. William M. Scholl College of Podiatric Medicine at Rosalind Franklin University of Medicine, 3333 Green Bay Road, North Chicago, Il 60064, USA

**ELIZABETH A. AYELLO**, Senior Adviser, The John A. Hartford Institute for Geriatric Nursing, New York University, The Steinhardt School of Education, Division of Nursing, 246 Greene Street, New York, NY 10003, USA

**JEAN-CLAUDE CASTÈDE**, Service des Brûlés, Hôpital Pellegrin, Place Amélie-Raba-Léon, 33076 Bordeaux cedex, France

**ROBERT H. DEMLING**, Professor of Surgery, Harvard Medical School, Director, Burn Center, Brigham and Women's Hospital, Boston, MA, USA

**ROLAND DE ROCHE**, Head of Pressure Ulcer Management Program and Consultant Plastic Surgeon, REHAB Basel, Rehabilitation Centre for Spinal Cord Injury and Brain Trauma, Im Burgfelderhof 40, 4025 Basel, Switzerland

**U. DIETZ**, Department of Plastic Surgery, University of Wuerzburg, Josef-Schneider-Str. 2, 97080 Würzburg, Germany

**KENNETH N. DOLYNCHUK**, Department of Surgery, Section of Plastic Surgery, University of Manitoba, 200–400 Taché Ave., Winnipeg Manitoba, CA R2H 3C3, USA

**E.L. DORMAND**, Department of Plastic Surgery, Radcliffe Infirmary, Woodstock Road, Oxford, Oxon OX2 8HE, United Kingdom

**ELOF ERIKSSON**, Brigham & Women's Hospital, Division of Plastic Surgery, 75 Francis Street, Boston, MA 02115, USA

**W. FLEISCHMANN**, Department of Trauma and Reconstructive Surgery, Klinikum Ludwigsburg-Bietigheim gGmbH, Riedstr. 12, 74321 Bietigheim-Bissingen, Germany

**N. FRASSON**, Centre Ster, Rééducation des Brûlés, 34240 Lamalou les Bains, France

**MICHAEL GOLD**, Gold Skin Care Center, 2000 Richard Jones Road, Suite 220, Nashville, TN 37215, USA

**FINN GOTTRUP**, University Center of Wound Healing, Department of Plastic Reconstructive Surgery, Odense University Hospital, 5000 Odense C, Denmark

**OLIVIER HEYMANS**, Head of Department, Plastic Durgeon, Service de Chirurgie Plastique, Maxillo-faciale et de la Main, CHU Sart Tilman, 4000 Liège, Belgique

**PER HOLSTEIN**, Copenhagen Wound Healing Center, Bispebjerg University Hospital, Bispebjerg Bakke 23, 2400 Copenhagen NV, Denmark

**RAYMUND E. HORCH**, Professor and Chief, Department of Plastic and Hand Surgery, University of Erlangen-Nürnberg, Krankenhausstraße 12, 91054 Erlangen, Germany

**DIANE L. KRASNER**, Wound & Skin Care Consultant, 212 East Market Street, York, PA 17403, USA

**DAVID LAVERTY**, Breckenridge Specialists Prof Bldg., 1313 Red River, Suite 200, Austin, TX, USA

**STEPHEN R. LAUTERBACH**, St. Joseph's Medical Center, 501 S. Buena Vista Street, Burbank, CA 91505, USA

**DAVID LEAPER**, Professorial Unit of Surgery, University Hospital of North Tees, Stockton-on-Tees, TS19 8PE, United Kingdom

**SYLVIE MEAUME**, Dermatologist and Geriatrician, Head, Department of Gerontology, Assistance Publique - Hôpitaux de Paris, Charles Foix Hospital, 7 avenue de la République, 94205 Ivry sur Seine, France

**JAMES MAHONEY**, Associate Professor, Department of Surgery, University of Toronto, St. Michael's Hospital, Division of Plastic Surgery, 30 Bond Street, Room 4-080 Queen Wing, Toronto, ON M5B 1W8, Canada

**STEFAN MEINERS**, Clinic for Surgery, Military Hospital Ulm, Oberer Eselsberg 40, 89081 Ulm, Germany

**ROLAND MOLL**, Department of Radiology, University of Wuerzburg, Oberdürrbacher Str. 6, 97080 Würzburg, Germany

**THOMAS A. MUSTOE**, Professor and Chief, Division of Plastic Surgery, Northwestern University Feinberg School of Medicine, Chicago, IL, USA

**NORBERT PALLUA**, Direktor der Klinik für Plastische Chirurgie, Hand- und Verbrennungschirurgie, Universitätsklinikum Aachen, Pauwelsstr. 30, 52074 Aachen, Germany

**SYLVIE PALMIER**, Wound Care Ambulatory Team, University Hospital, Montpellier, France

**T.R. PALSER**, Department of Plastic and Reconstructive Surgery, Radcliffe Infirmary, Woodstock Road, Oxford, United Kingdom

**RALF U. PETER**, Chairman, Hospital and Clinic of Vascular Surgery and Dermatology, Erhard-Groezinger-Str. 102, D-89134 Ulm-Blaustein, Germany

**G. PIVATO**, Institut de la Main, 6 Square Jouvenet, Paris – 75007s, France

PATRICIA PRICE, Wound Healing Research Unit, University of Wales, College of Medicine, United Kingdom

MARTIN C. ROBSON, Emeritus Professor of Surgery, University of South Florida, Tampa, Florida, Founding Director, Institute for Tissue Regeneration, Repair, and Rehabilitation, Department of Veterans Affairs Medical Center, Bay Pines, Florida, 3619 S.E. Cambridge Drive, Stuart, Florida 34997, USA

C. ROQUES, C.S.R.E Lamalou le Haut, 8 Place du Général de Gaulle, BP 10, 34240 Lamalou les Bains, France

KARSTEN SCHMIDT, Department of Surgery, Plastic- and Hand Surgery, University of Wuerzburg, Joseph-Schneider-Str. 2, 97080 Würzburg, Germany

K. SHOKROLLAHI, Department of Plastic Surgery, Radcliffe Infirmary, Woodstock Road, Oxford, Oxon OX2 8HE, United Kingdom

MALTE SYAMKEN, Clinic of Anaesthesiology, University of Wuerzburg, Oberdürrbacher Str. 6, 97080 Würzburg, Germany

F.R.H. TEMPELMAN, Burns Center, Department of Surgery, Red Cross Hospital, Beverwijk, The Netherlands

LUC TÉOT, Service des Brûles, Hôpital Lapeyronie, 391 Avenue Doyen Giraud, 34255 Montpellier Cedex, France

G.P.L. THOMAS, Department of Plastic Surgery, Radcliffe Infirmary, Woodstock Road, Oxford, Oxon OX2 8HE, United Kingdom

JARED TORKINGTON, Consultant Colorectal Surgeon, Cardiff and Vale NHS Trust, Llandough Hospital, Penlan Road, Vale of Glamorgen, CF64 2XX, United Kingdom

E.E. TREDGET, Firefighters' Burn Treatment Unit, Wound Healing Research Group, Division of Plastic and Reconstructive Surgery, Division of Critical Care, Department of Surgery, University of Alberta, Edmonton, Alberta, T6G 2B7, Canada

P. VOWDEN, Bradford Hospitals NHS Trust, Bradford Royal Infirmary, Duckworth Lane, Bradford, West Yorkshire BD9 6RJ, United Kingdom

CORINNA WICKE, Klinik für Allgemeine Chirurgie, Universitätsklinikum Tübingen, Hoppe-Seyler-Str. 3, 72076 Tübingen, Germany

A. WINDSOR, St. Mark's, Northwick Park Hospital, Watford Road, Harrow, Middlesex (London), HA1 3UJ, United Kingdom

ULRICH E. ZIEGLER, Department of Surgery, Plastic- and Hand Surgery, University of Wuerzburg, Joseph-Schneider-Str. 2, 97080 Würzburg, Germany

# I Background

# 1 The Pathophysiology of Acute Wounds

E.E. Tredget, A. Medina, J. Haik

## Introduction

Wound healing has been a concern of physicians through the ages and is still undergoing intense investigation and ongoing discovery. During human embryogenesis, dividing cells from discrete regions form complex organs and tissues that grow in size but maintain their unique highly organised architecture. The origin of cells that participate in wound repair are from cells located nearby in the skin as well as from the bone-marrow-derived peripheral blood cells. These cells are capable of entering sites of injured tissues, where they appear to contribute to wound repair; however, the process is complex and incompletely understood. Regeneration without scarring, as it is seen in the foetus during specific periods of gestation, differs substantially from adult wound repair, which can develop normal, insufficient or excessive scar. Wounds and their complications can be life-threatening, as well as frequently compromising function and appearance. However, through an increased understanding of the pathogenesis of the process at a molecular and cellular level the basis of future wound management will emerge, from which novel, new and exciting therapies will develop.

## Anatomy and Physiology of Normal Skin

The skin is more than an organ of external presentation in personal, social and sexual interactions in that it provides mechanical and immunological protection, participates in the body thermoregulation, delivers neurosensorial information to central nervous system, contributes to vitamin D synthesis and plays a role in the homeostasis of fluids, electrolytes and proteins. The skin consists of two layers, the epidermis and the dermis, which change in thickness according to age and anatomical location. The epidermis originates from the ectoderm layer and is primarily composed of epithelial cells, predominantly keratinocytes. Other skin-cell components are melanocytes, which are responsible for pigmentation and ultraviolet filtration, and Langerhans cells, which are involved in the immunological defense. Merkel cells are also present in the skin and act as mechanoreceptors. Keratinocytes are continuously turning over due to their growth, maturation and differentiation, which occur from a basal germinative layer to the skin surface. This process takes between 2 to 4 weeks and finishes with superficial desquamation. The skin also contains epidermal appendages such as hair follicles, sebaceous glands and sweat glands, located mainly in the dermis. They constitute important elements in tissue repair, providing additional sources of epithelial cells for repair of wounds.

**Table 1.** The source of cellular elements in wound healing

|  | Cell type | Origin |
|---|---|---|
| **Epidermis** | Keratinocytes | Skin ± bone marrow |
|  | Langerhans cells | Bone marrow |
|  | Merkel cells | Bone marrow |
|  | Melanocytes | Bone marrow |
|  | Keratinocyte stem cells | Hair bulb, basal layer of epidermis |
| **Dermis** | Fibroblast | Dermis ±? bone marrow |
|  | Fibrocyte, other mesenchymal stem cells | Bone marrow |
|  | Mast cells | Bone marrow |
|  | Lymphocytes | Bone marrow |
|  | Neutrophils | Bone marrow |
|  | Eosinophils | Bone marrow |
|  | Platelets | Bone marrow |

The dermis originates from the mesoderm, is thicker than the epidermal layer and is constructed predominantly of fibrous and connective tissue. The dominant cell is the fibroblast, which is involved in the production of extracellular matrix (ECM) proteins such as collagen and elastin, which undergo continuous remodelling to allow elasticity and tensile strength. The basic proteins of the skin also include glycosaminoglycans or proteoglycans, which are molecules consisting of a protein core with attached sugar chains of variable size. These chains make them negatively charged hydrophobic molecules which bind water, permitting dynamic nutrient exchange and inflammatory cell migration. Additionally, the dermis contains lymphatics, terminal nerve fibres with their specialised receptors and a vascular system organised in the dermal and subdermal plexus [1].

## Stages of Wound Healing

### Inflammatory Phase

Immediately following an acute tissue injury, there is a transient period of vasoconstriction that slows blood flow through injured tissue and facilitates haemostasis. This initial vasoconstriction is followed by active vasodilation. Exposed subendothelial collagen in the wound bed promotes platelet aggregation and activation of the complement system as well as the coagulation cascade via factor XII (Hageman factor), leading to amplification of preformed protein cascades of the innate immune system.

The final result of this complex sequence of cellular and biochemical events is the transformation of the connective tissue from a quiescent tissue to a region of intense cellular infiltration and subsequent protein synthesis designed to initiate wound repair. Coagulation products activate platelets that arrive during the first hours after tissue damage and initiate haemostasis via aggregation in the fibrin clot, where exocytosis of their α-granules [2] releases potent mitogens and growth factors [2] (Fig. 1). Platelet exocytosis is regulated by a number of signal-transducing molecules including the SNARE proteins [3], Sec1/Munc18 [4], protein kinase C [5], RABs family [6–10] and phospholipids [11]. Among the growth factors contained in their granules are platelet-derived growth factor (PDGF), transforming growth factor beta (TGF-β), platelet-derived angiogenic factor (PDAF), platelet-derived epidermal growth factor (PDEGF), platelet-derived epithelial growth factor (PDECGF), platelet factor 4 (PF-4), platelet activating factor (PAF), as well as β-thromboglobulin, fibrinogen, von Willebrand factor and β-thrombospondin [2, 12, 13]. PDGF released from platelets appears to be important in initiating the wound-healing process via chemotaxis of inflammatory cells such as neutrophils,

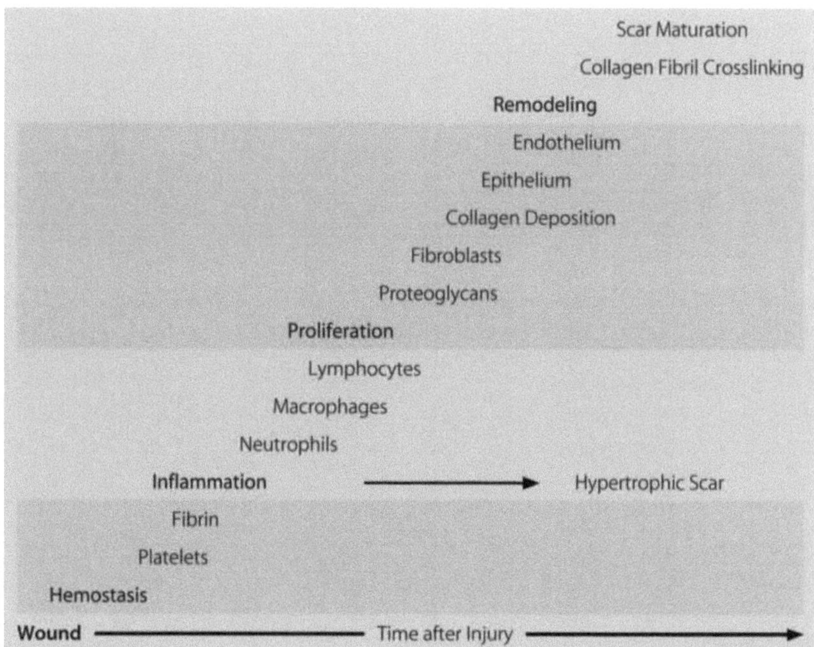


Fig. 1. The phases of normal wound repair follow an orderly sequence of events that are regulated by the chronological appearance of a number of different cell types over the course of healing. Prolonged activity or abnormal levels of fibrogenic cytokines released during the inflammatory phase may lead to fibroproliferative disorders. (With permission from [15])

monocytes and fibroblasts [14, 15], whereas, the PDGF released from macrophages appears to potentiate fibrogenesis. Platelets also contain high levels of insulin-like growth factor (IGF-1) which regulates immunity and inflammation, promoting migration of vascular endothelial cells [16].

The innate immune system is primarily a non-specific response to pathogenic agents which play a role in early recognition and clearance of debris and micro-organisms from the wound. Activated complement products such as C3a and C5a participate in the opsonisation process and increase vascular permeability. Neutrophils and monocytes are recruited to the injured site within 24 h of the injury by chemoattractant signals such as TGF-β, thrombin and ECM degradation products [17, 18]. Unlike platelets, neutrophils reside in the wound for prolonged periods and synthesise proteins, which amplify inflammation and promote tissue repair [12, 13, 16, 18]. Neutrophils enter the wound between 6 hours and 3 days later, to phagocytose red blood cells, bacteria and foreign material [11, 19–32], and release cytokines such as TNF-α, IL-1α and IL-1β. TNF-α promotes angiogenesis, glycos-aminoglycan synthesis and collagenase production by fibroblasts [20, 33]. Interestingly, secretion of TNF-α and monocyte chemoattractant protein-1 precedes monocyte recruitment to the injury [20], and releases GM-CSF that stimulates the function of neutrophils and macrophages in wound healing and the proliferation of keratinocytes [23, 34]. IL-1β up-regulates adhesion molecule expression by endothelial cells including ELAM-1, VCAM-1, and ICAM-1, and promotes the proliferation of fibroblasts and endothelial cells [33]. Both TNF-α and IL-1β are potent stimulators of monocytes, which are activated and differentiate into tissue macrophages that promote cell proliferation and ECM production [17]. Monocytes also release TNF-α and IL-1 and promote recruitment and activation of fibroblasts and other inflammatory cells [17, 32]. They participate in wound debridement by releasing collagenase, elastase and antimicrobial factors including nitric oxide and oxygen free radicals [17, 32]. Lymphocytes also arrive within the first few days after wounding as part of the acquired immune system and are activated when macrophages present antigens that lead to proliferation of antigen-specific T cells (CD4+). Activated T cells increase the expression of matrix metalloproteinase 1 (MMP-1), facilitating fibroblast migration and wound contraction, as well as producing gamma-interferon, which activates macrophages, inhibits collagen synthesis and generates T-cell differentiation during the immune response. Among the peripheral blood leukocytes attracted to the wound site, there is a small population (~0.5%) that becomes fibroblast-like cells called fibrocytes, reaching about 10% of the inflammatory cells that infiltrate the wound [33, 35–38]. These circulating fibrocyte precursors appear to interact with T cells, which stimulates early differentiation toward the fibrocyte phenotype before their migration to the injured area occurs [36]. These adherent, proliferating, spindle-shaped cells reach the wound within 24 h of injury, where the action of TGF-β appears to complete their maturation process [36, 38].

In the epidermis, keratinocytes respond to the nearby injury by detaching from neighbouring cells and the basement membrane, migrating towards the wound, where cell proliferation, stratification and differentiation occur until the wound is completely re-epithelialised.

### The Proliferative Phase

The proliferative phase of healing corresponds roughly to the period after the fourth post-injury day and lasts 2 to 4 weeks to re-establish functional and structural integrity in the injured tissue. Fibroblasts migrate to the inflammatory site where they have a crucial role in the creation of a stronger matrix from a transitional fibronectin scaffold [17]. They begin to enter the wound within 48–72 h along routes demarcated by fibrin fibres, and rapidly proliferate and undergo phenotypic changes to express contractile proteins. These cells produce collagen, elastin and glycosaminoglycans [32] for several weeks, and during this period endothelial cells form capillaries to deliver oxygen and nutrients necessary for the metabolic demands of wound closure [31]. These structures provide a mechanical substrate for epidermal cell migration across the wound surface. Collagen deposition increases its local level for weeks until a balance between synthesis and degradation is achieved [32]. Although many growth factors such as TNF-α, PDGF, IGF-1, EGF and IL-1 stimulate the synthesis of collagen, TGF-β1 appears to be the most important stimulator of fibrogenesis [39].

Under normal conditions, types I and III are the most abundant collagens in the ECM of the skin, where they are found in a 4:1 ratio [32, 40]. Initially in the tissue-repair process, fibronectin is degraded and substituted by type-III collagen, a more elastic and pliable isoform that provides adequate characteristics to increase local cellularity [17]. Thus, immature and hypertrophic scars present an increased content of type-III collagen, which can reach 33% of the total collagen content (2:1 ratio) [32]. Type-I collagen consists of two α1 chains and one α2 chain, and is present mainly in skin, tendon and bone [29]. Type-III collagen contains three α1 chains which are more highly hydroxylated, and is found in elastic tissues in skin and blood vessels [29]. These fibrillar collagens are produced as procollagens that, after removal of propeptides, form intra and intermolecular cross-links that stabilise the fibres and fibre bundles to increase the tissue tensile strength [30, 40]. During the first 3 to 4 weeks, the tensile strength of the wound increases in proportion to the collagen concentration. Afterwards, the strength increases more gradually as a result of ECM reorganisation and fibril cross-linking.

Glycosaminoglycans are molecules that contain a protein core coated by repeated disaccharide units (Fig. 2). Initially, the first glycosaminoglycan synthesised is hyaluronic acid. Within 2 weeks, chondroitin-4 sulphate and dermatan sulphate increase their levels. Finally, during the proliferation plateau, heparan sulphate appears [31, 32]. A core protein and covalently attached glycosaminoglycans chains form the heparan sulphate proteoglycan. The protein component of this molecule establishes the localisation on the cell surfaces or in the ECM, and the glycosaminoglycan component mediates interactions with numerous ligands (i.e. growth factors and adhesion molecules) [28]. Thus, modulation of heparan sulphate proteoglycan expression may be an essential regulatory step in cell proliferation and cell migration during wound healing [28].

During this transitional repair phase, the epithelial basal cells respond to the injury by detachment from other cells along the basement membrane, migration toward the wound and cellular differentiation and stratification until the wound is

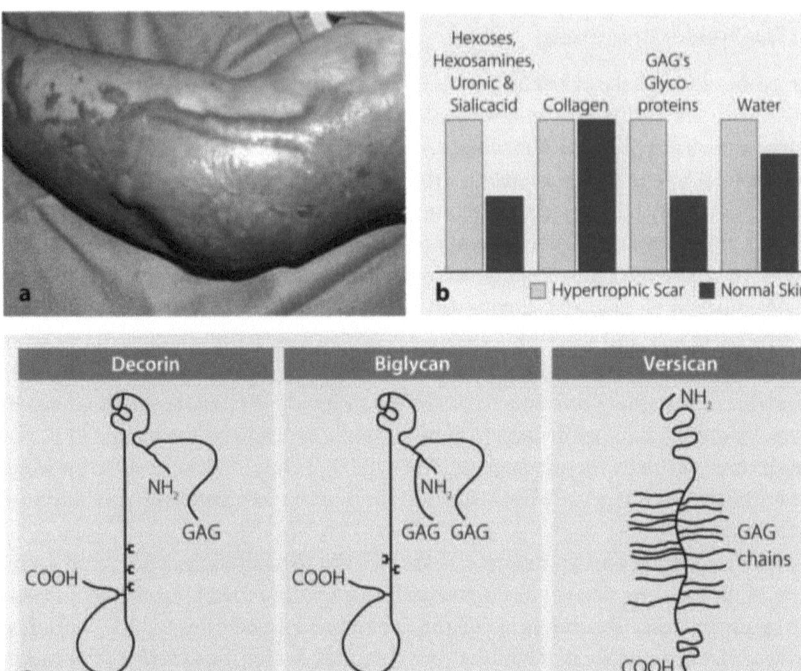

Fig. 2. a The expulsion of water from hypertrophic scar is depicted visually over this burn patient's elbow immediately following the removal of his silicone gel sheet and pressure garments. The expulsion of water is reversed rapidly if pressure is not maintained because of the continued presence of the glycosaminoglycan sugar chains that attract the water back into the region. b Extraction of normal (*light bar*) and hypertrophic (*dark bar*) scar tissue demonstrates an increased water content in hypertrophic scars relative to normal. This is probably caused, in part, by the hydrophilic glycosaminoglycans (GAGs). c Decorin and biglycan are small proteoglycans with one and two dermatan sulphate sugar chains, respectively. Versican is a large proteoglycan with as many as 30 glycosaminoglycan (GAG), thereby contributing significant rigidity to hypertrophic scars because of its hydrophilic properties (not drawn to scale). *NH₂* aminoterminis; *COOH* carboxyterminus. (With permission from Scott PG, Ghahary A, Tredget EE (2000) Molecular and cellular aspects of fibrosis following thermal injury. In: Thermal injuries. Hand Clinics 16: 271–287)

completely covered. During this process, the basal cells replace the mobilised cells by mitosis [32]. The basal layer of the epidermis appears to generate small electrical currents, which are an important biophysical control signal [41]. Basal cells are ordinarily interconnected by tight junctions. Following injury, the cells closest to the wound are lost, allowing current to flow, guiding nearby basal cells across the wound. As the migrating cells cover the wound and contact one another, contact inhibition occurs, tight junctions are re-established and current flow is retarded. Current magnitude is a function of wound size and the ability of cells to generate current. Factors that inhibit wound healing such as ischemia and oedema may do so by interfering with the ability of basal cells to generate current during the transitional repair phase of wound healing.

Re-epithelialisation begins at 24 h. Basal epithelial cells from the surrounding wound edges migrate as a sheet of cells extending lamellipodia along the advancing edge. Epithelialisation requires a conducive physiological environment, adequate nutrition and bacteriological control and, until the wound is epithelialised, wound inflammation persists. Wound re-epithelialisation down-regulates ECM formation. The wound is re-pigmented by migration of melanocytes from hair follicles. Desmouliere [42] illustrated that the number of myofibroblasts and vascular cells undergoing apoptosis increases as the wound closes. When granulation tissue persists, pathological scarring occurs. Thus, these myofibroblasts are involved in wound contraction and disappear by apoptosis when the wound is closed.

During the proliferative phase, fibroblasts are the predominant cell type and display heterogeneity [17, 35, 36] in cell shape, nuclear structure and organelle distribution, as well as proliferative capacity and response to stimuli [17]. The functional role of fibroblast subpopulations within a single injured tissue can differ very widely and may contribute to the broad spectrum of wound-healing response, from scarless foetal healing to hypertrophic scar and keloids in adult patients [17, 39]. The fibroblast donor source can also influence epidermal differentiation and regeneration time [43]. In burn patients, fibroblasts transform into $\alpha$-smooth muscle containing contractile myofibroblasts when derived from subcutaneous-derived fibroblasts as compared to dermal-derived fibroblasts, which express very little $\alpha$-smooth muscle actin ($\alpha$-SMA) [44]. Similarly, in myometrial and orbital fibroblasts, only Thy-1$^+$ fibroblasts (CD90 for human thymocytes) form myofibroblasts after induction with TGF-$\beta$ or platelet supernatants, whereas, the Thy-1$^-$ subgroup differentiated into lipofibroblasts [45, 46].

## Remodelling Phase

In normal or uncomplicated wound healing, the remodelling phase of injury typically begins 3 weeks after the injury. Collagen fibres establish a process of internal arrangement according to local mechanical forces and an improvement of the type-I to type-III collagen ratio appears. Additionally, continuous intramolecular and intermolecular cross-linking occurs and collagen bundles become more insoluble and resistant to enzymatic degradation. This process is highly regulated by collagenases and their inhibitors [17]. Matrix metalloproteinases (MMPs) are an important component of the remodelling process due to their capacity to cleave ECM proteins. Thus, matrix metalloproteinases control the ECM composition and facilitate cell migration. Moreover, they also have a function in the regulation of numerous growth factors, enzymes, cytokines, chemokines and cell receptors [26]. The remodelling stage also leads to a reduction in the level of hyaluronic acid and chondroitin-4 sulphate, as well as the local water content [32].

Fibroblasts and macrophages together form the basic processing unit of the remodelling phase. Active TGF-$\beta$, especially $\beta$1 isoform, induces a pro-fibrotic wound-healing phenotype with differentiation of fibroblasts into myofibroblasts [15, 47, 48] by the induction of phenotypic structural features resembling smooth-muscle cells including $\alpha$-SMA expression and intracellular attachments via desmosomes and maculae adherents [15, 32, 48, 49].

## Stem Cells for Wound Healing

### Local Tissue-Derived Stem Cells

Stem cells in the skin, as in any other tissues, are defined as cells that have clonogenic and self-renewing capabilities and that differentiate into cells with multiple lineages [50]. Adult epithelial stem cells in the skin are tissue-specific cells of the post-natal organism that are committed to differentiate but are capable of maintaining, generating and replacing the loss of terminally differentiated keratinocytes as part of normal turnover or after damage. They are located in the basal layer of the epidermis, in the bulge zone of the hair follicle and in sweat and sebaceous glands.

### Bone-Marrow-Derived Stem Cells

Recently, it has been recognised that adult stem cells are capable of "developmental plasticity" by forming tissue cells in solid organs that are functional and persist over time [51]. Krause and colleagues [52] demonstrated by limiting dilution techniques that single cells can differentiate into mature haemopoietic cells and into mature skin epithelial cells, suggesting that these circulating stem cells may play a role in homeostasis in solid organ tissue although the mechanism of recruitment is still unclear. Tissue injury and its subsequent local and systemic inflammatory signals may contribute to stem-cell recruitment. The presence of bone-marrow-derived cells in hepatic transplantation in the absence of histological hepatic damage suggests that the circulating cells collaborate in homeostasis and healing of local tissues [53, 54] such that when a rigorous demand for tissue repair exists that cannot be met by local stem cells, circulating stem cells may be triggered to differentiate into a specific injured tissue. Recently, it has been recognised that bone-marrow-derived circulating peripheral blood cells or fibrocytes possess not only typical antigen presenting and immunologic features of lymphocytes, but are also capable of entering injured tissue, where they appear to contribute to matrix formation through the synthesis of type-I collagen, fibronectin and various integrins [55].

## Growth Factors in Wound Healing

During the inflammatory phase of wound healing, the activation and release of growth factors are prerequisites to subsequent processes that include: angiogenesis, re-epithelialisation, fibroblast recruitment and proliferation, and matrix deposition. Angiogenesis is stimulated by endothelial chemoattractants and mitogens that include heparin, released by mast cells; fibroblast growth factor (FGF) and interleukin 8 (IL-8), released by neutrophils, macrophages and keratinocytes, and insulin-like growth factor I (IGF-I) released by macrophages [56]. The fibroblast recruitment,

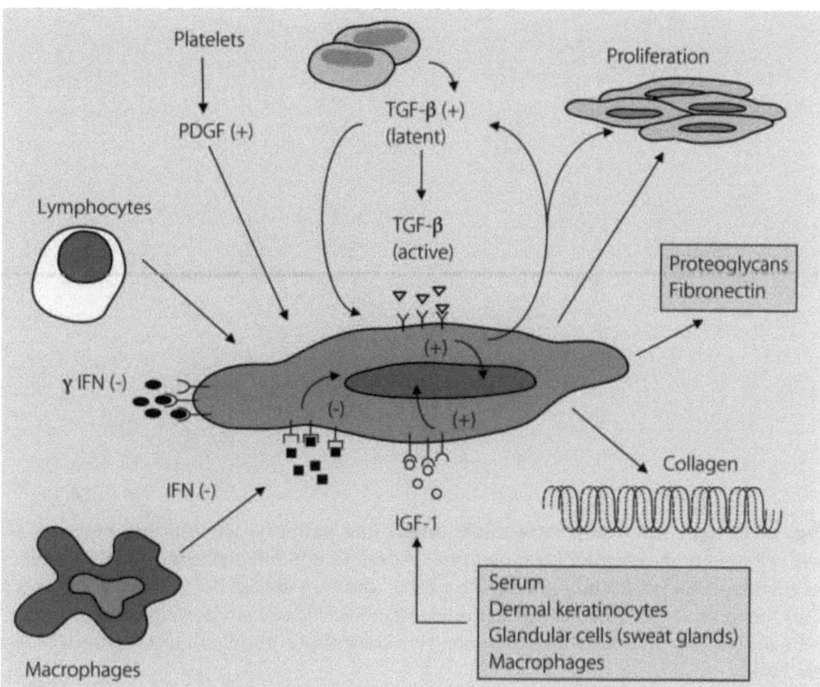


**Fig. 3.** Fibrogenic growth factors including TGF-β, PDGF and IGF-1 are involved in the development of fibroproliferative disorders with the interferons being potential inhibitors of matrix synthesis and fibroblast proliferation. (With permission from [15])

proliferation and production of ECM are influenced predominantly by the fibrogenic growth factors TGF-β, platelet-derived growth factor (PDGF), IGF-I, and basic fibroblast growth factor [57, 58]. These growth factors up-regulate the production of ECM proteins, increase the proliferation and/or migration of fibroblasts and inhibit the production of proteases required to maintain the balance between production and degradation. Among fibrogenic growth factors that have been identified, three have been implicated in the development of hypertrophic scarring: TGF-β, PDGF and IGF-I (Fig. 3).

TGF-β, a disulphide-bridged homodimeric protein, is a multifunctional cytokine that participates in numerous processes, including wound healing through an initial platelet activation within an hour after an injury [59], and a secondary activation several days later from lymphocytes [60], macrophages [37] and fibroblasts [61] with fibrogenic effects [59, 62]. The TGF-β family consists of at least five isoforms, which are highly conserved polypeptides that share 70–80% homology [63]. The synthesised TGF-β is released as a large latent complex, in an inactive form with a half-life of 90 min [57, 64]. TGF-β maturation (25 kDa) is reached by the action of plasmin, cathepsin D [63, 65], extreme pH, heat (80 °C for 10 min), proteases, glycosylation, exposure to reactive oxygen species, gamma irradiation, calpain, glucocorticoids, antiestrogens, vitamin D, retinoids [60, 61] and thrombospondin 1

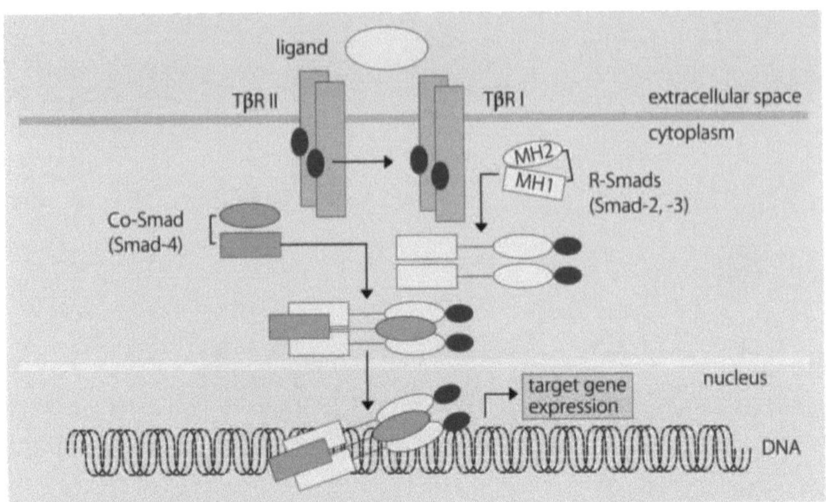

**Fig. 4.** TGF-β receptor and intracellular signalling pathway. The binding between TGF-β and cell membrane receptor promotes phosphorylation of intracellular signalling molecules. Regulatory Smads (-2 and -3) interact with a common modulator (Smad-4) or Co-smad. This Smad -3, -4/Co-Smad complex and protein SRA, is translocated into the nucleus. The I-Smads (-6 and -7) exert a negative autocrine control preventing phophorylation of regulator Smads

[66, 67]. The TGF-β superfamily has more than 40 members and binds to three types of cell-membrane receptors (TβRI, TβRII, and TβRIII) [68–70], which activate the complex system of intracellular signalling proteins of the Smad family [62, 68–70]. This intracellular system can be divided into three subgroups [62]. There are regulatory components that directly interact with cell-membrane receptors (R-Smads) [60, 62, 71–73], modulator components that serve as molecule adaptator for R-Smads (Co-Smad) [62, 73] and inhibitor components that exert a negative autocrine control on intracellular signalling (I-Smads) [73] (Fig. 4). Finally, a multimeric complex formed by R-Smads, Co-Smads and the facilitating protein SARA (Smad anchor for receptor activation) [60, 71–73] is translocated into the nucleus, where they bind to the promoter region to induce gene expression [62, 74] (Fig. 4). TGF-β acts as a chemoattractant for neutrophils, monocytes and fibroblasts [68–70]. It also increases the extracellular matrix production (i.e. collagen, fibronectin and glycosaminoglycans) and decreases its proteolysis [71, 72]. The promotion of collagen synthesis is due to an increase in fibroblast expression of mRNA for collagen types I and III. TGF-β also increases tissue inhibitors of the metalloproteinases (TIMPs) I and II, and α2-macroglobulin [48, 73, 75]. TGF-β inhibits proliferation of epithelial cells, and proliferation and differentiation of B and T cells. Finally, TGF-β increases its own autocrine production and secretion, increases the expression of several integrins and antagonises the action of proinflammatory cytokines (i.e. IL-1β, IL-2, IL-6, TNF-α and INF-γ) [36, 48, 60, 69, 72, 75]. TGF-β1 is the predominant isoform found in skin and in systemic circulation during wound healing

[67]. The stimulation of granulation tissue formation and an increase of connective tissue synthesis in vivo [25, 47, 49, 76] support the role of TGF-β in normal wound healing. However, the prolonged and excessive presence of TGF-β probably contributes to the development of hypertrophic scarring [3, 4, 25, 47, 49, 76, 77]. Further investigation is required into the relationship between the TGF-β isoforms, the release and activation of their binding proteins [78] and the synergistic/antagonistic interplay with other growth factors and with the ECM itself [42, 69].

Elevations of serum TGF-β have been found in burn patients with severe hypertrophic scarring [79] (see Fig. 2). Interestingly, high elevations of serum TGF β levels have been found to be predictive of the development of hepatic and pulmonary fibrosis in patients with breast cancer receiving ablative chemotherapy and bone-marrow transplant [67]. Additionally, Caver et al. have described the importance of elevated systemic TGF-β levels in an animal model of systemic lupus erythematosus (SLE) which were associated with an increase of their local level and the fibrotic and immunosuppressive effects [66]. This group also demonstrated that SLE patients had elevated TGF-β1 levels and suppressed neutrophil function during active disease periods, reverting back to normal with remission. These findings were consistent with the TGF-β transgenic models, where an enhanced expression of the TGF-β gene by the albumin promoter led to fibrosis in the liver and other tissues [80].

Platelet-derived growth factor (PDGF) is a heteromeric glycoprotein with a molecular weight of 30 kDa and with two chains (A and B) [81]. PDGF receptors are found on fibroblasts, vascular smooth-muscle cells and glial cells [81]. The exact mechanism of action of PDGF in tissue repair is not completely understood, but its activating effect over macrophages that release TGF-β and other growth factors is fundamental [82]. Furthermore, PDGF participates in the fibrogenesis through deposition of glycosaminoglycans and fibronectin, and stimulation of IGF-1 production in fibroblasts and endothelial cells [15]. In addition, IGF-1 elevates the production of TGF-β1, increasing the expression of TGF-β1 mRNA. On the other hand, TGF-β1 acts synergistically with IGF-1 in DNA synthesis and regulates IGF-1 production [83]. PDGF also has an association with thrombospondin-1 (TSP-1), which delays proteolytic degradation and promotes proliferative responses [84, 85]. PDGF is released into wounds early by platelets and then by infiltrating macrophages [86], fibroblasts [87], endothelial and epithelial cells [87]. PDGF also functions as a chemoattractant and mitogenic factor for fibroblasts [88, 89] and endothelial cells [90–92]. Although the abnormal persistence of PDGF has not been correlated with the development of hypertrophic scarring, the ability of this cytokine to modulate the production of IGF-I by fibroblasts [87] and endothelial cells [93] may indirectly contribute to fibrosis.

IGF-I acts as a mitogenic factor for fibroblasts, monocytes, endothelial cells and epithelial cells [94]. This collaborative effect has been demonstrated in in vivo wound-healing studies where the combination of PDGF and IGF-I resulted in a significant increase in epidermal and dermal synthesis relative to either growth factor applied alone [95]. Further enhancement of the effect of IGF-I can be seen following its association with IGF-I-specific binding proteins, which protect it from proteolytic degradation [96, 97]. The enhanced expression of IGF-I mRNA in hypertrophic scar tissue, its specific ability to increase expression of mRNA for type-I and type-III collagen and its ability to reduce release of collagenase – all suggest that IGF-I may play a role in hypertrophic scar formation [95, 98].

Basic fibroblast growth factor (bFGF) is a potent angiogenic agent that is produced by mesodermal and neuroectodermal cells. Following its release from these cells, the bFGF is stored along the basement membrane and in the extracellular matrix by binding to heparan sulphate [11]. The mast cell exocytosis also plays a role in the bFGF released during wound healing and angiogenesis [11].

## Foetal Wound Healing

Foetal wound healing during a selected period of gestation has been found to be a regenerative process which leads to minimal or no scarring rather than the normal post-natal wound healing, which typically yields a scar of varying quality [99]. Many studies have described differences between components and progression in foetal and adult skin wound healing, but it is still unclear which variables are critical in differentiating foetal or regenerative wound healing from post-natal wound healing. The foetal environment is characterised by a warm, sterile amniotic fluid that is rich in growth factors and extracellular matrix components such as hyalorunic acid (HA) and fibronectin. Morphologically, repaired foetal tissue consists mainly of hyaluronic acid, and has minimal proliferation of fibroblast and deposition of collagen. It forms a reticular pattern of extracellular matrix morphologically that resembles normal skin [17, 39]. Tissue oxygenation in the foetus is profoundly hypoxemic compared to post-natal tissue. In the foetal immune system, there is a lower inflammatory response due to few granulocytes in foetal wound healing. Macrophages are present but their role is uncertain [100]. As the foetus matures, the inflammation becomes more accentuated, resembling adult wound healing [101]. Amniotic fluid, that is rich in hyaluronic acid, can inhibit or stimulate fibroblast contraction in different animal models of wound healing. In addition, there are prominent and unique roles of several growth factors in foetal development, which may influence wound healing. For example, TGF-$\beta$ has been found in foetal wounds, where its expression is low and the tissue regeneration occurs without scar. With the application of exogenous TGF-$\beta$1 into the foetal wounds, it is possible to induce contraction and scarring [59]. However, the correlation between TGF-$\beta$ production and its isoforms, particularly TGF-$\beta$3, in the phenomenon of scarless foetal wound healing remains unclear.

In early foetal gestation, the small proteoglycan, decorin, is expressed in the skin in lower amounts than in late foetal gestation and adult patients [25]. This small leucine-rich proteoglycan produces modulation of TGF-$\beta$1 activity and regulates collagen assembly [15, 25, 60]. In the absence of decorin, uncontrolled TGF-$\beta$ activity appears to occur in association with fibrosis and scarring [76]. Decorin binds to fibrillar collagens (i.e. collagens I, II, III, V and XI), promoting lateral association of collagen fibrils that favour the formation of fibres and fibre bundles [15, 25, 76]. Fibromodulin is another significant component in the foetal environment. This is another proteoglycan that can act as a TGF-β ligand and potentially inhibit the TGF-β activity, where an inverse relationship between its expression and scarring appears to exist [27].

Other unique extracellular matrix proteins such as tenascin are known to be present earlier in foetal wounds, where they may be responsible for enhanced cell migration. This enhanced migration leads to a rapid epithelialisation of foetal wounds, thereby modulating deposition and organisation of extracellular matrix [102, 103].

## Wound Healing Following Thermal Injury

Following thermal injury, the skin is damaged to varying degrees depending on the intensity and duration of exposure. When thermal stimuli reach 40–44 °C, early denaturation of proteins and dysfunction of intracellular enzyme systems begins [104]. Cellular impairment is characterised by swelling of the cell membrane, loss of osmotic regulation and ultimately cell necrosis. Thus, coagulation necrosis generates a zone of coagulation where the barrier function of skin is lost [105] (Fig. 5). Necrotic cellular debris and denatured protein forms burn eschar, which represents a medium that facilitates bacterial growth [106]. Protein loss through the wound includes complement components, immunoglobulins [107–110] and clotting-related factors. Deeper and peripheral to the coagulation zone there exists the zone of stasis where blood flow is stagnant. In this transitional zone, there are questionably

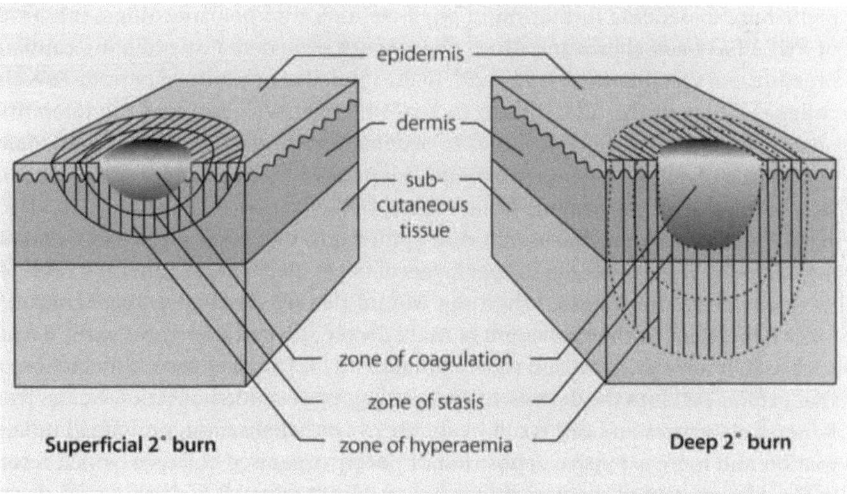


**Fig. 5.** Diagram depicting Jackson's three zones of burn injury showing the potential for conversion from a partial-thickness injury to a full-thickness injury when the zone of stasis progresses

viable cells that are less severely injured, that can evolve, over time, to either survive or progress to cell death. The transformation of the zone of stasis into burn eschar depends on the maintenance of the microvascular structures that may be injured as a result of direct injury of the blood vessels or by aggregation of platelets, granulocytes and deformed erythrocytes, and subsequent fibrin deposition [105]. This zone is very susceptible to additional insults such as dehydration, pressure, hypovolaemia, infection and electrolyte imbalance. The transformation of the zone of stasis into necrotic eschar can occur as early as the first hours after thermal injury [111], and cellular recovery in this zone can be achieved, under favourable conditions, within the first week [112] despite overlying damage to the epithelium.

The zone of hyperaemia is the outer region of the burn wound, which clinically is inflamed due to vasodilatation and increased blood flow, but exhibits minimal cell damage [105]. In normal wounds, oedema can be a positive mechanism contributing to the removal of bacteria and debris [113], whereas in burn wounds, oedema has a negative effect by compromising the oxygen delivery to already ischemic tissues [114]. Oedema appears soon after the injury due to more permeable tissue with increased leakage of plasma proteins to the interstitium [74, 115, 116]. The increased permeability is a direct result of capillary and venular endothelial cell damage [117] or secondary to chemical mediators such as histamine [70, 118], bradykinine [119, 120], oxygen free radicals [121] including nitric oxide and sensory peptides [122]. Increased leakage of interstitial fluid is a result of elevated capillary hydrostatic pressure [123], as well as vasodilatation due in part to histamine released from mast cells at the site of the injured tissue [124]. Inflammation in the burn wound also induces activation of phospolipase A [125], which converts the membrane phospolipids into prostaglandin precursor, arachidonic acid. This product leads to neutrophil activation in addition to components of the complement cascade [126], coagulation system and kinin/bradykinin cascade. Prostaglandins contribute to oedema formation in burn wounds, and pharmacologic inhibition of PGE2 has been shown to reduce the amount of oedema by reducing capillary pressure and vasodilatation [127–129]. In the immediate post-burn period, damaged collagen fibres in the interstitium increase the osmotic load and the interstitial oncotic pressure, which contributes to oedema formation [130, 131]. This oedema is maximal often by 12–24 h after injury, but persists at this level for 48–72 h before slow resolution of the oedema occurs thereafter.

In partial-thickness burns, rapid re-epithelialisation takes place when remaining epithelial cells, present in deeper layers of the epidermis and adnexal structures, re-epithelialise the wound. When the wound damage is deeper, regeneration is more dependent on the epithelium of more deeply situated structures in the dermis such as hair follicles, sweat and sebaceous glands [132]. In deep second-degree burns that extend well into the dermis, cell migration for re-epithelialisation occurs from adnexal structures and can result in slower re-epithelialisation, prolonged inflammation and more extensive deposition of poorly organised collagen, which results in the development of hypertrophic scarring. Recent research in deep second-degree and full-thickness burns has suggested that epithelial repair may also arise from stem cells derived from mesenchymal bone marrow-derived haematopoietic stem cells [51].

## Fibroproliferative Disorders of the Skin

### Hypertrophic Scar

Hypertrophic scarring and keloids are the result of an overproduction of all components of the extracellular matrix, including cells, collagen, elastin and proteoglycans [133]. Hypertrophic scars usually undergo some degree of regression with scar remodelling and maturation. The incidence of hypertrophic scars is highest in areas of higher skin tension and movement. Wounds oriented in the relaxed skin tension lines are mechanically shielded from stress by the adjacent intact collagen fibres and generally heal with less scar. Scar hypertrophy is more likely to occur following healing by secondary intention, particularly if more than 3 weeks were required to achieve epithelial closure [134]. Factors which cause local inflammation such as persistent irritation, acne, haematoma, foreign bodies in the wound, infection or wound dehiscence further predispose to hypertrophic scar. Systemic inflammation due to an infection at a remote site may also be an influential factor. Similarly, burn wounds involving the deep dermis that heal over a prolonged period of time develop hypertrophic scarring at high rates, independent of age, sex and racial background [135, 136](Fig. 6).

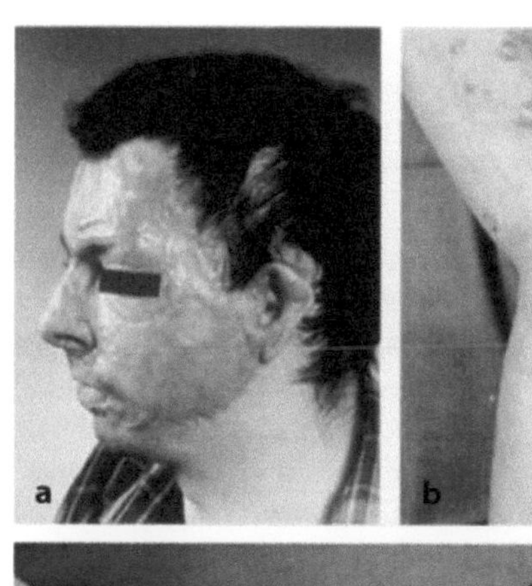
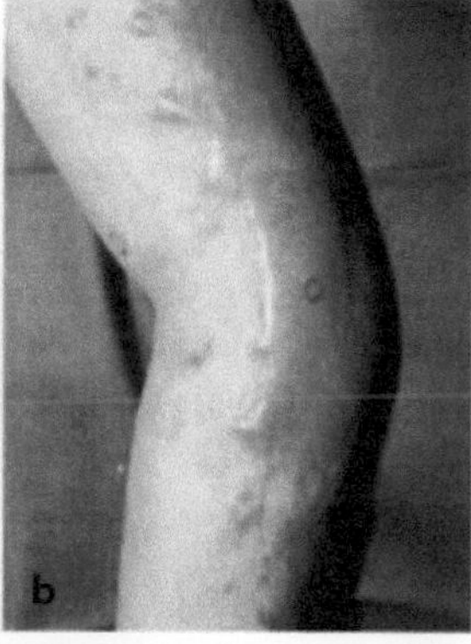
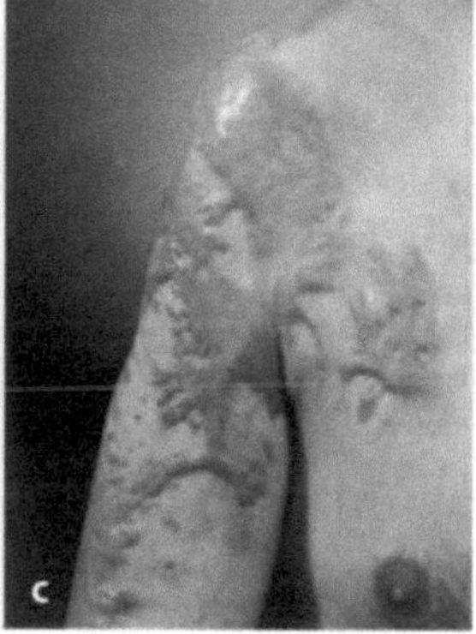
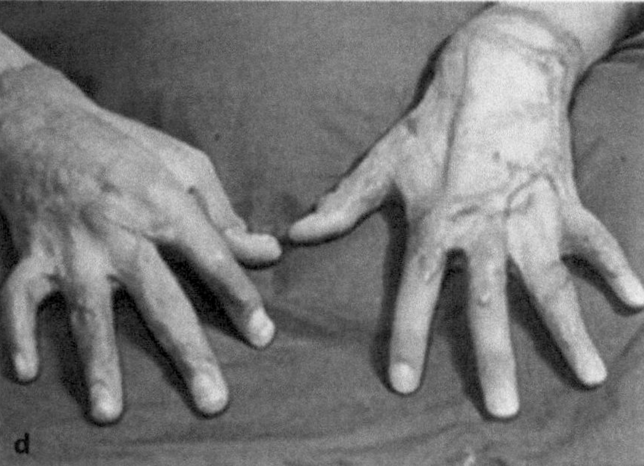

**Fig. 6.** Hypertrophic scarring in a 34-year-old white man 8 months following a 60% total body surface area burn involving the face, upper extremities and hands. (With permission from Scott PG, Ghahary A, Chambers MM, Tredget EE (1994) In: Biological basis of hypertrophic scarring. Adv Structural Biol 3: 157)

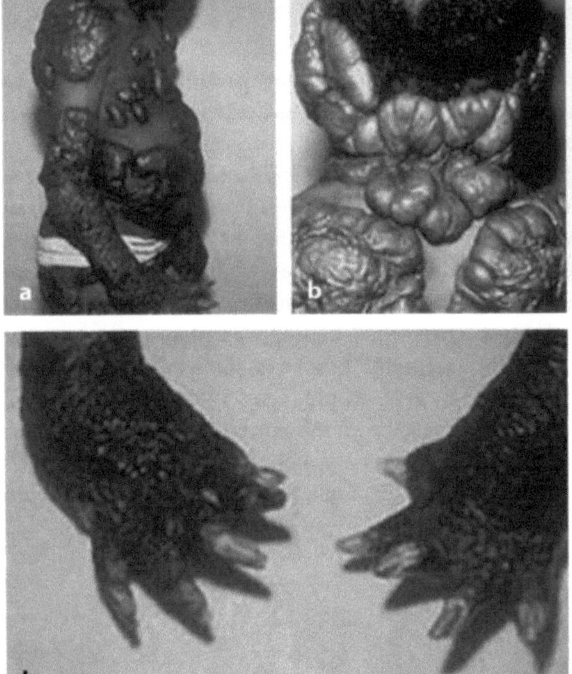

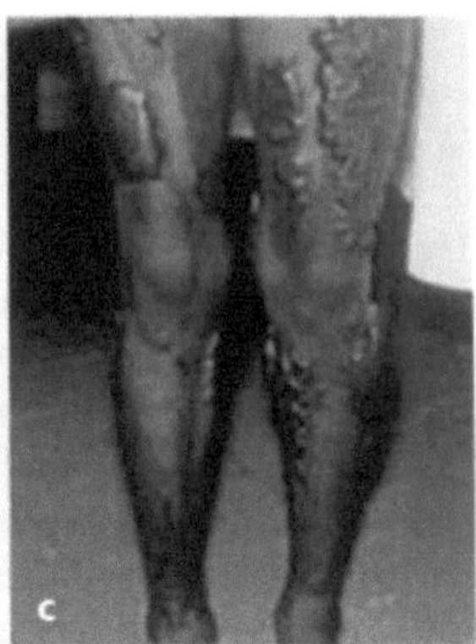

**Fig. 7.** A 12-year-old black child with severe keloids following a scald injury. (With permission from Scott PG, Ghahary A, Chambers MM, Tredget EE (1994) In: Biological basis of hypertrophic scarring. Adv Structural Biol 3: 157)

Ehrlich examined biopsies from patients with normal skin, normal scars, hypertrophic scars and keloids [137], and found that hypertrophic scars and keloids had increased density of blood vessels compared to normal scar and skin. Normal skin consisted of collagen fibres that were fine fibres arranged in a basket-like weave pattern, whereas hypertrophic scars contained collagen arranged in whorls or nodules that contained smooth-muscle actin-related myofibroblasts which were not present in keloids. The numbers of fibroblasts and myofibroblasts decreased during scar maturation and remodelling through apoptosis [138].

### Keloid Scars

Keloid scars are locally invasive and benign neoplastic scar tumours, which are hypocellular and contain broad, poorly retractile, pale-staining collagen bundles as compared to normal skin (Fig. 7). The normal fine fibrillar architecture is replaced by thick, irregular branched septal collagen bands [133]. Keloid fibroblasts manifest a loss of normal feedback in regulation of extracellular matrix production and respond more vigorously to the growth factors [135], although the binding affinities and receptor densities for growth factors are the same for keloidal and normal cells. This phenotypical difference suggests that the development of keloids occurs in a predisposing genetic background supporting the well-known familial predisposition [139, 140].

No direct correlations appear to exist between the magnitude of the skin injury and the size of the resultant scar/tumour. Many conditions that cause skin inflammation or disruption lead to keloid formation in these genetically susceptible individuals and the inciting injury can be so trivial as to be forgotten by the time the scar develops. Keloid scars often reach a specific size and remain unresolved for many years; however, the factors that limit the local scar growth have not been identified. Age plays a role in keloid development, in that children and young adults are more commonly affected; yet children who form keloids or hypertrophic scars are not necessarily predisposed to developing them later, whereas, in the geriatric population, the scar formation is generally less prominent. Keloids may undergo rapid growth during puberty and sudden increase in size and symptoms during pregnancy after years of apparent stability, suggesting that growth factors such as IGF-1 and other endocrine hormonal influences including oestrogen are important.

### Histologic and Biochemical Features of Hypertrophic and Keloid Scarring

Histological differences between scar tissue and normal skin include an increase in epidermal and dermal thickness, lack of epithelial ridges, minimal amounts of distinct collagen fibres and fibre bundles and the presence of whorls or nodules [141] (Fig. 8). Examination using immunohistochemistry shows that whorls in hypertrophic scarring contain fibroblasts positive for α-smooth muscle actin (α-SMA), randomly oriented collagen fibrils and small blood vessels. In contrast, keloids have few, if any, α-SMA positive fibroblasts and thick collagen fibres [142].

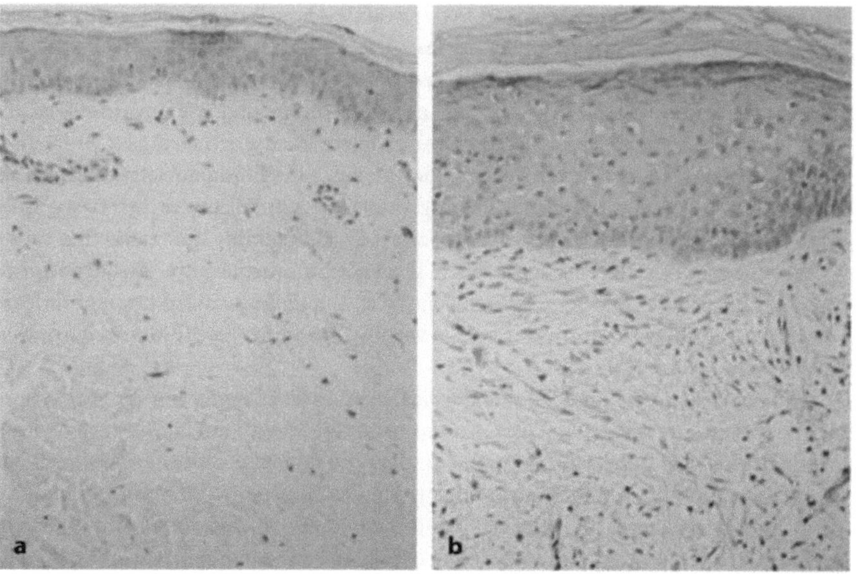


**Fig. 8a,b.** Hemotoxylin and eosin-stained sections of normal skin (**a**) and a hypertrophic scar (**b**)

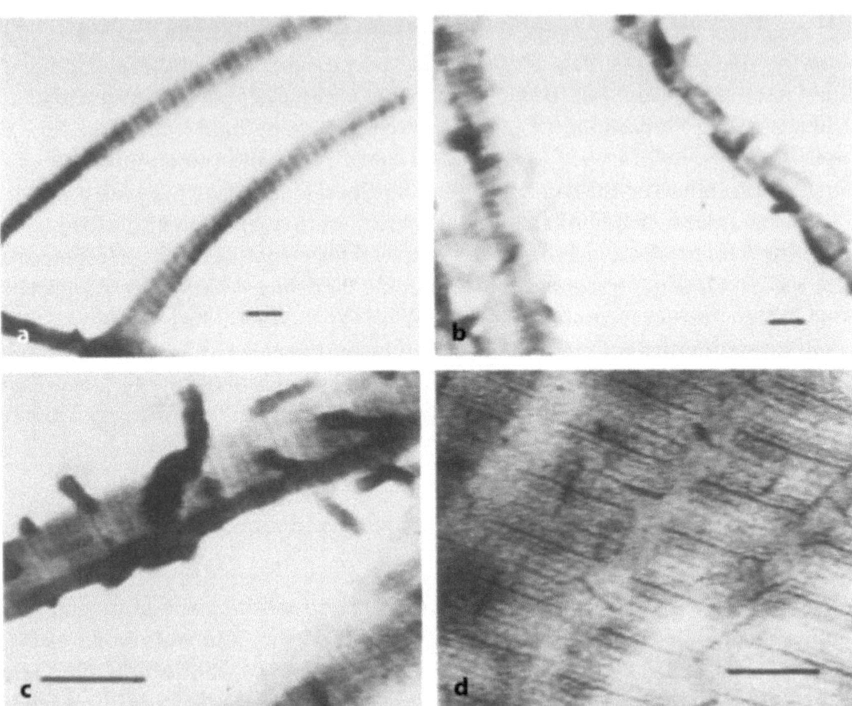

**Fig. 9a–d.** Scanning electron microscopic appearance of collagen fibrils (**a**), decorin binding using an antibody to the core protein of decorin to collagen fibrils (**b**), fibres (**c**) and fibre bundles (**d**) demonstrating the tightly packed pattern of assembly in the presence of decorin

Analysis of the proteoglycans in hypertrophic scars shows that decorin, a small molecular weight proteoglycan which may facilitate the resolution of fibrosis and inhibit the fibrogenic effects of TGF-β, decreases by 75% compared to normal skin. In contrast, levels of versican and biglycan, larger molecular weight proteoglycans with hydrophilic properties, are six times higher than normal [15, 47, 143–145] (Fig. 9). While the deficiency of decorin may increase the fibrogenic effects of TGF-β, the increased levels of versican and biglycan may contribute to the tissue bulk and rigidity by interference with the collagen fibril assembly and attracting water. As the scar matures, decorin returns to a level seen in normal skin. TGF-β co-localises with decorin [145], which is consistent with the theoretical function of decorin of facilitating the resolution of fibrosis through its ability to bind and neutralise TGF-β within the ECM [146].

Indications are that undesirable physical properties of hypertrophic scar are not a simple matter of excessive ECM protein production. Activated fibroblasts within hypertrophic scar appear to be unable to degrade collagen, and therefore, they inhibit their ability to remodel randomly oriented collagen into an organised matrix. Additionally, an increased level of TGF-β in the ECM, produced by fibroblasts or inflammatory cells, may account for the cellular and morphologic features in hypertrophic scar.

## The Cellular Basis of Hypertrophic Scarring

Fibroblasts from hypertrophic scar and normal dermal tissues taken from the same patient characterise abnormalities within connective tissue cells that produce the abnormal ECM [147–149] (Fig. 10). Fibroblast proliferation rates in keloids, hypertrophic scar and normal skin possess very similar doubling times, although similar studies in the past lacking the site-matched controls have reported differences in proliferation rates [134]. Analysis of a number of paired cell strains has shown that approximately half of the hypertrophic scar strains produce significantly more collagen in vivo. Additionally, mRNA for type-I collagen was increased in five of six strains compared to the normal skin fibroblasts [150]. Hypertrophic scar tissue showed an increase in the mRNA for proα2 [1] chain for type-I collagen and the proα1 [III] chains of type-III collagen [150] as was the level of fibronectin mRNA [151, 152].

Excessive matrix accumulation in hypertrophic scar can occur by increased synthesis of ECM proteins as well as by a reduction in matrix degradation (Fig. 11a and b). However, many hypertrophic scar fibroblast cell strains showed reduced mRNA for collagenase as well as net reductions in the ability to digest soluble collagen compared with their normal fibroblast pairs. These findings resemble those seen in scleroderma fibroblasts, suggesting that lack of collagenase activity is a frequent and consistent finding in dermal fibroproliferative disorders [153]. Hypertrophic scar fibroblasts also have a reduced ability to synthesise nitric oxide,

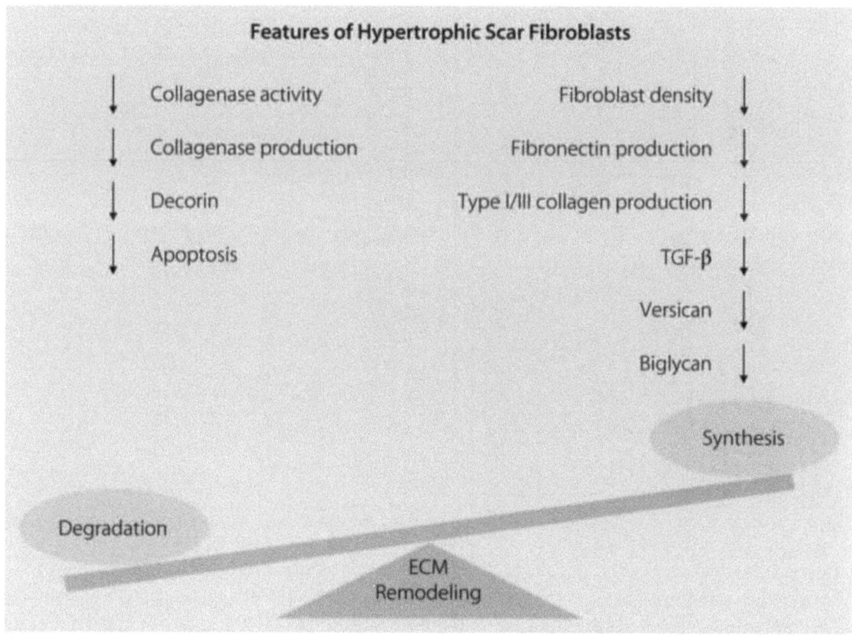


**Fig. 10.** The features of hypertrophic scar result in an imbalance in remodelling of the extracellular matrix, which leads to excessive synthesis and reduced degradation

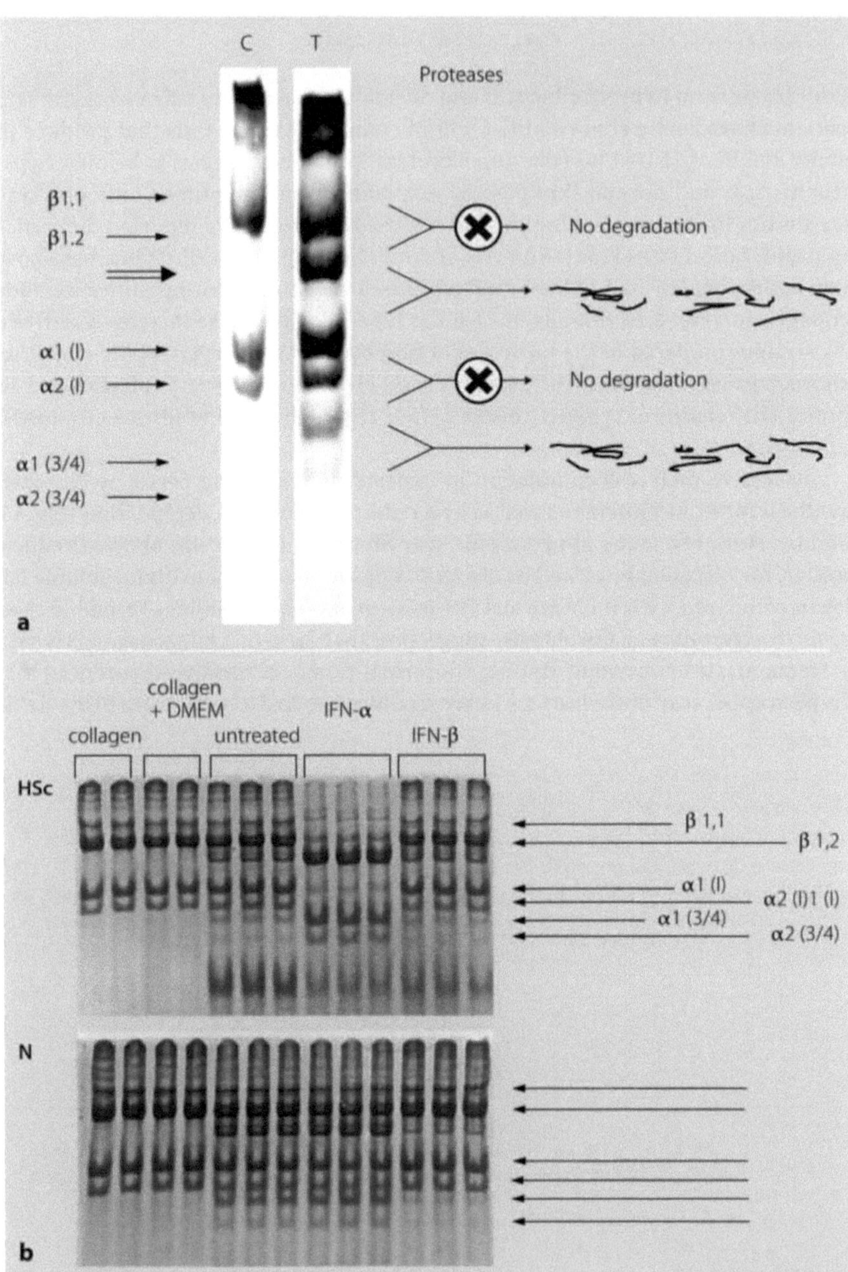



**Fig. 11. a** The effect of collagenase on collagen beta forms and alpha chains (α) which leads to the formation of α1 (3/4) and α2 (3/4) fragments of collagen in the treated lanes (*T*) of SDS-PAGE gel as compared to no enzyme in the control lane (*C*). **b** Collagenase activity in the conditioned media from fibroblasts from hypertrophic scar (HSc) and normal tissues (*N*) demonstrating increased collagen degradation in the normal fibroblasts as compared to HSc fibroblasts, which is restored in part by treatment of the fibroblasts with interferon α but not interferon γ

which has recently been found to be important in collagenase regulation [118]. As discussed previously, hypertrophic scarring fibroblasts also show a deficiency in synthesis of decorin, which normally promotes organised fibre formation and neutralises the fibrogenic effects of TGF-β. This underproduction of decorin combined with an overproduction of TGF-β may be an important mechanism in the formation of hypertrophic scarring given the fact that TGF-β mRNA and its protein are also synthesised in hypertrophic scar fibroblasts at higher levels than in normal fibroblasts taken from the same patient [15]. Treatment of normal fibroblasts with exogenous TGF-β stimulates fibroblast proliferation and DNA synthesis, increases production of collagen, fibronectin and tissue inhibitor of metalloproteinase (TIMP) I, as well as decreasing the expression of collagenase mRNA and enzyme activity. These phenotypic features of hypertrophic scar fibroblast can be reversed with the application of polyclonal TGF-β antibody [32, 70].

In addition, the circulating serum TGF-β may constitute an important mediator for tissue fibrosis. For example, the TGF-β is elevated in extensively burned patients and is associated with severe hypertrophic scarring after injury [15, 63]. Excessive fibrosis may also occur due to a failure in reduction of TGF-β receptor over-expression in fibroblasts during the inflammatory or remodelling processes [25, 70]; it regulates intracellular Smad cascade family and leads to overproduction of matrix proteins and their enzyme inhibitors at a genetic level [70]. TGF-β produces ECM accumulation of certain proteoglycans, increase in RNA translocation and transcription of fibroblast proteins (i.e. types-I, -III, -V collagen and fibronectin). It also increases proteinase inhibitors such as plasminogen activator inhibitor-1 (PAI-1) and tissue inhibitor of metalloproteinases (TIMPs) [48, 72], while decreasing matrix proteinases (i.e. collagenase, plasminogen activator).

Finally, although fibroblasts are the predominant cell present in hypertrophic scarring, mast cells are increased fourfold as compared to normal skin [154]. This higher mast-cell population may be important in stimulating extracellular matrix abnormalities, and histamine released from them contributes to the itchiness that is often associated with hypertrophic scarring [155].

## References

1. Williams WG (2002) Pathology of the burn wound. In: Herndon D (ed) Total burn care, 2nd edn. WB Saunders, Philadelphia, pp 514–522
2. Lemons PP, Chen D, Whiteheart SW (2000) Molecular mechanisms of platelet exocytosis: requirements for alpha-granule release. Biochem Biophys Res Commun 267: 875–880
3. Feng D et al. (2002) Subcellular distribution of 3 functional platelet SNARE proteins: human cellubrevin, SNAP-23, and syntaxin 2. Blood 99: 4006–4014
4. Polgar J, Chung SH, Reed GL (2002) Vesicle-associated membrane protein 3 (VAMP-3) and VAMP-8 are present in human platelets and are required for granule secretion. Blood 100: 1081–1083
5. Reed GL, Houng AK, Fitzgerald ML (1999) Human platelets contain SNARE proteins and a Sec1p homologue that interacts with syntaxin 4 and is phosphorylated after thrombin activation: implications for platelet secretion. Blood 93: 2617–2626
6. Logan MR, Odemuyiwa SO, Moqbel R (2003) Understanding exocytosis in immune and inflammatory cells: the molecular basis of mediator secretion. J Allergy Clin Immunol 111: 923–932; quiz 933

7. Chen M, Geng JG (2001) Inhibition of protein tyrosine phosphatases suppresses P-selectin exocytosis in activated human platelets. Biochem Biophys Res Commun 286: 831–838

8. Coorssen JR, Haslam RJ (1993) GTP gamma S and phorbol ester act synergistically to stimulate both Ca(2+)-independent secretion and phospholipase D activity in permeabilized human platelets. Inhibition by BAPTA and analogues. FEBS Lett 316: 170–174

9. Shotelersuk V, Gahl WA (1998) Hermansky-Pudlak syndrome: models for intracellular vesicle formation. Mol Genet Metab 65: 85–96

10. Heimann K et al. (1999) Specific isoforms of actin-binding proteins on distinct populations of Golgi-derived vesicles. J Biol Chem 274: 10743–10750

11. Walgenbach KJ et al. (2002) A potential role for mast cells in the of bFGF from normal myocytes during angiogenesis in vivo. J Invest Surg 15: 153–162

12. Knighton DR et al. (1986) Classification and treatment of chronic nonhealing wounds. Successful treatment with autologous platelet-derived wound healing factors (PDWHF). Ann Surg 204: 322–330

13. King SM, Reed GL (2002) Development of platelet secretory granules. Semin Cell Dev Biol 13: 293–302

14. Carter CA et al. (2003) Platelet-rich plasma gel promotes differentiation and regeneration during equine wound healing. Exp Mol Pathol 74: 244–255

15. Tredget EE et al. (1997) Hypertrophic scars, keloids, and contractures. The cellular and molecular basis for therapy. Surg Clin North Am 77: 701–730

16. Heemskerk VH, Daemen MA, Buurman WA (1999) Insulin-like growth factor-1 (IGF-1) and growth hormone (GH) in immunity and inflammation. Cytokine Growth Factor Rev 10: 5–14

17. Sempowski G et al. (1995) Fibroblast heterogeneity in the healing wounds. Wound Repair Regen 3: 120–131

18. Knighton DR et al. (1982) Role of platelets and fibrin in the healing sequence: an in vivo study of angiogenesis and collagen synthesis. Ann Surg 196: 379–388

19. Sylvia CJ (2003) The role of neutrophil apoptosis in influencing tissue repair. J Wound Care 12: 13–16

20. Heinrich SA et al. (2003) Elevated monocyte chemoattractant protein-1 levels following thermal injury precede monocyte recruitment to the wound site and are controlled, in part, by tumor necrosis factor-alpha. Wound Repair Regen 11: 110–119

21. Yamaguchi Y, Yoshikawa K (2001) Cutaneous wound healing: an update. J Dermatol 28: 521–534

22. Canturk NZ et al. (2001) The role of L-arginine and neutrophils on incisional wound healing. Eur J Emerg Med 8: 311–315

23. Canturk NZ et al. (2001) The relationship between neutrophils and incisional wound healing. Skin Pharmacol Appl Skin Physiol 14: 108–116

24. Syk I et al. (2001) Inhibition of matrix metalloproteinases enhances breaking strength of colonic anastomoses in an experimental model. Br J Surg 88: 228–234

25. Beanes SR et al. (2001) Down-regulation of decorin, a transforming growth factor-beta modulator, is associated with scarless fetal wound healing. J Pediatr Surg 36: 1666–1671

26. Stamenkovic I (2003) Extracellular matrix remodelling: the role of matrix metalloproteinases. J Pathol 200: 448–464

27. Soo C et al. (2000) Differential expression of fibromodulin, a transforming growth factor-beta modulator, in fetal skin development and scarless repair. Am J Pathol 157: 423–433

28. Tumova S, Woods A, Couchman JR (2000) Heparan sulfate proteoglycans on the cell surface: versatile coordinators of cellular functions. Int J Biochem Cell Biol 32: 269–288

29. Cameron GJ et al. (2002) Structure of type I and type III heterotypic collagen fibrils: an X-ray diffraction study. J Struct Biol 137: 15–22

30. Eriksen HA et al. (2002) Increased content of type III collagen at the rupture site of human Achilles tendon. J Orthop Res 20: 1352–1357

31. Kosir MA et al. (2000) Matrix glycosaminoglycans in the growth phase of fibroblasts: more of the story in wound healing. J Surg Res 92: 45–52

32. Rohrich RJ, Robinson JB (1999) Wound healing. Selected Readings in Plastic Surgery 9: 1–39

33. Chesney J et al. (1998) Regulated production of type I collagen and inflammatory cytokines by peripheral blood fibrocytes. J Immunol 160: 419–425

34. De Ugarte DA et al. (2002) Treatment of chronic wounds by local delivery of granulocyte-macrophage colony-stimulating factor in patients with neutrophil dysfunction. Pediatr Surg Int 18: 517–520

35. Chesney J et al. (1997) The peripheral blood fibrocyte is a potent antigen-presenting cell capable of priming naive T cells in situ. Proc Natl Acad Sci USA 94: 6307–6312

36. Abe R et al. (2001) Peripheral blood fibrocytes: differentiation pathway and migration to wound sites. J Immunol 166: 7556–7562

37. Grab DJ et al. (2002) A role for peripheral blood fibrocytes in Lyme disease? Med Hypotheses 59: 1–10

38. Yang L et al. (2002) Peripheral blood fibrocytes from burn patients: identification and quantification of fibrocytes in adherent cells cultured from peripheral blood mononuclear cells. Lab Invest 82: 1183–1192

39. Lee HG, Eun HC (1999) Differences between fibroblasts cultured from oral mucosa and normal skin: implication to wound healing. J Dermatol Sci 21: 176–182

40. Jussila T et al. (2002) Synthesis and maturation of type I and type III collagens in endometrial adenocarcinoma. Eur J Obstet Gynecol Reprod Biol 4449: 1–9

41. Canaday DJ, Lee RC (1991) Scientific basis for clinical applications of electric fields in soft tissue repair. In: Brighton CT, Pollack SR (eds) Electromagnetics in biology and medicine. San Francisico Press, San Francisico, CA, pp 275–291

42. Desmouliere A et al. (1995) Apoptosis mediates the decrease in cellularity during the transition between granulation tissue and scar. Am J Pathol 146: 56–66

43. Konstantinova NV et al. (1998) Artificial skin equivalent differentiation depends on fibroblast donor site: use of eyelid fibroblasts. Plast Reconstr Surg 101: 385–391

44. van den Bogaerdt AJ et al. (2002) The suitability of cells from different tissues for use in tissue-engineered skin substitutes. Arch Dermatol Res 294: 135–142

45. Koumas L et al. (2003) Thy-1 expression in human fibroblast subsets defines myofibroblastic or lipofibroblastic phenotypes. Am J Pathol 163: 1291–1300

46. Koumas L et al. (2001) Fibroblast heterogeneity: existence of functionally distinct Thy 1(+) and Thy 1(−) human female reproductive tract fibroblasts. Am J Pathol 159: 925–935

47. Nedelec B et al. (2000) Control of wound contraction. Basic and clinical features. Hand Clin 16: 289–302

48. Bauer BS et al. (2002) Latent and active transforming growth factor beta1 released from genetically modified keratinocytes modulates extracellular matrix expression by dermal fibroblasts in a coculture system. J Invest Dermatol 119: 456–463

49. Brown RA et al. (2002) Enhanced fibroblast contraction of 3D collagen lattices and integrin expression by TGF-beta1 and -beta3: mechanoregulatory growth factors? Exp Cell Res 274: 310–322

50. Weissman IL (2000) Stem cells: units of development, units of regeneration, and units in evolution. Cell 100: 157–168

51. Anderson DJ, Gage FH, Weissman IL (2001) Can stem cells cross lineage boundaries? Nat Med 7: 393–395

52. Krause DS et al. (2001) Multi-organ, multi-lineage engraftment by a single bone marrow-derived stem cell. Cell 105: 369–377

53. Theise ND et al. (2000) Liver from bone marrow in humans. Hepatology 32: 11–16

54. Theise ND et al. (2000) Derivation of hepatocytes from bone marrow cells in mice after radiation-induced myeloablation. Hepatology 31: 235–240

55. Chesney J, Bucala R (2000) Peripheral blood fibrocytes: mesenchymal precursor cells and the pathogenesis of fibrosis. Curr Rheumatol Rep 2: 501–505

56. Grant MB et al. (1993) Insulin-like growth factor I acts as an angiogenic agent in rabbit cornea and retina: comparative studies with basic fibroblast growth factor. Diabetologia 36: 282–291

57. Kovacs EJ, DiPietro LA (1994) Fibrogenic cytokines and connective tissue production. Faseb J 8: 854–861

58. Roberts AB, Sporn MB (1996) Transforming growth factor-beta. In: Lark RAF (ed) The molecular and cellular biology of wound repair. Plenum, New York, NY, pp 275–298

59. Branton MH, Kopp JB (1999) TGF-beta and fibrosis. Microbes Infect 1: 1349–1365

60. Zhu HJ, Burgess AW (2001) Regulation of transforming growth factor-beta signaling. Mol Cell Biol Res Commun 4: 321–330

61. Crawford SE et al. (1998) Thrombospondin-1 is a major activator of TGF-beta1 in vivo. Cell 93: 1159–1170

62. Shi Y (2001) Structural insights on Smad function in TGF-beta signaling. Bioessays 23: 223–232

63. Chan T et al. (2002) Development, characterization, and wound healing of the keratin 14 promoted transforming growth factor-beta1 transgenic mouse. Wound Repair Regen 10: 177–187

64. Grainger DJ, Mosedale DE, Metcalfe JC (2000) TGF-beta in blood: a complex problem. Cytokine Growth Factor Rev 11: 133–145

65. Yang L et al. (2001) Healing of burn wounds in transgenic mice overexpressing transforming growth factor-beta 1 in the epidermis. Am J Pathol 159: 2147–2157

66. Miao WM et al. (2001) Thrombospondin-1 type 1 repeat recombinant proteins inhibit tumor growth through transforming growth factor-beta-dependent and -independent mechanisms. Cancer Res 61: 7830–7839

67. Yehualaeshet T et al. (1999) Activation of rat alveolar macrophage-derived latent transforming growth factor beta-1 by plasmin requires interaction with thrombospondin-1 and its cell surface receptor, CD36. Am J Pathol 155: 841–851

68. Miyazono K, Kusanagi K, Inoue H (2001) Divergence and convergence of TGF-beta/BMP signaling. J Cell Physiol 187: 265–276

69. Govinden R, Bhoola KD (2003) Genealogy, expression, and cellular function of transforming growth factor-beta. Pharmacol Ther 98: 257–265

70. Chin GS et al. (2001) Differential expression of transforming growth factor-beta receptors I and II and activation of Smad 3 in keloid fibroblasts. Plast Reconstr Surg 108: 423–429

71. Roberts AB (1999) TGF-beta signaling from receptors to the nucleus. Microbes Infect 1: 1265–1273

72. Mori Y, Chen SJ, Varga J (2000) Modulation of endogenous Smad expression in normal skin fibroblasts by transforming growth factor-beta. Exp Cell Res 258: 374–383

73. Attisano L et al. (2001) The transcriptional role of Smads and FAST (FoxH1) in TGFbeta and activin signalling. Mol Cell Endocrinol 180: 3–11

74. Brouhard BH, Carvajal HF, Linares HA (1978) Burn edema and protein leakage in the rat. I. Relationship to time of injury. Microvasc Res 15: 221–228

75. Ghahary A, Tredget EE, Shen Q (1999) Insulin-like growth factor-II/mannose 6 phosphate receptors facilitate the matrix effects of latent transforming growth factor-beta1 released from genetically modified keratinocytes in a fibroblast/keratinocyte co-culture system. J Cell Physiol 180: 61–70

76. Sayani K et al. (2000) Delayed appearance of decorin in healing burn scars. Histopathology 36: 262–272

77. Polgar J, Reed GL (1999) A critical role for N-ethylmaleimide-sensitive fusion protein (NSF) in platelet granule secretion. Blood 94: 1313–1318

78. Flaumenhaft R et al. (1999) Proteins of the exocytotic core complex mediate platelet alpha-granule secretion. Roles of vesicle-associated membrane protein, SNAP-23, and syntaxin 4. J Biol Chem 274: 2492–2501

79. Tredget EE et al. (1998) Transforming growth factor-beta in thermally injured patients with hypertrophic scars: effects of interferon alpha-2b. Plast Reconstr Surg 102: 1317–1328; discussion 1329–1330

80. Sanderson N et al. (1995) Hepatic expression of mature transforming growth factor beta 1 in transgenic mice results in multiple tissue lesions. Proc Natl Acad Sci USA 92: 2572–2576

81. Takehara K (2000) Growth regulation of skin fibroblasts. J Dermatol Sci 24 [Suppl 1]: S70–77

82. Ghahary A et al. (2000) Mannose-6-phosphate/IGF-II receptors mediate the effects of IGF-1-induced latent transforming growth factor beta 1 on expression of type I collagen and collagenase in dermal fibroblasts. Growth Factors 17: 167–176

83. Ghahary A et al. (1998) Induction of transforming growth factor beta 1 by insulin-like growth factor-1 in dermal fibroblasts. J Cell Physiol 174: 301–309

84. Krishnaswami S et al. (2002) Thrombospondin-1 promotes proliferative healing through stabilization of PDGF. J Surg Res 107: 124–130

85. Rabhi-Sabile S et al. (1996) Proteolysis of thrombospondin during cathepsin-G-induced platelet aggregation: functional role of the 165-kDa carboxy-terminal fragment. FEBS Lett 386: 82–86

86. Shimokado K et al. (1985) A significant part of macrophage-derived growth factor consists of at least two forms of PDGF. Cell 43: 277–286

87. Antoniades HN et al. (1991) Injury induces in vivo expression of platelet-derived growth factor (PDGF) and PDGF receptor mRNAs in skin epithelial cells and PDGF mRNA in connective tissue fibroblasts. Proc Natl Acad Sci USA 88: 565–569

88. Scher CD et al. (1979) Platelet-derived growth factor and the regulation of the mammalian fibroblast cell cycle. Biochim Biophys Acta 560: 217–241

89. Seppa H et al. (1982) Platelet-derived growth factor in chemotactic for fibroblasts. J Cell Biol 92: 584–588

90. Bernstein LR, Antoniades H, Zetter BR (1982) Migration of cultured vascular cells in response to plasma and platelet-derived factors. J Cell Sci 56: 71–82

91. Ross R et al. (1974) A platelet-dependent serum factor that stimulates the proliferation of arterial smooth muscle cells in vitro. Proc Natl Acad Sci USA 71: 1207–1210

92. Ross R, Vogel A (1978) The platelet-derived growth factor. Cell 14: 203–210

93. Clemmons DR, Van Wyk JJ (1985) Evidence for a functional role of endogenously produced somatomedin-like peptides in the regulation of DNA synthesis in cultured human fibroblasts and porcine smooth muscle cells. J Clin Invest 75: 1914–1918

94. Barreca A et al. (1992) In vitro paracrine regulation of human keratinocyte growth by fibroblast-derived insulin-like growth factors. J Cell Physiol 151: 262–268

95. Ghahary A et al. (1996) Collagenase production is lower in post-burn hypertrophic scar fibroblasts than in normal fibroblasts and is reduced by insulin-like growth factor-1. J Invest Dermatol 106: 476–481

96. Camacho-Hubner C et al. (1992) Identification of the forms of insulin-like growth factor-binding proteins produced by human fibroblasts and the mechanisms that regulate their secretion. J Biol Chem 267: 11949–11956

97. Jones JI et al. (1993) Extracellular matrix contains insulin-like growth factor binding protein-5: potentiation of the effects of IGF-I. J Cell Biol 121: 679–687

98. Ghahary A et al. (1995) Enhanced expression of mRNA for insulin-like growth factor-1 in post-burn hypertrophic scar tissue and its fibrogenic role by dermal fibroblasts. Mol Cell Biochem 148: 25–32

99. Mast BA et al. (1992) Scarless wound healing in the mammalian fetus. Surg Gynecol Obstet 174: 441–451

100. Longaker MT, Bouhana KS, Harrison MR (1994) Wound healing in the fetus: Possible role for inflammatory macrophages and transforming growth factor-beta isoforms. Wound Repair Regen 2: 104

101. Longaker MT, Adzick NS (1991) The biology of fetal wound healing: a review. Plast Reconstr Surg 87: 788–798

102. Whitby DJ et al. (1991) Rapid epithelialisation of fetal wounds is associated with the early deposition of tenascin. J Cell Sci 99: 583–586

103. Luomanen M, Virtanen I (1993) Distribution of tenascin in healing incision, excision and laser wounds. J Oral Pathol Med 22: 41–45

104. Moritz AR, Henriquez FC (1947) Studies of thermal injury II. The relative importance of time and surface temperature in the causation of cutaneous burns. Am J Pathol 23: 695–720

105. Jackson DM (1953) The diagnosis of the depth of burning. Br J Surg 40: 588–596

106. Pruitt BA Jr, Moncrief JA (1967) Current trends in burn research. I. J Surg Res 7: 280–293

107. Heggers JP, Heggers R, Robson MC (1982) The immunological deficit encountered in thermal injury. J Am Med Tech 44: 99–102

108. Heggers JP et al. (1980) Evaluation of burn blister fluid. Plast Reconstr Surg 65: 798–804

109. Waxman K et al. (1987) Protein loss across burn wounds. J Trauma 27: 136–140

110. Jelenko C 3rd, Ginsburg JM (1971) Water-holding lipid and water transmission through homeothermic and poikilothermic skins. Proc Soc Exp Biol Med 136: 1059–1062

111. Zawacki BE (1987) The local effects of burn injury. In: Boswick JA (ed) The art and science of burn care. Aspen, Rockville, MD

112. Zawacki BE (1974) Reversal of capillary stasis and prevention of necrosis in burns. Ann Surg 180: 98–102

113. Warden G (1987) Immunological response to burn injury. In: Boswick JA (ed) The art and science of burn care. Aspen, Rockville, MD

114. Remensnyder JP (1972) Topography of tissue oxygen tension changes in acute burn edema. Arch Surg 105: 477–482

115. Arturson G (1979) Microvascular permeability to macromolecules in thermal injury. Acta Physiol Scand Suppl 463: 111–122

116. Arturson G, Soeda S (1967) Changes in transcapillary leakage during healing of experimental burns. Acta Chir Scand 133: 609–614

117. Cotran RS (1965) The delayed and prolonged vascular leakage in inflammation. II. An electron microscopic study of the vascular response after thermal injury. Am J Pathol 46: 589–620

118. Robson MC, Smith DJ, Heggers JP (1987) Innovations in burn wound management. In Habal MB (ed) Advances in plastic and reconstructive surgery. Year Book, Chicago, IL

119. Rohrich R, Robinson J (1999) Selected Readings in Plastic Surgery 9 (3): 1–40

120. Demling RH (1987) Pathophysiology of burn injury. Trauma, Clinical Care and Pathophysiology, ed. J.D. Richardson. 1987, Chicago, IL: Year Book.

121. Hatherill JR et al. (1986) Thermal injury, intravascular hemolysis, and toxic oxygen products. J Clin Invest 78: 629–636

122. Siney L, Brain SD (1996) Involvement of sensory neuropeptides in the development of plasma extravasation in rat dorsal skin following thermal injury. Br J Pharmacol 117: 1065–1070

123. Pitt RM et al. (1987) Analysis of altered capillary pressure and permeability after thermal injury. J Surg Res 42: 693–702
124. Douglas WW (1985) Histamine and 5-hydroxytrytamine (serotonin) and their antagonists. In: Gilman AG et al.(eds) The pharmacological basis of therapeutics. Macmillan, New York, NY
125. Arturson MG (1985) The pathophysiology of severe thermal injury. J Burn Care Rehabil 6: 129–146
126. Fjellstroem KE, Arturson G (1963) Changes in the human complement system following burn trauma. Acta Pathol Microbiol Scand 59: 257–270
127. Anggard E, Arturson G, Jonsson CE (1970) Efflux of prostaglandins in lymph from scalded tissues. Acta Physiol Scand 80: 46A–47A
128. Arturson G, Hamberg M, Jonsson CE (1973) Prostaglandins in human burn blister fluid. Acta Physiol Scand 87: 270–276
129. Heggers JP et al. (1980) Histological demonstration of prostaglandins and thromboxanes in burned tissue. J Surg Res 28: 110–117
130. Lund T et al. (1989) Mechanisms behind increased dermal imbibition pressure in acute burn edema. Am J Physiol 256: H940–948
131. Leape LL (1970) Initial changes in burns: tissue changes in burned and unburned skin of rhesus monkeys. J Trauma 10: 488–492
132. Zawacki BE (1974) The natural history of reversible burn injury. Surg Gynecol Obstet 139: 867–872
133. Linares HA, Larson DL (1976) Elastic tissue and hypertrophic scars. Burns 3: 407
134. Deitch EA et al. (1983) Hypertrophic burn scars: analysis of variables. J Trauma 23: 895–898
135. Cohen IK, McCoy BJ (1980) The biology and control of surface overhealing. World J Surg 4: 289–295
136. Doong H (1997) Alteration of fibroblast cell shape and induction of procollagenase synthesis by calcium channel blockers, calmodulin inhibitors, and protein kinase C inhibitors. The University of Chicago
137. Ehrlich HP et al. (1994) Morphological and immunochemical differences between keloid and hypertrophic scar. Am J Pathol 145: 105–113
138. Nedelec B et al. (2001) Myofibroblasts and apoptosis in human hypertrophic scars: the effect of interferon-alpha2b. Surgery 130: 798–808
139. Omo-Dare P (1975) Genetic studies on keloid. J Natl Med Assoc 67: 428–432
140. Bloom D (19556) Heredity of keloids; review of the literature and report of a family with multiple keloids in five generations. NY State J Med 56: 511–519
141. Dinarello CA, Wolff SM (1993) The role of interleukin-1 in disease. N Engl J Med 328: 106–113
142. Fulton JE Jr (1995) Silicone gel sheeting for the prevention and management of evolving hypertrophic and keloid scars. Dermatol Surg 21: 947–951
143. Cromack DT, Porras-Reyes B, Mustoe TA (1990) Current concepts in wound healing: growth factor and macrophage interaction. J Trauma 30 [Suppl 12]: S129–133
144. Gan JL et al. (1996) Microwave heating in the management of postmastectomy upper limb lymphedema. Ann Plast Surg 36: 576–580; discussion 580–581
145. Gold MH (1994) A controlled clinical trial of topical silicone gel sheeting in the treatment of hypertrophic scars and keloids. J Am Acad Dermatol 30: 506–507
146. Griffith BH (1966) The treatment of keloids with triamcinolone acetonide. Plast Reconstr Surg 38: 202–208
147. Aggeler J, Frisch SM, Werb Z (1984) Changes in cell shape correlate with collagenase gene expression in rabbit synovial fibroblasts. J Cell Biol 98: 1662–1671
148. Ahn ST, Monafo WW, Mustoe TA (1989) Topical silicone gel: a new treatment for hypertrophic scars. Surgery 106: 781–786; discussion 786–787
149. Arnold HL Jr, Grauer FH (1959) Keloids: etiology, and management by excision and intensive prophylactic radiation. Arch Dermatol 80: 772–777
150. Hoffman S (1982) Radiotherapy for keloids. Ann Plast Surg 9: 265
151. Katz BE (1995) Silicone gel sheeting in scar therapy. Cutis 56: 65–67
152. Ketchum LD et al. (1966) The treatment of hypertrophic scar, keloid and scar contracture by triamcinolone acetonide. Plast Reconstr Surg 38: 209–218
153. Kischer CW, Shetlar MR, Shetlar CL (1975) Alteration of hypertrophic scars induced by mechanical pressure. Arch Dermatol 111: 60–64
154. Kischer CW, Bailey JF (1972) The mast cell in hypertrophic scars. Tex Rep Biol Med 30: 327–338
155. Kischer CW, Shetlar MR, Chvapil M (1982) Hypertrophic scars and keloids: a review and new concept concerning their origin. Scan Electron Microsc 4: 1699–1713

# Pathophysiology of Chronic Wounds

M.C. ROBSON

## Introduction

The normal response to tissue injury is a timely and orderly reparative process that results in sustained restoration of anatomical and functional integrity [1]. Wound repair, however, is not a simple linear process but rather a complex integration of dynamic interactive processes involving cell–cell and cell–matrix interactions mediated by humoral messengers [2, 3]. Unencumbered, these processes follow a specific time sequence or chronology [2]. Although the timing of the various processes is usually orderly, it is not mutually exclusive and there is a varying overlap in time [3, 4].

Because wound healing is dynamic and the various processes involved in repair ideally proceed in an orderly and timely manner, it is clear that time is an important variable in wound repair [3, 4]. Clinically, categorisation of wounds as acute or chronic has been based on timeliness of healing [5]. The importance of factoring time into wound repair becomes clear when one realises that one of the goals of wound treatment is to accelerate healing [6].

## Definition of the Chronic Wound

The scheme of cellular processes and humoral mediators can be applied to all wounds [3] (Fig. 1). When a wound proceeds through an orderly and timely process and results in a sustained restoration of anatomical and functional integrity, it is labelled an acute wound [1]. Conversely, a chronic wound is one that has failed to proceed through an orderly and timely process to produce anatomical and functional integrity, or has proceeded through the repair process without establishing a sustained anatomical and functional result [1]. Simply stated, wounds may be classified as those that repair themselves or can be repaired in an orderly and timely process (acute wounds) and those that do not (chronic wounds) [1,3].

## Excessive Inflammation of Chronic Wounds

The various cellular processes in the wound-healing scheme are mediated by arachidonic acid metabolites, cytokines, growth factors and matrix metalloproteinases (MMPs) [4]. Because the individual cellular processes appear to be capable of func-

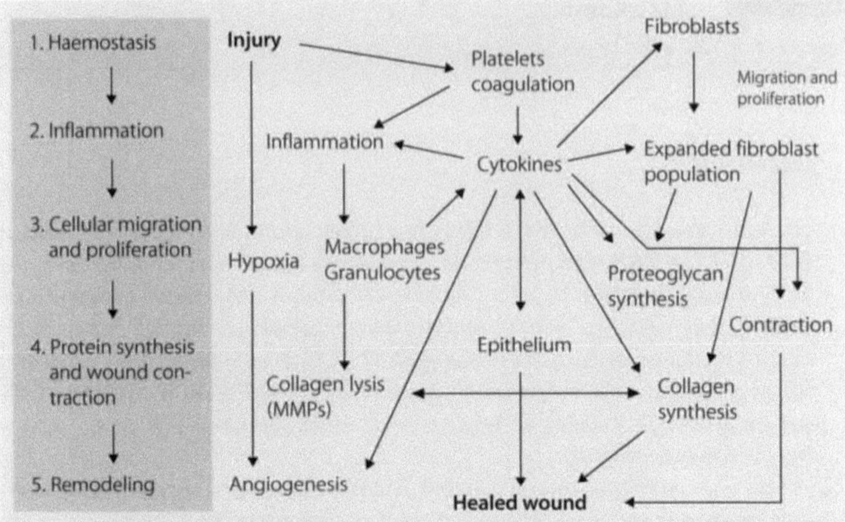



**Fig. 1.** The scheme of cellular processes and humoral mediators that results in wound repair. When a wound proceeds through the scheme in an orderly and timely manner, acute wound healing occurs. (Reprinted with permission from Monaco JL, Lawrence WT (2003) Acute wound healing: an overview. Clin Plast Surg 30: 2)

tioning in both acute and chronic wounds, the implication is that an impairment or imbalance in inflammatory mediators, cytokines, growth factors and/or MMPs in wounds promotes the establishment and maintenance of chronic wounds [3, 7] (Fig. 2). When fluids from chronic wounds are compared with those from acute

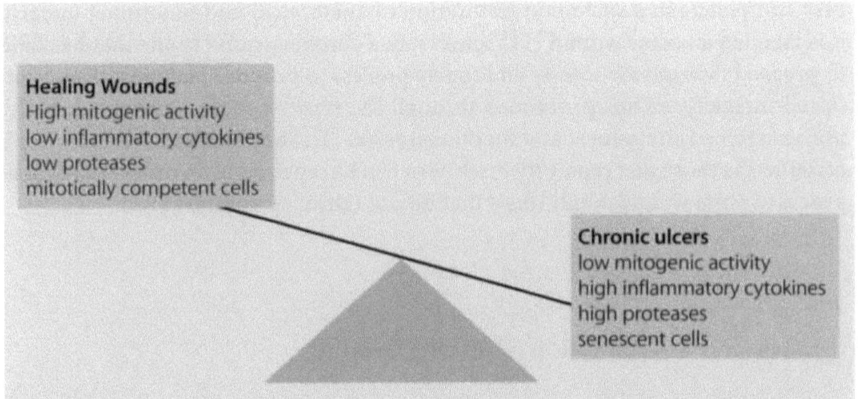



**Fig. 2.** An imbalance in favour of inflammatory cytokine mediators, proteases, low mitogenic growth factors and non-proliferating cells results in establishment and maintenance of chronic wounds. (With permission from [11])

wounds, it has been demonstrated that chronic wounds have elevated proinflammatory cytokines, high MMP activity, decreased levels of natural tissue inhibitors to MMPs (TIMPs) and diminished growth-factor activity [5, 8, 9, 10].

## Final Common Pathway for the Failure of Wounds to Heal

Outwardly, chronic wounds appear to be rather heterogenous [8]. Integumentary chronic wounds such as pressure ulcers, venous stasis ulcers, diabetic neuropathic ulcers and ischemic ulcers are each characterised by a unique set of causal factors and patient characteristics [4, 5]. Yet there have been postulated a common origin and a final common pathway for the failure of wounds to heal [4]. The common chronic wounds of the integument and soft tissues resulting in indolent ulcers are similar in that each is characterised by one or more persistent inflammatory stimuli: repeat trauma, ischemia or bacterial contamination [8]. These conditions lead to an ongoing proinflammatory stimulus instead of the self-limited proinflammatory stimulus present in acute wounds [4, 11]. The final common pathway activated by this prolonged inflammatory stimulus has been documented accurately as excess secretion of the proinflammatory cytokines such as tumour necrosis factor alpha (TNF-$\alpha$) and interleukin one beta (IL-1$\beta$), which synergistically increase production of MMPs while reducing the synthesis of TIMPs [10]. The elevated levels of MMPs rapidly degrade proteins that are necessary for wound healing, including growth factors, cytokines and their receptors, and extracellular matrix proteins [9, 12]. Degradation of growth factors and their receptors limits the progression of the wound-healing cascade by eliminating the mediators of the cascade [10]. Progression through the wound-healing scheme is thereby impaired, and the wound fails to heal [4].

## Inflammatory Stimuli Lead to Wound Chronicity

Each of the inflammatory stimuli (repeated trauma, ischemia and infection) are detrimental to healing and lead to wound chronicity. Wound healing begins at the time of wounding. Therefore, the initial traumatic event is beneficial and sets in motion the various processes of repair. Coagulation, platelet accumulation and release, and neutrophil and monocyte recruitment are all necessary to initiate the cascade. However, repeated trauma with a persistent stimulus for inflammation results in continual recruitment and activation of neutrophils and monocytes, resulting in development of a chronic inflammatory lesion [13]. Repeated or continuous injury results in the progression of the injured cells to necrosis [14].

Necrotic tissue present in a wound has several deleterious effects on tissue repair [15]. Wound bacteria use necrotic debris as a nutrient source, increasing the likelihood of invasive wound infection [4]. Metabolites of cell membrane eicosanoids released from dying cells can be toxic to adjacent normal cells [14, 16]. Necrotic debris within the wound may also establish a mechanical barrier against the influx of wound repair cells or humoral mediators from the surrounding tissue. Tissue proteases released by necrotic cells can degrade wound-growth factors, thus preventing the initiation of growth factor-dependent healing pathways [17].

## Role of Ischemia/Hypoxia in Delayed Healing

Clinical observation for a long time has shown that ischemic tissue does not heal well. Tissue perfusion is impaired as a consequence of many disorders, including a central low flow state due to shock or congestive heart failure, peripheral vascular disease, hypothermia, vasospastic diseases and peripheral venous hypertension [4]. The reduced peripheral capillary perfusion results in a low tissue oxygen tension that is associated with delayed wound healing and increased wound infections when a critical $PaO_2$ level is reached [18].

Oxygen is a critical element in the healing of wounds [19]. Cellular proliferation during angiogenesis, fibroplasia and epithelialisation proceeds at a more rapid pace in response to higher oxygen levels [18, 20–22]. Bacterial killing by phagocytic cells is also an oxygen-dependent process [23]. The oxygen-dependent processes of healing begin to fail as the tissue oxygen pressure ($pO_2$) levels fall below 40 mmHg [4]. Generally, a wound $pO_2$ below 30 mmHg implies that there may be insufficient oxygen for healing. Below 10 mmHg, oxygen is deficient, and growth factors have little chance of directing repair mechanisms for cells in wounds [24]. Severe ischemia/hypoxia can inhibit all wound-healing processes [20, 25].

## Excessive Bacteria Burden Impedes Wound Repair

Wound infection is probably the most common reason for impaired wound healing and wound chronicity [15, 26]. A definition of wound infection or excessive bacterial burden is important. All open wounds may be considered contaminated but not necessarily infected. For a wound to be infected, an imbalance must exist between the offending organisms and the host immune barriers such that tissue invasion and rising microbial colony counts occur [4]. For this reason, quantitative bacteriologic counts of the wound tissue provide a useful guide to the degree of wound contamination. When the bacterial burden approaches one million ($10^6$) organisms per gram of tissue or if any invasion by beta haemolytic streptococci occurs, healing will most often be impeded [26].

Each of the processes in the wound-healing scheme has been demonstrated to be inhibited by high levels of bacteria [27]. There are several mechanisms by which the excessive bacteria impair tissue repair. Infection prolongs the inflammatory phase of normal wound healing, induces the increased expression of tissue proteases leading to destruction of surrounding tissue, delays epithelialisation and collagen deposition and disrupts the progression of the inflammatory, proliferative and re-modelling phases of acute tissue repair [4]. There is a persistent production of in-flammatory mediators such as prostaglandin E2 and thromboxane and steady ingress of neutrophils, which release cytotoxic enzymes and free oxygen radicals. This produces localised thrombosis, which can lead to tissue hypoxia, bringing about further bacterial proliferation and tissue destruction [11, 14].

## Degradation of Growth Factors and Their Receptors

Inappropriately elevated tissue proteases stimulated by excessive bacteria may di-gest wound growth factors and membrane receptor sites necessary for the normal stimulation of cells involved in tissue repair [7, 12]. When bacterial species com-monly colonising wounds were mixed with growth-factor mediators of the healing cascade in vitro, the bacteria were demonstrated to cleave the complex molecules and degrade and inactivate growth factors [28]. Bacteria in the presence of tissue cells such as fibroblasts appeared to act synergistically to further degrade the growth factors. This may have been due to further production of harmful proteases and MMPs when the bacteria were in contact with the tissue cells. Receptors for several growth factors have also been reported to show decreased expression in chronic wounds [29, 30, 31]. Interestingly, high levels of bacteria did not affect the function of keratinocyte growth factor-2 (KGF-2) receptors [31].

## Cell-Cycle Arrest as the Mechanism of Chronicity

How the various factors such as trauma, ischemia, infection, prolonged inflamma-tion, excessive neutrophil, protease, MMP activity and decreased growth-factor levels actually result in wound chronicity has only recently become clear. Any event in the wound-repair process, from cell proliferation to cell migration, involves cell-cycle activity [32]. The cell cycle can be perceived as a clock that regulates ac-tivities of cell division and multiplication (Fig. 3). One full revolution of the clock culminates in the formation of two genetically identical daughter cells to assist in wound repair [32]. Normally, in intact skin, most cells are relatively inactive and are docked in a state of quiescence known as G0. Upon injury, as the healing cascade is activated, platelet factors are released to stimulate proliferation and the migration of inflammatory and other connective tissue cells that proliferate in wound repair.

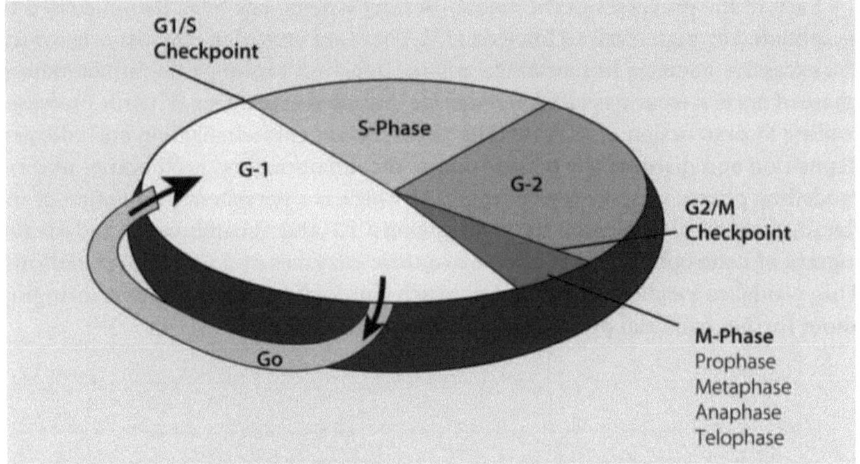

**Fig. 3.** The cell cycle can be perceived as a clock that regulates activities of cell division and multiplication. In normal uninjured skin, most fibroblasts are in a state of quiescence, designated G0. On injury, fibroblasts become activated by growth factors, when available, that initiate competence in G1. Cyclins, inhibitors and other factors help cells progress to the G1/S checkpoint to allow cells to progress through the cycle. (With permission from [32])

To be effective, growth factors must be released at certain threshold concentrations [32]. Such mitogen levels are necessary to activate the cells out of quiescence (G0) and instill competence for cell division [33].

Platelet-derived growth factor (PDGF) and fibroblast growth factor (FGF) are competence growth factors and have the ability to initiate the signal transduction pathway for cells to respond to additional stimuli known as progression factors [34]. Progression factors stimulate cellular competence to synthesise proteins and specific enzymes required for DNA replication [34–36]. Recognised progression factors are the insulin-like growth factors (IGFs) and epidermal growth factor (EGF) [32, 34, 36]. If growth factor titres are below the necessary threshold, competence is not achieved, and cells remain quiescent in G0.

## Growth Factor Deficiency as the Cause for Cell Cycle Arrest

As has been discussed, when wounds have prolonged inflammatory stimuli and continuous high titres of MMPs, there is a deficiency of growth factors in the wound. This deficiency could be absolute or relative, due to decreased production or secretion, more rapid breakdown, or trapping or binding of the growth factors so as to prevent their effective use in the healing processes [4]. Using the ELISA technique on retrieved chronic wound fluid it was demonstrated the PDGF, bFGF, EGF and transforming growth-factor beta (TGF-β) levels were markedly decreased compared to acute wounds [37]. Even when growth factors are not lacking, they may not be effectively available to the wound for healing [38]. In venous stasis ulcers, macromolecular leakage – specifically fibrinogen, alpha macroglobulin and albumin – leads to binding of these substances to growth factors, making them unavailable to the repair process [39]. These extravasated macromolecules scavenge not only growth factors but certain signal molecules involved in promoting wound repair [40]. This type of trapping of growth factors has also been reported in diabetic ulcers [38]. In instances in which the integrity of the growth factors is compromised or cell receptors are altered or absent, the released mitogenic signal is below the necessary threshold. As a result, wound cells are unable to become competent and subsequently become arrested in the cell cycle [32].

## Role of Cyclins and Cyclin-Dependent Kinases (CDKs) in Cellular Arrest

In addition to insufficient growth factors to drive the cell cycle, negative influences created by the continuous insults from inflammatory agents, proteases, metalloproteinases, low oxygen and increased radicals are factors that short-circuit the cell cycle by damaging the DNA and decreasing the nutrients required for DNA replication. Movement through phases of the cell cycle is orchestrated by cyclin-dependent kinases (CDKs) and regulatory subunits called cyclins [41–43]. These cyclin proteins activate CDKs to appropriate substrates to execute key steps in the cell-cycle process. Cycling cells enter and leave the cycle in association with synthesis and degradation of each cyclin at specific times [44]. Further control of the cell cycle is achieved through CDK inhibitors, which are involved in promoting differentiation, maintenance of terminal differentiation and regulation of the checkpoints within the cell cycle [45–47]. CDK inhibitors function by binding CDKs in the cyclin/CDK complexes. Although moderate concentrations of these inhibitors are positive regulators of cyclin D-dependent kinases, over-expression induces cell-cycle arrest [48].

## Prolonged Inflammatory Stimuli and the Cell Cycle

The exact manner in which pro-inflammatory cytokines affect the cell cycle is not yet clear. However, it has been shown that chronic wound fluid inhibits proliferation of fibroblasts and decreases the level of cylins while increasing the level of cyclin inhibitors [49]. Chronic wound fluid contains pro-inflammatory cytokines such as IL-1$\beta$ and TNF-$\alpha$ at levels 100 times higher than acute wound fluid [12]. If young human diploid fibroblasts are repeatedly stimulated with non-cytotoxic and non-proliferative doses of IL-1 and TNF-$\alpha$, increased percentages of cells with senescent morphology are observed, suggesting cell-cycle arrest [50]. Presently, studies are underway to evaluate the influence of prolonged inflammation as a direct cause of cell-cycle arrest.

## Evidence Linking Cell-Cycle Arrest to Chronicity

The cellular contribution of wound repair is a matter of numbers [32]. Three processes that produce increases in cell numbers are:

1. a shortening of the cell cycle (cells divide more frequently),
2. more cells becoming active in the cell cycle by decreasing the number of cells in G0, and
3. a decrease in the rate of cell death [51].

If the proportion of actively stimulated cells is sufficient to affect the proportion of cells arrested in the cell cycle or lost to necrosis, the wound exhibits repair and healing [32]. Conversely, when the number of cells in the arrested state increases, repair cannot proceed at the normal rate and wound chronicity occurs.

The indirect evidence of the final common pathway to decreased growth-factor activity, cell-cycle arrest and wound chronicity is overwhelming, as has been discussed. Recently, direct evidence has been reported in a four-arm clinical trial of chronic pressure ulcers. Wound fluid and tissue samples were collected longitudinally from patients enrolled in a four arm, blinded, prospective, randomised, placebo-controlled clinical trial comparing topical administration of granulocyte macrophage-colony stimulating factor (GM-CSF), bFGF, and sequential treatment with GM-CSF followed by bFGF over a 35-day period. Details of the clinical trial and results have been published previously [52]. In the trial, an 85% decrease in wound volume over 35 days was chosen as indicative of good healers, intermediate healers were defined as having 50–85% decrease in volume and poor healers were defined as having a decrease in volume of less than 50% [53]. Metalloproteinases in the wound (MMP-2 and MMP-9) correlated directly with the ability to heal the wound. Prior to treatment, the levels of MMP-2 and MMP-9 were higher in patients who proved to be poor or intermediate healers compared with patients who proved to be good healers. Conversely, tissue inhibitors of metalloproteinases (specifically TIMP-1) were low in poor and intermediate healers and higher in good healers. The MMP-9/TIMP-1 ratio on day 0 was fourfold higher in patients whose pressure ulcers healed poorly at the end of the study, and approximately twofold higher in patients whose pressure ulcers healed intermediately, compared to patients who healed well ($p<0.05$) [53]. This study provides the strongest data yet supporting the hypothesis that elevated levels of pro-inflammatory cytokines and proteinases, especially MMPs, contribute to the failure of wounds to heal.

In the same clinical trial fibroblasts were evaluated for cell-cycle arrest or cell-cycle progression. Using antibodies for cell markers, p21 was used as a marker for non-proliferation and proliferating cell nuclear antigen (PCNA) was a marker for cell proliferation [54]. Fibroblasts demonstrating co-localisation of both antigens were considered arrested in the cell cycle. At day 0, biopsies from the chronic pressure ulcers demonstrated that the fibroblast nuclei were stained in decreasing order by antibodies to p21, p21/PCNA, and PCNA [55]. The p21 labelling suggested that most of the cells were senescent or quiescent. When wounds were stimulated to heal by exogenous application of single or sequential growth factors, there was a decreasing number of p21 positive cells and an increasing proportion of PCNA-labelled cells [54, 55]. These data suggest that when growth factors are deficient in chronic wounds, the cell cycle is arrested, and when growth factors are added, chronicity is overcome, wound fibroblasts are stimulated to progress through the cell cycle and wound healing can occur.

There are additional problems that can occur to impair normal healing [4, 56]. These include poor nutrition, diabetes mellitus, chronic renal failure, immuno-deficiency syndromes, jaundice, age, radiation, cancer and medication/drugs among other factors. Although the exact mechanisms by which each of these factors shifts the wound-healing trajectory to the right towards chronicity have not been totally elucidated, many of these conditions have associated hypoxia or increased inflammatory states. Others predispose the wound to infection [57]. Still others directly inhibit cell proliferation, DNA synthesis and protein synthesis [4,57].

## Linking Molecular/Cellular Abnormalities to Clinical Observations

The elevated levels of inflammatory cytokines and proteases, along with low levels of mitogenic activity and the poor response of cells in chronic wounds, have led to the concept that the molecular environment of chronic wounds must be rebalanced to levels seen in acute healing wounds [11]. In most cases it is not possible to apply the principles of acute wound healing to chronic wounds without considering the biochemical environment of the latter. The management of chronic wounds needs to be freed from the acute wound model to optimise their clinical management [58]. Clinicians have labelled this approach of attempting to rebalance the molecular environment leading to chronicity as wound-bed preparation [58]. At a meeting of international wound experts held in France in June 2002, the clinical components of wound bed preparation along with the underlying cellular environment at each stage of wound repair were summarised [11]. The paradigm of wound-bed preparation is a simple way to link clinical observations to the underlying molecular, chemical and cellular abnormalities discussed in this chapter (Fig. 4). It also helps clinicians link their clinical interventions, attempting to shift repair of chronic wounds toward a more normal healing trajectory to the effects at a cellular level that were responsible for the underlying wound chronicity. Only by fully comprehending the molecular and cellular abnormalities responsible for the pathophysiology of chronic wounds will one be able to design interventions to optimise wound bed preparation and allow the chronic wound to heal in a more orderly and timely manner.

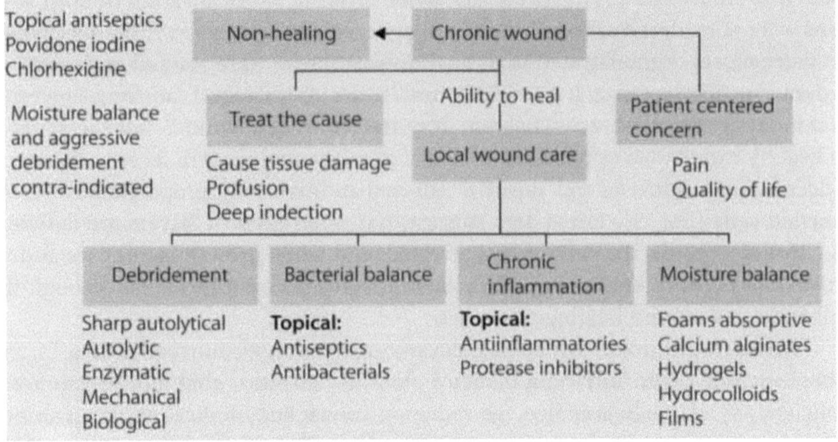


**Fig. 4.** Paradigm for preparing the wound bed. (With permission from [11])

## References


1. Lazurus GS, Cooper DM, Knighton DR, Margolis DJ, Pecoraro RE, Rodeheaver G, Robson MC (1994) Definitions and guidelines for assessment of wounds and evaluation of healing. Arch Dermatol 130: 489–493
2. Clark RAF (1993) Biology of dermal wound repair. Dematol Clin 11: 647–666
3. Robson MC (2003) Cytokine manipulation of the wound. Clin Plast Surg 30: 57–65
4. Robson MC, Steed DL, Franz MG (2001) Wound healing: biologic features and approaches to maximize healing trajectories. Curr Prob Surg 38: 61–140
5. Nwomeh BC, Yager DR, Cohen IK (1998) Physiology of the chronic wound. Clin Plast Surg 25: 341–346
6. Robson MC, Hill DP, Woodske ME, Steed DL (2000) Wound healing trajectories as predictors of effectiveness of therapeutic agents. Arch Surg 135: 773–777
7. Yager DR, Nwomeh BC (1999) The proteolytic environment of chronic wounds. Wound Rep Regen 7: 433–441
8. Mast BA, Schultz GS (1996) Interactions of cytokines, growth factors, and proteases in acute and chronic wounds. Wound Rep Regen 4: 411–420.
9. Tarnuzzer RW, Schultz GS (1996) Biochemical analysis of acute and chronic wound environments. Wound Rep Regen 4: 321–325
10. Trengove NJ, Stacey MC, MacAuley S, Bennett N, Gibson J, Burslem F, Murphy G, Schultz G (1999) Analysis of the acute and chronic wound environments: the role of proteases and their inhibitors. Wound Rep Regen 7: 442–452
11. Schultz GS, Sibbald G, Falanga V, Ayello EA, Dowsett C, Harding K, Romanelli M, Stacey MC, Teot L, Vanscheidt W (2003) Wound bed preparation: a systematic approach to wound management. Wound Rep Regen 11: 1–28
12. Yager DR, Chen SM, Ward SI, Olutoye OO, Diegelmann RF, Cohen IK (1997) Ability of chronic wound fluids to degrade peptide growth factors is associated with increased levels of elastase activity and diminished levels of protease inhibitors. Wound Rep Regen 5:23–32
13. Wahl LM, Wahl SM (1992) Inflammation. In: Cohen IK, Diegelmann RF, Lindblad WJ (eds) Wound healing, biochemical and clinical aspects. WB Saunders, Philadelphia, pp 40–62
14. Robson MC, Heggers JP (1992) Eicosanoids, cytokines, and free radicals. In: Cohen IK, Diegelmann RF, Lindblad WJ (eds) Wound healing, biochemical and clinical aspects. WB Saunders, Philadelphia, pp 292–304

15. Robson MC (1988) Disturbances in wound healing. Ann Emerg Med 17: 1274–1278

16. Robson MC (1989) The immediate and delayed damage following soft tissue trauma. In. Zarins C (ed) Essays in surgery. Churchill Livingstone, New York, pp 153–158

17. Lawrence WT (1992) Clinical management of nonhealing wounds. In: Cohen IK, Diegelmann RF, Lindblad WJ (eds) Wound healing, biochemical and clinical aspects. WB Saunders, Philadelphia, pp 541–561

18. Hunt TK, Pai MP (1971) Effect of varying oxygen tensions on healing of open wounds. Surg Gynecol Obstet 135: 561–567

19. Lavan FB, Hunt TK (1990) Oxygen and wound healing. Clin Plast Surg 17: 463–472

20. Zamboni WA, Browder LK, Martinez JA (2003) Hyperbaric oxygen and wound healing. Clin Plast Surg 30: 67–75

21. Knighton DR, Silver IA, Hunt TK (1981) Regulation of wound healing angiogenesis – effect of oxygen gradients and impaired oxygen concentration. Surgery 90: 262–269

22. Whitney JD (1989) Physiologic effects of tissue oxygenation in wound healing. Heart and Lung 18: 466–474

23. Knighton DR, Halliday B, Hunt TK (1986) Oxygen as an antibiotic: a comparison of the effects of inspired oxygen concentration and antibiotic administration on in vivo bacterial clearance. Arch Surg 121: 191–195

24. Robson MC, Mustoe TA, Hunt TK (1998) The future of recombinant growth factors in wound healing. Am J Surg 176 [Suppl]: 80S–82S

25. Niinikoski J, Hunt TK (1995) Oxygen and healing wounds: tissue-bone repair enhancement. In: Oriani G, Marroni A (eds) Handbook on hyperbaric medicine, 1st edn. Springer New York, pp 485–508

26. Robson MC (1997) Wound infection: a failure of wound healing caused by an imbalance of bacteria. Surg Clin N Amer 77: 637–650

27. Robson MC, Stenberg BD, Heggers JP (1990) Wound healing alterations caused by infection. Clin Plast Surg 17: 485–492

28. Payne WG, Wright TE, Ko F, Wheeler C, Wang X, Robson MC (2003) Bacterial degradation of growth factors. J Appl Res 3: 35–40

29. Hasan A, Murata H, Falabella A, Ochoa S, Zhou L, Badiava E, Falanga V (1997) Dermal fibroblasts from venous ulcers are unresponsive to the action of transforming growth factor beta 1. J Dermatol Sci 16: 59–66

30. Agren MS, Steenfos HH, Dabelsteen S, Hansen JB, Dabelsteen E (1999) Proliferation and mitogenic response to PDGF-BB of fibroblasts isolated from chronic venous leg ulcer is ulcer-age dependent. J Invest Dermatol 112: 463–469

31. Robson MC, Wright TE, Ko F, Connolly KM, Halpern W, Payne WG (2003) Genomics-based KGF-2 (Repifermin) and its receptors function effectively in infected wounds. J Appl Res 3: 97–103

32. VandeBerg JS, Robson MC (2003) Arresting cell cycles and the effect on wound healing. Surg Clin N Amer 83: 509–520

33. Soprano KJ (1994) WI-38 cell long term quiescence model system: a valuable tool to study molecular events that regulate growth. J. Cell Biochem 54: 405–414

34. Morgan CJ, Pledger WJ (1992) Fibroblast proliferation. In: Cohen IK, Diegelmann RF, Lindblad WJ (eds) Wound healing, biochemical and clinical aspects. WB Saunders, Philadelphia pp 63–76

35. Schafer KA (1998) The cell cycle: a review. Vet Pathol 35: 461–478

36. Svoboda ME, Van Wyk JJ, Klapper DG, Fellows RE, Grissom FE, Schlueter RJ (1980) Purification of somatomedin-C from human plasma, chemistry and biologic properties, partial sequence analysis, and relationship to other somatomedins. Biochemistry 19: 790–797

37. Cooper DM, Yu EZ, Hennessey P, Ko F, Robson MC (1994) Determination of endogenous cytokines in chronic wounds. Ann Surg 219: 688–692

38. Robson, MC, Smith PD (2001) Topical use of growth factors to enhance healing. In: Falanga V (ed) Cutaneous wound healing. Martin Dunitz, London, pp 379–398

39. Falanga V, Eaglstein WH (1993) The trap hypothesis of venous ulceration. Lancet 341: 1006–1008

40. Falanga V, Grinnell F, Gilchrist B, Maddox YT, Moshell A (1994) Workshop on the pathogenesis of chronic wounds. J Invest Dermatol 102: 125–127

41. Assoian RK (1997) Control of the G1 phase cyclin-dependent kinases by mitogenic growth factors and the extracellular matrix. Cytokine Growth Factor Rev 8: 156–170

42. Sherr CJ, Matsushima H, Kato J-Y, Quelle DE, Roussel MF (1994) Control of G1 progression by mammalian D-type cyclins. In: Hu VW (ed) The cell cycle regulators, targets, and clinical applications. Plenum Press, New York, pp 17–23

43. Morgan DO (1995) Principles of CDK regulation. Nature 374: 131–134
44. Ludlow JW, Glendening CL, Livingston DM, DeCarprio JA (1993) Specific enzymatic dephosphorylation of the retinoblastoma protein. Mol Cell Biol 13: 367–372
45. Bohmer RM, Scharf E, Assoian RK (1996) Cytoskeletal integrity is required throughout the mitogen stimulation phase of the cell cycle and mediates the anchorage dependent expression of cyclin D1. Mol Biol Cell 7: 101–111
46. Browne JP, Wei W, Sedivy JM (1997) Bypass of senescence after disruption of p21 C1P1/WAF1 gene in normal diploid human fibroblasts. Science 277: 831–834
47. Campisi J (1999) Replicative senescence and immortalization. In: Stein GS, Baserga R, Denhardt DT (eds) The molecular basis of cell cycle and growth control. Wiley-Liss, New York, pp 348–373
48. Sherr CJ, Roberts JM (1999) CDK inhibitors: positive and negative regulators of G1-phase progression. Genes Dev 13: 1501–1512
49. Seah CC, Phillips T, Park H-Y (2001) The First Annual Young Investigator's Award. Modulation of cell cycle regulatory proteins by chronic wound fluid. Wounds 13: 136–142
50. Schwarz DA, Lindblad WJ, Rees RS (1995) Altered collagen metabolism and delayed healing in a novel model of ischemic wounds. Wound Rep Regen 3: 204–212
51. Baserga R (1999) Introduction to the cell cycle. In: Stein GS, Baserga R, Dehnardt DT (eds) The molecular basis of cell cycle and growth control. Wiley-Liss, New York, pp 1–14
52. Robson MC, Hill DP, Smith PD, Wang X, Meyer-Siegler K, Ko F, VandeBerg JS, Payne WG, Ochs D, Robson LE (2000) Sequential cytokine therapy for pressure ulcers: clinical and mechanistic response. Ann Surg 231: 600–611
53. Ladwig GP, Robson MC, Liu R, Kuhn MA, Muir DF, Schultz GS (2002) Ratios of activated matrix metalloproteinase-9 to tissue inhibitor of matrix metalloproteinase-1 in wound fluids are inversely correlated with healing of pressure ulcers. Wound Rep Regen 10: 26–37
54. VandeBerg JS, Smith PD, Haywood-Reid PL, Munson AB, Soules KA, Robson MC (2002) Influence of single and sequential cytokine therapy on the cell cycle of pressure ulcer fibroblasts. J Appl Res 2: 11–19
55. VandeBerg JS, Smith PD, Haywood-Reid PL, Munson AB, Soules KA, Robson MC (2001) Dynamic forces in the cell cycle affecting fibroblasts in pressure ulcers. Wound Rep Regen 9: 19–27
56. Burns JS, Mancoll JS, Phillips LG (2003) Impairments to wound healing. Clin Plast Surg 30: 47–56
57. Williams JZ, Barbul A (2003) Nutrition and wound healing. Surg Clin N Amer 83: 571–596
58. Falanga V (2000) Classifications for wound bed preparation and stimulation of chronic wounds. Wounds Rep Regen 8: 347–352

# Control of Infection

D. Leaper, A. Melling

## Introduction

Health-care-related infection, also known as hospital-acquired or nosocomial infections, are common, expensive to health services and increase patient morbidity and length of stay. The huge rise in day-case surgery and early discharge from hospital has not been associated with an increase in support and trained services within primary care. Surgical site (wound) infections (SSIs) and chronic wound infections have almost their entire cost transferred to primary health care, where there may often be inappropriate management.

There are many aspects to infection control which do not involve the surgery of wound care. These are listed in Table 1 and are not discussed further. All health-care staff should be cognisant of infection control and follow local protocols in prevention. Surgeons and ancillary staff must practice the preventative steps which can be undertaken perioperatively to prevent SSIs; the factors involved are many (see list below).

**Table 1.** Health-care-related infectious clinical conditions

|  | Infection | Agent |
| --- | --- | --- |
| **Those principally affecting patients:** | Deep and superficial surgical site infection | – |
|  | Colonisation/infection of chronic wounds | MRSA in particular |
|  | Urinary tract infection | Usually catheter-related |
|  | Respiratory tract infection | e.g. ventilator-associated pneumonia |
|  | Central vascular catheter infection | Mostly CNS organisms |
|  | Acquired gastrointestinal infections | e.g. Clostridium diffi-cile, VRE, Norwalk virus, Shigella/Salmonella |
|  | Transmissible spongiform encephalopathy | e.g. CJD |
|  | Immune deficiency syndrome (AIDS, cancer, steroids, etc. | e.g. CMV, fungal infection, TB, pneumocystitis |

**Table 1.** *Continued*

|  | Infection | Agent |
|---|---|---|
| Those principally affecting health-care workers: | Needle-stick related | – |
|  | Hepatitis B and C, HIV | Only hep B immuni-sation available |

### Peri-Operative Risk Factors for SSI

- Evidence-based factors
  - Handscrub and skin preparation
  - Antibiotic prophylaxis
  - Shaving and handwashing
  - Long pre-operative hospital stay
  - Long operation
  - Nutritional status
  - Bowel preparation
  - Dehydration or shock
  - Foreign bodies in wound
  - Peri-operative blood transfusion
  - Theatre or ward environment (and disciplines)
  - Immunosuppression (metabolic, steroids, cancer, HIV)
  - Patient temperature
- Unproven or uncertain (but usually observed) factors
  - Surgical technique (which cannot be measured)
  - Pre-operative antiseptic shower
  - Wound guards
  - Wound drapes
- Incise drapes (impregnated or not)
  - Dressings
  - Sutures, clips and tapes
  - Masks and gowns
  - Surgical gloves
  - Theatre cleaning between cases (although logical)
  - Number of people in theatre

Infection control and surveillance of health-care-related infections can reduce incidence by up to one third. However, their surveillance has a relatively low priority to the infection control team (ICT) of a hospital. The introduction of comparative data (league tables) for surgeons and institutions may change this. The ICT is made up of an infection control doctor (usually a microbiologist) and nurses (dedicated specialists) with an infection control committee, with representatives from management, support services and clinical specialities. The ICT has equally important educational and advisory roles and are responsible for implementing national guidance.

## Basic Principles of Infection Control in Relation to Wounds

- Elimination/reduction of environmental organisms (including patients' endogenous organisms)
- Prevention of cross-infection
- Optimisation of patient's host defences (e.g. attention to nutrition and use of antimicrobials)

These factors relate to both surgical or traumatic wounds as well as to open chronic wound healing by secondary intention when patients are admitted to hospital.

Elimination/reduction of environmental organisms (including patients' endogenous organisms). It has been repeatedly said that effective hand-washing between each patient contact (strictly observed in the operating theatre but not as scrupulously in hospital wards or outpatient departments) is probably the single most important factor in the prevention of contamination leading to direct or cross-infection. Hand-washing should follow an agreed protocol, which should be strictly checked. For general use, hand-washing with soap and effective hand drying with disposable paper towels is adequate, although a hand rub with alcoholic preparations is probably as good and is more acceptable. In the operating theatre skin preparation with an aqueous (surgical team) or alcoholic (patient) antiseptic is conventional. Antiseptics in common use are shown in Table 2; some have other uses.

Skin "scrubbing up" should not be a prolonged affair. For the first case on an operating list it is necessary to clean the nails with a scraper and a scrubbing brush.

**Table 2.** Antiseptics in use for skin preparation and wound care

| Name | Presentation | Uses | Comments |
| --- | --- | --- | --- |
| Chlor-hexidine, Hibiscrub | Alcoholic 0.5%, Aqueous 4% | Skin preparation, surgical scrub; in dilute solutions in open wounds | Has cumulative effect, effective against Gram-positive organisms and relatively stable in presence of pus and body fluids |
| Povidon-eiodine Betadine | Alcoholic 10%, Aqueous 7.5% | Skin preparation, surgical scrub; in dilute solutions in open wounds | Safe, fast-acting, broad spectrum. Some sporicidal activity. Antifungal. Iodine is not free but combined with polyvinyl-pyrrolidone (povidone) |
| Cetrimide Savlon | Aqueous cationic surfactant | Hand-washing | Active against Gram-positive organisms. Pseudomonas spp. may grow in stored contaminated solutions. Quaternary ammonium compounds have good detergent action (surface active agent) |
| Alcohols | 60 or 70% ethyl, isopropyl | Skin preparation | |

**Table 2.** *Continued*

| Name | Presentation | Uses | Comments |
|---|---|---|---|
| Hypochlorites, Eusol, Milton | Aqueous preparations | Instrument and surface cleaning (debriding agent in open wounds?) | Should be reserved for use as a disinfectant |
| Hexachlorophene | Aqueous bisphenol | Hand-washing | Active against Gram-positive organisms. Systemic absorption may lead to neurotoxicity with repeated or extensive use in babies |
| Triclosan, Aquasept, Manusept | Aqueous phenolic preparations, 2%, 0.5% | Hand-washing | Similar activity to hexachlorophene, no toxicity described in neonates. Alternative to povidone-iodine and chlorhexidine |

Cleaning the arms to the elbows in a systematic fashion for 4–5 min with an aqueous antiseptic such as 4% chlorhexidine or 7.5% povidone iodine is all that is required. Between cases a 2–3-min antiseptic wash is sufficient. Overdoing scrubbing has the same effect as shaving undertaken too long before surgery; the trauma produces more organisms to migrate to the skin surface and if the skin is damaged, organisms can multiply and risk an increase of infection. Preparation of patients' skin requires the antiseptic to dry for optimal effect. One application can reduce surface organisms by as much as 95%. When using alcoholic antiseptics skin should also be dried before diathermy is used.

Other methods of reducing patients' endogenous organisms and SSIs include antibiotic prophylaxis, which is not described further here (Table 3).

**Table 3.** Use of prophylactic antibiotics to reduce SSIs

| Type of surgery – wound classification | Antibiotic prophylaxis | Infection rate (SSIs) |
|---|---|---|
| Clean (e.g. hernia, varicose veins) | Controversial | Controversial[a] may be >10% |
| Clean prosthetic (e.g. hip or vasculosurgery) | 1–3 doses against *Staphylococcus aureus*, CNS, AGNB | 1–2% |
| Clean contaminated (open cholecystectomy) | 1 dose against enterococci enterobacteria | Reduction from 20% to <10% |
| Contaminated (e.g. elective colorectal surgery) | 1–3 doses against enterobacteriacea + anaerobes | Reduction from 50% to 15–20% |
| Dirty (e.g. faecal peritonitis) | Antibiotic treatment required for 5 days + (broad spectrum) | Reduction from >60% to <40% |

## Operating Theatre, Equipment and Discipline

A safe, comfortable working environment should be provided for staff and patients, adjacent to A&E, surgical wards, radiology and ICU. The highest aseptic and antiseptic ideals should be observed. Management should be strictly controlled by multidisciplinary representation on a Theatre Users' Committee which liaises with the Infection Control Team. Most theatres are "zoned" from clean to dirty; this relates to movement of personnel as well as theatre ventilation, which directs airflow from aseptic to less critical areas. Transfer of infection from one patient to another during surgery is uncommon, but it is sensible to place patients known to be colonised, with MRSA for example, at the end of a list.

A safe range of temperature (20–22 °C) and humidity (40–60%) to avoid electrostatic sparks should accompany appropriate ventilation to reduce airborne bacteria and anaesthetic gases. Plenum ventilation is filtered air pumped in from ceiling, to leave via side vents (baffles) in the walls. Twenty air changes/hour is suitable for most operations. Ultraclean air with laminar flow can be used for prosthetic surgery, particularly hip replacements, with high-efficiency filters and up to 300 air changes/hour. Exhaust-ventilated, bacteria-proof operating suits can further reduce contamination, although the use of prophylactic antibiotics and UV radiation may be as good. Microbiological sampling should be carried out regularly for optimum performance. In ultraclean air theatres air sampled within 300 mm of the wound should contain <10 cfu/m$^3$, which can be as low as <1 cfu/m$^3$ if occlusive clothing is used.

Theatre linen should be an effective barrier to organisms but remain comfortable and antistatic, with a low risk of shed particles. Specialised disposable linen is required when operating on a patient with a transmissible viral risk. This is impermeable and waterproof but can feel uncomfortable and hot. The use of masks has been shown to be unrelated to SSIs but should be practised in prosthetic operations and to protect the operating staff, as gloves do, when there is a viral risk. The use of hoods is aesthetic, but also advisable, particularly in prosthetic operations. Eyewear is becoming mandatory to protect staff, but footwear must have impermeable, non-slip, antistatic soles. Overshoes, just like sticky mats at the operating theatre's entrance, do not reduce microbial contamination.

There are many types of sterilisation. Heat is used as steam under pressure for maximum penetration (autoclave). Three min at 134 °C (2.2 bar) is suitable for heat-resistant instruments, gowns, drapes and swabs. Irradiation is used by manufacturers of disposable instruments such as sutures, syringes and single-use surgical equipment. Sterilisation solutions are used for delicate instruments, such as endoscopes, but are toxic. Sterilisation involves the destruction of all organisms and spores, whereas disinfection used in theatres and wards for cleaning purposes can only reduce their number. Some disinfectants, such as the hypochlorites, are toxic to human tissues and should be replaced by antiseptics (see Table 2) for this use. All antiseptics are rapidly inactivated by contact with body fluids and tissues.

## Prevention of Cross-Infection

Medically qualified staff are the worst offenders of cross-infection risk. They may underestimate by a factor of eight the number of times they wash their hands. Nevertheless, cross-infection in the ward is uncommon but can be potentially serious with organisms such as MRSA. The same principles of asepsis and antisepsis should, whenever possible, be observed as those seen in the operating theatre. Some hospitals refuse the transfer of patients unless they are certified as being MRSA-free. When a potentially dangerous infection is acquired by a patient who cannot go home, then isolation and barrier nursing need to be instituted. Equally, when a member of staff has an infectious focus, such as a skin abscess, he/she should not be at work. Patients and staff who are colonised by resistant organisms need identification to prevent their contact with patients at risk.

## Optimisation of Patient's Host Defence

Patient factors which contribute to an increased risk of SSI are shown below. These patients are also at an added risk of opportunistic pathogens. Host defences can be improved by judicious timing of surgery and control of underlying illness. However, the patient with cancer who has had a recent 30% body weight loss may not respond to prolonged ineffective attempts to improve nutrition; nor is the patient presenting with faecal peritonitis likely to benefit from prolonged resuscitation and antibiotic therapy when emergency surgery and source control are the key to reducing the risk of mortality and morbidity, including SSI.

### Patient Factors for Increased Risk of SSI

- Malnutrition (recent weight loss, obesity)
- Metabolic disease (diabetes, renal and liver failure)
- Immunosuppression (steroids, cancer, AIDS, oncology therapies)
- Colonisation and translocation in the GI tract
- Poor perfusion (systemic shock or local ischaemia)
- Presence of foreign body
- Patient temperature
- Previous surgery

## References


1. Williams JD, Taylor EW (eds) (2003) Infection in surgical practice. Arnold, London, UK, pp 10–29
2. Leaper DJ, Harding KG (1998) Wounds. Biology and management. Oxford Medical Publications, Oxford, UK
3. Schein M, Marshall JC (2003) Source control. Springer, Berlin Heidelberg New York Tokyo
4. Leaper DJ (2004) Wound infection. In: Russell RCG, Williams NS, Bulstrode CJK (eds) Bailey and Love's short practice of surgery, 24th edn. Arnold, London, UK (in press)
5. Centers for Disease Control and Prevention (1999) Guidelines for prevention of surgical site infections. Am J Infect Control 27: 97–134
6. Melling AG, Ali B, Scott EM, Leaper DJ (2001) The effects of preoperative warming on the incidence of wound infection after clean surgery. Lancet 358: 876–880
7. Leaper DJ, Melling AG (2002) Antibiotic prophylaxis in clean surgery: clean non-implant wounds. J Antimicrob Chemother 13 (special issue 1): 96–101

# Radiotherapy and Wounds

E.L. Dormand, P.E. Banwell, T.E.E. Goodacre

## Introduction

Radiotherapy has been used for over a 100 years to treat certain cancers, either as a curative, adjuvant or palliative treatment. Although radiation therapy is used to kill cancerous cells, it also results in damage to healthy cells, which leads to a variety of acute and long-term complications. Side effects may be due to radiation-induced DNA mutations, cell death within irradiated organs, ischaemia due to the effects of radiation on small blood vessels or due to perturbed inflammatory and repair responses. The skin is particularly affected with atrophy, soft-tissue fibrosis and microvascular damage.

Wound-healing problems are long-term sequelae of radiotherapy, characterised by decreased wound strength, decreased collagen deposition and decreased angiogenesis. These problems may lead to delayed or non-healing ulceration (radiation ulcers), superimposed infection, carcinogenesis and acosmesis. Furthermore, these effects have significant implications when surgical intervention is considered.

Current radiotherapy protocols aim to minimise radiation damage to normal tissue by fractionating the radiation dose and protecting normal tissue either physically or pharmacologically. Radiotherapy is targeted by modelling radiation beams to the tumour using recent advances in imaging and computer technology (3-D conformal radiotherapy and intensity-modulated radiation therapy) or by inserting radioactive implants directly into the tumour (internal radiotherapy/brachytherapy). However, some radiation damage to normal tissue is inevitable and may be a serious problem for surgical procedures. The damaged tissue is a poor substrate for reconstructive surgery and poor wound healing may complicate usually straightforward operations. This chapter explores the underlying pathophysiology of radiation damage and the implications for surgeons.

## Pathophysiology of Radiation Injury

The normal response to traumatic cell injury is a complex cascade involving haemostasis, inflammation, proliferation of granulation tissue, restitution and remodelling. Many of these stages are affected in radiation-induced injury [1, 2]. The ordered sequence of events is interrupted by repetitive radiation damage during fractionated radiotherapy. At first, normal tissue is irradiated, but subsequent radiation doses are applied to damaged, pre-irradiated tissue, resulting in on-going cellular regeneration and increasingly amplified inflammation. Damage may progress for many years after the course of radiotherapy (Fig. 1).

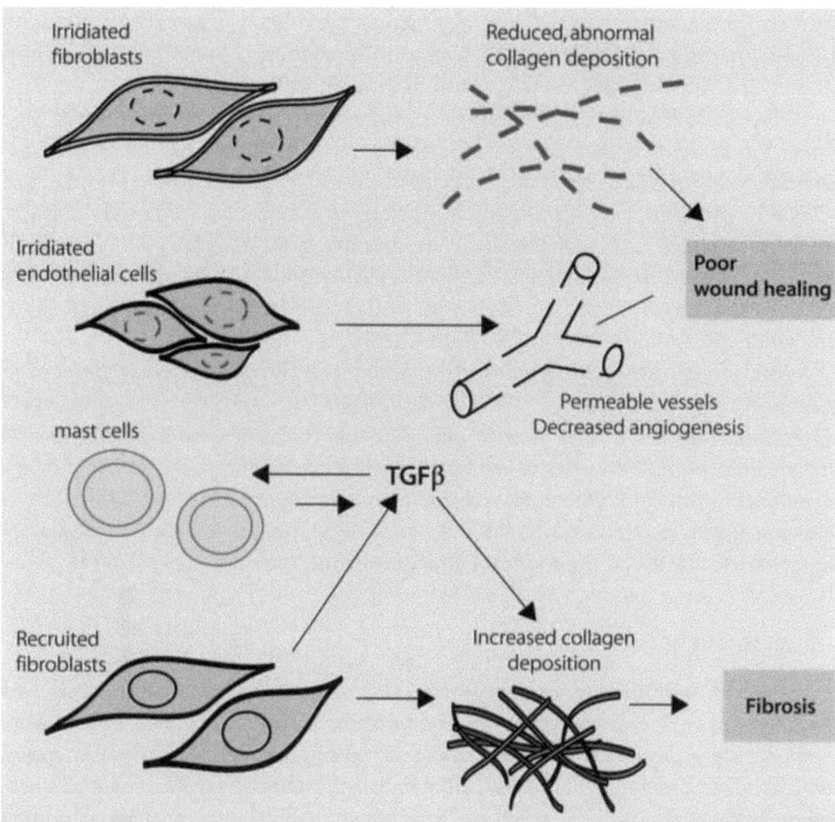


**Fig. 1.** Tissue damage due to radiotherapy. Radiation-damaged endothelial cells and fibroblasts lead to impaired wound healing. TGFβ1 is thought to be a major determinant of radiation fibrosis, recruiting and stimulating local fibroblasts to permanently synthesise and deposit collagen

## Early Inflammation

Radiation-induced DNA, protein and membrane damage lead to cell death by apoptosis. As with most forms of traumatic injury, the coagulation cascade is rapidly activated by radiation, partly due to free radical inactivation of anti-coagulatory factors. Radiation-induced apoptosis of endothelial cells, coupled with their slow proliferation, results in increased vascular permeability and vessels denuded of endothelium which are susceptible to thrombosis, intimal proliferation and eventually obliteration.

The acute inflammatory response after physical trauma is triggered by stress-sensitive kinases and transcription factors. Pro-inflammatory cytokines are synthesised, such as tumour necrosis factor alpha (TNFα), interleukin (IL)-1, IL-8 and interferon gamma (IFNγ) [1]. Inflammation is terminated as a result of the short half-life of these cytokines, and the action of anti-inflammatory cytokines such as transforming growth factor beta (TGFβ), IL-4, IL-10 and IL-13. Following radiation injury, however, inflammation does not resolve adequately, due to overproduction of pro-inflammatory cytokines, resulting in perturbed cell–cell and cell–matrix interactions, uncontrolled matrix accumulation and fibrosis [3].

Nitric oxide (NO) is a major player in early inflammation, promoting collagen deposition in the wound. NO is synthesised by macrophages and fibroblasts and is diminished in irradiated wounds, compared to non-irradiated wounds [4]. Reduced NO is also thought to be responsible for poor wound healing in diabetic patients, which may be further exacerbated by radiotherapy. Lymphocyte synthesis of TNFα and IFNγ, which prevent collagen deposition, is increased in irradiated wounds so that the early balance of secreted factors leads to poor collagen deposition at the time when collagen is essential for wound strength.

Radiation-induced epithelial injury results in inflammatory responses in the underlying supportive tissue. After a period of growth arrest, re-epithelialisation is initiated. However, if there is additional damage to the basement membrane, the formation of granulation tissue is delayed and does not form as effectively following radiation injury. Reduced expression of matrix metalloprotease 1 (MMP1) in post-irradiation granulation tissue has been reported to reduce cell migration, angiogenesis and tissue remodelling, thus retarding the healing process [5].

### Late Healing

Late effects of radiotherapy include fibrosis, necrosis, atrophy, vascular damage and carcinogenesis. The extracellular matrix composition is perturbed as a result of complex interactions between microvascular injury, damaged fibroblasts, altered TGFβ levels and mast cell activity. Collagen is the main extracellular matrix component in the skin and is secreted by fibroblasts. Extracellular matrix components are degraded by tissue MMPs which are inhibited by specific tissue inhibitors of metalloproteases (TIMPs). In irradiated wounds, collagen synthesis by fibroblasts and degradation by MMPs are both increased, leading to long-term accumulation of cross-linked type-I collagen in irradiated skin [6].

Radiation-induced microvascular injury may cause long-term reduced blood flow to the tissues and ischaemic damage leading to fibrosis, necrosis or atrophy. Radiation-induced phenotypic changes to the endothelial cells induce increased expression of TNFα and platelet-derived growth factor (PDGF), with down-regulation of NO synthase and thrombomodulin, all of which can stimulate events leading to fibrosis [1]. Endothelial cell expression of inter-cellular adhesion molecules such as I-CAM1 and E-selectin is also disrupted during and following radiotherapy [7]. Radiation-induced vessel damage is thought to lead to ischaemia and has been blamed for the long-term effects of radiation injury. However, a recent study showed that irradiated tissues are not hypoxic, suggesting that other factors may be involved in long-term damage, such as permanent changes in fibroblasts [8].

Fibroblast dysfunction following radiotherapy may result in poor wound healing and/or skin fibrosis. Poor wound healing results from defective collagen deposition by irradiated fibroblasts, including decreased collagen synthesis and deposition, or deposition of defective collagen. Irradiated fibroblasts exhibit subcellular changes, altered cell adhesion molecule and cytokine expression, decreased collagen gene expression and a reduced proliferative ability. Injection of normal, syngeneic fibroblasts into an irradiated wound results in normal wound healing [9]. A reactive fibrosis may also result following radiation damage due to over-recruitment and stimulation of local fibroblast progenitors. Fibroblasts recruited to the site of radiation injury exhibit increased proliferation, increased synthesis and deposition of extracellular matrix components, reduced collagenolytic activity due to increased TIMP expression, and increased TGF$\beta$1 expression [10].

The TGF$\beta$ family is important for all aspects of wound healing [11]. There are three mammalian isoforms, differing ratios of which lead to scarring and fibrosis. The family members and their receptors are up-regulated in irradiated wounds [12]. TGF$\beta$ family members have many roles which can contribute to fibrosis, including chemotaxis of mast cells, fibroblasts, monocytes and macrophages, proliferation and stimulation of fibroblasts, enhancing collagen and extracellular matrix molecule deposition, inhibition of collagenase and extracellular matrix degradation and inhibition of epithelial cell growth [1]. TGF$\beta$1 levels are elevated in endothelial cells and fibroblasts long after radiotherapy and TGF$\beta$1 is thought to be a major factor inducing radiation fibrosis [13].

## Specific Problems for Surgery

### Radiation Ulcers

Non-healing radiation ulcers may arise at any time following radiotherapy, and up to decades later [14]. Radiation ulcers are associated with considerable morbidity, including infection, pain, acosmesis, psychological distress, reduced quality of life and mortality due to overwhelming infection. Radiation ulcers may be treated conservatively, with wound dressings, antibiotics, Gentian Violet and hyperbaric oxygen, or with surgical attempts at wound closure. Skin grafts and local flaps have not been successful for the treatment of radiation ulcers; however, there have been good results importing vascularised myocutaneous and omental flaps. Complication rates are high, however, due to viable flaps not taking to the irradiated ulcer bed, resulting in partial or total flap loss, or thrombosis. A recent study of free-tissue transfer flaps reported a 40% complication rate, including problems with pedicle thrombosis when recipient vessels were within the irradiated zone [15].

There is still controversy as to whether radiation damage directly affects the risk of free-flap loss after reconstructive surgery. A study of free-flap survival in head and neck reconstructions found that the failure rate for irradiated versus non-irradiated patients was not significantly different; infection and lag time between radiotherapy and surgery did significantly affect the outcome [16]. Although complications are more common in irradiated tissue, it has been suggested that this might be due to confounding factors such as infection [17]. Indeed, the choice of free-flap techniques has been postulated to be the most important factor affecting outcome [18]. Special care is necessary when planning and performing reconstructive surgery on previously irradiated tissue.

### Breast Cancer Surgery

Late-stage breast cancer is usually treated by mastectomy and adjuvant radiotherapy. Following mastectomy, the breast may be reconstructed with silicone implants, tissue expanders or autologous reconstruction, either immediately after the mastectomy, or electively at a later time. Immediate breast reconstruction, following skin-sparing mastectomy, has been found to have superior aesthetic results to delayed reconstruction [19]. However, the effects of radiotherapy on wound healing may lead to an inhospitable environment for a reconstructive flap, resulting in wound dehiscence and acosmetic results.

Recent long-term studies have found that adjuvant radiotherapy results in worse long-term outcomes for immediate reconstruction. A retrospective evaluation of the results of immediate transversus rectus abdominis musculocutaneous flap (TRAM) with post-operative radiotherapy found that although flap transfer was successful, it was difficult to achieve good cosmesis, with unpredictable volume, contour and symmetry loss following post-operative radiotherapy [20]. A longer term study with 3–5 years follow-up concluded that although there was no difference in early complications following an immediate or delayed TRAM, late complications such as fat necrosis, volume loss and flap contracture were considerably increased in patients who had had immediate reconstruction and post-operative radiotherapy [21]; 28% of patients in the immediate TRAM group required an additional flap to correct deformity. Similar results, with decreased aesthetic scores, have been found for irradiated versus non-irradiated deep inferior epigastric perforator flaps [22]. This study also found that patients who smoked or were obese were at higher risk of complications. In summary, it appears that there are fewer complications and better cosmetic results if reconstruction is delayed when radiotherapy is necessary.

Early-stage breast cancer is usually treated by lumpectomy and radiotherapy. However, if this is unsuccessful, a salvage mastectomy is necessary and reconstructive surgery may be requested. It is generally accepted that previous radiotherapy adversely affects the outcome of implant-based breast reconstruction, leading to skin-flap ischaemia, poor skin expansion, implant extrusion, capsular contracture and poor cosmesis. However, autologous breast reconstruction may be successful in previously irradiated patients, despite higher complication rates than in non-irradiated patients. More recent techniques of skin-sparing mastectomy have also been successful in previously irradiated patients, although only in patients with reasonably good-quality irradiated breast skin [23]. Breast reconstruction and radiotherapy are clearly not incompatible, but require careful consideration of the patient, timing and type of reconstruction.

### Soft-Tissue Sarcoma Surgery

Adult soft-tissue sarcomas are rare but problematic mesenchymal malignancies. Extensive local invasion involving muscles, vessels and nerves can lead to substantial loss of function if the tumour is completely excised. Metastases are also a problem, via haematogenous spread. Management is a balance between controlling local tumour and distant metastases while preserving maximal function of the limb. Peri-operative radiotherapy has been found to give better local control of the tumour than surgery alone and allows for more conservative surgery to preserve as much limb function as possible [24]. However, pre- or post-operative radiotherapy may lead to wound-healing problems and the need for reconstructive surgery in radiation-damaged tissue. Pre-operative radiotherapy has been preferred since lower doses of radiation are required. However, recent studies suggest that post-operative radiotherapy results in lower rates of wound complications and so is preferable when possible [25].

Specific radiotherapy targeting reduces damage to the surrounding tissues and loss of function. Advances in the conformal planning of external beam radiotherapy have enabled careful modelling of the radiation specifically to the sarcoma, avoiding surrounding structures [26]. Advances in brachytherapy techniques have also enabled high doses of radiation to be delivered specifically to the tumour, modelled to avoid surrounding critical structures [27]. Hyperthermia has been used to try to augment the response to radiotherapy; however, although it appears to improve local control, it does not improve metastases or long-term survival rates [28]. More effective adjuvant therapies would be useful to further reduce the damage to surrounding tissues.

## Head and Neck Cancer Surgery

Surgery and radiotherapy for head and neck tumours often result in deformity due to large soft- or hard-tissue defects that need reconstructive surgery. Defects have been repaired by musculocutaneous flaps [29] or by prosthetic implants [30]. One of the most serious long-term effects of radiotherapy to the head and neck is osteoradionecrosis of the mandible, which can lead to orocutaneous fistulae, exposed mandible, pathological fractures and considerable pain. Progression of osteoradionecrosis is reduced by prolonged courses of intravenous antibiotics and hyperbaric oxygen [31]. Attempts at reconstruction using bone grafts have had poor results but, in contrast, reconstruction with free vascularised bone (fibula, iliac crest or serratus anterior/rib flaps) has resulted in good functional and cosmetic results [32].

The Marx protocols combine hyperbaric oxygen therapy with aggressive surgical debridement and microvascular reconstruction to treat osteoradionecrosis [33]. Hyperbaric, but not normobaric, oxygen has an angiogenic effect, inducing increased vascular density in the treated tissue. Protocols for staging the osteoradionecrosis to determine the appropriate combinations of hyperbaric oxygen and surgical treatment have cure rates of up to 95%. The incidence of osteoradionecrosis of the mandible has also decreased as prophylaxis has been developed. Preventative measures have been determined such as limiting the total and fractional radiation doses, shielding the bone when possible and pre-radiation dental evaluations and extractions [31]. The value of aggressive oral and dental hygiene following radiotherapy has also been appreciated.

## New Strategies for Wounds Following Radiotherapy

Although irradiated tissue is more difficult to repair surgically, surgery is not contra-indicated and there are many reports of success. Increased complication rates necessitate careful consideration of the patient and the type of reconstruction. The type of flap, use of non-irradiated vessels and microvascular free-tissue transfer may all contribute to a successful outcome. Complications must be predicted and treated appropriately if they arise.

There is ongoing research into potential methods for specifically targeting radiotherapy to the tumour to avoid radiation damage to healthy tissue. Cancerous cells may be sensitised to radiation damage by chemicals such as platinum agents, taxanes and cyclooxygenase-2 inhibitors or hypothermia. Conversely, healthy tissue may be protected from radiation damage by agents such as amifostine, the anti-oxidant mitochondrial enzyme Mn-SOD and the erythropoietin analogue epoetin alfa [34]. More specific methods of targeting internal radiotherapy are also being investigated, using radioimmunotherapy or microsphere delivery techniques.

Exciting progress is being made identifying factors involved in causing and healing radiation-induced damage. This research is leading to opportunities for limiting radiation damage, promoting wound healing after irradiation or preventing radiation-induced fibrotic reactions [35]. Preliminary studies in animal models of radiation-induced injury have found that topical application of some of the growth factors involved in normal healing promote free-flap survival and wound healing after radiation damage. Inhibition of TGFβ is also being attempted to improve wound healing in radiation-damaged tissue [36]. Other interventions such as fibroblast or stem-cell injection into irradiated wounds and the use of artificial skin substitutes are also being investigated.

## Conclusions

Radiotherapy may complicate surgical procedures in many ways. Surgical excision of tumours combined with adjuvant radiotherapy may be complicated by the immediate inflammatory effects of radiation which lead to poor wound healing, dehiscence and breakdown. Immediate reconstructive procedures may also be jeopardised in radiation-damaged tissue. The long-term effects of irradiation, including fibrosis and microvascular damage, may complicate later surgical procedures in irradiated tissue even many years after the radiotherapy. There is still potential for reduction of radiation damage to normal tissue during radiotherapy.

Current strategies to prevent radiation damage to healthy tissue include novel targeted radiation delivery methods and pharmaceutical agents to protect normal cells from radiation damage. Research into the cellular and molecular basis of radiation damage is discovering opportunities to prevent progressive fibrosis and damage of previously irradiated tissue, and revealing interventions to promote successful wound healing. This is an exciting area of research which has huge implications for surgery involving irradiated wounds.

## References

1. Denham JW, Hauer-Jensen M (2002) The radiotherapeutic injury – a complex "wound". Radiother Oncol 63: 129–145
2. Stone HB, Coleman CN, Anscher MS, McBride WH (2003) Effects of radiation on normal tissue: consequences and mechanisms. Lancet Oncol 4: 529–536
3. Herskind C, Bamberg M, Rodemann HP (1998) The role of cytokines in the development of normal-tissue reactions after radiotherapy. Strahlenther Onkol 174 [Suppl 3]: 12–15
4. Schaffer M, Weimer W, Wider S, Stulten C, Bongartz M, Budach W, Becker HD (2002) Differential expression of inflammatory mediators in radiation-impaired wound healing. J Surg Res 107: 93–100
5. Gu Q, Wang D, Gao Y et al. (2002) Expression of MMP1 in surgical and radiation-impaired wound healing and its effects on the healing process. J Environ Pathol Toxicol Oncol 21: 71–78
6. Sassi M, Jukkola A, Riekki R, Hoyhtya M, Risteli L, Oikarinen A, Risteli J (2001) Type I collagen turnover and cross-linking are increased in irradiated skin of breast cancer patients. Radiother Oncol 58: 317–323
7. Handschiel J, Prott FJ, Sunderkotter C, Metze D, Meyer U, Joos U (1999) Irradiation induces increase of adhesion molecules and accumulation of b2-integrin-expressing cells in humans. Int J Radiation Oncology Biol Phys 45: 475–481
8. Rudolph R, Tripuraneni P, Koziol JA (1994) Normal transcutaneous oxygen pressure in skin after radiation therapy for cancer. Cancer 74 : 3063–3070
9. Dantzer D, Ferguson P, Hill RP, Keating A, Kandel RA, Wunder JS, O'Sullivan B, Sandhu J, Waddell J, Bell RS (2003) Effect of radiation and cell implantation on wound healing in a rat model. J Surg Oncol 83: 185–190
10. Rodemann PH, Bamberg M (1995) Cellular basis of radiation-induced fibrosis. Radiother Oncol 35: 83–90
11. O'Kane S, Ferguson MW (1997) Transforming growth factor betas and wound healing. Int J Biochem Cell Biol 29: 63–78
12. Schultze-Mosgau S, Wehrhan F, Rodel F, Amann K, Radespiel-Troger M, Grabenbauer GG (2003) Transforming growth factor-beta receptor-II up-regulation during wound healing in previously irradiated graft beds in vivo. Wound Repair Regen 11: 297–305
13. Martin M, Lefaix J, Delanian S (2000) TGF-beta1 and radiation fibrosis: a master switch and a specific therapeutic target? Int J Radiat Oncol Biol Phys 47: 277–279
14. Landthaler M, Hagspiel HJ, Braun-Falco O (1995) Late irradiation damage to the skin caused by soft X-ray radiation therapy of cutaneous tumors. Arch Dermatol 131: 182–186
15. Gurlek A, Miller MJ, Amin AA, Evans GR, Reece GP, Baldwin BJ, Schusterman MA, Kroll SS, Robb GL (1998) Reconstruction of complex radiation-induced injuries using free-tissue transfer. J Reconstr Microsurg 14: 337–340
16. Mulholland S, Boyd JB, McCabe S (1993) Recipient vessels in head and neck microsurgery: radiation effect and vessel access. Plast Reconstr Surg 92: 628–632
17. Kroll SS, Robb GL, Reece GP, Miller MJ, Evans GR, Baldwin BJ, Wang B, Schusterman MA (1998) Does prior irradiation increase the risk of total or partial free-flap loss? J Reconstr Microsurg 14: 263–268
18. Kroll SS, Schusterman MA, Reece GP, Miller MJ, Evans GR, Robb GL, Baldwin BJ (1996) Choice of flap and incidence of free flap success. Plast Reconstr Surg 98: 459–463
19. Grotting JC, Beckenstein MS, Arkoulakis NS (2003) The art and science of autologous breast reconstruction. Breast J 9: 350–360
20. Tran NV, Evans GR, Kroll, SS Baldwin BJ, Miller MJ, Reece GP, Robb GL (2000) Postoperative adjuvant irradiation: effects on transverse rectus abdominis muscle flap breast reconstruction. Plast Reconstr Surg 106: 313–317

21. Tran NV, Chang DW, Gupta A, Kroll SS, Robb GL (2001) Comparison of immediate and delayed free TRAM flap breast reconstruction in patients receiving postmastectomy radiation therapy. Plast Reconstr Surg 108: 78–82

22. Rogers NE, Allen RJ (2002) Radiation effects on breast reconstruction with the deep inferior epigastric perforator flap. Plast Reconstr Surg 109: 1919–1924

23. Disa JJ, Cordeiro PG, Heerdt AH, Petrek JA, Borgen PJ, Hidalgo DA (2003) Skin-sparing mastectomy and immediate autologous tissue reconstruction after whole-breast irradiation. Plast Reconstr Surg 111: 118–124

24. O'Sullivan B, Ward I, Catton C (2003) Recent advances in radiotherapy for soft-tissue sarcoma. Curr Oncol Rep 5: 274–281

25. O'Sullivan B, Davis AM, Turcotte R et al. (2002) Preoperative versus postoperative radiotherapy in soft-tissue sarcoma of the limbs: a randomised trial. Lancet 359: 2235–2241

26. Robinson MH, Bidmead AM, Harmer CL (1992) Value of conformal planning in the radiotherapy of soft tissue sarcoma. Clin Oncol (R Coll Radiol) 4: 290–293

27. Ballo MT, Lee AK (2003) Current results of brachytherapy for soft tissue sarcoma. Curr Opin Oncol 15: 313–318

28. Prosnitz MD, Maguire P, Anderson JM et al. (1999) The treatment of high-grade soft tissue sarcomas with preoperative thermoradiotherapy. Int J Radiation Oncology Biol Phys 45: 941–949

29. Butler CE, Lewin JS (2004) Reconstruction of large composite oromandibulomaxillary defects with free vertical rectus abdominis myocutaneous flaps. Plast Reconstr Surg 113: 499–507

30. Misiek DJ, Chang AK (1998) Implant reconstruction following removal of tumors of the head and neck. Otolaryngol Clin North Am 31: 689–725

31. Costantino PD, Friedman CD, Steinberg MJ (1995) Irradiated bone and its management. Otolaryngol Clin North Am 28: 1021–1038

32. Ioannides C, Fossion E, Boeckx W, Hermans B, Jacobs D (1994) Surgical management of the osteoradionecrotic mandible with free vascularised composite flaps. J Craniomaxillofac Surg 22: 330–334

33. Cronje FJ (1998) A review of the Marx protocols: prevention and management of osteoradionecrosis by combining surgery and hyperbaric oxygen therapy. SADJ 53: 469–471

34. Grdina DJ, Murley JS, Kataoka Y (2002) Radioprotectants: current status and new directions. Oncology 63 [Suppl 2]: 2–10

35. Moulder JE (2003) Pharmacological intervention to prevent or ameliorate chronic radiation injuries. Semin Radiat Oncol 13: 73–84

36. Martin M, Lefaix J, Delanian S (2000) TGF-beta1 and radiation fibrosis: a master switch and a specific therapeutic target? Int J Radiat Oncol Biol Phys 47: 277–290

# The Sequelae of the Cutaneous Radiation Syndrome

R.U. PETER

## Relevance of Cutaneous Radiation Injuries Following Accidental Exposure

The probability of cutaneous injury by nuclear weapons or dispersed nuclear material has, in contrast to post cold-war euphoria, considerably increased during the past 13 years. This is in part due to a temporary loss of control over nuclear material including uncontrolled deployment, in part to an increasing capability and apparent willingness of terrorist and other criminal groups to use such material for their purposes. A relatively recent danger emerges from the development of so-called robust nuclear earth penetrators (RNEPs) to destroy very deep bunkers, which may be used in future in "conventional" wars, and which without doubt will cause contamination with short-ranging radioactive nuclides. These nuclides again will affect the skin primarily. In summary, the probability of cutaneous radiation exposures with, in part, extremely high absorbed doses (< 60 Gy) with concomitantly survivable bone marrow doses has increased.

## Pathophysiology of Cutaneous Radiation Reactions

Ionising radiation leads to long-term impairment of various physiological functions, which have been reported for several decades. With regard to skin injuries, however, recent scientific progress has slightly altered previous concepts of the pathophysiology of cutaneous radiation injuries, with a decisive impact on diagnosis, treatment and follow-up.

In contrast to older concepts, ionising radiation does not only affect the proliferative capacity of cutaneous or epidermal stem cells, but modulates also the communicative network of epidermal keratinocytes, dermal fibroblasts and circulating and resident immunocompetent cells, such as Langerhans cells, dermal dendritic cells and both neutrophilic and eosinophilic granulocytes and lymphocytes. The concept of the cutaneous radiation syndrome (CRS), as it was coined a decade ago [1], thus combines anti-proliferative effects with those of local inflammatory reactions, occurring in a characteristic temporal pattern: in the initial phase, a couple of hours after irradiation (p. i.), a transient and inconsistent erythema may occur – the prodromal erythema, which may additionally be associated with an itching sensation. In this early phase, a transcriptional acitivation of pro-inflammatory cytokines such as interleukin (IL)-1, 3, 5, 6, and tumour necrosis factor alpha in keratinocytes and of chemokines such as IL-8 and eotaxin both in epidermal keratinocytes and dermal fibroblasts induces induction of adhesion molecules like ICAM-1 on keratinocytes and dermal endothelial cells as well as V-CAM and E-selectin on endothelial cells [2–4], and is identifiable both in vitro and in vivo. This transcriptional activation of pro-inflammatory cytokines leads to a liberation of anti-inflammatory cytokines on the other side, most importantly TGF-beta-1. As long as there is an equilibrium between pro- and anti-inflammatory processes, a clinically asymptomatic condition, denominated latency phase results. The duration of this latency phase and the intensity of the subsequent clinical sequelae depends on the damage induced by radiation exposure, and is thus, within certain margins, dose-dependent. Some days to a couple of weeks later, the manifestational stage may occur. In this stage, intense reddening, blistering and ulceration of the irradiated site will be discernible. At this stage the tissue destruction, specifically of the upper epidermal layer, associated with a capillaritis and a vasculitis of the dermal venules and arterioles and an infiltrate of neutrophil and eosinophil granulocytes leads to a complex wound, that may either be confined to the epidermis and upper dermis or may well penetrate through the subcutaneous fatty tissue to the musculature. Subepidermal blistering is a result of both apoptotic and necrotic breakdown of epidermal tissue. Following this stage, a vasculitis of the deep dermal and subcutaneous blood vessels results in a bluish red stain of the affected skin [5]. In consequence, all these processes result in considerable tissue damage, which is, however, not present from the onset but develops due to the described inflammatory reactions, for which the radiation exposure may serve as an initiating spark.

In contrast to thermal burns or consequences of cutaneous contamination with chemical toxic agents, these wounds do not develop immediately, but evolve over several days to weeks, dependent on the initial radiation intensity and the individual's radiation sensitivity.

With a latency of 3 months to 2 years, a dermal and subcutaneous fibrosis may occur at the site of radiation exposure. This fibrosis, progressive by its nature, may be very prominent and lead to complete disappearance of the subcutaneous fatty tissue, so that in advanced cases a direct continuation from the dermis to the underlying muscle fascia will be identified.

In this phase, a scarce perivascular infiltrate composed primarily of cd4+ lymphocytes can be seen histologically.

Transforming growth factor beta-1 is, in this phase, heavily transcriptionally activated. This is the result of a cascade-like activation of smad transcription factors [19].

Several years to decades after exposure, chronic sequelae like severe xerosis (dryness) of the skin due to loss of sebaceous and sweat glands, alopecia and increased transepidermal water loss result in an increased vulnerability of the skin, often leading to secondary ulceration [6]. Neoplastic transformation with squamous and basal cell carcinomas, sometimes preceded by radiation keratoses, may develop over several years at the irradiated site. This aspect of accidental exposure, however, is often over-estimated. Based upon published literature and our own experience in treatment and follow-up of accident survivors, secondary malignancies generally do not occur in the areas of maximum exposure and severe clinical consequences, but rather in locations without any signs of deterministic effects, which would correspond to absorbed single doses between 1 and 10 Gy (Table 1).

**Table 1.** Stages of the cutaneous radiation syndrome (according to Second Consensus Development Conference on the Management of Radiation Injuries, Bethesda Md. 1993)

| Stage | Name and onset | Symptoms | Old synonyms |
|---|---|---|---|
| I | Prodromal (24–72 h) | Transient erythema, itch | Early erythema |
| II | Manifestational (days to 4 weeks) | Intense erythema/dry scales Blisters, erosions, pain Ulcerative necrosis | Main erythema/ radiodermatitis/dry-moist desquamation/radionecrosis |
| III | Subacute (4–6 weeks) | Subcutaneous vasculitis | (Dusky mauve erythema in pig skin model) |
| IV | Chronic (3 months to 2 years) | Epidermal keratosis, atrophy, subcutaneous fibrosis, telangiectasias, ulceration | Chronic radiodermatitis radioderma, late ulceration, radiation scar |

## Clinical Features and Diagnostic Difficulties of the CRS

The effects of physical damage to skin generally result in a common final development; once tissue integrity has been dissolved, it is impossible to discriminate between a thermal burn, a chemical toxic reaction, or a radiation injury. It is the time sequence of events that makes the difference in the acute phase. In the chronic stage, it is the progressive nature of radiation fibrosis which distinguishes this reaction from scarring of a thermal burn or a severe toxic reaction to a chemical agent. It may be considered as the characteristic trait of the CRS that the reactions occur in a delayed pattern. This implies that the clinical reactions after an accidental exposure may remain unnoticed, and the patient presents only a couple of days or even weeks later with the symptoms of the manifestational stage. It may then be extremely difficult to identify the reaction as a cutaneous radiation syndrome – a feature that has occurred globally in almost every major radiation accident in the past 15 years. The prodromal erythema, as it is transient in nature, may easily be overlooked. If there is a suspicion of local cutaneous exposure to ionising radiation, the prodromal erythema should be searched for and documented, ideally by photography. Though extent and intensity of the prodromal erythema are not predictive of the intensity of the manifestational or chronic stage to be expected, they give valuable information as to where the maximum of the clinical reaction will occur.

Physical and, in most instances, biologic dosimetry is generally grossly overestimated with respect to its relevance for the clinical management of the CRS, apart from the fact that it may prove that an exposure has, in fact, occurred. The reason for this is the basic circumstance that a clinically relevant cutaneous radiation reaction must be the result of an extremely inhomogeneous partial body exposure, mostly with short-ranging nuclides, as clinically relevant cutaneous reactions will generally be expected beyond a single dose of 15 Gy. A total body exposure with deeply penetrating radiation of that dose would be lethal due to the development of the bone marrow and/or gastrointestinal radiation syndrome. On the other hand, a local exposure of such a dose at, for example, the upper thighs, would not necessarily create a major alteration of tooth enamel or a total body counter, which might be used for physical dosimetry. A bone-marrow count or searching for chromosomal alterations of lymphocytes may in this case also not reveal major alterations, as they will rather reflect an average of the bone marrow or lymphocytes of the whole organism. Therefore, though recently it could be proven by multicolour fluorescence in situ hybridisation (M-FISH) that irradiated human dermal fibroblasts reveal chromosomal aberrations comparable to irradiated lymphocytes, the diagnosis of CRS remains a clinical one.

During the manifestational and subacute stage the extent of tissue involvement, but not necessarily damage, can be detected by high-frequency ultrasound and magnetic resonance imaging (MRI). The latter method can be combined with contrast enhancement by injected gadolinium, which, however, gives only a hint to the extent of the inflammatory reaction, but does not mean that the imaged tissue is also necrotic. This has important therapeutic implications, as, in contrast to older concepts, not the whole tissue should be surgically resected.

An additional non-invasive method to reveal the extent of cutaneous involvement in the manifestational and subacute stage is thermography, which has been used with success in a variety of accidents (J.M. Cosset, pers. comm.).

In the chronic stage, fibrosis is the predominant symptom which causes additional distress to the patient, as it may lead to further tissue breakdown (late ulceration), mechanical impairment of members and joints, and to muscular atrophy. It can be quantified by both high-frequency ultrasound and MRI. Epidermal atrophy, pigmentary changes and focal radiation keratoses together with an increased epidermal water loss and a severe xerosis contribute to a highly vulnerable skin, which requires continuous support and follow-up.

Teleangiectasias, though generally a cosmetic problem, may become a nuisance to the patient: if they are very extensive, the resulting cutaneous hyperaemia leads to burning sensations in the affected areas.

## Diagnostic and Therapeutic Consequences

Although much research has been carried out in the past few decades to identify unequivocal indicators for a radiation exposure incident and to discriminate it from other physical effectors, to date a really specific indicator has not been found. Recently, our group could identify chromosomal deletions and translocations in primary irradiated human skin fibroblasts identical to those which have for long been described in lymphocytes, which may well serve as an indicator for partial body exposure at a time when clinical signs of CRS have not yet appeared. This may open a new window of opportunity for causal-oriented treatment of cutaneous radiation injuries at an early stage.

In the prodromal stage of CRS, anti-histamines and topical anti-pruriginous preparations may be used. Anti-histamines do not only act against itch, but also reduce induction of adhesion molecules on keratinocytes and endothelial cells and thus help prevent or attenuate initiation of the vicious circle which finally leads to the manifestational stage.

The latency phase between prodromal erythema and manifestational stage, which is by definition without clinical symptoms, is the optimal phase for secondary prophylaxis: due to the substantial inflammatory component of the manifestational stage, medium- to high-dose systemic glucocorticosteroids (methylprednisolone equivalent of 0.5–1.5 g/kg body-weight/day) should be combined with effective topical anti-inflammatory treatment with class-III to class-IV steroids. Whether there is a place for the new topical anti-inflammatory drugs like topical tacrolimus and pimecrolimus, which is theoretically very probable, remains to be determined in practice [7].

Once the manifestational stage has developed, an additional threat is presented by bacterial, fungal and viral infections. Repeated swabs in order to identify this superinfection as early as possible and to monitor the efficacy of antibiotic treatment are necessary. The indication of antibiotic prophylaxis will mainly depend on additional symptoms like radiation-induced bone-marrow suppression or a simultaneously occurring gastrointestinal syndrome.

Blisters, if sterile, should be punctured, but not removed, as long as they are intact. In the case of necrosis, thorough but cautious debridement should be carried out, which, apart from using a conventional scalpel, can sometimes be better achieved by using an ErYag laser or a high-pressure water scalpel (own unpublished data).

Topical treatment comprises the application of wet dressings, later alginates and hydrocolloids. Growth factors like PDGF (Regranex) and KGF (not yet formally approved) may be used to foster granulation and epithelialisation; they will, however, require thorough bacterial decontamination of the surface defects in order to be effective. Surgical procedures require a defined analysis of the extent of disease by MRI and high-frequency (20 MHz) ultrasound. In the case of positive MRI, anti-inflammatory treatment with 0.5–1 mg of methylprednisolone is warranted prior to surgical excision, in order to avoid too extensive a resection.

If cutaneous and muscular layers are affected and surgical resection is unavoidable, temporary coverages with the synthetic skin equivalent Integra® have proven very effective (M. Carsin, personal communication). If further granulation has been reached, closure with full-thickness or split skin grafts as well as with cultured and reconstituted skin are possible.

In the subacute stage, heparinisation to prevent sludging of dermal and subcutaneous vessels additionally to anti-inflammatory treatment has been claimed to be helpful.

In the chronic stage, fibrosis is the predominant clinical problem. In contrast to former guidelines, which considered radiation fibrosis an entity which was impossible to treat by means other than surgery, a variety of different options have been developed in the past few years for conservative treatment of radiation fibrosis.

Apart from bovine Mn superoxidedismutase [9], which is for obvious reasons not available at present, an oral administration of Pentoxifylline (400 mg t.i.d.) and vitamin E (400 mg q.d.), initially reported as a case description [10], has been proven effective in a controlled trial [11] on patients suffering from fibrosis after radiation therapy.

In an open trial both on survivors of the Chernobyl radiation accident as well as on five patients suffering from cutaneous fibrosis after radiation therapy [11–15], subcutaneous injection of interferon gamma (Imukin) has been demonstrated to reduce pre-existing fibrosis to almost normal values. These options should be carefully considered before excision of larger fibrotic plaques and streaks.

Radiation keratoses are focal tight keratotic lesions, indicating an increased cornifying activity of epidermal keratinocytes. In some instances, these keratoses present pre-cancerous lesions, though few data exist about the factual quantitative component of transformation. In any case of clinical doubt, excisional biopsy and histologic assessment of lesions to exclude squamous cell carcinoma should be performed.

Teleangiectasias may be effectively treated with argon, diode or dye lasers, without any relevant side effects or sequelae (own unpublished observations).

Basal cell and squamous cell carcinomas are long-term stochastic sequelae of cutaneous radiation exposure, which may occur in areas which did not necessarily show any symptoms of CRS immediately after exposure [16], in contrast to malignant melanoma, which has never conclusively been demonstrated to follow cutaneous radiation over-exposure [17]. As latencies may be years and decades, a long-term, if not life-long follow-up of radiation-exposed patients is necessary.

## References


1. Peter RU (1996) the cutaneous radiation syndrome. In: MacVittie T, Browne D, Weiss J (eds) Advances in the treatment of radiation injuries. Elsevier, Oxford, pp 237–240
2. Beetz A, Peter RU, Ried C, Ruzicka T, Michel G (1996) Uniform induction of TNF α and IL-8 in human keratinocytes by ionizing radiation is accompanied by nonuniform regulation of corresponding receptors. J Europ Acad Dermatol Venerol 7: 188–190
3. Behrends U, Peter RU, Hintermeier-Knabe R, Eißner G, Holler E, Bornkamm GW, Caughman SW, Degitz K (1994) Ionizing radiation induces human intercellular adhesion molecule-1 in vitro. J Invest Dermatol 103: 726–730
4. Heckmann M, Douwes K, Peter R, Degitz K (1998) Vascular activation of adhesion molecule mRNA and cell surface expression by ionizing radiation. Exp Cell Res 238: 148–154
5. Hopewell JW (1990) The skin: Its structure and response to ionizing radiation. Int J Radiat Biol 57: 751–773
6. Peter RU, Braun-Falco O, Kerscher M, Birioukov A, Hacker N, Peterseim U, Ruzicka T, Konz B, Plewig G (1994) Chronic cutaneous damage after accidental exposure to ionizing radiation: the Chernobyl experience. J Am Acad Dermatol 30: 719–723
7. Gottlöber P, Krähn G, Peter RU (2000) Das kutane Strahlensyndrom: Klinik, Diagnostik und Therapie. Hautarzt 51: 567–574
8. Gottlöber P, Bezold G, Weber L, Gourmelon P, Cosset JM, Baehren W, Peter RU (2000) The radiation accident in Georgia: clinical appearance and diagnostics of cutaneous radiation syndrome. J Am Acad Dermatol 42: 453–458

9. Delanian S, Baillet F Huart J et al. (1994) Successful treatment of radiation induced fibrosis using liposomal Cu-Zn superoxide dismutase: Clinical trial. Radiother Oncol 32: 12–20

10. Lefaix JL, Delanian S, Vozenin MC et al. (1999) striking regression of subcutaneous fibrosis induced by high doses of gamma rays using in a combination pentoxifylline and a-tocopherol: An experimental study. Int J Radiat Oncol Biol Phys 43: 839–847

11. Gottlöber P, Krähn G, Korting HC, Stock W, Peter RU (1996) Treatment of cutaneous radiation fibrosis with Pentoxyfilline and Vitamin E – a case report [in German]. Strahlenther Onkol 172: 34–38

12. Peter RU, Gottlöber P, Krähn G, Nadejina N, Braun-Falco O, Plewig G (1999) Gamma-interferon in survivors of the Chernobyl power plant accident- new therapeutic option for radiation induced fibrosis. Int J Radiat Oncol Biol Phys 45: 147–152

13. Gottlöber P, Steinert M, Bähren W, Weber L, Gerngroß H, Peter RU (2001) Interferon-gamma in patients with cutaneous syndrome after radiation therapy. Int J Rad Oncol Biol Phys 47: 159–166

14. Duncan MR, Berman B (1985) Gamma-interferon is the lymphokine and beta-interferon the monokine responsible for inhibition of fibroblast collagen production and late but not early fibroblast proliferation. J Exp Med 162: 516–527

15. Gurujeyalakshmi G, Giri SN (1995) Molecular mechanisms of antifibrotic effect of interferon gamma in bleomycin-mouse model of lung fibrosis: Down regulation of TGF-ß and procollagen I and III gene expression. Exp Lung Res 21: 791–808

16. Gottlöber P, Steinert M, Weiss M et al. (2001) The fate of local radiation injuries: 14 years of follow-up after the Chernobyl accident. Radiation Res 155: 409–416

17. Peter RU, Gottlöber P, Nadeshina N, Krähn G, Plewig G, Kind P (1997) Radiation lentigo: a distinct cutaneous lesion after accidental radiation exposure. Arch Dermatol, 133: 209–211

18. The Radiation accident in Lilo (2001) Special publication of the International Atomic Energy Agency. The Agency, Vienna

19. Reisdorf P, Lawrence DA, Sivan V, Klising E, Martin MT (2001) Alteration of transforming growth factor-beta1 response involves down-regulation of Smad3 signaling in myofibroblasts from skin fibrosis. Am J Pathol 159: 263–272

# 6 Surgical Debridement

J. Mahoney, J. Ward

## Introduction

Surgical debridement is the most important aspect of wound-bed preparation and management. The word surgical implies the most direct form of debridement. This involves the removal of compromised tissue with precise, sharp surgical instruments using appropriate surgical technique. Debridement is the removal of foreign material and devitalised or significantly compromised tissue that impedes or prevents wound healing. Surgical debridement can be considered in conjunction with other forms of debridement and surgical interventions, such as incision and drainage.

## Applied Anatomy and Physiology

Before performing any surgical procedure, it is important to consider the anatomy of the skin, its underlying tissues and the changes that occur following injury. A completely necrotic area can be excised; however, special care should be taken when treating partially necrotic areas or normal tissue planes. The skin varies in thickness in different parts of the body and has an underlying subcutaneous or a fatty tissue layer of variable depth that is attached by vertically oriented fibres connected to the underlying longitudinally oriented fascia layers. Within the subcutaneous layer run the small blood vessels and sometimes larger veins (1–3 mm). This layer also carries the cutaneous nerves that supply sensation to the skin. Beneath the deeper longitudinal fascia lie muscle, tendons, larger blood vessels and nerves. The fascia acts like an envelope around these deeper structures and provides protection from infection. Once these envelopes are violated, the enclosed structures can become exposed to the external environment including bones, joints and tendons, which have poor blood supply and, when exposed to air, will become desiccated and even necrotic, requiring debridement. These structures need to be carefully considered.

As we age, the skin becomes thinner and weaker, increasing the potential for injury from minor forms of trauma. The pretibial (shin) area is particularly prone to tearing from blunt injury. Structural and physiologic alterations may also occur in diseases such as diabetes and vasculitis, as well as with the use of drugs such as anticoagulants and steroids. Poor blood supply (ischemia) to the area can prevent healing, and optimisation of the blood supply is critical prior to debridement. All the negative factors affecting wound healing should be considered and minimised either prior to or in conjunction with debridement.

## Acute Wounds

There are different traumatic wound mechanisms that require surgical debridement on an acute basis. In addition to wound cleansing, washing and irrigation, the actual cutting back of the wound margin to create a healthier edge may be necessary. Contaminated irregular or ischemic wound margins may need to be resected to optimise the healing process, allowing approximation for uncomplicated primary healing. This becomes more important after a crush or avulsion, where in addition to trauma of the surface skin, the attachments to the underlying tissue are violated, leading to variable degrees of ischemia and possible skin and soft-tissue necrosis. Other forms of acute trauma such as burns can also damage skin to a variable degree. Surgical debridement to healthy tissue should be considered when full-thickness skin loss is anticipated. High-velocity penetrating injuries can cause extensive injury to the deep soft tissues not evident on surface examination. The knowledge and understanding of the different mechanisms, their potential damage to tissue, and the underlying structures including nerves, blood vessels and tendons, are important in planning debridement.

## Chronic Wounds

A chronic wound is defined as a wound that is not progressing or has stopped healing. Necrotic, compromised tissue can be the source of this delay and must therefore be removed. Wounds that have been healing for a time will have varying degrees of progress involving scar formation, contraction and epithelialisation. These processes become less active in chronic wounds. Bacterial colonisation and infection often play a significant role in delay. They require investigation, and debridement with a tissue biopsy can be helpful. Similarly, deterioration in a wound with visible progression of necrosis needs a diagnosis and debridement with biopsy should be considered.

## General Aspects of Wound Management

Acute traumatic wounds are usually contaminated and delay in treatment (more than 24 h) increases the risk of wound infection following closure. As outlined, cleaning the wound with gentle washing, irrigation and debridement is appropriate. However, in addition, surgical debridement can be considered so that these wounds can also be repaired. Acute wounds that have been left open to heal by secondary means (contraction and epithelialisation) may fall into the chronic category based on their time to heal (>4 weeks, lack of progression in wound size). In certain circumstances, surgical debridement involving the complete removal of the wound bed can lead to converting a chronic contaminated wound into a clean wound which can be considered for closure. This approach can provide a significantly shorter healing time that otherwise would have not been possible.

Other forms of mechanical debridement implying the application of a mechanical instrument can help clean the wound. Brushes, pusatile irrigation techniques and newer ultrasound device are available; however, surgical debridement is still the most effective and rapid way to achieve preparation of the wound bed.

## Setting and Instrumentation

As the frequency and complexity of wounds is increasing, the requirements for debridement become greater and a careful assessment of the resources required is needed: appropriate setting for the procedure, the need of anaesthesia and the experience of the person performing the debridement. A discussion of the proposed procedure with the patient and its effect on wound management should be performed and documented.

Debridement can be performed safely in the clinic or office setting, providing there are suitable instruments and appropriate lighting. The surgeon performing the debridement should position the patient in a way that allows easy access to the wound. Anaesthesia needs to be considered in patients who have sensation. Topical local anaesthetics may be helpful but infiltration with local anaesthetics is more effective. Patients who are insensate are easier in this regard, but distinguishing healthy from compromised tissue is more difficult. Older patients who have sensation may benefit from staged procedures, involving gentle serial debridement minimising discomfort or pain. Sedation may also be helpful. Anticipate potential complications, such as bleeding, and have appropriate resources readily available.

## Technique

Surgical debridement can be performed by one person. Anaesthesia, appropriate draping the area, separating it from the environment and cleaning the surrounding skin or wound using a poviodine-iodine preparation are performed. Usually one hand will support or stretch the tissue to be debrided or it can be held with an instrument such as a forceps. The other hand will use a sharp instrument such as a scalpel or scissors to debride or cut. A toothed thumb forceps and sharp serrated iris scissors are usually the most versatile. Scalpels require care in their use, particularly when cutting into thick eschar. Going too deep is quite easy; the thick hard eschar suddenly gives way to the underling healthy tissue. Additional instruments such as haemostats may be required to control bleeding. Ronguers are helpful in debriding bone. Consider performing the procedure in the operating room when surgical reconstruction is required, an assistant is needed or increased complexity, requiring surgical retractors or other instruments such as electrocautery, is anticipated.

## Technical Tips for Clinic or Bedside Debridement

Excision of obviously necrotic tissue is usually performed by gradually working from the definitely necrotic toward the healthier periphery, paying attention to the appearance of healthy potentially sensate tissue that bleeds. Consider preserving partially viable tissue. It can be left and debrided at a second stage. Staged debridement is particularly applicable in the deeper tissue layers such as with acute pressure sores where the extent of necrosis is initially indistinct. The larger blood vessels are frequently still patent and can be cut in areas of partial necrosis. Extending the debridement to the beginning of bleeding is a way to reduce the risk of bleeding that can be difficult to control.

In circumstances where the actual depth of tissue injury is uncertain, using the blade parallel to the surface of the skin and excising through the skin by shaving laterally in layers is helpful. This may be very important on the dorsal surface of a toe or finger, as once the tendons or bones are exposed to the external environment, desiccation and contamination may follow.

## Complications

Surgical debridement is a procedure that carries some risk. It may fail to achieve the goals of reducing the bacterial colonisation or preparing the wound bed for healing. Certain medical conditions are notorious for the poor response to debridement, for example, the arterial disease, vasculitis and pyoderma gangrenosum. Specific problems can be encountered with a sharp invasive technique; the first and foremost is bleeding. Bleeding can usually be controlled with direct pressure. A variety of topical agents can be helpful where generalised small point bleeding or oozing is seen. When larger pulsatile flow is not controlled with pressure for 5 min, grasping the bleeding point with an instrument such as a haemostat, and electrocoagulation or ligation is necessary. In chronic wounds where the tissue consistency can be softer, which makes the localisation of bleeding difficult, over-sewing with a suture can be helpful. Infection can be minimised with the appropriate use of antibiotics, particularly in patients who are immune or vascularly compromised. For example, an intact dry black eschar secondary to pressure in an ischemic limb can be left until the vascular reconstruction is performed to increase the capacity of the wound to heal after debridement.

Once the wound has been debrided, it is important to consider the alternatives to obtain definitive wound closure. In acute traumatic wounds, wound closure is preferred. In some chronic wounds following wound-bed excision debridement, immediate definitive wound closure can be achieved. In others, however, this may not be feasible, so healing by secondary intention is the option.

A variety of different dressing strategies should be considered following surgical debridement. In clean open acute wounds, maintenance of a moist environment while minimizing infection is important. When debridement is not complete, or the presence of a significant bacterial load is suspected, the short-term use of dilute antiseptics – such as poviodine-iodine, hygeol, acetic acid or silver dressings – can be helpful. Monitoring the appearance of the wound, quality and quantity of drainage are required. Once clean, the wound management should shift to techniques to maximise the healing potential of the wound bed.

## References

1. Dolynchuk KN (2001) Debridement. In: Krasner DL, Rodeheaver GT, Sibbald RG (eds) Chronic wound care: a clinical source book for healthcare professionals, 3rd edn. HMP Communications, Wayne, PA, pp 385–390
2. Smith L (1989) Histopathologic characteristics and ultrastructure of aging skin. Cutis 43: 414

# Use of High-Pressure Waterjets in Wound Debridement

S. Palmier, C. Trial

## Introduction

One of the main factors in wound healing is the prevention of infection. Necrotic tissues develop quickly in chronic wounds. Debridement is needed in order to remove necrotic tissue and fibrin, and some authors have advocated rapid management of all that stands in the way to growth of the granulation tissue. This step, which remains difficult for most nurses and of little interest for most surgeons, has to be detailed, as new techniques permit natural closure to develop under good conditions with less surgical techniques.

Several techniques are proposed for debridement today: surgical, chemical, mechanical and enzymatic. Each of these is more or less adapted to a specific case and may be efficient, feasible, necessary or not, depending on the availability of the different solutions. A combination of these different methods will often be necessary. New dressings, even if they are more powerful in absorbing exudates, are not always suitable and mechanical debridement still represents the faster way to remove large amounts of necrotic tissues.

New methods using pulsed water have been were introduced in the past two decades, the high-pressure water-jet representing the most sophisticated method at present proposed. We will focus our interest on two different devices, Debritom and Versajet.

### Debritom (Amtech Medaxis)

#### Technical Description of the Device

As seen in Fig. 1, this equipment is composed of a high-pressure command unit, a metallic tube linked to the hand piece and a pressure air bottle. The pump aspirates NaCL (0.9%), which is directed through the high-pressure tube to the hand piece. The pressure can vary by adaptating the working distance or using a pressure-regulation system (from 0 to 800 bar). This equipment can be transported easily to different sites.

The liquid is ejected distally to the hand piece through the nozzle. Cutting, dissecting and washing can be carried out on demand, and shifting from one to the other is very easy. This system can therefore be used as a powerful bistouri if needed.

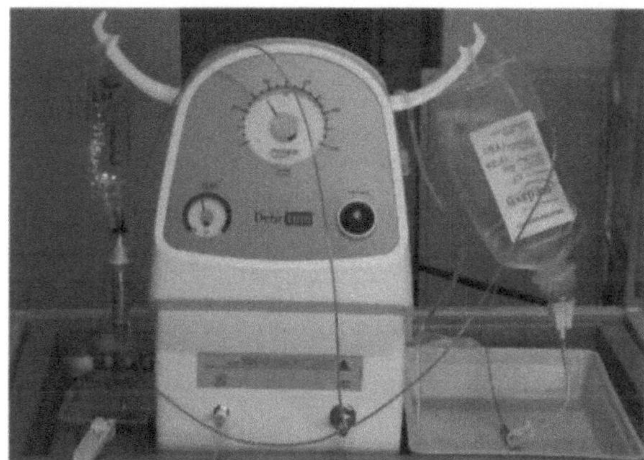

**Fig. 1.** Debritom

## Clinical Observations

Debritom was recently evaluated in Montpellier CHU during a period of 3 months on 30 chronic wounds (22 scars, 7 leg ulcers and 1 diabetic foot) in 17 patients. The results show an noticable reduction of necrotic tissue and fibrin and a better appearance of wounds after only two treatments (interval 2 to 3 days). The mean pressure used was about 300 bar during each application (Figs. 2 and 3).

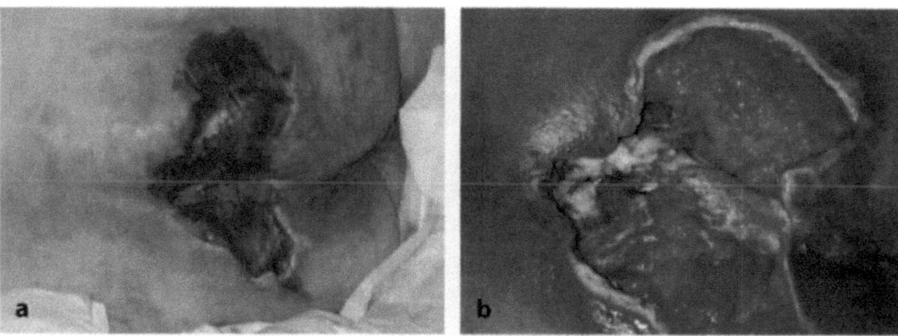

**Fig. 2.** Sacral pressure ulcer after two treatments with Debritom

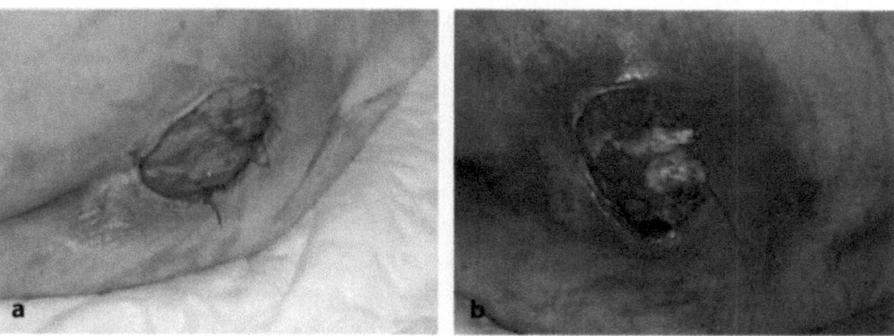

**Fig. 3.** Sacral pressure ulcer after the first Debritom treatment

## Results

**Interest.** The use of these new techniques shows that their main use is against fibrin, with considerable success: half the fibrin was eliminated in eleven wounds after the first treatment and all the fibrin and necrotic tissue were eliminated after two or three applications. (Two or three treatments are necessary at intervals of 2 to 8 days. More time between the two interventions seems to favour fibrin production.) Slight blood spotting appeared after the first use, showing blood-flow stimulation.

Debritom can be useful to treat cavity wounds even if the access aperture is small.

Debridement is often very painful, especially in leg ulcers. In this treatment, the water-jet seems to generate less pain than classical mechanical debridement using scalpel and curette. Traditional local anaesthetic methods (subcutaneous injection or cream) are often sufficient to obtain considerable pain reduction, allowing treatment in arteritic wounds.

**Disadvantages.** Risks from waste projection are important. The risk of infectious dissemination is probably as important for the nurse as for the surrounding surfaces!

The cost is high because disposable material is used: hand pieces, tubes etc. With Debritom a disinfectant solution must be used and sterile clothing for the nurse, which add to time and money difficulties.

## Versajet (Smith & Nephew)

### Technical Description of the Device

The equipment consists of a high-pressure command unit which pressurises the NaCl (without pressure air bottle), and a disposable hand piece. Waste water and debridement products are sucked up by the nozzle of the hand piece and transferred to a waste container (less risk of projection).

The maximal pressure is 827 bar. Pressure can only be regulated by adjusting the hand piece.

Three different working angles are available as hand pieces, allowing the geometry to be adapted to different wounds. The angle of the hand piece relative to the tissue determines the effect: when the operating window is parallel to the tissue, precise excision and aspiration are possible, but when the operating window is directed obliquely to the tissue, wound irrigation and contaminant removal are the primary effects (Fig. 4).

Because of this configuration, Versajet cannot be compared to a bistouri but looks more like a curette (the cutting of black necrotic tissue is thus not always possible and has to be carried out previously).

Versajet was evaluated in Philadelphia on 25 patients suffering from numerous wounds. Specifically, Versajet was used to treat traumatic wounds and burns, resect necrotic muscle and debride decubitus pressure ulcers (Fig. 5).

In all cases, debridement could be performed rapidly using this device alone.

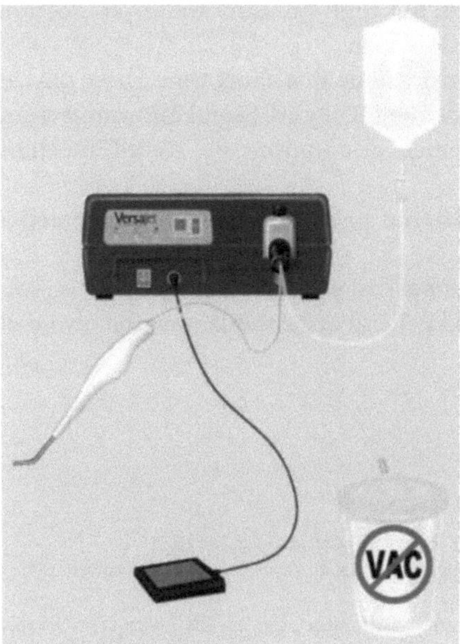

**Fig. 4.** Versajet

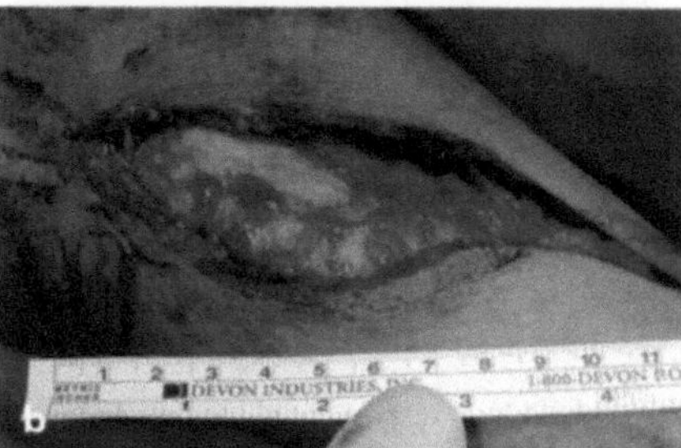

**Fig. 5.** Traumatic wound before and after using Versajet

## Results

**Interests.** The benefit lies in the ability to effect surgical debridement while at the same time providing lavage. Tissue excision is precise, avoiding damage to healthy tissue or vasculature.

Versajet requires significantly less irrigant than traditional lavage techniques, confines the irrigant to the wound area and provides immediate fluid evacuation. Pain management is an important factor, similar with both Debritom or Versajet.

**Disadvantages.** Due to the construction of the hand piece, if the wound is full of black necrotic tissue, debridement must be done with a classic bistouri as a first step and Versajet will be useful as a second.

The high cost of this technique is similar to that of Debritom because of the use of disposable material.

## Conclusion

The two systems are very intuitive devices, allowing operative debridement to progress in the same manner as traditional approaches. Little formal training is needed since the surgeon or nurse is not required to learn any new operative principles: the only requirement is mastery of a new instrument, not a new procedure.

First evaluations have to be continued, but high-pressure water-jets seem to permit debridement to be shortened with less pain.

By helping removal of fibrin and necrotic tissue in a short time, these devices have substantially simplified wound debridement. They are useful for wound cleaning, permitting granulation tissue development and limiting the risk of infections in the wound bed.

They permit a radical debridement with less pain. Fibrin can be eliminated in two or three dressings.

Even if each treatment is expensive, the total cost of wound management is probably interesting because heavy surgery and general anaesthesia are often avoided.

## References


1. Teot L (1999) La détersion des plaies. Journal des Plaies et Cicatrisations 3: 7–12
2. Bradley M, Cullum N, Shelder T (1999) The debridement of chronic wound: a systematic review. Les Hydrogels. Journal des Plaies et Cicatrisations. 3: 1–90
3. Morgan D, Hoelscher J (2000) Pulsed lavage: promoting comfort and healing home care. Ostomy/ Wound Management 46: 44–49
4. Kammerlander G, Gutermuth O, Eberlein T (2000) Débritom in wound care: clinical observations. May 2000

# Autolytic Debridement

P. Vowden

## Introduction

The principles of modern chronic wound care are based on two assumptions: firstly that a moist wound environment is necessary for wound healing to occur and secondly that debris, necrotic tissue and eschar are barriers to wound healing. The use of debridement, that is the removal of necrotic tissue from the wounds, is largely based on expert opinion rather than on evidence derived from randomised controlled clinical trials.

## Management of Autolytic Debridement

Autolytic debridement occurs naturally in all wounds [1] and is the process by which necrotic tissue and debris is removed from the wounded area. The process relies upon the activity of leukocytes and the presence of endogenous proteolytic enzymes within wound fluid and is thus dependent on the local wound environment, in particular the state of wound hydration but also the wound temperature, pH and enzymatic co-factor availability. Bacterial proteases also contribute to the process of debridement [2]. The process is slow and delayed by ageing, malnutrition and chronic diseases where protease levels and cellular activity in the wound may be decreased [3].

Before undertaking any form of therapy to enhance natural autolytic debridement, a full wound-management plan must be established. This plan should include defined aims, measurable endpoints and a realistic timeline. Debridement of necrotic tissue is not always appropriate; for example, in an ischaemic limb, stable dry eschar (gangrene) should generally not be rehydrated or debrided until vascular perfusion has been restored.

Debridement can be undertaken using a number of different methods [4, 5]. Each method has advantages and disadvantages (see the following list for an analysis of those relating to autolytic debridement). Surgical debridement is, for example, rapid, but it requires equipment and skill that may not be readily available, and has the potential in unskilled hands to damage healthy tissue. Autolytic debridement is by contrast slow, yet the skills and dressings necessary to apply this technique are widely available.

### Autolytic Debridement

- Advantages
  - Selective, removing only necrotic tissue
  - Painless
  - Easy to use
  - Can be combined with other methods of debridement
  - Suitable for most wounds and patients
  - Cost effective
  - Widely available in all care settings
- Disadvantages
  - Slow
  - Possible risk of maceration to surrounding skin

Frequently, complex wounds require the sequential application of one or more debridement method in order to maximise the healing potential of a specific wound. Debridement should therefore be regarded as a dynamic ongoing process [6]; in many cases the wound enters a maintenance phase of debridement where dressings designed to enhance the natural autolytic process function well as they also provide an ideal environment for moist wound healing.

Some of the potential complications of autolytic debridement include over-hydration and maceration of the surrounding skin. This is particularly the case where there is an inappropriate dressing selection or in the presence of high exudate output where contact dermatitis is also a risk [7, 8]. In these situations exudate production should be reduced as part of dressing-assisted autolytic debridement.

The choice of dressing used for autolytic debridement will be determined by the state of the wound bed, the exudate level and the bacterial load, patient preference, dressing availability and staff skill and availability.

## Choice of Dressing

Dressings that may enhance autolytic debridement include:

### Gel-Formation Dressing

Hydrocolloids and hydrogels are most suitable for wounds with a low to moderate volume exudate. These dressings can rehydrate necrotic tissue and eschar. Alginate [9] and hydrofibre [10, 11] dressings are suitable when debriding wounds with moderate to high volume and viscosity exudate. The dressing takes up fluid to form a gel and holds it within the dressing but in contact with the wound surface, facilitating autolytic debridement.

### Absorptive Dressings

These dressings consist of foam or a pad with a primary non-adherent wound contact layer, and can handle moderate to high volumes of fluid. These dressings do not rehydrate necrotic tissue but assist autolytic debridement by maintaining a moist environment at the wound bed while reducing the risk of wound margin maceration and are suitable to use with moderate- to high-volume exudating wounds.

### Capillary Action Dressings

Although the main function of these dressings is to conduct fluid away from the wound surface, some authors have used them to assist in the debridement process [12]. These dressings have been shown to be effective in moderate- to high-volume, low- to moderate-viscosity exudating wounds [13]. Cadexomer beads can function in a similar way and have also been shown to be effective debridement agents [14].

### Bacterial Control Dressing

Iodine [14] and silver-containing products can, because of their antiseptic or antimicrobial action, reduce the bacterial load [9] while assisting with the natural process of autolytic debridement. Such dressings are suitable for moderately to heavily exudating (high-volume and viscosity) wounds with evidence of heavy bacterial colonisation or overt infection. The slow release of antimicrobials from some products reduces the need for frequent dressing changes.

### Topical Negative Pressure (TNP) Devices

These devices, which are suitable for high-volume, low- to high-viscosity exudate wounds, have been suggested to reduce bacterial load [15]. They remove bacterial toxins, MMPs and other toxic chemicals from the wound environment, facilitating debridement.

## Conclusion

Autolytic debridement is the most commonly performed method of wound debridement and its simplicity means that it is generally a safe technique available to all health-care professions involved in wound management. Evidence supporting its clinical and cost effectiveness is lacking, but expert opinion favours its widespread use. It is, from the patient's perspective, acceptable, and from the nursing perspective the obvious first choice as a debridement method. A wide range of wound-care products are available that assist the natural process of autolytic debridement and this means that a suitable product is available for most wounds. However, its ease of use and the ready availability of products does not mean that it is always the most appropriate debridement technique, as other factors such as the site and nature of the wound, the urgency of debridement and the presence of infection may require the use of alternative, more rapid debridement methods.

## References


1. Thomas AM, Harding KG, Moore K (1999) The structure and composition of chronic wound eschar. J Wound Care 8: 285–287
2. Baharestani M (1999) The clinical relevance of debridement. In: Baharestani M et al. (eds) The clinical relevance of debridement. Springer, Berlin Heidelberg New York Tokyo
3. Himel H (1995) Wound healing: focus on the chronic wound. Wounds. 7 [Suppl A]: 70A–77A
4. Vowden KR, Vowden P (1999) Wound debridement. Part 1: Non-sharp techniques. J Wound Care 8: 237–240
5. Vowden KR, Vowden P (1999) Wound debridement. Part 2: Sharp techniques. J Wound Care 8: 291–294
6. Vowden P, Vowden K (2002) Wound bed preparation (WBP). World Wide Wounds
7. Cutting KF, White RJ (2002) Maceration of the skin and wound bed. 1: Its nature and causes. J Wound Care 11: 275–278
8. Nielsen A (1999) Management of wound exudate. J Community Nurs 13: 27–34
9. Stewart J (2002) Next generation products for wound management. World Wide Wounds
10. Foster L, Moore P (1997) The application of a cellulose-based fibre dressing in surgical wounds. J Wound Care 6: 469–473
11. Robinson BJ (2000) The use of a hydrofibre dressing in wound management. J Wound Care 9: 32–34
12. Lisle J (2002) Debridement of necrotic tissue and eschar using a capillary dressing and semi-permeable film dressing. Br J Community Nurs 7: 29–30, 32, 34
13. Deeth M (2002) Review of an independent audit into the clinical efficacy of VACUTEX. Br J Nurs 11 [Suppl 12]: S60, S62–66
14. Iodine and Wound Physiology (1995) A symposium. 5th Annual Meeting of the European Tissue Repair Society. European Tissue Repair Society, Padua, Italy
15. Morykwas MJ, Argenta LC, Shelton-Brown EI, McGuirt W (1997) Vacuum-assisted closure: a new method for wound control and treatment: animal studies and basic foundation. Ann Plast Surg 38: 553–562
16. Thomas S, Andrews A (1999) The effects of hydrogel dressings on maggot development. J Wound Care 8: 75–77
17. Bradley M, Cullum N, Sheldon T (1999) The debridement of chronic wounds: a systematic review. Health Technol Assess 3: iii–iv, 1–78

# III Wound Preparations and Treatment

# 9

# Wound-Bed Preparation – Promotion of Granulation Tissue

U.E. Ziegler, U.A. Dietz, K. Schmidt

## Introduction

The understanding of the pathophysiological processes in chronic wounds, as compared to acute wounds, is still very limited. Different concepts of treatment have therefore resulted from this knowledge. Recently, the term wound-bed conditioning has been focused on the fact that, to achieve an accelerated healing, especially chronic wounds need a more intensive treatment than acute wounds. The role of wound-bed preparation or the status of the wound bed as influencing prediction for the healing process has not yet been completely determined. Considered retrospectively, inadequate wound-bed conditioning is one of the reasons why some of the modern therapies, such as growth factors or skin substitution, fail. Wound-bed conditioning enables the clinician to eliminate extensive wound-healing barriers and to stimulate the wound-healing process.

## Wound-Bed Conditioning as Strategy

It is difficult to establish general guidelines for the preparation of the wound bed since we have to deal on the one hand with different wound entities and, on the other hand, with wound-specific, patient-specific and socio-economic problems (good wound care). In addition, the wound-healing process itself is an extremely complicated system with complex cellular interactions.

Wound-bed conditioning as a strategy makes it possible to understand and to treat the different aspects of wound therapy including its individual elements without neglecting the final goal (e.g. wound closure). Industry also follows this treatment concept, so that new dressings for patients and practitioners are continually being developed. However, reliable published and sufficiently evaluated studies (also evidence-based) seldom exist for this strategy of treatment.

Up to now, wound-bed conditioning has meant wound debridement. In acute wounds, surgical debridement [6], including the removal of necrotic tissue and bacteria, results in unproblematic healing. This is not the case in chronic wounds, which need more than surgical debridement to achieve healing. In chronic wounds, tissue infection is more likely (e.g. diabetic foot ulcer, ulcer in arterial occlusive disease) and an increased amount of exudate is observed, obviously associated with an increased number of proteases and therefore hindering wound healing.

Thus, wound-bed conditioning in chronic wounds followed by incomplete coverage or healing *per secundam* plays an important role in wound therapy, together with the causal therapy of the ulcer (e.g. control of diabetes, compression therapy, relief etc.).

Wound-bed conditioning means total wound management in order to enhance endogenous healing or to augment the efficiency of other therapeutic methods [7].

The goals of local wound-bed conditioning are stimulation of:

- angiogenesis,
- new formation of collagene,
- re-epitheliasation,
- wound contraction and cell growth.

Periulcerous surrounding skin is one of the clinical signs for the efficacy of this treatment (own experience). The most important measures to achieve well-vascularised granulation tissue or healing are:

- removal of necroses and wound coating (debridement),
- creating a bacterial balance on the wound surface (germ reduction/elimination),
- management of exudate,
- wound-edge activation.

## Management of Necrosis and Wound Coating

### Sharp Debridement

At present, sharp debridement before changing the dressing, as well as moist wound treatment to optimise the wound bed, are established measures in treating chronic wounds in order to achieve correction of the wound matrix [6]. Sharp and enzymatic debridement are considered to be the most effective methods to remove necrotic tissue, eschars and bacteria from the wound surface. Local perfusion can be improved immediately, the risk of infection reduced significantly, and minor bleeding results in the release of different cytokines which influence the onset of repair processes positively [6].

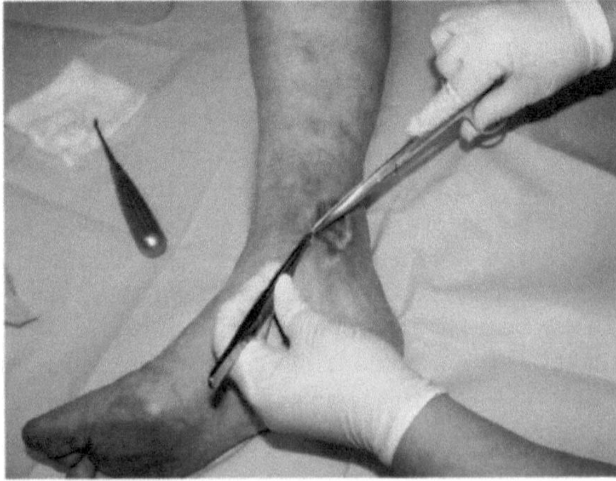

**Fig. 1.** Wound debridement with shears and surgical tweezers

Depending on the local findings, sharp debridement is carried out with the "sharp" spoon, a ring abrasor, scalpel or shear (Fig. 1), the different methods having advantages and disadvantages in respect to pain, the patient's psyche, handling and efficacy. Newer but also more expensive methods, such as the removal of wound coating by ultrasound or waterjet, are available. Their efficacy is very high and pain must be individually relieved, depending on the local findings or the patient.

### Anaesthesia in Sharp Debridement

To treat pain during surgical debridement, an anaesthetic gel (Emla), infiltration anaesthesia (local anaesthesia) or block anaesthesia (foot block [29], midfoot block or toe block) are recommended, depending on the individual patient. Accompanying analgetics or sedatives can be administered. In the case of expansive local findings, risk patients, severe systemic infections or extremely anxious patients, the anaesthesiologist in the operating theatre should choose the right form of anaesthesia (e.g. narcosis, spinal anaesthesia) [25].

### Maggot Treatment (Lucilia sericata)

The removal of moist necroses by using maggots is meanwhile an established method in Germany [22, 26]. Enzymatic liquor is secreted and then re-absorbed by the maggot. A selective differentiation between healthy and sick tissue takes place, which is sometimes quite difficult in surgery.

Practitioners appreciate not only the biologically debriding effect of the maggots but also the antimicrobial effect, since almost sterile wound conditions after treatment exist. A third advantage of maggot secretion is the effect of wound healing in the sense of an induction of the re-epithelialisation. This effect has been known for many centuries [16].

Indications for a maggot therapy are rich and fixed tissue residues with and without surrounding infection. In special localisations maggots are more appropriate than surgical abrasion by the wound therapist. At the calcaneus, dorsum, in deep bags of the forefoot and the metatarsus, as well as on ulcerations of the achilles' tendon (own indications), 100 to 200 sterile grubs (usually 2 days old) are set on the necroses and left there for 2–3 days, either loose or in a biobag. For free maggots a special dressing technique is necessary, e.g. stripes of hydrogel round the ulcer to keep the maggots on the wound. An additional dressing with activated carbon, used as odour filter, can be applied as a bad odour occurs during treatment. Psychological factors in the patient have to be considered, and the order has to be organised in time. At present, maggot therapy is not sufficiently cost-effective.

### Enzymatical Debridement

The removal of fibrinous and necrotic parts from the wound can also be done by enzymatic ointments. In our opinion, such a method will only be indicated if after sharp debridement further debriding effects are necessary or if contra-indications for a sharp debridement exist (e.g. tendency to bleeding, heavy pain, logistical problems) [6, 31]. Of the enzymatic ointments available today, only proteolytic enzymes appear to be useful and, among them, only the bacterial collagenase (*Clostridium histolyticum*) [13]. Enzymes work only in a moist and warm environment, so that an appropriate secondary dressing has to be applied. Furthermore, frequent dressing change is necessary, which might be a logistic problem and is often problematic for the patient.

### Autolytical Debridement

Similarly to the case of enzymatically debriding substances, it is difficult to determine the importance of autolytical therapeutics based on the existing data. Hydrogels, hydrocolloids, xerogels and alginates etc. have different clinically debriding characteristics; they are used successfully, also in combination, as supporting therapeutics in chronic wounds [30]. They produce a moist environment, and macrophages, leukocytes and endogenously proteolytical enzymes are activated in a highly selective process, so that necrotic tissue and coating of differing colour and origin can be removed, thereby having a supportive effect on the granulation tissue in each of the wound-healing phases [14].

## Management of the Bacterial Balance

### Bacterial Colonisation and Wound Healing

The terms contamination (mere existence of bacteria on the wound without bacterial reproduction), colonisation (reproduction of pathogen bacteria on the wound without reaction in the host) and infection (classically local and systemic signs of an infection in the host) describe a classification of the local condition of the wound in order to start an appropriate treatment [5, 23].

The term critical colonisation has been introduced because many chronic wounds are presented in such a stage (depending on further different parameters), and it describes the transitional stage from colonisation to infection, in the sense of a threatening infection.

Not only the number of bacteria but also the pathogenic virulence, the amount of necrotic material and the immunisation of the host seem to be important in chronic wounds. According to Falanga, these are the critical variables which may lead to an infection [7].

The clinical signs of wound infection and delayed wound healing in chronic wounds (apart from classical parameters such as reddening, swelling etc.) are:
- increased exudation,
- increased pain,
- (dark) red, fragile (soft) granulation tissue slightly bleeding when touched
- bad-smelling wound basis/granulation tissue,
- increased changes of the skin in peri-ulcerous regions (dermatitis),
- non-reactive wound basis and wound edge,
- recurrent necrosis and coatings.

Until a few years ago, bacterial colonisation played an insignificant role in treatment of chronically problematic wounds. Growing understanding of the microbiological processes at the wound surface in the interstitial and intracellular area has resulted in conceiving new products to reduce the number of bacteria in chronic wounds.

Classifying infected, contaminated and colonised wounds is possible; however, the question remains to what extent several bacterial species are actually the cause of wound-healing defects or whether additional parameters might be responsible.

Various studies have shown a clear correlation between the number of bacteria on the wound surface and increased wound-healing defects [17, 23]; others reach no consensus [2, 12,24]. All the studies on anaerobic and aerobic cultures in chronic wounds have included only a few patients, had no differentiated classification and carried out no deep wound biopsy.

In chronic wounds, we have to deal with at least two different pathogens of the Gram-positive and the Gram-negative region in most of the cases (*Staphylococcus aureus*, streptococci, *Pseudomonas aeruginosa*, colibacillus) [4]; from acute wounds usually only one species is isolated [3].

## Bacterial Screening of Chronic Wounds

Different techniques are possible to determine the bacterial situation in chronic wounds (quantitative biopsy, quantitative smear, semi-quantitative smear, rapid slide technique, irrigation-aspiration technique, molecular methods). Today, because of the costs and practicability, only a semi-quantitative smear and the consequent tests are performed in chronic wounds [9]. However, our own studies using this method show no definite relationship between the number of isolated species and the amount of bacteria in a clinically clear infection of diabetic ulcer [21]. Therefore, we recommend the determination of bacterial species and their number only on primary treatment, before starting a systemically antibiotic therapy or if the wound healing is arrested.

Considering the data so far published on quantitative biopsy and wounds, it can be observed that the experimental inoculation of wounds with $10^8$ pathogens/g tissue leads to more complications in wounds. Furthermore, apart from the bacterial type of pathogen, a wound-healing defect can be induced with $10^5$–$10^6$ (or even more) pathogens/g and, especially with streptococci, even a small number of bacteria can lead to an infection.

The existence of a so-called biofilm on the wound surface, the patient's immunological situation, the amount of existing necrotic material and the virulence of the bacterial species seem to be more important than the mere number of bacteria:

$$\text{risk of infection} = \frac{\text{number of bacteria} \times \text{virulence}}{\text{immunological resistance}}$$

(immunological resistance: individual variables of infection and immunological function).

## Local and Systemic Factors Influencing the Risk of Wound Infection

The amount of necrotic material on the wound is one of the local factors which can hamper wound healing. Clinically, surgical debridement is the most important method to promote wound healing and to prevent infection, as necrotic tissue is an important variable of infection. Depending on the virulence and number of bacteria, different amounts of exudate can be observed. Less exudation on the moist wound surface is an indication for good wound healing. Furthermore, the biochemistry of the wound and cellular dysfunction in the repair process are significant local factors for the development of wound infection.

Systemic risk factors in the development of wound infection are a badly adjusted diabetes mellitus, anaemia, malnutrition, circulatory and coagulation disturbances, as well as an immunosuppressive treatment.

## Biofilm on Chronic Wounds

In antibiotic therapy, changed temperatures and a shift of osmolarity on the wound surface, antiseptics, alcohol or stationary treatment lead to a situation of external stress, which stimulates certain bacterial species to produce biofilm (Fig. 2). Biofilm is a matrix made of lipopolysaccharids which are produced by the bacteria; however, not all species are able to produce biofilm.

Biofilm production functions as self-protection for the bacterial colonies whereby single bacteria react with bacterial species. Biofilm-positive colonies of the parent bacteria can then change their genetic structure at a chromosomal level to differing variants [10, 15]. It is highly probable that biofilm production results in an extremely solid adhesion of biofilm with the wound surface, similar to that found in catheter systems or in artificial joint prostheses. This biofilm seems to greatly promote wound-healing defects, and must be removed mechanically (debridement). In the same way, anti-bacterial silver dressings seem to be able to break through this biofilm and probably hamper the development and interaction of wound-healing barriers.

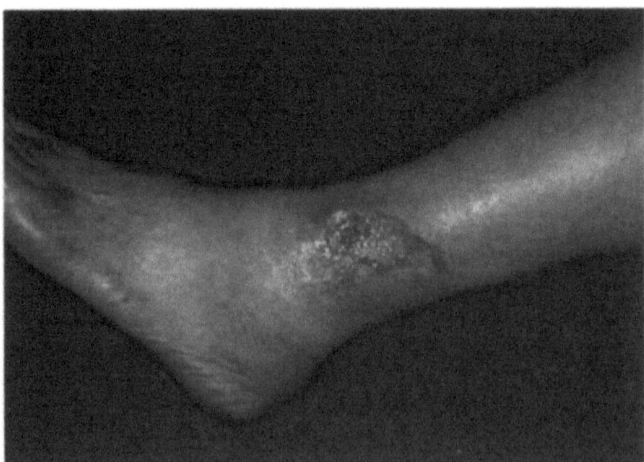

**Fig. 2.** Biofilm with chronic ulcer and scleroderma

Although it has so far not been possible to obtain clear results concerning biofilm production on the wound surface in chronic wounds, the clinical application of a biofilm destroyer such as mechanical debridement and anti-microbial substances seems to be useful (according to current knowledge). The combination of debridement and vacuum-sealing techniques also seems to destroy biofilm on the wound surface and is one of the clinically most effective methods of wound-bed conditioning. Further studies are urgently needed to discover the function of biofilm in delayed wound healing.

## Management of Wound Exudate

During the past years, an increasing number of studies on wound liquid has broadened the pathophysiological understanding of wound-healing defects. Most studies have dealt with chronically venous ulcers. Compared to acute wounds, chronic wound liquid on the wound bed indicates a hypoxic and proteolytic situation, followed by proliferation or blocking of key cells, such as keratinocytes, fibroblasts and endothelial cells of the extra-cellular matrix [11, 27]. Increased expression of inflammatory mediators und proteases can also be observed, which might lead to an arrest of wound healing [1, 19, 28]. The clinical data published so far have a small number of patients (in most cases between 10 and 15 patients) and none of the biochemical wound analyses is complete or has been exactly evaluated; it is therefore not possible to develop final clinical treatment regimes, not least because the extreme heterogeneity in the individual ulcerations is an added complication.

However, the increased amount of exudate on the wound surface is an indication for a wound-healing defect, triggered, for example, by an increased bacterial level with or without infection, oedema or necrosis. Clinically, the attempt should be made to minimise the exudate, but maintain a consistent wound treatment.

During the treatment, indirect and direct regimes are used. Indirect exudate management is performed by anti-inflammatory agents (e.g. silver preparations) and antiseptics [23]. Direct management consists of compression therapy, vacuum sealing or other highly adsorbent dressings, such as alginates, foam dressings etc.

## Wound-Edge Activation – Epithelialisation

Wound-edge activation plays an important role in local wound treatment. Removing coatings and necroses and stabilising the surrounding skin can re-establish dermal function by re-epithelialisation. In acute wound healing, a defined process takes place on a molecular/cellular level, enabling dermal wound occlusion. It is well known that in diabetic wounds this healing process is halted in the proliferative phase, thereby creating a non-reactive wound situation. Metabolic processes in extra-cellular matrix proteins (e.g. fibronectin) prevent the growth of fibroblasts, and appropriate growth factors are not produced or are insufficiently available. Local hypoxy at the wound due to decreased local perfusion prevents this normal wound-healing process, as has been proved by different studies [8].

## Wound Dressings, Wound Therapeutics

In the year 2000, Sibbald et al. developed generally binding guidelines for the Canadian Wound-Healing Society. These guidelines were presented in a table [23] from which the right dressing system can be chosen according to the colour of the wound bed and the granulation tissue. As already mentioned above, an individual adaptation of the right dressing system is absolutely necessary and can therefore not always be standardised.

Meanwhile, many different therapeutics are commercially available. The expected amount of exudate can be determined by anamnesis and inspection of the last wound dressing in order to choose the right form for the new dressing. To choose the suitable dressing for an individual wound situation, it is necessary to answer the following questions:

- After sharp debridement, is a debriding or rather a granulation-promoting dressing necessary (hydrocolloids, alginates, hydrogels, collagenases etc.)?
- How much exudate must be adsorbed by the dressing until the next possible change of dressing to prevent dermal maceration from taking place (alginates, hydrocolloids, sponges, foams etc.)?
- Is an additional antiseptic/antibacterial treatment necessary to create a bacterial balance (antiseptics/silver dressings)?

## Wound Documentation

Falanga describes the current wound-bed situation on dressing change in simple numbers and letters [7] by considering granulation, exudate and the infection:
- granulation: A = 100%, B = 50–100%, C = <50%
- exudate: 1 = minimum, 2 = medium, 3 = maximum
- infect: k = none, d = threatening/beginning, i = infect, s = other

Which debridement, wound cleansing, dressing, dressing material, dressing interval or supplementary methods is used can be additionally and easily documented; this is suited to domestic or ambulant health care. We use the wound net [20] for an exact computer-assisted documentation, but, out of practical considerations, add the short criteria of Falanga to our data.

## Conclusion

Treatment of wounds has seen extensive changes over the past 15–20 years. Although no evidence-based data exist, a differentiated therapy regime is used in chronic wounds. Correspondingly, different dressing systems are commercially available today and are being used successfully, as our understanding of wound-healing biology is continually growing. The tightrope walk between clinical experience and proven procedures will still remain in the near future. Patients profit from the concept of wound-bed conditioning; however, moist wound treatment, debridement, bacterial control and exudate management have not yet been established everywhere in Germany. The numerous individual factors which have to be taken into consideration are often rejected (good wound care) and the complexity in the treatment of chronic wounds has been appreciated sufficiently by the health-care system.

We must insist on standards in wound healing and wound care, as well as on the establishment of appropriate training centres.

## References

1. Agren MS, Eaglstein WH, Ferguson MWJ et al. (2000) Causes and effects of the chronic inflammation in venous leg ulcers. Acta Derm Venereol 210 [Suppl]: 3–17
2. Annoni F, Rosina M, Chiurazzi D, Ceva M (1989) The effects of a hydrocolloid dressing on bacterial growth and the healing process of leg ulcers. Int Angiol 8: 224–228
3. Bowler PG, Davies BJ (1999) The microbiology of acute and chronic wounds. Wounds 11: 72–78
4. Davis CE, Wilson MJ, Hill KE, Stephens P, Hill M, Harding KG, Thomas DW (2001) Use of molecular techniques to study microbial diversity in the skin: Chronic wounds reevaluated. Wound Repair and Regeneration 9: 332–340
5. Dow G, Browne A, Sibbald RG (1999) Infection in chronic wounds: Controversies in diagnosis and treatment. Ostomy/Wound Management 45: 23–40
6. Dräger E, Winter H (1999) Surgical debridement versus enzymatic debridement – benefits and drawbacks. In: Baharestani M et al. (eds) The clinical relevance of debridement. Springer, Berlin Heidelberg
7. Falanga V (2000) Classification for wound bed preparation and stimulation of chronic wounds. Wound Rep Reg 8: 347–352
8. Falanga V, Qian SW, Danielpour D et al.(1991) Hypoxia upregulates the synthesis of TGF-beta 1 by human dermal fibroblasts. J Invest Dermatol 97: 634–637
9. Gilchrist B, Reed C (1989) The bacteriology of chronic venous ulcers treated with occlusive hydrocolloid dressings. Br J Derm 121: 337–344
10. Götz F (2002) Staphylococcus and biofilms. Molecular Microbiology 43: 1367–1378
11. Grinell F, Zhu M (1996) Fibronectin degradation in chronic wounds depends on the relative level of elastase alpha1-proteinase inhibitor, and alpha2-macroglobulin. J Invest Dermatol 106: 335–341
12. Hannson C, Hoborn J, Moller A, Swanbeck G (1995) The microbioal flora in venous leg ulcers without clinical signs of infection. Acta Derm Venereol (Stockh) 75: 24–30
13. Jung W, Winter H (1998) Considerations for the use of clostridial collagenase in clinical practice. Clin Drug Invest 15: 245–252
14. Kennedy Kl, Tritch DL (1997) Debridement. In: Krasner D, Kane D (eds) Chronic wound case: A clinical source book for healthcare professionals, 2nd ed. Wayne PA: Health Management Publications, Inc, pp 336–343

15. Krimmer V, Merkert H, v.Eif C, Frosch M, Eulert J, Löhr J, Hacker J, Ziebuhr W (1999) Detection of Staphylococcus aureus and Staphylococcus epidermidis in Clinical Samples by 16S rRNA-Directed In Situ Hybridization. J Clin Microbiol 2667–2673.

16. Livingston SK, Prince LH (1932) The treatment of chronic osteomyelitis with special reference to the use of maggot active principle. J Am Med Assoc 98: 1143–1149

17. Majewski W, Cybulski Z, Napierala M et al. (1995) The value of quantitative bacteriological investigations in the monitoring of treatment of ischaemic ulcerations of lower legs. Int Angiol 14: 381–384

18. Mekkes J (2000) Autolytic debridement. In: Cherry GW, Harding KG, Ryan TJ (eds) Wound bed preparation. International Congress and Symposium Series 250, The Royal Society of Medicine Press, London

19. Nwomeh BC, Yager DR, Cohen IK (1998) Physiology of the chronic wound. Clin Plast Surg 25: 341–356

20. Pfeffer E, Coerper S, Riediger H, Becker HD, Köveker G, Hopt UT, Verein Wundnetz e.V. (2001) Die Vernetzung chirurgischer Wundzentren mit Hilfe eines neuen EDV-Dokumentationssystems. Chirurg 72: 1458–1463

21. Schmidt K, Debus ES, Jeßberger S, Ziegler UE, Thiede A (2000) Bacterial population of chronic crural ulcers: is there a difference between the diabetic, the venous, and the arterial ulcer? VASA 29: 62–70

22. Sherman RA, Hall MJ, Thomas S (2000) Medicinal maggots: an ancient remedy for some contemporary afflications. Annu Rev Entomol 45: 55–81

23. Sibbald RG, Williamson D, Orsted HL, Campbell K, Keast D, Krasner D, Sibbald D (22000) Preparing the wound bed – Debridement, bacterial balance and moisture balance. Ostomy Wound Management 46: 14–35

24. Steer JA, Papini RP, Wilson AP, Mgrouther DA, Parkhouse N (1996) Quantitative microbiology in the management of burn patients. II. Relationship between bacterial counts obtained by burn wound biopsy culture and surface alginate swab culture, with clinical outcome following burn surgery and change of dressings. Burns 22: 177–181

25. Téot L (2000) Surgical and shrap debridement. In: Cherry GW, Harding KG, Ryan TJ (eds) Wound bed preparation. International Congress and Symposium Series 250, The Royal Society of Medicine Press, London

26. Thomas S, Jones M, Shutler S, Jones S (1996) Using larvae in modern wound management. J Wound Care 5: 60–69

27. Trengove NJ, Langton SR, Stacey MC (1996 Biochemical analysis of wound fluid from non-healing and healing chronic leg ulcers. Wound Rep Reg 4: 234–239

28. Wysocki AB, Staiano-Coico L, Grinell F (1993) Wound fluid from chronic leg ulcers contains elevated levels of metalloproteinases MMP-2 and MMP-9. J Invest Dermatol 101: 64–68

29. Ziegler UE, Schmidt K, Breithaupt B, Debus ES, Thiede A (2000) Minoramputationen am Fuß – ambulantes Operieren mittels Fußblock-Leitungsanästhesie. Krankenpflege Journal 38: 282–286

30. Ziegler UE, Schmidt K, Keller HP, Thiede A (2003) Behandlung chronischer Wunden mit einer Kalzium-Zink-Mangan-Alginatauflage. MMW-Fortschritte der Medizin 1: 19–26

31. Ziegler UE (2000) Enzymatic debridement. In: Cherry GW, Harding KG, Ryan TJ (eds) Wound bed preparation. International Congress and Symposium Series 250, The Royal Society of Medicine Press, London

# Cleansing and Cleansers

ELIZABETH A. AYELLO

## Introduction

Wound-bed preparation is "the management of a wound to accelerate endogenous healing or to facilitate the effectiveness of other therapeutic measures" [1]. Wound cleansing is a vital component of preparing the wound bed. It should be done initially and with each dressing change. Wound cleansing removes wound exudate, dressing residue, foreign materials, topical agents and metabolic wastes, which is necessary for getting the wound bed ready for healing to occur.

## Definition and Indications

Removing wound exudate in chronic wounds reduces one of the burdens that interfere with the healing process. Research has supported the idea that chronic wound exudate or fluid is biochemically different from acute wound fluid [2]. There is a decrease in mitogenic cellular activity in chronic wounds while acute wounds promote DNA synthesis [3–5]. Chronic wound fluid has high levels of pro-inflammatory cytokines, which keep the wound in the inflammatory phase [2, 4]. The high levels of matrix metalloproteinases (MMPs) in chronic wound fluid destroy or alter the newly formed matrix [6–11]. Fibroblast proliferation is also inhibited in chronic wound fluid [3]. Because of these inhibitory effects on wound healing, action by the clinician must be taken to remove the exudate and put the chronic wound in the best state for healing to occur.

Wound cleansing is defined as "a process that removes these less adherent inflammatory contaminants from the wound surface and renders the wound less conducive to microbial growth" [12]. It includes selecting both the correct solution and the mechanical method of delivering that solution to the wound bed without causing trauma to the wound bed. In making these decisions, clinicians must weigh the benefits of cleaning the wound, and thus removing surface debris and contaminants, against the risks of trauma to the wound bed from the cleaning process. Minimising chemical Cland mechanical trauma is an important goal in wound cleansing. Chemical trauma can occur if the chemicals in the wound-cleaning fluids are toxic to the wound tissue. Mechanical trauma can occur from the amount of pressure with which the wound-cleaning fluid is delivered. Because the science of wound cleansing is limited, some practice recommendations are based on historical practice and/or expert consensus.

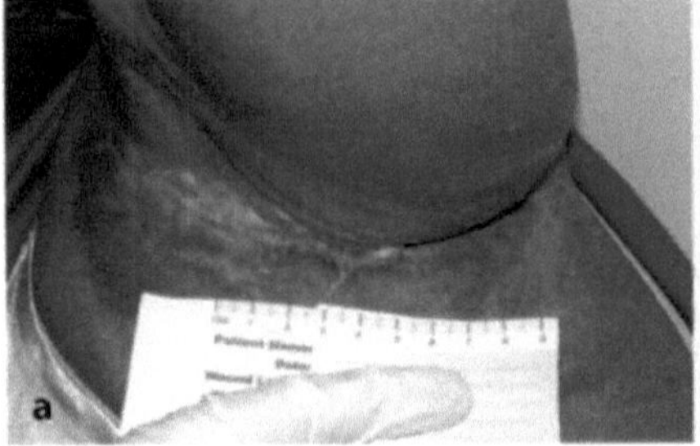
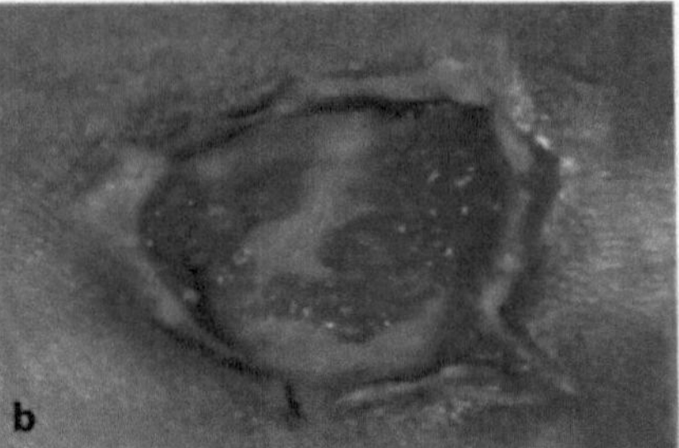

**Fig. 1. a** Acute wound of axilla, **b** chronic wound

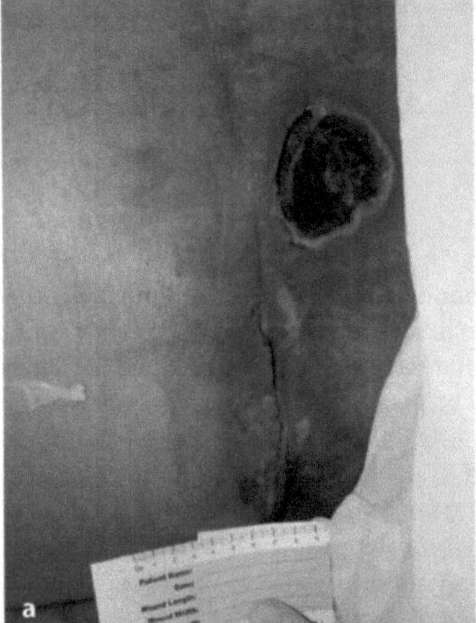
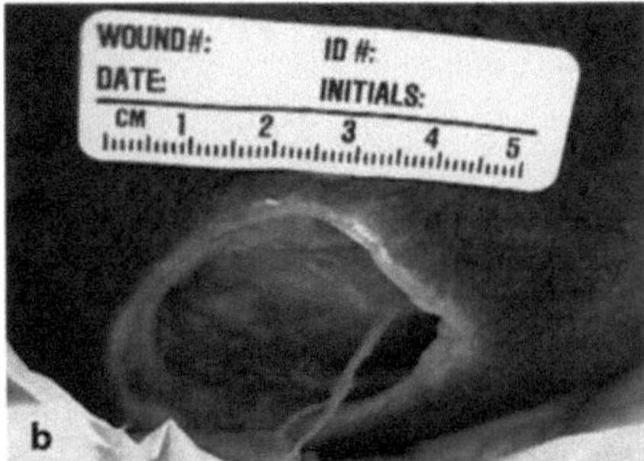

**Fig. 2. a** Chronic wound – needs debridement. **b** This wound with stringy slough needs cleansing and debridement

Wound cleansing is indicated for removing debris and organisms that are on the wound surface (Fig. 1). Once the bacteria have adhered to the wound bed (Fig. 2), then surface cleansing is not enough and some method of debridement is required. (see section II of this volume for discussion of ways to perform debridement).

## Cleansing Solutions

Saline (0.9% sodium chloride) is widely used to clean wounds. Isotonic saline is considered safe and adequate for cleansing most chronic wounds. When not available commercially, saline solution can be made by adding two teaspoons of non-iodised salt to 1 liter of boiling water. Allow the solution to cool before using it. Since the fluid has only brief contact with the wound, water (without any contaminants), although not isotonic, may also be used. When comparing two groups of emergency-room patients with wounds, Angeras and colleagues [13] found a lower infection rate (5.4%) in wounds irrigated with tap water compared to 10.3% in wounds irrigated with sterile saline.

Commercially available wound cleansers, which have surface-active agents, can also be used to clean wounds. Do not confuse wound cleansers with skin cleansers, as they are very different solutions. Skin cleansers are meant to be used on intact skin and not in open wounds.

When selecting the cleansing solution, it is important for the clinician to consider the total patient care plan. For example, if an enzymatic debriding agent is also being used on the wound, it is imperative to select the right cleansing solution that is compatible with it. Some solutions will inactive certain enzymes, so they should not be used if that particular enzymatic debriding agent is also being applied to the wound. Use the following chart as a guide for wound cleansing when enzymatic debriding agents are part of your patient's treatment plan:

Collagenase:
- Can use
  - Saline
  - Water
  - Hydrogen peroxide
  - Dakin's solution
  - Hydrogen peroxide
- Do not use
  - Detergents
  - Heavy metals (silver, mercury)

Papain urea:
- Can use
  - Saline
  - Water
- Do not use
  - Hydrogen peroxide
  - Heavy metal salts (lead, silver, mercury)

Detergents are chemicals that reduce surface tension. While detergents can have a positive or negative charge, only those that have no charge at all (non-ionic) are not harmful to cells. Wound cleansers may be especially useful for wounds with a large amount of debris. The surface-active agents (surfactants) in these cleansers break the chemical bonds that hold wound contaminants to the wound surface.

Clinicians sometimes confuse wound cleansers with skin cleansers. This is an important distinction since wound cleansers are not the same as skin cleansers. Skin cleansers are often designed to remove urinary or faecal contamination from intact skin. Given their strength and toxicity to cells, skin cleansers should not be used in wounds.

When selecting a wound cleanser, its cleaning capacity should be compared against its toxicity to cells. Although a standardised method of comparing wound cleansers is lacking, there is some evidence basis for clinical decision-making. Most studies have been done in vitro under controlled conditions with, at times, contrasting results. Studies do suggest that there is a wide range in the relative toxicity of these cleansers. Toxicity tables have been published elsewhere [14, 15]. Foresman and colleagues [15] evaluated the relative toxicity of wound and skin cleaners by their effect on PMNs. For most wound cleansers, the toxicity indices ranged from 10 to 1000 while skin cleansers were 10 000 or above. Wright and Orr [16] also evaluated the toxicity of wound cleansers on human fibroblasts and white blood cells. Results found that constant clenz and saf-clens were significantly less ($p<0.005$) cytotoxic to fibroblasts in vitro compared to other wound-cleanser products (Cara-Klenz, ultra-klenz, Shur-Clens). A deviation from the manufacturer's recommended pH for Shur-Clens is given as the explanation for the difference in this study's findings compared to the Foresman et al. [15] study.

Some clinicians erroneously believe that in order to clean the wound bed, all organisms must be killed. Historically, these clinicians used antiseptics to clean wounds in the hope of preventing wound infection. Antiseptics destroy the cell walls in the bacteria but unfortunately also in non-bacterial cells such as fibroblasts and macrophages. Almost a 100 years later, later evidence supports Fleming's [17] work that antiseptics cannot kill bacteria within tissue. When antiseptics are used with wound cleansers, the toxicity indices for the wound cleansers are then raised to 10 000, leaving the benefit of this addition to the cleansing regime questionable [18]. Despite this, the use of antiseptic solutions persists in clinical practice. Even though povidone iodine, sodium hypochlorite and acetic acid are cytotoxic, some clinicians have used these diluted solutions as cleansing agents when wound debridement and infection control rather than cleansing are the goal. A comprehensive review of the research on human and animal wounds by Drosou et al. [19] concluded:

- Antiseptics are effective against a broader range of bacteria than antibiotics.
- Antiseptics are less likely to create resistant bacteria.
- Povidone iodine showed conflicting results, with some studies showing a decrease in bacterial counts and others with no effect. A 10% povidone-iodine solution showed histological evidence of tissue toxicity.
- Acetic acid decreased bacterial burden in in vivo studies.
- Cadexomer iodine (in ointment or dressing form which releases iodine slowly into the wound) consistently showed decreased bacterial counts and accelerated wound healing in humans.
- Silver compounds effectively reduced bacterial burden without negative effects on wound healing. Some in vivo studies showed accelerated wound healing.
- Due to its effervescent positive effect, hydrogen peroxide may be useful in removing debris from wounds, but has little effect on wound healing or bacterial control.

Since antiseptic solutions are toxic to cells, and their effectiveness in healing needs to be established, they should not be used for routine wound cleansing [20]. Antibiotics, rather than antiseptics, may be required for infected wounds.

## Cleansing Delivery Methods

It is not enough to just pick the correct wound-cleansing solution. It is equally important to select a safe way of getting the appropriate cleansing solution to the wound bed that will minimise wound trauma. These methods of wound cleansing include irrigation, scrubbing and showering.

### Wound Irrigation

Irrigation is "cleansing by a stream of fluid, preferably saline" [14]. Effective wound cleansing will occur when the hydraulic force created by the fluid stream is greater than the adhesive force that is holding the debris on the wound surface. The system used to deliver the irrigation solution does matter!

The right amount of pressure is critical. Too low a pressure will not adequately clean the wound while too high a pressure can cause tissue injury along with removal of contaminants. The work by Beltran et al. [21] provides evidence that a bulb syringe has an irrigation impact of 2 psi and therefore may not have enough pressure to adequately cleanse the wound [14]. Conversely, too high an irrigation pressure can cause soft tissue damage. In Europe and the United States, clinical guidelines about wound cleansing for pressure ulcers have been recommended (see following list). Both the EPUAP and the American AHRQ clinical practice guidelines recommend 4 to 15 psi as safe and effective irrigation pressures for cleansing wounds (Fig. 3).

### Recommendations: Wound Cleansing for Pressure Ulcers

- European Pressure Ulcers Advisory Panel (EPUAP) [22]:
    1. Cleanse wounds as necessary with tap water or with water, which is suitable for drinking, or with saline (strength of evidence = C)
    2. Use minimal mechanical force when cleansing or irrigating the ulcer. Showering is appropriate. Irrigation can be useful for cleaning a cavity ulcer (C)
    3. Antiseptics should not routinely be used to clean wounds but may be considered when bacterial load needs to be controlled after clinical assessment. Ideally, antiseptics should only be used for a limited period of time until the wound is clean and surrounding inflammation reduced (C)
- Agency for Health Care Policy and Research (AHCPR) [14]:
    1. Cleanse wounds initially and at each dressing change (strength of evidence = C)
    2. Use minimal mechanical force when cleansing the ulcer with gauze, cloth, or sponges (C)
    3. Do not clean ulcer wounds with skin cleansers or antiseptic agents [e.g. povidone iodine, iodophor, sodium hypochlorite solution (Dakin's solution), hydrogen peroxide, acetic acid] (B)
    4. Use normal saline for cleansing most pressure ulcers (C)

> 5. Use enough irrigation pressure to enhance wound cleansing without causing trauma to the wound bed. Safe and effective ulcer irrigation pressures range from 4 to 15 psi (B)
> 6. Consider whirlpool treatment for cleansing pressure ulcers that contain thick exudate, slough or necrotic tissue. Discontinue whirlpool when the ulcer is clean (C)

Because as the syringe size increases, the pressure decreases, while as the needle size increases, the pressure increases, the right combination of syringe size and needle size is required to provide a safe and effective irrigation method. By using a 35-ml syringe with a 19-gauge needle, saline is delivered to the wound at 8 psi. Longmire et al. [23] provide evidence to support the use of this system. In their study of emergency room patients, there was statistically significant less wound inflammation and infection in wounds cleansed with a needle and syringe compared to wounds cleaned with a bulb syringe.

Some clinicians have used a screw cap with an irrigating tip on a 250-ml soft plastic bottle of normal saline to clean wounds. The bottle must be squeezed full force, so an acceptable cleaning pressure of 4.5 to 5.0 psi can be achieved [24].

Pulsatile and continuous battery-powered commercially available irrigation systems are also now available. The evidence base for these products is being built. As with any intervention, it is important for clinicians to use the equipment properly and follow the manufacturer's guidelines. When using pressurised irrigation, the clinician needs to wear protective clothing, gloves and eyewear. Splash shields can also reduce splatter (see Key Points for Wound Irrigation below). Use only those systems designed for use in wounds. Do not substitute irrigation systems intended for dental cleaning; their pressures are too high (over 50 psi) and cause damage to wound tissue.

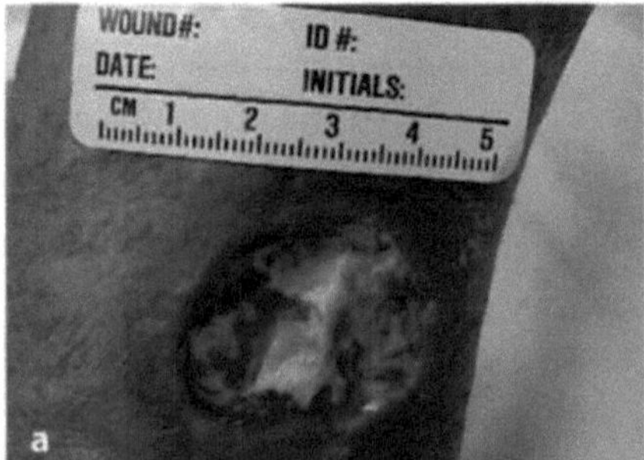
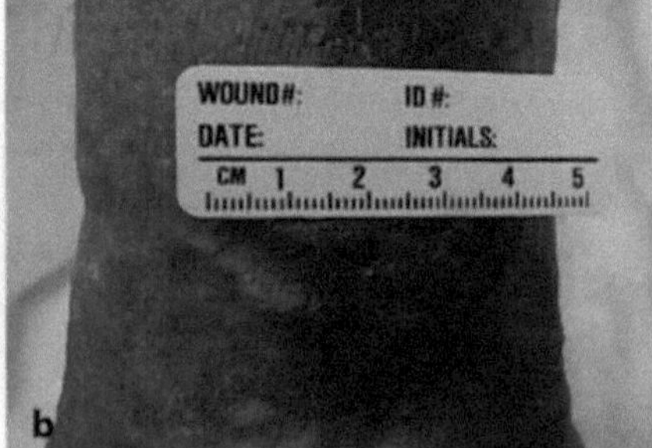

**Fig. 3. a** Person with venous leg ulcer at initial presentation. **b** Same venous ulcer healed after 4 months' treatment with antimicrobial dressing and layer-compression bandaging system

**Key Points for Wound Irrigation**

- Read directions for the equipment. Ask yourself: are you at the appropriate application distance?
- Use an adequate quantity of a safe irrigation solution.
- Warm the solution to body temperature.
- Consider the need for analgesia: ask the patient if there is pain that needs to be managed with this intervention.
- Protect yourself and the patient – be aware of splashback and splatter.

### Scrubbing and Showering

Scrubbing devices, when properly used, can increase the efficacy of wound-cleansing solutions. If the clinician scrubs too hard, this increased force can cause an unnecessary trauma to the wound tissue. Although the available evidence is limited, it suggests that cleaning wounds with coarse sponges rather than smooth sponges makes them more susceptible to infection [25]. Best practice is to use less pressure with the lowest coarseness-scrubbing device that will effectively clean the wound.

Clinicians also need to consider the direction of cleaning the wound. Wounds are usually either cleaned from top to bottom, working outward from the incision in parallel lines, or in circles beginning from the centre of the wound and working outwards.

Showering has been used for wound cleansing. This is especially useful for ulcers in the perinanal and trunk areas as well as extensive metastatic wounds that erupt on the skin in some palliative care patients. Frequent showering with large amounts of water will help reduce the bacterial burden on the wound surface, and provide physical and psychological benefits to patients with fulgating wounds [26]. Tell the patient not to aim the shower water directly at the wound, but instead, to direct the water above the ulcerated area so that it gently trickles down over the wound without too much force. Some patients may prefer a hand-held shower device.

### Summary

Wound cleansing is a vital part of preparing the wound bed for healing. Consideration of the right solution, delivered with the right equipment and the right pressure, as well as using the right technique are important steps in clinical decision-making for evidence-based wound care. Regular cleaning with a non-cytotoxic solution with sufficient, safe force to remove surface contaminants is required.

## References

1. Schultz GS, Sibbald G, Falanga V et al. (2003) Wound bed preparation: a systematic approach to wound management. Wound Repair Regen 11 [Suppl 2]: S1–S28
2. Schultz GS, Mast BA (1998) Molecular analysis of the environment of healing and chronic wounds: cytokines, proteases, and growth factors. Wounds 10 [Suppl F]: 1F–11F
3. Bucalo B, Eaglestein WH, Falanga V (1993) Inhibition of cell proliferation by chronic wound fluid. Wound Repair Regen 1: 183–186
4. Harris IR, Yee KC, Walters CE et al. (1995) Cytokine and protease levels in healing and non-healing chronic venous leg ulcers. Exp Dermatol 4: 342–349
5. Katz MH, Alvarez, AF, Kirsner RS et al. (1991) Human wound fluid from acute wounds stimulates fibroblast and endothelial cell growth. J Am Acad Dermatol 25: 1054–1058
6. Bullen EC, Longaker MT, Updike DL et al. (1995) Tissue inhibitor of metalloproteinases-1 is decreased and activated gelatinases are increased in chronic wounds. J Invest Dermatol 104: 236–240
7. Yager Dr, Zhang LY, Liang HX et al. (1996) Wound fluids from human pressure ulcers contain elevated matrix metalloproteinase levels and activity compared to surgical wound fluids. J Invest Dermatol 107: 743–748
8. Rogers AA, Burnett S, Moore JC et al. (1995) Involvement of proteolytic enzymes, plasminogen activators, and matrix metalloproteinases in the pathology of pressure ulcers. Wound Repair Regen 3: 273–283
9. Rao CN, Lidein DA, Liu et al. (1995) Alpha 1-antitrypsin is degraded and non-functional in chronic wounds but intact and functional in acute wounds: the inhibitor protects fibronectin from degradation by chronic wound fluid enzymes. J Invest Dermatol 105: 572–578
10. Wysocki AB, Staiano-Coico L, Grinnell F (1993) Wound fluid from chronic leg ulcers contains elevated levels of metalloproteinases MMP-2 and MMP-9. J Invest Dermatol 101: 64–68
11. Grinnell F, Zhu M (1996) Fibronectin degradation in chronic wounds depends on the relative levels of elastase, alpha 1-proteinase inhibitor, and alpha 2-macroglobulin. J Invest Dermatol 106: 335–341
12. Gardner SE, Frantz RA (2004) Wound Bioburden. In: Baranoski S, Ayello EA (eds) Wound care essentials: practice principles. Lippinkott Williams & Wilkins, Springhouse, pp 91–116
13. Angeras MH, Brandberg A, Falk A, Seeman T (1992) Comparison between sterile saline and tap water for the cleaning of acute traumatic soft tissue wounds. Eur J Surg 158: 347–350
14. Bergstrom N, Bennett MA, Carlson C E et al. (1994) Treatment of pressure ulcers. Clinical Practice Guideline, No. 15. Rockville, MD: U.S. Department of Health and Human Services. Public Health Service Agency for Health Care Policy and Research. AHCPR Publication No. 95–0652
15. Foresman PA, Payne DS, Becker D, Lewis D, Rodeheaver GT (1993) A relative toxicity index for wound cleansers. Wounds 5: 226–231
16. Wright RW, Orr R (1993) Fibroblast cytotoxicity and blood cell integrity following exposure to dermal wound cleansers. Ostomy/Wound Management 39: 33–36, 38, 40
17. Fleming A (1919) The action of chemical and physiological antiseptics in a septic wound. Br J Surg 7: 99–129
18. Hellewell TB, Major DA, Foresman PA, Rodeheaver GT (1997) A cytotoxicity evaluation of antimicrobial and non-antimicrobial wound cleansers. Wounds 9: 15–20
19. Drosou A, Falabella A, Kirsner RS (2003) Antiseptics on wounds: An area of controversy. Wounds 15: 149–166
20. European Pressure Ulcer Advisory Panel (EPUAP) (1999) Guidelines on treatment of pressure ulcers. EPUAP Rev 1: 1–6
21. Beltran KA, Thecker JG, Rodeheaver GT (1994) Impact pressures generated by commercial wound irrigation divices (unpublished research report) University of Virginia Health Science Center, Charlottesville
22. Fletcher J (2001) Updating the EPUAP pressure ulcer prevention and treatment guidelines. EPUAP Rev 3: 78–82
23. Longmire AW, Broom LA, Burch J (1987) Wound infection following high-pressure syringe and needle irrigation (letter). Am J Emergency Med 5: 179–181
24. Maklebust J, Sieggreen MY (2001) Pressure ulcers: Guidelines for prevention and management, 3rd edn. Springhouse, Springhouse, PA
25. Rodeheaver GT, Smith SL, Thacker JG, Edgerton, MT, Edlich RF (1975) Mechanical cleaning of contaminated wounds with a surfactant. Am J Surg 129: 241–245
26. Bauer C, Gerlach MA, Doughty D (2000) Care of metastatic skin lesions. J WOCN 27: 247–251

# Control of Exudate and Periwound Skin Care

D.L. KRASNER

## Introduction

Exudate and periwound skin problems, either alone or in combination, are often early signs of some underlying pathology or complication in the surgical wound. Common causes include infection, impending dehiscence, fistulae and recurrent malignancy. There are times when exudate or periwound skin problems can be anticipated; in such cases, strategies can be taken early on to minimise additional complications. For example, skin sealants or moisture barriers can be used on periwound skin before it breaks down from exudate. A faecal pouch can be applied to an incontinent patient directly in the operating room to prevent faecal contamination of a new staple line following, for example, a myocutaneous flap repair of a sacral pressure ulcer.

Exudate and periwound skin conditions can be anxiety-provoking and distressful for patients, their families and care-givers, as well as for members of the health-care team. They are often a source of significant pain [1] and can diminish quality outcomes. Mismanagement of these problems by members of the health-care team may significantly increase anxiety and mistrust. This chapter will review strategies for controlling exudate and for periwound skin care in the surgical wound. Many of these techniques are applicable to other acute wounds and chronic wounds as well. By assessing and addressing these problems early on, wound deterioration can often be minimised and quality of life can be enhanced, including reduced pain and suffering. Sometimes, further surgery will be required to address the underlying aetiology. At other times, it may be determined that the wounds are non-healable [2], and a palliative pathway [3, 4] will have to be followed. In all of these cases, following a careful assessment, goals and plans of care to manage exudate and periwound skin conditions must be delineated in order to maximise wound healing whenever possible, decrease pain, improve self-image and enhance quality of life.

## Assessment

Careful assessment of the exudate and the condition of the periwound skin is the essential first step to good management. The characteristics of the exudate, including colour, odour, consistency and quantity, can serve as clues to the underlying cause. Changes in these parameters can be markers of deterioration or improvement. The well-trained nose can pick out the scent of *Pseudomonas* in exudate. The observant eye can observe the early, subtle signs of candidasis in the colour and texture changes of periwound skin.

Experience can be the best guide in anticipating the problems commonly associated with a particular surgery, monitoring for it and intervening rapidly at the first signs (e.g. peristomal skin erosion following retraction of a colostomy stoma). In open wounds, the colour of the wound bed, as well as the presence of foreign bodies, can give clues to the underlying cause. In closed wounds, looking carefully at the dressing that has just been removed is often an invaluable information source. Dressings can give clues to the level of exudate; exudate strike-through suggests that either the type of dressing material or the frequency of dressing changes needs to be re-evaluated. Location of the wound and gravity play important roles in exudate management. The management scheme that was working well to control exudate when the patient was bed-bound may need to be re-assessed and re-evaluated once the person begins to get out of bed and/or ambulate.

Falanga, in writing on wound-bed preparation, has developed a staging system for wound-bed preparation that includes the amount of wound exudate as one of the critical aspects to be evaluated [5]. Falanga suggests that, once validated, this system could be used to judge wound preparedness and to correlate it with the ultimate outcome of complete wound closure.

## Exudate Management

The following products can be especially useful during the prevention phase, when it is anticipated that the wound might be exudative, but the process has not yet begun:

- Skin sealants (select the non-stinging varieties)
- Moisture barrier creams or ointments
- Ostomy-type geletin-pectin skin barriers

Once a wound has started exudating, the management strategy should address cleansing or irrigation, debridement of any devitalised tissue, and primary and/or secondary dressings to control the exudate. Careful consideration should be given to debridement of necrotic tissue (eschar or slough), since bacteria can proliferate in necrotic tissue, increasing the risk of infection, increased exudate and periwound skin breakdown. So, even in palliative wounds where healing is not necessarily the desired outcome, debridement of devitalised tissue might be considered in order to obviate infection, exudate and periwound skin breakdown [6, 7].

Primary dressings run the gamet from no absorption (e.g. transparent films) to maximal absorption (e.g. calcium alginates and hydrofibres). The trick is to match the proper level of absorbency with the level of exudate so that the wound does not stay too soppy wet or become overly dessicated. For exudate control the following dressing types, alone or in combination, with or without antimicrobials, are most useful (listed from least absorptive to most absorptive):

- Gauze
- Hydrocolloids
- Foams
- Alginates
- Hydrofibres

When exudate cannot be contained by these dressings or when exudate and odour combine to create management problems, ostomy pouches (drainable ostomy for purulent or faecal exudate, urostomy for most liquid exudate) or wound pouches designed specifically for this purpose should be considered. Not only does such equipment save time and money in the long run, it can also protect periwound skin and enhance quality of life for the patient. Pouching has infection control benefits when the exudate is potentially infective (e.g. MRSA or blood) and can also enable the health-care team to get a truly accurate assessment of the quantity of the exudate.

Devices, such as the vacuum-assisted closure device (the VAC, KCI, San Antonio, Texas), can be employed to control exudate and speed wound healing when the previously mentioned measures fail. Certain wounds, such as draining fistulae and deeply infected wounds, may be contra-indicated, however. The reader is referred to discussions of the VAC in other chapters of this book as well as those published elsewhere [8].

## Other Considerations

### Odour Control

Odour from the exudate is frequently due to its source in the body (e.g. the faecal odour of a faecal fistula) or the degree of colonisation or infection. Careful identification of the cause of the odour should direct management. Control measures may include one or more of the following:

- Odour-reducing charcoal dressings
- Pouching (instead of dressings) to contain odour
- Room deodorisers, especially kitty-litter in a basin under the bed shaken daily, stick deodorants, non-aerosol spray deodorants or scented candles at home
- Topical medication in the wound bed to reduce odour (for example, metronidazone gel or crushed tablets topically in a fungating wound) [3]
- Systemic medications to control odour (e.g. chlorophyll tablets to reduce faecal fistula odour)
- Systemic medications to control deep wound infections and their associated odour (e.g. antibiotics, antimicrobials)
- Systemic medications to decrease output (e.g. antidiarrheals or somatostatin for a small-bowel fistula

### Pain Management

There are many reasons for pain associated with exudate: the irritating nature of the exudate itself, pressure from copious exudate on nerve endings in the wound bed, breakdown of the periwound skin. Assessment of the actual cause of the pain should direct the interventions. Control measures may include one or more of the following:

- Cleansing with normal saline or a speciality wound cleanser (avoid skin cleansers and topical antiseptics that can sting or burn)
- Gentle cleansing with low irrigation pressures (8 to 15 psi). Note that in certain situations cleansing or pulsed lavage can reduce pain and provide comfort; in other situations it can increase pain. It is best to ask the patient.
- Topical anaesthetics or analgesia
- Re-evaluation of the dressing procedures to maximise exudate absorbency and minimise friction and trauma

### Bleeding

Bleeding or bloody exudate is a common problem that requires attention not only to containment but also to infection control. Bleeding may derive from a friable tumour, a bleeding fistula or may be due to bleeding wound margins due to trauma on dressing removal or secondary to local infection. Control measures may include one or more of the following:

- Gentle care
- Soaking dressings (or showering) prior to dressing removal in order to reduce trauma
- Use of moist wound healing, so tissue does not dessicate and bleed further
- Use of non-adherent dressings, such as silicon contact layer dressings, hydrogels, impregnated fine-mesh gauze, moisture-retentive dressings
- Pouching (instead of dressings) to contain the bloody drainage
- Use of haemostatic agents, such as calcium alginates, haemostatic foams, liquid thrombin
- Careful positioning and/or splinting
- Contact, airborne or droplet precautions may be required

In certain situations, especially with bleeding malignancies, ligation or cauterisation of the bleeder and/or oral antifibrinolytics, radiation therapy and embolisation may be needed to achieve haemostatis. For fungating malignant tumours that continue to bleed, chemotherapy or radiation therapy may be needed to shrink and control the tumour.

### Copious Exudate

Increasing drainage is often a sign of bacterial imbalance, infection or wound deterioration [9]. When current strategies start to require interventions every hour or two, a different management strategy should be considered. For example, if strike-through of a super-absorbent alginate rope dressing occurs every 2 h, pouching the wound is a cost-effective, time-efficient alternative [10]. Control measures may include one or more of the following:

- Innovative, cost-effective containment devices, such as adult briefs or pieces of baby diapers
- Pouching (instead of dressings)
- Systemic medications to decrease output (e.g. antidiarrheals for a faecal fistula or somatostatin for a small-bowel fistula)
- Contact, airborne or droplet precautions may be required

When these control measures are no longer adequate, repeat surgery must be considered. So, for example, re-siting a leaking gastrostomy tube or reconstructing a retracted stoma – while requiring another surgery – in the long run might be the most effective and efficient intervention in certain situations.

## Periwound Skin Care

Periwound skin problems are due to many factors, most commonly:

- **Dressing-related causes,** such as skin stripping from tapes, tape blisters, skin tears, contact dermatitis, allergy
- **Device-related causes,** such as leaking tubes or drains, vascular access device sites or friction or pressure from the devices themselves
- **Site-related causes,** such a skin folds (dark moist sites predispose to rashes, especially candidiasis)
- **Exudate-related causes,** such as fistulas, wounds with drainage that denudes or erodes the skin
- **Other causes,** such as maceration from sweating or incontinence
- Any **combination** of the above

Careful assessment of the cause(s) of the periwound skin condition will direct the plan of care and the associated interventions.

## Prevention

Many periwound skin problems can be anticipated and prevented, which provides the most efficient and cost-effective outcome. Orders should be written for careful routine cleansing and drying of periwound skin as well as appropriate preventive strategies that might include:

- Skin sealants (select the non-stinging variety)
- Moisture barrier creams and ointments

- Exudate control (e.g. with dressings or pouches)
- Control of incontinence with incontinence cleansers, moisture barriers or adult briefs or faecal collectors

A distinction should be made between those cleansers that can be used on intact skin (skin cleansers) and those that are formulated to be used with broken skin or wounds (saline, wound cleansers) [11]. Antiseptics, such as, for example, povidone-iodine and Dakin's solution, can be extremely painful on denuded or eroded periwound skin and should be avoided. Whenever possible, one should also avoid using products that contain sensitisers or allergens, such as lanolin, fragrances and colophany.

## Other Management Strategies

In addition to the prevention strategies outlined above, the following additional strategies may be useful:

- Speciality skin barrier creams and ointments formulated for this purpose
- Non-adherent contact layers, such as silicon
- Use of antifungal creams or ointments PRN. *Candida* is the most common periwound rash encountered in most settings. Antifungal powers work well under breasts, axillae and around stomas under ostomy pouches. Antifungal creams and ointments are useful at other sites.
- Use of topical steroids to control inflammation

## Other Considerations

### Pain Management

Pain from denuded or eroded periwound skin can be severe [12]. In many cases, it can be relieved by covering exposed nerve endings with moisture-retentive dressings, ointments or creams. Topical anaesthetics, such as 2% lidocaine gel or EMLA, can offer significant relief of pain. Topical steroids can be used to reduce inflammation as needed.

### Pruritus

Pruritus or itching is commonly associated with periwound skin problems, especially:

- Contact dermatitis or allergy
- Rashes, candidiasis being the most common
- Reactions to chemotherapy or radiation therapy

Control measures may include one or more of the following strategies:
- Avoiding skin dryness that can increase itching by moisturizing the skin with water-soluble lotions or emollients
- Adequate fluid intake to maintain skin hydration
- Humidifying the environment
- Topical medications, such as steroids or topical antifungals, PRN
- Systemic medications, including antihistamines and tranquilisers PRN

### Securing Tapes and Dressings

When periwound skin is irritated, denuded or eroded, securing tapes and dressings becomes especially challenging. The goal should be to avoid pain and further trauma to the periwound skin. One or more of the following management strategies may be useful:
- Use of saline- or water-moistened gauze or non-stinging adhesive removers to gently break the seal and remove adhesive tapes and dressings
- Soaking adherent tapes and dressings with saline or water prior to removal (or showering to soak the dressing off)
- Selection and use of less traumatic tapes, such as dressing-retention sheets
- Use of innovative secondary dressings to secure primary dressings, such as transparent films, contouring bandages, tubular bandages, mesh, binders, clothing, so as to avoid tapes altogether
- Reducing the frequency of dressing changes (e.g. moving from every shift wet-to-dry gauze dressings to three times a week moisture-retentive dressings)

### Conclusion

Prevention is the best intervention for managing wound exudate and for controlling periwound skin problems. Anticipatory interventions can go a long way in preventing the painful and costly sequela of these situations. If problems do arise, careful attention to exudate management and periwound skin care reduces pain, enhances quality of life and builds confidence in the wound-healing team.

### References

1. Krasner DL (2004) Wound pain management: A hyperbaric perspective. In: Sheffield PJ (ed) Wound care practice. Best Publishing, Flagstaff AZ (in press)
2. Krasner D, Sibbald RG (1999) Nursing management of chronic wounds: Best practices across the continuum of care. Nurs Clin N Am 34: 933–953
3. Belcher AE, Selekof J (2001) Skin care for the oncology patient. In: Krasner D, Rodeheaver G, Sibbald RG (eds) Chronic wound care: A clinical source book for healthcare professionals, 3rd edn. HMP Communications, Wayne PA, pp 711–720

4. Rolstad BS, Nix D (2001) Management of wound recalcitrance and deterioration. In: Krasner D, Rodeheaver G, Sibbald RG (eds) Chronic wound care: A clinical source book for healthcare professionals, 3rd edn. HMP Communications, Wayne PA, pp 731–742

5. Falanga V (2000) Classifications for wound bed preparation and stimulation of chronic wounds. Wound Repair Regen 8: 347–352

6. Barton P, Parslow N (2001) Malignant wounds: holistic assessment and management. In: Krasner D, Rodeheaver G, Sibbald RG (eds) Chronic wound care: a clinical source book for healthcare professionals, 3rd edn. HMP Communications, Wayne PA, pp 699–710

7. Haisfield-Wolf ME, Rund C (1997) Malignant cutaneous wounds: a management protocol. Ostomy/Wound Management 43: 56–66

8. Krasner DL (2002) Managing wound pain in patients with vacuum-assisted closure devices. Ostomy/Wound Management 48: 38–43

9. Schultz GS, Sibbald RG, Falanga V et al.(2003) Wound bed preparation: a systematic approach to wound management. Wound Repair Regen 11 [Suppl 2]: S1–S28

10. Faller NA, Beitz JM (2001) When a wound is not a wound: Tubes, drains, fistulae, and draining wounds. In: Krasner D, Rodeheaver G, Sibbald RG (eds) Chronic wound care: a clinical source book for healthcare professionals, 3rd edn. HMP Communications, Wayne PA, pp 721–729

11. Rodeheaver G (2001) Wound cleansing, wound irrigation, wound disinfection. In: Krasner D, Rodeheaver G, Sibbald RG (eds) Chronic wound care: a clinical source book for healthcare professionals, 3rd edn. HMP Communications, Wayne PA, pp 369–383

12. Hofman D, Ryan T, Arnold F et al. (1997) Pain in venous leg ulcers. J Wound Care 6: 222–224

# Topical Negative-Pressure Therapy in Wound Management

G.P.L. Thomas, P.E. Banwell

## Introduction

Topical negative pressure therapy (TNP) is the application of a local sub-atmospheric pressure across a wound [1]. It is a novel non-pharmacological physical method of promoting wound healing. TNP has found a routine role in acute wound management, the down-staging and temporisation of complex trauma prior to surgery, in chronic wound treatment and in the management of patients with a poor operative risk [2]. The evidence base for TNP is rapidly expanding, although it has been considered controversial in some quarters [2, 3].

## Development

Surgical practice has long recognised that healing is promoted by removing fluid collections from a wound site in the post-operative period while maintaining a moist environment. In addition, the observation that tissue growth responds positively to applied mechanical forces (a permutation of Wolff's Law), as in osteogenic distraction and soft-tissue expansion, has led to a variety of negative-pressure wound-therapy systems being designed [4–9]. The philosophies underpinning the early development of TNP differed subtly between North American and European groups. The North American approach was principally concerned with developing a therapy for managing difficult, complex wounds, with an emphasis on improving granulation-tissue formation, exudate management, infection control and wound closure [10, 11]. The European concept of TNP can be characterised as a therapy designed for managing acute high-energy contaminated injuries where haemostasis and infection control are at a premium [12]. From the mid 1990s the majority of published research examining TNP has focused on the use of purpose-built programmable vacuum pumps. These devices deliver a predetermined and programmable negative pressure across a wound surface in a planned – either cyclical or constant – manner. This facility has encouraged a more structured and scientific examination of TNP and produced a body of research with negative pressure devices at its core. Within the literature and clinical practice a number of synonyms for TNP [1] are presently in use, including: sub-atmospheric pressure [10], vacuum-sealing technique (VST) [12], sealed surface wound suction (SSS), vacuum-assisted closure (VAC), vacuum pack [13], negative pressure dressing and foam suction dressing [2, 14].

## Dressing and Components

The TNP dressing essentially consists of an open-pored foam dressing (Fig. 1), of polyurethane ether or polyvinyl alcohol, which is shaped to fit the wound and sealed within it using an adhesive semi-occlusive dressing. A negative pressure is then delivered across the wound bed via a drainage tube embedded within the foam and connected to a negative-pressure device [1]. Adjacent but separate wounds may be served by a single negative-pressure device in series or parallel [15].

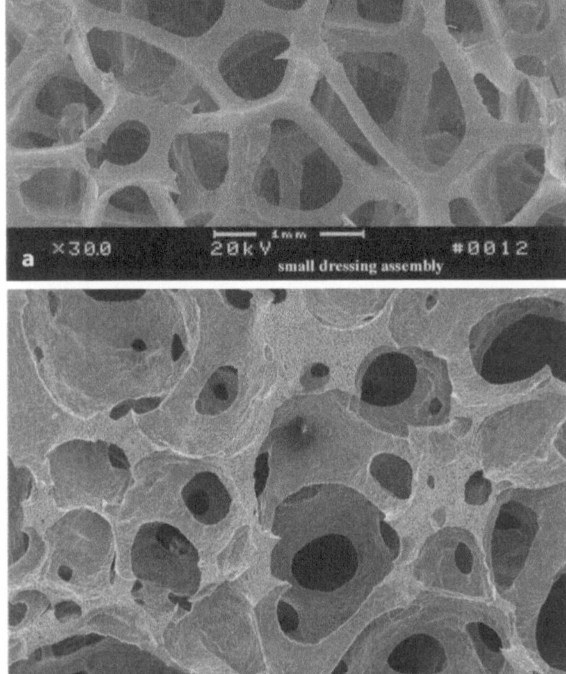


**Fig. 1a,b.** Electron micrographs of foam dressings illustrating the open pore appearance in polyurethane ether (a) and polyvinylalcohol (b)

The foam dressing partially collapses on application of negative pressure, yet transmits an even distribution of vacuum across the wound bed. The pressure and extent of the vacuum experienced at the wound interface are dependent upon the foam structure and deformation under negative pressure and any interposed dressing [12, 16].

The adhesive semi-occlusive dressing maintains the low-pressure environment, retains moisture at the wound and protects from external contamination. In addition, the dressing is gas-permeable, allowing oxygen diffusion and so preventing anaerobic conditions, and thus flora, from prevailing [17].

The recommended parameters for TNP are based on experimental studies that deliver a negative pressure of 125 mmHg to a standard wound [1]. Notably in an experimental acute wound swine model (using polyurethane foam) granulation-tissue formation was significantly impaired in low (25 mmHg) and high (500 mmHg) negative pressures as compared to a pressure of 125 mmHg [18]. Elevated negative pressures (125–175 mmHg) may be used with polyvinyl alcohol foams as opposed to 125 mmHg with polyurethane dressings [19]. Lower pressures (50–75 mmHg) are advised in treating chronic ulcers, where pain may well be a limiting factor [1, 19], although if tolerated, then pressures should be increased to 125 mmHg [15]. Split skin grafts are successfully secured with generally lower negative pressures [20, 21].

Duration of therapy is determined by achieving predetermined goals. Such goals are necessarily indication-specific. No maximum duration for TNP has been identified, providing resources, patient compliance and clinical progress support further therapy. Indeed, prolonged use beyond 20 weeks, with resulting wound healing, is reported [22], but is not recommended.

TNP can be applied immediately following injury or wound debridement [23]. Dressings are changed routinely at between 48 and 72 h, although more frequently in contaminated infected wounds [15, 17, 24]. In clean, stable wounds dressings may be changed as infrequently as once every 5 days [23, 25].

---

**Recommended Regimes (Adapted from [1])**

- Negative Pressure
  - 50–75 mmHg, titrate to 125 mmHg: Chronic ulcers, especially leg ulcers
  - 50–125 mmHg: Skin grafts
  - 125 mmHg: All other wounds, polyurethane foam
  - 125–175 mmHg: All other wounds, polyvinyl alcohol foam
- Cycle
  - Constant for 48 h, then intermittent (5 min on/2 min off)
- Dressing Changes
  - 48 h then every 4 to 5 days: Most wounds
  - 48-hourly or less: Infected wounds
  - 4–5 days: Clean wounds

## Mechanism of Action

The original work of Morkywas and Argenta in 1997 demonstrated significantly increased granulation-tissue formation in wounds treated with TNP as against control wounds created in vivo in a pig model [10]. Needle-probe laser Doppler studies revealed markedly elevated blood flow in wounds treated with an intermittent regimen. Wounds inoculated with bacteria showed a significant drop in counts by day 5, from $10^8$ to $>10^{5,}$ in TNP wounds, while controls achieved this only by day 11. TNP also increased the survival of ischaemic random pattern flaps. It is these observations that established the thesis that TNP has multimodal mechanisms of action (Fig. 2).

### Enhanced Dermal Perfusion

Human studies that have applied negative pressure to uninjured skin have shown immediate increases in local blood flow [26–28]. In excised wound models this increase is pressure-dependent, and higher negative pressures (400 mmHg) depress blood flow [10]. It is also dependent on pressure loading. With constant negative pressures the response is transient (5 to 7 min) but maintained in cyclical loading to a fourfold increase over baseline flow rates [10]. Deep dermal wound models also demonstrate increased dermal perfusion in response to TNP, even following a delay of treatment [29]. Enhanced dermal perfusion may result from increasing the hydrostatic pressure gradient along an arteriole, by reducing end-arteriolar, venous and extravascular hydrostatic pressures and thus directly drawing blood down the vessel [1]. Although an attractive proposition, this conflicts with some physiological evidence. Skagen and Henriksen demonstrated in a series of xenon washout studies vasoconstriction and increased vascular resistance in the presence of even low topical negative pressures (40 mmHg) in fit human volunteers [26]. An alternative hypothesis is suggested in wound models whereby the putative action of TNP is shown in reducing tissue oedema directly and indirectly by removing osmotically active molecules and mediators, thus preventing microvascular compromise [10, 30]. This improves dermal perfusion in treated wounds as against controls.

### Oedema and Exudate Control

Clinical and experimental series report significant volumes of exudate removal and oedema reduction in TNP-treated wounds. However, as yet there are no quantitative studies to support this or reveal definite reductions in interstitial tissue fluid volumes. TNP both directly suctions fluid from the wound and eliminates factors that promote oedema [2]. TNP-treated burn wounds have been observed to contain remarkably less denatured collagen than controls [30], and osmotically active denatured collagen is considered to be a key causative factor in burns oedema [31].

Chronic wound and burn exudate contains raised concentrations of proteolytic enzymes and growth factors [32, 33] which in vitro suppress keratinocyte, fibroblast and endothelial cell proliferation [34, 35]. High levels of these biochemicals have

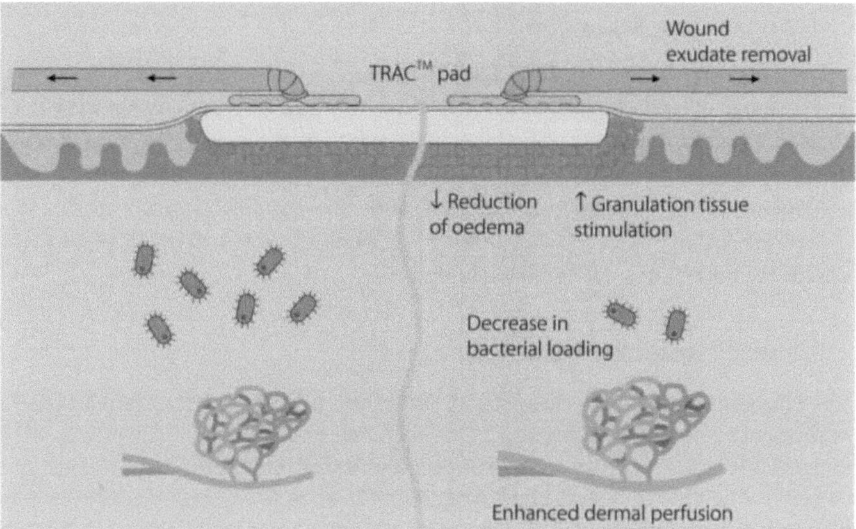


**Fig. 2.** Diagrammatic illustration of the mechanisms of action of TNP (courtesy of the Oxford Wound Healing Society)

been reported in wound fluid removed by TNP during treatment [36–38]. Thus, TNP may modify the wound environment by reducing inhibitory factor concentrations and so promoting healing [1].

## Mechanical Stress Induction of Granulation Tissue

TNP exerts a shear mechanical stress across a wound during treatment. It is recognised that mechanical stress modulates soft-tissue repair, and, in particular, angiogenesis [39–42]. Whether this significantly influences healing in TNP is presently under investigation (Fig. 3).

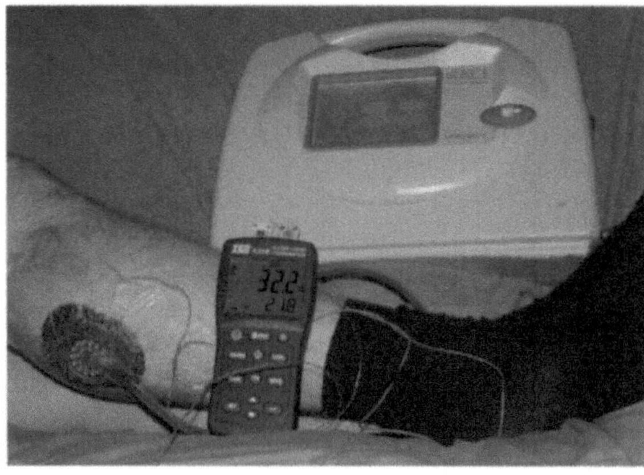

**Fig. 3.** Research into TNP is essential. Here, investigators are measuring the effect of TNP on blood flow and temperature

### Reverse Tissue Expansion

The collapse and shrinkage of the TNP foam dressing in response to a closed negative pressure exerts a mechanical shear force not only across the wound but also extends to surrounding healthy tissues, drawing them towards the wound. This action is analogous to the tissue stretching observed in the technique of soft-tissue expansion. Tissue-expanded skin demonstrates increased mitotic activity and improved vascularity [43, 44]. It is hypothesised that this will be demonstrated also in tissues surrounding a TNP-treated wound [2].

### Granulation-Tissue Formation

The original experimental work of Morykwas and Argenta demonstrated increases in granulation-tissue volume in TNP-treated wounds of 63.3% (continuous TNP) and 103.4% (cyclical TNP) when compared with controls [10]. Similar significant increases in granulation tissue have been found in an ischaemic rabbit ear full-thickness excision wound model [45]. These findings are borne out in clinical observations and the prospective randomised controlled trial of Joseph et al. found that in chronic wounds treated with TNP granulation tissue formation occurred in 64% versus inflammation and fibrosis in 81% of controls [46].

### Bacterial Colonisation

TNP has been repeatedly shown to decrease bacterial colonisation rates in wounds in both experimental and clinical settings [10, 16, 47–49]. It remains unclear whether this is due to the direct removal of organisms or via rendering the wound environment less accommodating to bacterial colonisation through removal of exudate and improved tissue perfusion [1]. In clinical practice, TNP is a useful adjunct to debridement in rapidly controlling infected wounds [50].

### Tissue Salvage

TNP appears to rescue compromised wound tissue in the peripheral zone of injury. Experimental models using random pattern skin flaps of excessive length to breadth ratio revealed that those flaps treated with TNP both before and after lifting survived significantly better than controls [10]. Likewise, TNP applied within 12 h following a partial-thickness burn, inflicted upon a swine model, significantly reduced the depth of cell death within the wound [30]. Less inflammatory cells and cellular debris were also found in the TNP-treated wounds. In an animal study mimicking doxorubicin extravasation injury, modelled by injecting doxorubicin repeatedly intradermally into pigs, TNP prevented chronic ulcer formation in all treated wounds, while ulcers occurred in 10 of 16 control wounds [51]. Tissue salvage is considered to be effected by removing toxic and proinflammatory factors, reducing oedema and inhibiting progression to a deteriorating wound environment.

## Clinical Indications

Topical negative-pressure therapy was initially developed to control difficult, often chronic, wounds with the aim of increasing patient comfort, decreasing patient morbidity and decreasing cost and duration of hospitalisation [11]. However, in the first large series of over 300 cases published in 1997, 10% were acute wounds and 31% sub-acute wounds [11]. Several series now exist [16, 45, 46, 52–54].

### Acute Wounds

TNP is highly efficacious in the management of trauma [11, 16]. Exposed bone, tendon and neurovascular bundles are rapidly encroached upon and covered by granulation tissue in fit patients, while contamination and infection are controlled [2, 55]. Dressings may be applied immediately following injury or debridement [23].

Early wound debridement and vascularised tissue coverage of exposed bone within 72 h remains the gold standard management of open fractures. However, TNP may permit temporisation of open fractures beyond 72 h pending definitive soft-tissue cover [2, 56]. Open long-bone fractures, both chronic and acute, will respond to TNP. Both may be down-staged, with granulation tissue encasing exposed inner and outer bony cortices over 2 to 9 weeks of treatment, depending on the size of the defect [2]. Complex open trauma has been managed over an extended period with TNP, in one series for a mean of 19 days, prior to tissue cover [57]. This practice of delayed soft-tissue cover remains controversial.

In cases of significant soft-tissue loss following adequate debridement, TNP application for 2 or more weeks will control bacterial colonisation and generate profuse granulation tissue. This converts a technically challenging wound into one that requires only split skin graft or local flap cover of open granulation tissue. Tissue loss from the foot, exposed tendons, tissue loss in gunshot wounds and degloving injuries are good candidates [2, 58–61].

Distal wounds of extremities can present peculiar difficulties for flap cover due to excessive bulk, impaired lymphatic drainage, poor colour match and chronic instability. TNP provides an alternative with the prospect of better functional and aesthetic outcomes [2].

Prolonged TNP with resulting wound down-staging also presents an alternative to flap cover of a wound in patients with significant comorbidity, in situations where the necessary surgical skills are not available, or where patient beliefs (e.g. Jehovah's Witnesses) render major surgery potentially life-threatening.

Burns may also be treated with TNP. In the acute phase it is of particular benefit in unstable patients where definitive coverage may be delayed and repeated dressing changes interrupt intensive care therapy. Burn wound progression, documented by Jackson in 1953 [62], is also inhibited with the timely application of TNP, resulting in more superficial wounds [30].

### Surgical Wounds

#### The Open Abdomen

The open abdomen is an uncommon but significant entity arising from abdominal wound dehiscence, necrotising fasciitis of the abdominal wall or laparostomy, for trauma, sepsis and abdominal compartment syndrome. Therapeutic approaches to the open abdomen by necessity initially control the wound, containing abdominal contents and preventing infection, and must subsequently promote wound closure without hernia formation.

TNP has revolutionised management [63–68]. It obviates the need for deep tension sutures or the use of prosthetic meshes and, unlike previous therapies, such as the Bogota Bag, prosthetic mesh closure, Wittman patch or vacuum pack, TNP actively removes exudate and provides quantitative analysis of third-space fluid losses. It also facilitates fascial closure with robust wound healing reducing hernia occurrence. In superficial wounds, dressing foam is applied directly to the intact fascia, while in deep wounds with exposed viscera or in complex cases where a fistula is present an interposed dressing inserted between foam and wound bed is required [2] (Fig. 4).

#### Post-Sternotomy Infection

Post-sternotomy infection remains a significant cause of morbidity following elective cardiac surgery. A number of series support the use of TNP with debridement in successfully managing deep infections, post-sternotomy mediastinitis and sternal osteomyelitis, either eventual healing through secondary intent or with delayed definitive flap closure [69–72].

Patients treated with TNP are reported to have significantly fewer dressing changes, fewer final flap procedures and reduced hospital stays as against those undergoing conventional treatment [73]. Further, the partially collapsed foam of the TNP dressing acts to splint the two elements of the divided sternum, improving ventilation and reducing pain.

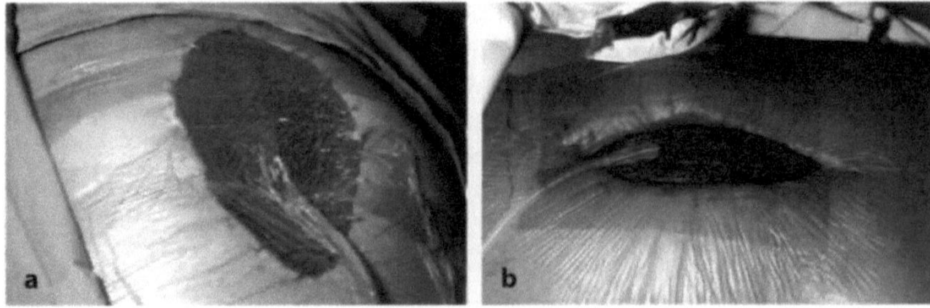

**Fig. 4a,b.** TNP is now the gold standard in the management of open abdominal wounds

### Skin-Graft Fixation

TNP dressings provide firm fixation of a skin graft to its bed following the wound contour, eliminating shearing, removing fluid collections and inhibiting infection. These are the optimal conditions for graft-take, and graft survival rates of more than 90% are reported using this technique [20, 74–77]. Graft-take may well be more rapid with TNP [19]. TNP is also effective in managing graft-donor site complications such as exposed tendons following free radial forearm flap harvest [78].

## Chronic Wounds

### Pressure Ulcers

Pressure ulcers are commonly present in aged and infirm patients and those suffering from debilitating neurological disease. In such patients, significant co-morbidity and associated impaired wound healing often precludes reconstructive surgery. TNP is an effective and safe definitive treatment of pelvic and trochanteric pressure ulcers. It delivers enhanced wound healing with less hospital admissions and expense when compared to previous non-surgical therapies [79–83]. Dressing changes twice a week reduce patient discomfort and nursing demands [2] and encourage extended management within the community. TNP is also valuable in optimising ulcer wound beds in those selected cases where surgery is planned [83].

When applying a TNP dressing to pressure ulcers it is necessary to de-roof the ulcer to enable the dressing to entirely fill the defect and thus permit circumferential granulation to occur. Osteomyelitis of bone involved in pressure ulcers has been shown to resolve in some cases following TNP [82]. Ulcers that extend to the anus or genitalia are at risk from contamination, although the TNP occlusive dressing will provide protection if an adequate seal is maintained. Faecal diversion should be considered [2]. Heal pressure ulcers respond to TNP although granulation over exposed calcaneum is slow [2].

### Complex Diabetic Wounds

An increasing body of evidence is being amassed that TNP is more effective than traditional dressings in managing diabetic ulcers, in terms of nursing demands, costs, patient comfort and in improving outcome [22, 54, 84–86].

### Vascular Ulcers

Large venous ulcers will respond to TNP, although results vary and prolonged treatment is to be expected. TNP arguably has no impact on arterial ulcers and those with significant arterial deficiency and persistent local ischaemia [22]. Further, the foam dressing may cause localised necrosis of any underlying skin. Experimentally, ischaemic human limbs show no improvement in skin microcirculation during or following negative pressure (115 mmHg) therapy [87]. Also, high-negative pressures are recognised as impairing healing in healthy tissues [18] and it is probable that in arterial ischaemic tissue injurious pressure will be lower.

### Wound Infection

The fundamental tenets of surgical practice – debridement, irrigation, microbiological sampling, appropriate antimicrobial therapy and the establishment of adequate tissue perfusion – remain central to the management of chronic wound infections. However, infected wounds and osteomyelitis, besides post-sternotomy sternal infections, have been successfully treated with TNP [55, 88, 89]. In refractory and complex wounds where tissue salvage is a priority the regular instillation of antiseptics and topical high-dose antibiotics (Instillation Therapy) in combination with TNP may prove a useful adjunct to surgery [89].

**Indications for Topical Negative Pressure Therapy**

- Acute
  - Trauma:
    - Temporisation of open fractures
    - Delaying surgical procedures
    - Tissue loss
    - Infected traumatic wounds
    - Complex trauma in unfit patients
    - Exposed metalwork
  - Burns:
    - Post-excision wound cover
    - Split skin graft fixation
    - Skin substitutes
- Postsurgical
  - Sternal dehiscence:
    - Superficial wound infection
    - Sternal osteomyelitis
    - Mediastinitis
  - Open abdomen:
    - Abdominal dehiscence
    - Compartment syndrome
  - Skin graft fixation:
    - Donor and graft site
- Chronic
  - Pressure ulcers
    - Ischial
    - Sacral
    - Trochanteric
  - Leg ulcers
    - Diabetic
    - Venous
  - Wound infection

## Contra-Indications

There are no established absolute contra-indications to TNP. However, it must be applied to a prepared wound bed free of infected, sloughing or necrotic tissue. It is inadvisable to apply TNP over an open joint. Application over a tumour is theoretically hazardous, although it may be considered in palliative wound control [1]. Particular caution is recommended when considering TNP in cases with a

- coagulopathy or
- over an open peritoneal or pleural space.

## Complications and Cessation of Therapy

### Pain

Pain in TNP may arise as direct result of the negative pressure applied across a wound or during dressing changes. Pain is more probable in chronic wounds and ulcers treated with TNP. Reduction of negative pressures will reduce symptoms, and once pain has subsided, pressures can be titrated back towards the therapeutic target [1, 11]. Pain during dressing changes results from the avulsion of new tissue intimately involved in the foam dressing [2]. This may be lessened by syringing saline with or without local anaesthetic down the drainage tube in advance of a dressing change [2]. Also, tissue in-growth into the foam dressing is prevented by interposing a non-adherent porous dressing between the wound bed and foam [8, 19, 20].

Pain also, of course, may herald other local complications including pressure necrosis from the drainage tube or progressive local infection.

### Failure in Response to TNP

Improvement in the wound should be expected within 7 or 8 days of commencing therapy or following two to three dressing changes [2]. If this is not the case, then the indication for TNP and all other local and patient factors needs to be reviewed. Inadequate wound debridement, ongoing infection and a catabolic patient state are common culprits. Over-frequent dressing changes may lead to a paradoxical regression in granulation tissue formation [1].

### Infection

TNP has the potential to significantly alter wound bacterial flora and clinical sepsis from wound infection has been reported [90]. Wound flora can be monitored by culturing successive wound aspirates and should therefore be considered. Frank pus in the dressing or collection canister is an absolute indication to halt treatment [2].

### Haematoma and Haemorrhage

The occurrence of wound haematoma or bleeding into the dressing or collection tube demands immediate investigation and cessation of treatment until the cause has been identified and corrected [2].

## Benefits

The principle benefits of TNP are improved rates of wound healing, reduction in complication occurrences, especially wound infection, and a reduced frequency of dressing changes. These tend to significant cost savings during therapy and need to be offset against the expense of the TNP device and dressings. The Weinberg Group, Inc. performed a cost-effectiveness analysis of TNP in 1999 in the USA. Data was sourced from clinicians, Medicare charges and health-care providers. TNP proved to have lower long-term costs than standard wound-care methods [91]. The potential for TNP treatment of chronic wounds in the community is enormous. The decrease in dressing change frequency reduces community nursing demands, so permitting more patients to be managed by a single nursing team. This, in turn, reduces nursing-related hospital admissions and, with more resources available, should facilitate more rapid discharge back into the community, benefiting clinicians and patients alike. One study has ascertained that the cost of treating heal pressure ulcers in the community was 38% less with TNP than with saline-soaked gauze dressings [81].

## Future

Ongoing TNP research continues to investigate the subcellular, cellular and biochemical response of wounds to negative pressure. Ongoing clinical trials will further tailor clinical practice and refine treatment protocols.

Advances in technology are having a profound impact on TNP both in delivering more powerful and compact mobile suction devices and in providing microprocessor driven systems, such as the TRAC. TRAC systems enable constant monitoring of the local wound environment by providing real-time feedback between the foam/wound interface. Presently, this is limited to measuring pressures only, but is likely to incorporate further diagnostic and therapeutic modalities in the future. Remote management via integrated modems is an exciting prospect for community-based therapy.

The structure and composition of the TNP foam dressing appears to influence wound behaviour. A better understanding of foam material science and foam/wound interactions will lead to new materials for dressings. Impregnated foams containing growth factors or antibacterial agents, for example silver, offer a further attractive method of altering the wound environment.

Finally, the novel field of combination therapy involving TNP is only beginning to be explored but holds out the possibility of new treatments that include tissue engineering, direct delivery of drugs and growth factors and micro-management of the wound environment [2].

## References


1. Banwell PE (1999) Topical negative pressure therapy in wound care. J Wound Care 8: 79–84
2. Banwell PE, Teot L (2003) Topical negative pressure (TNP): the evolution of a novel wound therapy. J Wound Care 12: 22–28
3. Greer SE (2000) Whither subatmospheric pressure therapy? Ann Plas Surg 453: 332–334
4. Fox JW 4th, Golden GT (1976) The use of drains in subcutaneous surgical procedures. AM J Surg 132: 673–674
5. Fay MF (1987) Drainage systems: their role in wound healing. AORN J 46: 442–455
6. Brock WB, Barker DE, Burns RP (1995) Temporary of open abdominal wound: the vacuum pack. Am Surg 61: 30–35
7. Shaer WD (2001) Inexpensive vacuum-assisted closure employing a conventional disposable closed suction drainage. Plas Recon Surg 107: 292–293
8. Masters J (1998) Reliable, inexpensive and simple suction dressings. Br J Plas Surg 51: 267
9. Strover AE, Thorpe R (1997) Suction dressings: a new surgical dressing technique. J R Coll Surg Edin 42: 119–121
10. Morykwas MJ, Argenta LC, Shelton-Brown EI, McGuirt W (1997) Vacuum-assisted closure: a new method for wound control and treatment: animal studies and basic foundation. Ann Plas Surg 38: 553–562
11. Argenta LC, Morykwas MJ (1997) Vacuum-assisted closure: a new method for wound control and treatment: clinical experience. Ann Plas Surg 38: 563–576
12. Fleischmann W, Becker U, Bischoff M, Hoekstra H (1995) Vacuum sealing: indication technique and results. Eur J Orthop Surg Trauma 5: 37–40
13. Smith LA, Barker DE, Chase CW, Somberg LB, Brock WB, Burns RP (1997) Vacuum pack technique of temporary abdominal closure: a four-year experience. Am Surg 63: 1102–1107
14. Evans D, Land L (2001) Topical negative pressure for treating chronic wounds: a systemic review. Br J Plas Surg 54: 238–242
15. Short B, Claxton M, Armstrong DG (2002) How to use VAC therapy on chronic wounds. Podiatry Today, July 2002
16. Mullner T, Mrkonjic L, Kwasny O, Vecsei V (1997) The use of negative pressure to promote the healing of tissue defects: a clinical trial using the vacuum sealing technique. B J Plas Surg 50: 194–199
17. Mendez-Eastman S (2001) Guidelines for using negative pressure wound therapy. Adv Skin Wound Care 14: 314–322
18. Morykwas MJ, Faler BJ, Pearce DJ, Argenta LC (2001) Subatmospheric pressure on the rate of granulation tissue formation in experimental wounds in swine. Ann Plast Surg 47: 547–551
19. Genecov DG, Schneider AM, Morykwas MJ et al. (1998) A controlled subatmospheric pressure dressing increases the rate of skin graft donor site re-epithelialisation. Ann Plas Surg 40: 219–225
20. Schneider AM, Morkywas MJ, Argenta LC (1998) A new and reliable method of securing skin grafts to the difficult recipient bed. Plast Recon Surg 1024: 1195–1198

21. Banwell PE (1998) Skin graft fixation. Br J Oral Maxillofac Surg 36: 480–481
22. Clare MP, Fitzgibbons TC, McMullen ST, Stice RC, Hayes DF, Henkel L (2002) Experience with the vacuum assisted closure negative pressure technique in the treatment of non-healing diabetic and dysvascular wounds. Foot Ankle Int 23: 896–901
23. Banwell PE (1998) Negative pressure therapy: a new concept in wound healing. Association of Surgeons in Training Book 1998/9. Rowan Group, London
25. Cooper SM (2000) Topical negative pressure. Int J Derm 39: 892–898
26. Skagen K, Henriksen O (1983) Changes in subcutaneous blood flow during locally applied negative pressure to the skin. Acta Physiol Scand 117: 411–414
27. Fentem PH, Matthews JA (1970) The duration of the increase in arterial inflow during exposure of the forearm to sub-atmospheric pressure. J Physiol Lond 2102: 65–66
28. Banwell PE, Jones S, Evison D et al. (2002) Topical negative pressure modulates dermal microvascular blood flow dynamics and temperature profiles at the wound-dressing interface. J Wound Care (submitted)
29. Banwell PE, Morkywas MJ, Jennings DA et al. (2000) Dermal microvascular blood flow in experimental partial thickness burns: the effect of topical sub-atmospheric pressure. J Burn Care Rehabil 21: 161
30. Morykwas MJ, David LR, Schneider AM, Whang C, Jennings DA, Canty C, Parker D, White WL, Argenta LC (1999) Use of subatmospheric pressure to prevent progression of partial-thickness burns in a swine model. J Burn Care Rehabil 201: 15–21
31. Lund T, Wiig H, Reed DK (1986) Acute post burn edema: role of strongly negative interstitial fluid pressure. Am J Physiol 255: 1069–1074
32. Wysocki AB, Staiano-Coico L, Grinnell F (1993) Wound fluid from chronic leg ulcers contains elevated levels of metalloproteinases MMP-2 and MMP-9. J Invest Derm 101: 64–68
33. Yager DR, Nwomeh BC (1999) The proteolytic enviroment of chronic wounds. Wound Rep Regen 76: 433–441
34. Bucalo B, Eaglstein WH Falanga V (1993) Inhibition of cell proliferation by chronic wound fluid. Wound Rep Regen 1: 181–186
35. Falanga V (1992) Growth factors and chronic wounds: the need to understand the microenviroment. J Derm 19: 667–672
36. Banwell PE (2002) Novel perspectives in wound care: Topical negative pressure therapy. Eur Tiss Rep Soc Bull 92: 49–50
37. Buttenschoen K, Fleischmann W, Haupt U, Kinzl L, Buttenschoen DC (2001) The influence of vacuum assisted closure on inflammatory tissue reactions in the postoperative course of ankle fractures. Foot Ankle Surg 7: 165–173
38. Gustafsson R, Johnsson P, Algotsson L et al. (2002) Vacuum-assisted closure therapy guided by C-reactive protein level in patients with deep sternal wound infection. J Thorac Cardiovasc Surg 1235: 895–900
39. Urschel JD, Scott PG, HTG Williams (1988) The effect of mechanical stress on soft and hard tissue repair; a review. Br J Plas Surg 41: 182–186
40. Ryan TJ, Barnhill RL (1983) Physical factors and angiogenesis in development of the vascular system. Ciba Foundation Symposium 100. Pitman Books, London
41. Ichioka S, Shibata M, Kosaki I et al. (1997) Effects of shear stress on wound healing in the rabbit ear chamber. J Surg Res 721: 29–35
42. Sumpio BE, Banes AJ, Levin LJ et al. (1987) Mechanical stress stimulates aortic endothelial cells to proliferate. J Vasc Surg 6: 252–256
43. Olenius M, Dalsgaard, CJ, Wickmann M (1993) Mitotic activity in expanded human skin. Plas Reconstr Surg 91: 213–216
44. Cherry GW, Austad E, Pasyk K et al. (1983) Increased survival and vascularity of random pattern flaps elevated in controlled expanded skin. Plas Reconstr Surg 72 : 680–687
45. Fabian TS, Kaufman HJ, Lett ED, Thomas JB, Rawl DK, Lewis PL, Summitt JB, Merryman JI, Schaeffer D, Sargent LA, Burns RP (2000) The evaluation of subatmospheric pressure and hyperbaric oxygen in ischaemic full thickness wound healing. Am Surg 66: 1136–1143.
46. Joseph E, Hamori CA, Bergman S, Roaf E, Swann NF, Anastasi GW (2000) A prospective randomized trial of vacuum-assisted closure versus standard therapy of chronic non-healing wounds. Wounds 12: 60–67
47. Fleischmann W, Lang E, Russ M (1997) Treatment of infection by vaccum sealing. Unfallchirurg 1004: 301–304

48. Giovanni UM, Demaria R, Teot L (2001) Benefits of negative pressure therapy in infected surgical wounds after cardiovascular surgery. Wounds 132: 82–87

49. Obdeijn MC, de Lange MY, Lichtendahl DH, de Boer WJ (1999) Vacuum-assisted closure in the treatment of poststernotomy mediastinitis. Ann Thorac Surg 686: 2358–2360

50. Avery CM, Harrop C (2002) Rapid healing of MRSA infection at the suprafascial radial donor site. Int J Oral Maxillofac Surg 31: 318–321

51. Morykwas MJ, Kennedy A, Argenta JP, Argenta LC (1999) Use of subatmospheric pressure to prevent doxorubicin extravasation ulcers in a swine model. J Surg Oncol 72: 14–17

52. Avery C, Pereira J, Moody A, Whitworth I (2000) Clinical experience with the negative pressure wound dressing. Br J Oral Maxillofac Surg 38: 343–345

53. Wanner MB, Schwarzl F, Strub B, Zaech GA, Pierer G (2003) Vacuum-assisted wound closure for cheaper and more comfortable healing of pressure sores: a prospective study. Scand J Plast Reconstr Surg Hand Surg 37: 28–33

54. McCallon SK, Knight CA, Valiulus JP, Cunningham MW, McCulloch JM, Farinas LP (2000) Vacuum-assisted closure versus saline-moistened gauze in the healing of postoperative diabetic foot wounds. Ostomy Wound Manage 46: 28–32

55. DeFranzo AJ, Argenta LC, Marks MW, Molnar JA, David LR, Webb LX, Ward WG, Teasdall RG (2001) The use of vacuum-assisted closure therapy for the treatment of lower-extremity wounds with exposed bone. Plast Reconstr Surg 108: 1184–1191

56. Labler L, Oehy K (2002) [Vacuum sealing of problem wounds] Swiss Surg 8: 266–272.

57. Herscovici Jr D, Sanders RW, Scaduto JM, Infante A, DiPasquale T (2003) Vacuum-assisted wound closure (VAC Therapy) for the management of patients with high-energy soft tissue injuries. J Orthop Trauma 17: 683–688

58. Meara JG, Guo L, Smith JD, Pribaz JJ, Breuing KH, Orgill DP (1999) Vacuum-assisted closure in the treatment of degloving injuries. Ann Plast Surg 42: 589–594

59. DeFranzo AJ, Marks MW, Argenta LC, Genecov DG (1999) Vacuum-assisted closure for the treatment of degloving injuries. Plast Reconstr Surg 104: 2145–2148

60. Josty IC, Ramaswamy R, Laing JH (2001) Vacuum-assisted closure: an alternative strategy in the management of degloving injuries of the foot. Br J Plast Surg 54: 363–365

61. Banwell PE, Evison D, Whitworth IM (2002) Vacuum therapy in degloving injuries of the foot: technical refinements. Br J Plast Surg 55: 264–366

62. Jackson DM (1953) The diagnosis of the depth of burning. Br J Surg 40: 588–596

63. Cro C, George KJ, Donnelly J, Irwin ST, Gardiner KR (2002) Vacuum-assisted closure system in the management of enterocutaneous fistulae. Postgrad Med J 78: 364–365

64. Garner GB, Ware DN, Cocanour CS, Duke JH, McKinley BA, Kozar RA, Moore FA (2001) Vacuum-assisted wound closure provides early fascial reapproximation in trauma patients with open abdomens. Am J Surg 182: 630–638

65. Erdmann D, Drye C, Heller L, Wong MS, Levin SL (2001) Abdominal wall defect and enterocutaneous fistula treatment with the vacuum-assisted closure (VAC) system. Plast Reconstr Surg 108: 2066–2068

66. Bonnamy C, Hamel F, Leporrier J, Fouques Y, Viquesnel G, Le Roux Y (2000) Use of the vacuum-assisted closure system for the treatment of perineal gangrene involving the abdominal wall. Ann Chir 125: 982–984

67. Alvarez AA, Maxwell GL, Rodriguez GC (2001) Vacuum-assisted closure for cutaneous gastrointestinal fistula management. Gynecol Oncol 80: 413–416

68. Kercher KW, Sing RF, Matthews BD, Heniford BT (2002) Successful salvage of infected PTFE mesh after ventral hernia repair. Ostomy Wound Manage 48: 40–42

69. Domkowski PW, Smith ML, Gonyon DL Jr, Drye C, Wooten MK, Levin LS, Wolfe WG (2003) Evaluation of vacuum-assisted closure in the treatment of poststernotomy mediastinitis. J Thorac Cardiovasc Surg 126: 386–390

70. Luckraz H, Murphy F, Bryant S, Charman SC, Ritchie AJ (2003) Vacuum-assisted closure as a treatment modality for infections after cardiac surgery. J Thorac Cardiovasc Surg 125: 301–305

71. Fleck TM, Fleck M, Moidl R, Czerny M, Koller R, Giovanoli P, Hiesmayer MJ, Zimpfer D, Wolner E, Grabenwoger M (2002) The vacuum-assisted closure system for the treatment of deep sternal wound infections after cardiac surgery. Ann Thorac Surg 74: 1596–1600

72. Doss M, Martens S, Wood JP, Wolff JD, Baier C, Moritz A (2002) Vacuum-assisted suction drainage versus conventional treatment in the management of poststernotomy osteomyelitis. Eur J Cardiothorac Surg 22: 934–938

73. Song DH, Wu LC, Lohman RF, Gottlieb LJ, Franczyk M (2003) Vacuum assisted closure for the treatment of sternal wounds: the bridge between debridement and definitive closure. Plast Reconstr Surg 111: 92–97

74. Blackburn JH 2nd, Boemi L, Hall WW, Jeffords K, Hauck RM, Banducci DR, Graham WP 3rd (1998) Negative-pressure dressings as a bolster for skin grafts. Ann Plast Surg 40: 453–457

75. Scherer LA, Shiver S, Chang M, Meredith JW, Owings JT (2002) The vacuum assisted closure device: a method of securing skin grafts and improving graft survival. Arch Surg 137: 930–933

76. Chang KP, Tsai CC, Lin TM, Lai CS, Lin SD (2001) An alternative dressing for skin graft immobilization: negative pressure dressing. Burns 27: 839–842

77. Avery C, Pereira J, Moody A, Gargiulo M, Whitworth I (2000) Negative pressure wound dressing of the radial forearm donor site. Int J Oral Maxillofac Surg 29: 198–200

78. Greer SE, Longaker MT, Margiotta M, Mathews AJ, Kasabian A (1999) The use of subatmospheric pressure dressing for the coverage of radial forearm free flap donor-site exposed tendon complications. Ann Plast Surg 43: 551–554

79. Baynham SA, Kohlman P, Katner HP (1999) Treating stage IV pressure ulcers with negative pressure therapy: a case report. Ostomy Wound Manage 45: 28–32, 34–35

80. Azad S, Nishikawa H (2002) Topical negative pressure may help chronic wound healing. BMJ 4: 1100

81. Philbeck TE Jr, Whittington KT, Millsap MH, Briones RB, Wight DG, Schroeder WJ (1999) The clinical and cost effectiveness of externally applied negative pressure wound therapy in the treatment of wounds in home healthcare Medicare patients. Ostomy Wound Manage 45: 41–50

82. Ford CN, Reinhard ER, Yeh D, Syrek D, De Las Morenas A, Bergman SB, Williams S, Hamori CA (2002) Interim analysis of a prospective, randomized trial of vacuum-assisted closure versus the healthpoint system in the management of pressure ulcers. Ann Plast Surg 49: 55–61

83. Coggrave M, West H, Leonard B (2002) Topical negative pressure for pressure ulcer management. Br J Nurs 11 [Suppl 6]: S29–36

84. Clare MP, Fitzgibbons TC, McMullen ST, Stice RC, Hayes DF, Henkel L (2002) Experience with the vacuum assisted closure negative pressure technique in the treatment of non-healing diabetic and dysvascular wounds. Foot Ankle Int 23: 896–901

85. Armstrong DG, Lavery LA, Abu-Rumman P, Espensen EH, Vazquez JR, Nixon BP, Boulton AJ (2002) Outcomes of subatmospheric pressure dressing therapy on wounds of the diabetic foot. Ostomy Wound Manage 48: 64–68

86. Armstrong DG, Boulton AJ, Banwell PE (2004) The management of complex diabetic wounds: the role of topical negative pressure. In: Banwell PE (ed) z. Spires Publishing, Oxford

87. Ubbink DT, van der Oord BM, Sobotka MR, Jacobs MJ (2000) Effects of vacuum compression therapy on skin microcirculation in patients suffering from lower limb ischaemia. Vasa 29: 53–57

88. Moch D, Fleischmann W, Westhauser A (1998) [Instillation vacuum sealing – report of initial experiences] Langenbecks Arch Chir Suppl Kongressbd 115: 1197–1199

89. Fleischmann W, Russ M, Westhauser A, Stampehl M (1998) [Vacuum sealing as carrier system for controlled local drug administration in wound infection] Unfallchirurg 101: 649–654

90. Chester DL, Waters R (2002) Adverse alteration of wound flora with topical negative-pressure therapy: a case report. Br J Plast Surg 55: 510–511

91. Weinberg Group Inc (1999) Technology assessment of the V.A.C. for in-home treatment of chronic wounds. Weinberg Group, Washington, DC, p 61

# Maggot Debridement

W. Fleischmann

## Introduction

When the orthopaedic surgeon William S. Baer presented his method and results of maggot therapy in 1931 [1], his focus of interest was bone and soft tissue infection. He disinfected the eggs of the fly *Phaenicia sericata* and was thus able to produce maggots without bacterial contamination. This happened before the introduction of antibiotics into medicine. Later, it was mainly the work of Ronald Sherman which enlarged the scope of indications to chronic wounds, like stasis ulcers and bed sores [2]. At that time, clinical emphasis was on the problem of impaired wound healing as found in diabetic patients [3].

## Mode of Action

Maggots in wounds cause some mechanical irritation due to their sharp mouth hooks and spicules. This is believed to stimulate wound healing. More important, maggots ingest and thus kill bacteria and secrete digestive enzymes into the wound which contain growth factors, antiseptic substances and proteases. The high proteolytic activity results in liquefying of necrotic tissue, the food source of maggots [4].

## Indications

Maggots may be used in acute and chronic wound infections, osteomyelitis, burns and chronic wounds. Especially diabetic wounds respond well to maggot therapy, whereas unsatisfactory results are to be expected in ischemic lesions due to an arterial occlusive disease [5].

## Adverse Effects and Risks

Sometimes maggots are the cause of pain and skin irritation. They should be applied with caution in the event of exposed bowels or vessels. There might be a certain risk of the development of intestinal fistula or haemorrhage. As larval secretions do not inhibit the growth of some *Pseudomonas* and *Proteus* strains in the case of contamination, maggot therapy should be interrupted for some time and suitable antiseptics applied intermittently.

## Maggot Dressings

For many years, mechanical irritation of wound surfaces by the movement of maggots was believed to be one of the most important factors for the stimulation of wound healing. Consequently, maggots were put directly into the wound. From the beginning, most maggot dressings consisted of a mesh which covered the wound and was glued to the skin, sometimes with an additional stripe of foam rubber. Crawling in the wound, the maggots were thus confined to a cage which was made up from the wound surface and the mesh [1, 6]. Later, Sherman published a more refined dressing technique for the application of maggots to wounds (Figs. 1 and 2). It consisted of a hydrocolloid sheet glued around the wound edges. The netting covered the wound and was fixed to the hydrocolloid with adhesive tape [7]. Thomas et al. [9] described a mesh which was formed like a sleeve or a bag, similar to the construct of Fine and Alexander. In difficult wound locations, e.g. on the feet, the bag could be pulled over the affected extremities and the maggots.

It was a new finding that maggots do not lose their beneficial effect on wound healing if applied to the wound in a porous pouch that resembled a tea bag [8]. Maggots' secretions and dissolved nutrients of the wound were able to pass through the walls of the bags, which consisted of a nylon netting or an open cell membrane. The growth of maggots was more or less the same whether enclosed in bags or applied directly to the wound. Stimulation of wound healing also showed no striking difference between both dressing techniques. Thus, it could be deduced that the mechanical effect of maggots on wound healing was less important than the action of their secretions. In daily use both dressing methods are used, i.e. application of maggots directly to the wound surface or separated by a porous membrane. With regard to patients' comfort, ease of maggot application, hygiene and aesthetics, the maggot pouch dressing revolutionises maggot therapy (Fig. 3).

## Surgical Strategy

In superficial defect wounds like stasis and diabetic ulcers or some bed sores, a mechanical macro-debridement (scalpel etc.) should be performed as a first measure to reduce the time of treatment. Maggots are then used for micro-debridement and as antiseptic agents. A septic bone or deep soft-tissue focus should be completely removed before applying maggots. If this is impossible, the infected tissue is exten-

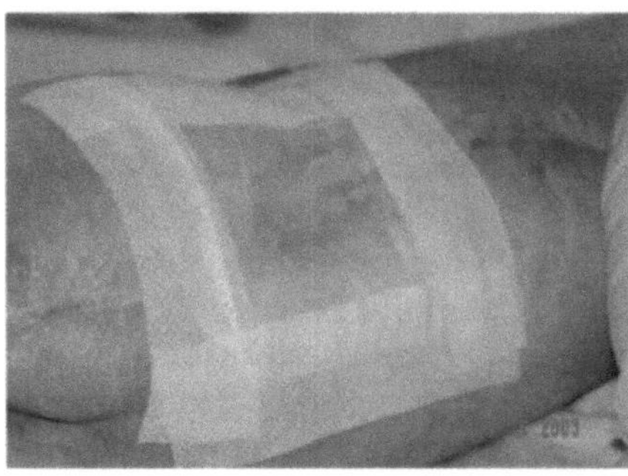

**Fig. 1.** Dressing technique as described by Sherman (primary dressing)

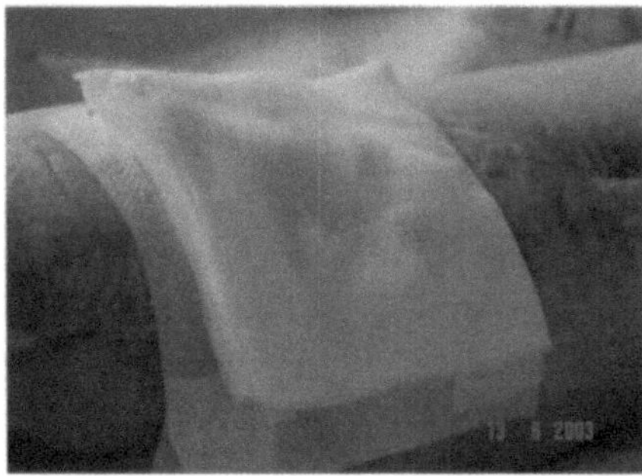

**Fig. 2.** The primary dressing is covered by moist gauzes (secondary dressing)

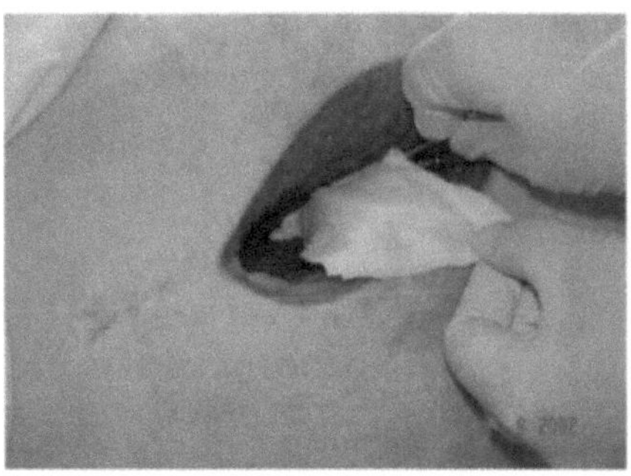

**Fig. 3.** A containment pouch with spacer and maggots is introduced into a deep wound

sively exposed by tissue incisions or excisions to give the maggots and their secretions enough space to do their work. To prevent suffocation of the maggots, either textile spacers or polyvinyl-alcohol sponges are used to keep the wound edges apart. Profuse wound secretions need to be drawn off with drainage systems. For the survival of the maggots in particularly deep wounds special drains for ventilation purposes may be necessary. Having achieved a clean wound by maggot therapy, vacuum dressings may be applied for exsudate management. External skin expansion may be used for rapid closure of remaining wound defects.

## Organisation

Maggots are applied directly to the wound, which takes approximately 20 min, or enclosed in a porous containment bag, which is much easier and done in 5 min. The life span of maggots is limited, and after 4–5 days in the wound they have to be removed. For logistic reasons it is good to define 2 days of the week for the application and removal of maggot dressings, e.g. Tuesday and Friday. Thus, the producer of the maggots knows in advance when to deliver. Costs of transportation are reduced by treating all patients on the same day. Out-patients have to be informed to keep the dressings moist, otherwise the maggots will die.

## Final Remarks

Maggots are not a universal remedy. In acute wound infections a vacuum dressing (VAC Instill) will get rid of the infection much faster than the maggots. In chronic bone infections, surgery is often necessary to get the maggots down to the septic area. Chronic stasis ulcers need a surgical fasciectomy if they do not show a tendency to heal after approximately four cycles of maggot therapy. Ischemic wounds should be examined for the possibility of revascularisation before any other therapy starts. Maggots are an excellent low-risk tool for the treatment of infected and chronic wounds, given that it is embedded in a good concept of interdisciplinary wound management.

## References


1. Baer WS (1931) The treatment of chronic osteomyelitis with the maggot (larva of the blowfly. J Bone Joint Surg 13: 438
2. Sherman RA (2002) Maggot versus conservative debridement therapy for the treatment of pressure ulcers. Wound Repair Regen 10: 208–214
3. Sherman RA (2003) Maggot therapy for treating diabetic foot ulcers unresponsive to conventional therapy. Diabetes Care 26: 446–451
4. Fleischmann W, Grassberger M, Sherman R (2004) Maggot therapy. Thieme, Stuttgart New York
5. Fleischmann W, Russ M, Moch D, Marquardt C (1999) Biosurgery – Maggots, are they really the better surgeons? Chirurg 70: 1340–1346
6. Fine A, Alexander H (1934) Maggot therapy – Technique and clinical application. J Bone Joint Surg 16: 572–582
7. Sherman RA (1997) A new dressing design for use with maggot therapy. Plast Reconstr Surg 100: 451–456
8. Grassberger M, Fleischmann W (2002) The BioBag-A new device for the application of medicinal maggots. Dermatol 204: 306
9. Sherman RA, Hall JR, Thomas S et al. (2000) Medicinal maggots: an ancient remedy for some contemporary afflictions. Annu Rev Entomol 45: 55–91

# IV Surgical Interventions in Wounds



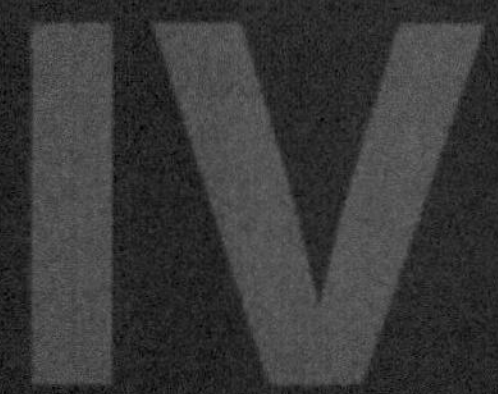

M. Syamken, H. Trautner, U. Schwemmer

Reduction of peri-operative risk and prevention of deterioration of the trophic situation in wounds has to be the aim of peri-operative management in wound care.

## General Status

The peri-operative risk of a patient depends substantially on his intercurrent diseases. Pre-existing diseases may lead to an increased peri-operative morbidity and mortality depending on extent and severity. The aim of peri-operative management is to optimise the patient's condition in the time available before surgery (this may vary widely between emergency and elective surgery). Peri-operative morbidity in non-cardiac surgery is mainly due to cardiovascular complications [4, 11]. Therefore, peri-operative risk evaluation is crucial to avoid these adverse events [7].

In patients above the age of 40 years, the ECG is a basic investigation, often providing hints for cardiovascular diseases. Stress testing and, in special cases, stress echocardiography or scintigraphy can detect significant coronary artery disease. Other diagnostic procedures like echocardiography, chest X-ray, routine scintigraphy, halter ECG or halter blood-pressure measurement do not add information to the peri-operative risk assessment, although these techniques might be very relevant in evaluating other co-existing diseases (heart failure; valve lesions, in particular aortic stenoses etc.) and can be useful to improve medical treatment preoperatively (e.g. normalisation of blood pressure) [16].

## Ischaemic Heart Disease

Ischaemic heart disease is today the most frequent cause of morbidity and mortality in men over 40 years and women over 50 years [12]. Pre-operative assessment of asymptomatic patients is of a particular importance since ischaemic heart disease is identified as the main source of peri-operative complications. Peri-operative risk increases after a history of myocardial infarction. The more recently myocardial infarction has occurred, the higher is the risk of perioperative reinfarction [14, 17, 18]. Thus selected surgery should be generally postponed until 6 months after infarction and instable angina pectoris has to turn into a stable angina pectoris unless it is urgent. Blood pressure has to be normalised, tachycardia has to be avoided by β-blockade, and angina pectoris has to be treated by reducing cardiac pre-load.

Demands of anaesthetic management are: close monitoring, avoidance of tachycardia and bradycardia, maintenance or normotension or slight hypotension and careful choice of anaesthetic agent. β-blockade should be maintained, and this requires care in fluid replacement and concurrent drug application.

## Cardiac Failure

Apart from ischaemic heart disease, cardiac failure is significant as a risk factor for peri-operative morbidity and mortality [6]. Compensatory conditions of heart failure can turn to decompensation during anaesthetic and surgical procedures. Underlying risk of heart failure has to be cleared up, and treatment introduced or improved before surgery.

Hypertension has to be treated with the aim of normalising blood pressure. Conditions of ischaemic heart diseases have to be optimised by control of blood pressure, heart rate and reduction of pre-load. Drug therapy of valvular heart defect and cardiomyopathy has to be improved [10]. Retention of water has to be treated with diuretics under close monitoring of electrolytes. Glycosides are indicated when atrial fibrillation occurs, but not in normal systolic ventricular function [4].

## Hypertension

Untreated hypertension is associated with increased peri-operative risk [18]. Major problems include severe variation of blood pressure, cerebrovascular accident, myocardial infarction and renal failure. Hypertension is identified as an important cardiovascular risk factor. Cardial, cerebral and renal manifestation of hypertension leads to an increased peri-operative risk [2].

Anti-hypertensive therapy has to be optimised. If hypertension is an unexpected peri-operative finding or treatment is insufficient, surgery should be delayed, if possible. Drug therapy has to be continued throughout the peri-operative period (except diuretics and long-acting ACE inhibitors).

## Arrhythmias

Arrhythmias may indicate underlying cardiac disease and can influence haemodynamics effectively. Tachycardia can lead to increased myocardial oxygen consumption and a reduced coronary perfusion by shortening of diastole. Bradycardia reduces coronary perfusion by a decreased cardiac output. Both mechanisms can lead to increased cardiac morbidity and mortality. Thus, underlying arrhythmia has to be identified and treated sufficiently. Arrhythmias have to be treated in the peri-operative period, if they are to be haemodynamically effective [3].

Atrial fibrillation is a strong indication for therapy with glycosides. If tachycardia persists after treatment with glycosides, β-blockers or calcium antagonists can be beneficial. Electrical cardioversion has to be considered in the early phase of atrial fibrillation [4].

## Diabetes Mellitus

Peri-operative management has to consider the type of diabetes and anti-diabetic therapy. Peri-operative blood-glucose control needs to be tight. Resultant diseases and their end-organ pathology have to be carefully assessed and optimised conditions created [15]. Elective surgery has to be carried out only in well-prepared adjustment of anti-diabetic therapy. Regional anaesthesia should be preferred due to the improved trophical situation. Patients with diabetes should be planned as the first point in a surgical programme, because of the lower risk of metabolic instabilities. Oral anti-diabetics have to be withdrawn at pre-operative night and morning. Long-acting oral anti-diabetics and metformin (danger of lactate acidosis) have to be stopped 3 days before surgery. Insulin has to be withdrawn at pre-operative morning [1, 13].

## COPD

Airway obstruction resulting from bronchoconstriction, bronchial oedema and hypersecretion of mucus can lead to pulmonary atelectasis and pneumonia if sputum is not cleared. Hypoxaemia, hypercapnia and dyspnoea caused by chronic airway obstruction increase the perioperative risk [8].

In the peri-operative period detection and treatment of active airway infection should be carried out with antibiotic therapy [20]. Treatment of airway obstruction with bronchodilatators ($β_2$-agonists and aminophylline) can be extended with steroids in the peri-operative phase if necessary [19]. the condition of biventricular failure resulting from concurrent ischemic heart disease and cor pulmonale should improved by therapy with diuretics, nitrates or glycosides.

## Improvement of Trophical Situation in Wounds

The aim of peri-operative management in wound care is to avoid decrease of vascular perfusion or oxygen delivery. Severe pain in the post-operative period causes vasoconstriction and increased oxygen consumption in the wound and leads to a deterioration of wound healing [9]. Thus effective peri-operative pain management plays a substantial role. Analgesic therapy can be carried out by systemic application of non-opioids or opioid analgesics or by regional anaesthesia techniques [5].

Although no difference in peri-operative severe morbidity or mortality had been seen on comparing anaesthesia techniques, a sympathetic block may result from regional anaesthesia. This may lead to an increased perfusion of tissue and improved trophic conditions in wounds. Regional techniques acting into the post-operative phase and analgesic effect can develop in the most painful period after surgery. Thus methods using catheters for continued application of local anaesthetics should be considered for blockade of pain in the peri-operative period.

## Conclusion

Reduction of peri-operative risk by improving conditions of concurrent diseases and effective analgesic therapy to avoid deterioration of trophical situation in wounds must be the aim of peri-operative management in wound care. These aims must be achieved in an interdisciplinary manner, with close cooperation between surgeons and anaesthetists.

## References

1. Alberti KGMM, Thomas BJB (1970) The management of diabetes during surgery. Br J Anaesth 51: 693
2. Alexander JP (1991) Management of hypertension. In: Dundee J, Clarke RSJ, McCaughey W (eds) Clinical anaesthetic pharmacology. Churchill Livingstone, Edinburgh
3. Bennett DH (1985) Cardiac arrhythmias. Practical notes on interpretation and treatment. Wright, Bristol
4. Böhm M (1997) Die präoperative kardiale Risikoabschätzung und Diagnostik. Die Sicht des Kardiologen. Anaesthesist [Suppl] 46: S85–S95
5. Brodner G, Pogatzki E, Van Aken H (1997) Ein modernes Konzept zur postoperativen Schmerztherapie. Anaesthesist [Suppl 2] 46: S124–S131
6. Foster E, Davis K, Carpenter J, Abele S, Fray D (1986) Risk of noncardiac operation in patients with defined coronary artery disease: the coronary artery surgery study (CASS) registry experience. Ann Thorax Surg 41: 42–50
7. Goldman L (1994) Assessment of perioperative cardiac risk. N Engl J Med 330: 707–709
8. Grant IS (1994) Anaesthesia and respiratory disease. In: Nimmo WS, Rowbotham DJ, Smith G (eds) Anaesthesia, 2nd edn. Blackwell, London
9. Grond S, Lehmann KA (1994) Auswirkungen des postoperativen Schmerzes auf die Rekonvaleszenz. In: Lehmann KA (ed) Der postoperative Schmerz, 2nd edn. Springer, Berlin Heidelberg New York, S 121–147

10. Jung J, Schreiber JU (2003) Current treatment of chronic heart failure. Anaesthesist 52: 612–618
11. Mangano DT, Biebuyck JF, Phil D (1990) Perioperative cardiac morbidity. Anesthesiology 72: 153–184
12. Mangano DT, Goldman L (1995) Preoperative assessment of patients with known or suspected coronary disease. N Engl J Med 333: 1750–1756
13. McAnulty GR, Robertshaw HJ, Hall GM (2001) Anesthetic management of patients with diabetes mellitus. Eur J Anaesthesiol 18: 277–294
14. Rao TK, Jacobs KH, El-Etr AA (1983) Reinfarction following anesthesia in patients with myocardial infarction. Anesthesiology 59: 499–505
15. Scherpereel PA, Tavernier B (2001) Perioperative care of diabetic patients. Eur J Anaesthesiol 18: 277–294
16. Smith MS, Muir H, Hall R (1996) Perioperative management of drug therapy. Clinical considerations. Drugs 51: 238–259
17. Steen PA, Tinker JH, Tarhan S (1978) Myocardial reinfarction after anesthesia and surgery. JAMA 239: 2566–2570
18. Stone J, Foex P, Sear J, Johnson L, Khambatta H, Triner L (1988) Risk of myocardial ischemia during anesthesia in treated and untreated hypertensive patients. Br J Anaesth 61: 675–679
19. Symreng T, Karlberg BE, Kagedal B, Schildt B (1981) Physiological cortisol substitution of long-term steroid treated patients undergoing major surgery. Br J Anaesthesia 53: 949–953
20. Thoracic Society (1993) Guidelines for the management of asthma: a summary. Br Med J 306: 776–782

# Dressings for Chronic and Acute Wounds

S. MEAUME

## Introduction – Background to Healing in a Moist Environment

Since antiquity, dressings have formed an integral part of the art of treating wounds. Earlier than 2000 B.C., Sumerian writings described dressings based on plants, mud, milk, wine, beer, oil and flour. In 1550 B.C., the Egyptians used plant fibres for their absorbent qualities, as well as honey and fats, inventing the first greasy dressings. They often used bandages as a means of holding these dressings in place. The same products were indeed used over subsequent centuries. In the 19th century, Semmelweis, Pasteur and Lister participated in the development of antiseptics and thought they could prevent infection by keeping a wound as dry as possible: at that time, the purpose of dressings was therefore to absorb and eliminate all traces of exudate and moisture. This concept was finally called into question by the studies of Winter [46] and Hinman [17] during the 1960s, who demonstrated again what the Egyptians had known already: the beneficial effects of a moist environment on healing. During the second half of the 20th century, it was technological advances in polymers, adhesives and textiles which were the source of intensive research and development into modern dressings. Thus the introduction of hydrocolloids represented a real revolution in the treatment of all types of wounds. However, for some heavily exuding wounds, they do not enable the optimum control of exudate. It is, then, necessary to use more absorbent polymers: alginates, foams or hydrofibres. Similarly, some little-exuding wounds require an input of moisture, which today is possible thanks to the development of hydrogel dressings.

Today, when treating a wound, efforts must be made to avoid superinfection, eliminate necrotic tissue, control exudate, encourage granulation and not prevent epidermisation. Modern dressings make it possible to ensure these different phases in an optimum fashion. However, none of these dressings is truly active in healing, and no significant difference has been demonstrated versus the reference treatment, which consists in ensuring a moist environment for the wound through the use of plain dressings soaked in physiological saline. The principal dressings available for use today are thus mainly aimed at not preventing the natural healing process, without accelerating it.

## The Principal Properties of Modern Dressings

Modern dressings:
- Can assist in the cleansing and sloughing of chronic wounds, which should primarily be mechanical (cutting with scissors or a lancet).
- Maintain a moist environment conducive to healing. They thus favour the natural phenomena of healing and particularly the phases of granulation and epithelialisation. They absorb exudates to prevent maceration around the wound or, on the contrary, provide moisture if the wound is dry.
- Protect the wound from external infection and trauma.
- Are designed not to adhere to the wound and thus reduce pain when dressings are changed.

## Criteria Governing the Choice of Dressing

A dressing should be chosen according to different criteria, of which the principal are:
- appearance of the wound bed: necrosis, fibrin which needs to be cleansed or granulation and epithelialisation which must be preserved,
- quantity of exudate,
- appearance of the skin around the wound,
- cavity wound or not,
- cost,
- odour,
- compliance of the patient,
- allergies, intolerance of products previously applied.

## The Performance Expected of a Modern Dressing

Certain qualities are required for a dressing:
- **Capacity for absorption.** For example, polyurethane films are not at all absorbent, while alginates or hydrofibres are highly absorbent. Hydrocolloid and foam dressings exhibit intermediate absorption capacities. Interfaces, greasy dressings and hydrogels are little or not absorbent.
- **Capacity for moisturising.** Hydrogels are the dressings most suited to the treatment of dry wounds. Occlusive dressings make it possible to preserve the natural moisture existing in a wound (hydrocolloid or foam dressings, films).

- **Adhesiveness.** The use of an adhesive dressing depends on the quality of the skin around the wound. For fragile skins, notably around leg ulcers, non-adhesive dressings are available: alginate, hydrofibre, interface, foam dressings, for example. However, in some cases, adhesiveness may be a property which is sought in a dressing: for use on some parts of the body, for example (heels, elbows, sacrum). Other dressings with a non-adhesive centre and an adhesive border are also available, as are those coated with silicone with selective micro-adhesiveness.
- **Conformability.** Thin hydrocolloid dressings, anatomically shaped hydrocolloid and foam dressings (especially for heels, elbows, the sacrum) are appropriate for different anatomical sites of wounds. Hydrogels, alginates in the form of rope or ribbon, foam pads or hydrocolloid paste can fill cavity wounds.
- **Ability to absorb odours.** Cleanliness of charcoal dressings.
- **Ability to control the growth of micro-organisms.** Examples are charcoal, silver or alginate dressings.

## Regulations Governing Modern Dressings and Their Reimbursement

Dressings and biomaterials used to cover wounds are not usually categorised as drugs. They are medical devices and they are subject to CE labelling. The requirements in terms of their manufacture and safety are virtually identical to those prevailing for drugs, but the level of proof of efficacy does not, for most of these devices, require the implementation of large-scale, controlled, randomised, clinical studies. For most products, their reimbursement for outpatient use is possible, but this varies depending on the country.

## Different Categories of Dressings and Biomaterials

### Hydrocolloids (HC)

**Presentation and Composition.** Hydrocolloid dressings (HC) are available in the form of:
- dressing cut in squares of various sizes, thin dressing (more or less transparent) (Fig. 1) or more absorbent dressing;
- paste to fill cavity wounds before covering them with a dressing.

Some presentations are designed as a function of the morphology of the areas where pressure sores are often found (heels, sacrum, elbows).

The inner layer of all HC dressings is absorbent. It is composed of carboxymethyl cellulose (CMC) sodium, enclosed in an elastic and adhesive mass which in some cases contains pectin or gelatine of porcine origin. A film and/or polyurethane foam, or unwoven fabric, constitute the outer layer.

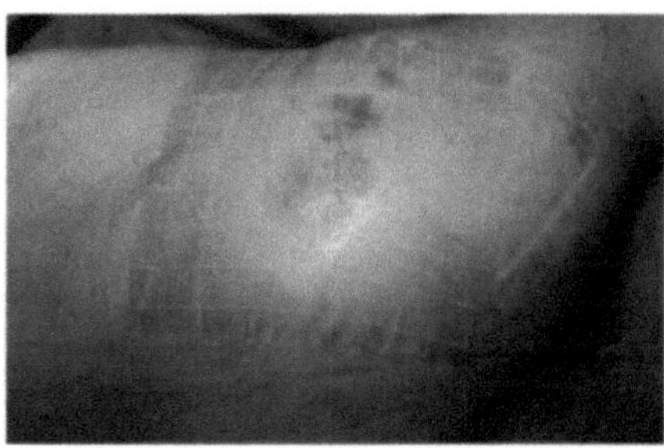

**Fig. 1.** Thin hydrocolloid dressing

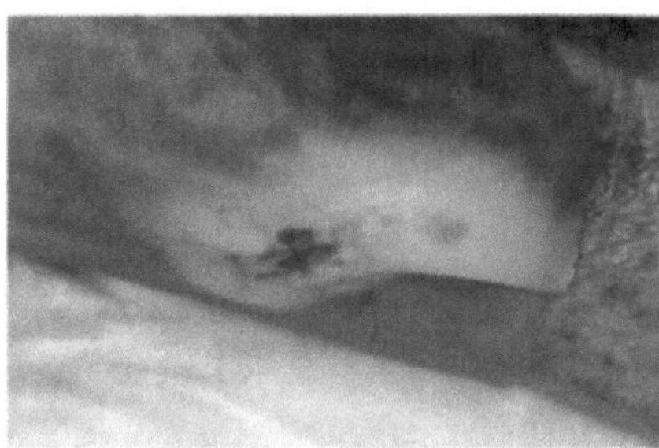

**Fig. 2.** Saturated hydrocolloid dressing after 4 days in place

**Method of Use.** The sheet is applied directly to the area of the wound, after cleansing with physiological saline or water, with the dressing overlapping 2–3 cm onto the surrounding skin, to which it adheres. In some sites, and in the case of heavily exuding wounds, and particularly during a cleansing phase, it is preferable to cover the sheet with a secondary dressing which can absorb the excess exudate after a few days, and hold the sheet in position if the wound is in a friction zone. For less heavily exuding wounds, transparent sheets can replace thick sheets. The rate of dressing changes is between a few days and a week, depending on the amount of exudate. The dressing should be changed only when the HC is "saturated" and/or the sheet is already partially detached from the skin (Fig. 2).

**Indications.** Numerous studies have demonstrated the value of using HC in the treatment of pressure sores [1, 48], leg ulcers [7, 13, 15, 31], wounds in diabetics [2], first- and second-degree superficial burns [16, 47], particularly in children, donor graft sites, excision of pilonidal sinus [42], other acute wounds [22, 45], areas of skin biopsy [30, 34] and dermatological diseases such as epidermolysis bullosa [11] and scleroderma [27] to protect and treat damaged areas of skin.

**Advantages.** Used only on spontaneously moist wounds, these dressings respect the bacterial cycle of the slough which is characterised by a gradual replacement of Gram – germs by Gram + microflora [35]. They maintain a warm and moist environment favourable to healing. They can be used at all stages of healing, from cleansing to epidermisation. The film covering the sheet protects the wound from outside bacterial contamination (incontinence) and allows patients to take a shower. Because HC does not adhere to a wound, dressing changes are practically painless.

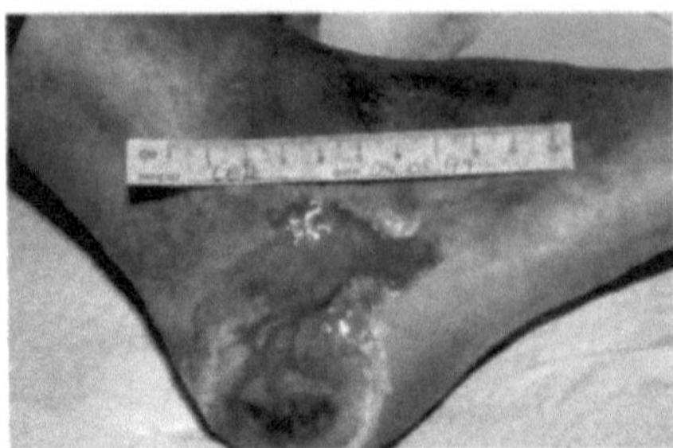

**Fig. 3.** Disintegration of hydrocolloid dressing: substance resembling pus

**Disadvantages.** Because it disintegrates in contact with exudate, CMC changes into a substance which resembles pus (Fig. 3). Doctors, nurses, patients and their families must be informed of the normal nature of this appearance, particularly since this fluid is usually very foul-smelling. Maceration may be observed around the wound when it is exuding heavily. A change should then be made to more absorbent dressings.

Although they have been widely used for many years, HC only rarely cause contact eczema. The rare published cases correspond to sensitisation to the adhesive (colophane) or more rarely to other components. The onset of erythema or petechial eruption around the wound should not be a cause for concern: this usually signifies a non-allergic irritant reaction, related to excessively frequent dressing changes.

**Contra-Indications.** HC are not indicated in the case of wholly dry wounds, nor should they be used for clinically infected wounds, which is the case for any occlusive dressings.

### Polyurethane Films

**Presentation and Composition.** These films are made up of a transparent polyurethane (PU) membrane coated on one side with hypoallergenic adhesive. Available in a variety of sizes, they are presented on a stiff backing which helps with their application.

**Method of Use.** They are applied either directly to a wound, with the film overlapping beyond it onto previously dried peripheral skin, or on top of another dressing, where they then constitute a secondary dressing to ensure the occlusion and isolation of the wound. They thus can be used as secondary dressings on alginates, hydrogels or hydrocellular dressings, or on ordinary gauze. They can also be used as surgical drapes for incision, or as a dressing to hold central catheters or peripheral venous lines in place.

**Indications.** PU films are endowed with the remarkable qualities of semi-permeable membranes. Permeable to oxygen and water vapour, they prevent maceration; impermeable to water and bacteria, they maintain moisture while at the same time preventing outside bacterial contamination. They ensure the physical protection of wounds against friction and soiling. Different studies have demonstrated their value as a primary dressing in superficial burns [29], donor graft sites [4] and skin tears [38] or in chronic wounds such as low-grade pressure ulcers [32].

**Advantages.** They adhere to healthy skin but not to a wound. For open wounds, these dressings maintain a moist environment favourable to healing and thus prevent the formation of a scab. Transparent, they allow visual checks on the wound. They are supple and very adaptable.

**Contra-Indications.** These films should not be used on heavily exuding, infected wounds.

## Alginates

**Presentation and Composition.** These polymers are mainly and sometimes wholly composed of alginic acids (calcium alginate) obtained from brown seaweed (laminar). They are endowed with considerable absorbent potential and gel more or less in contact with exudate (depending on their composition in manuronic and guluronic acids), which enables them not to adhere to a wound (Fig. 4). They are sometimes mixed with CMC, in varying percentages. They are commercially available in the form of dressings of different sizes and ribbon which is well suited to packing cavity wounds.

**Indications.** Generally acknowledged as haemostatic, they are therefore used for haemorrhagic wounds, although alginates are now also indicated in the treatment of heavily exuding wounds, mainly at the debridement stage or if bleeding exists. In particular, they are indicated in maxillofacial surgery [45], donor graft sites [5, 10, 21, 36], pressure sores [6, 37] and diabetic foot ulcers [3].

**Methods of Use.** Before use, the dressing needs to be cut approximately to the dimensions of the wound, but can extend beyond it onto peripheral skin without danger, which may make dressing changes easier. The wound is cleaned with physiological saline and then the alginate dressing is placed dry on the wound, covered with a secondary dressing and fixed with an elastic bandage, a film or an adhesive. When the wound is not exuding heavily, it is also possible to soak the alginate dressing in physiological saline and then cover it with a polyurethane film in order to maintain a moist environment and prevent it from adhering to the wound.

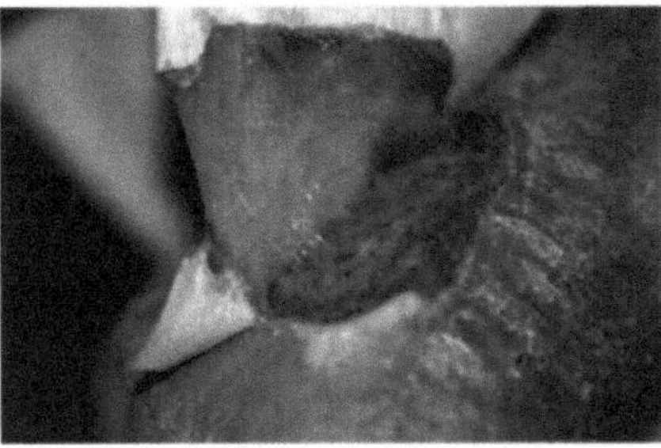

**Fig. 4.** Alginate dressing on leg ulcer

The dressing is changed depending on the abundance of exudate: daily during the cleansing phase, every 2 or 3 days during granulation. The dressing can be removed from the wound in a single movement or be rinsed with physiological saline to eliminate the gelled dressing.

**Advantages.** The very high absorbent potential of alginates represents their principal quality. Indicated during the cleansing and granulation stages, particularly for heavily exuding wounds, they do not adhere to the wound and maintain a moist environment favourable to healing. It is possible to use them on infected wounds, on condition that they are not covered with an occlusive dressing but just with pads of gauze.

**Disadvantages.** They constitute only primary dressings and need to be covered with another dressing.

**Contra-Indications.** Dry or moderately exuding wounds are not an indication for alginates.

### Hydrofibre

**Presentation and Composition.** At present there is only one representative of this new type of dressing, Aquacel, which is made up of non-woven fibres of pure HC (sodium CMC) and presented in the form of sheets and ribbon.

**Method of Use.** It is a highly absorbent dressing which can be used almost like an alginate. After cleansing the wound with physiological saline, the dressing should be applied, overlapping onto the skin around the wound or not. For cavity wounds, ribbon dressing should be used for preference. In all cases, the dressing should then be covered with a secondary dressing (HC sheet, film or gauze dressing, e.g. in the case of infected wounds). The interval between dressing changes varies, depending on the abundance of exudate and the type of secondary dressing. Under an HC sheet, it can usually be left in place for 3 to 5 days (Fig. 5).

**Indications.** On the surface of a wound, Aquacel interacts immediately with exudate to form a cohesive gel, creating a moist environment favourable to healing while controlling excess fluid. Like alginates, this product is indicated during the cleansing and granulation of exuding wounds. Controlled studies have been performed essentially in the treatment of pressure sores and leg ulcers, but also in the treatment of burns [44].

**Advantages.** This dressing does not adhere to a wound and can be changed painlessly.

**Disadvantages.** This substance can only be used as a primary dressing and needs to be covered with a secondary dressing, which increases the cost of care. However, because it can be left in place for longer, the cost of treatment with hydrofibre is lower than with some alginates.

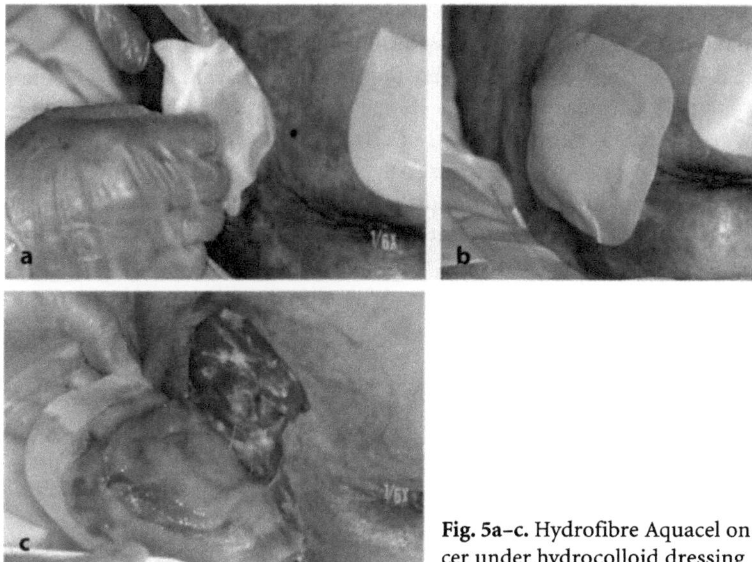

**Fig. 5a–c.** Hydrofibre Aquacel on pressure ulcer under hydrocolloid dressing

**Contra-Indications.** Dry wounds or low exuding wounds should not be dressed with hydrofibre.

### Foam Dressings

**Forms, Presentations and Composition.** These dressings are made up of a hydrophilic layer, usually of polyurethane, combined with a film or outer layer which is impermeable to liquids, and in some cases, has a hypoallergenic adhesive backing (Fig. 6). Some dressings are thus adhesive all over, while others have only an adhesive border, and others are non-adhesive. Dressings of different sizes and shapes are commercially available, and can be used for different wound sites (e.g. sacrum, heels) and for cavity wounds. Less absorbent forms have recently been introduced on the market ("lite" forms) for more superficial and less exuding wounds. Absorbent silicone dressings (Mépilex) have an inside silicone surface which can stick to the skin around the wound thanks to a patented technology (Safetac) enabling micro-ad-hesiveness to hold the dressing in place, or even reposition or remove it

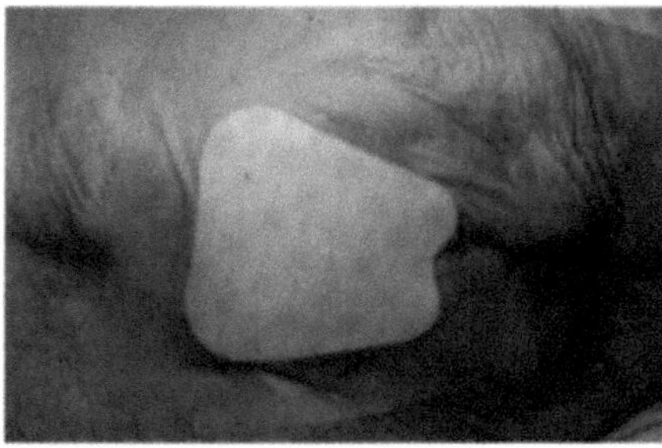

**Fig. 6.** Hydrocellular dressing on sacral pressure ulcer

without pain and without damaging the peripheral skin. The central part of the superabsorbent dressing (Cellosorb) is a lipocolloid interface, another patented substance which is made of woven polyurethane impregnated with a mixture of vaseline and carboxymethyl cellulose (CMC). In contact with the wound, a thin layer of gel forms which enables painless dressing changes. Hydroabsorbent dressings (Cutinova) are similar to hydrocellular dressings, even though their appearance is closer to a hydrocolloid, but they do not disintegrate in the wound in contact with exudate and they do not contain any CMC.

**Method of Use and Choice of Foam Dressing.** After cleansing the wound with physiological saline or water, the dressing should be cut to a size a few centimetres larger all round the wound. In their non-adhesive form, these dressings can be used even if the skin around the wound is not entirely healthy (contact dermatitis, irritation, maceration). They are then held in place by a secondary dressing (pad, multi-layer dressing and extensible band). When they can be borne, the adhesive forms can be used as primary and secondary dressings. However, at certain sites, it is preferable to cover them with a protective dressing to prevent excessive friction, which may detach them. The rate of dressing changes depends on the quantity of exudate, ranging from about 3 to 8 days.

**Indications.** These absorbent dressings maintain moisture in the wound, respect its ecosystem and prevent contamination by external micro-organisms when they are occlusive (adhesive forms). They are indicated when the wound is already partially cleansed, but particularly at the granulation stage and until complete epithelialisation. Studies have been performed in the context of leg ulcers and pressure sores [23, 24, 49], donor graft sites [12] and skin tears [38]. Numerous other types of wounds also represent indications: diabetic foot ulcer, surgical wounds (ingrowing toenails, etc.).

**Advantages.** These dressings are very comfortable, and prevent the odours which may be experienced with HC, as there is no disintegration of the dressing. It is possible to take a shower while wearing an adhesive foam dressing. Dressing changes are painless because the dressing never adheres to the wound, even if it is low-exuding.

**Disadvantages.** The absorption capacity of foam dressings is insufficient for heavily exuding wounds. Peripheral maceration may then be observed. With adhesive types, rare cases of allergy have been reported. Irritation due to the adhesive is also possible, if adhesive foam dressings are changed too often. Non-adhesive foam dressings require the use of a secondary dressing to hold them in place, and they are not occlusive.

**Contra-Indications.** Like hydrocolloid dressing, these should not be chosen in the case of dry or low-exuding secreting wounds.

## Hydrogels

**Presentation and Composition.**  Hydrogels are insoluble polymers with hydrophilic sites, containing more than 80% water. The most commonly used polymer at present is CMC. The dressings take the form of a translucent sheet or amorphous gel, which is more or less cohesive, colourless or pale yellow. When in a sheet form, the quantity of water they can release into the wound depends on their thickness. Gel forms appear to be the most effective in releasing moisture into wounds.

**Method of Use.**  The CMC-based gel is applied in a thick layer to a previously cleansed wound (Fig. 7). It is necessary to use a secondary dressing, which may be an hydrocolloid or polyurethane film. Classic gauze pads are not indicated as the water in the hydrogel is then absorbed by the secondary dressing and does not enter the wound. A period of several days can be allowed between dressing changes (3 to 4 days).

**Indications.**  Designed for use on drier wounds, hydrogels are used for the cleansing and healing of wounds emitting little or no exudate. They are amongst the most efficient products in softening a plaque of necrosis in the case of a pressure sore, and can advantageously replace pads soaked in physiological saline, which need to be changed three times a day.

Multicentre, randomised studies on hydrogels have been published in the context of pressure sores [9], leg ulcers, donor graft sites and burns.

**Advantages.**  Hydrogels supply moisture to wounds which are not spontaneously exuding, thus allowing healing in a moist environment.

**Disadvantages.**  Hydrogels do not have a very high potential for absorption and favour maceration of the edges of wounds.

**Contra-Indications.**  Heavily exuding wounds should not be treated with hydrogels.

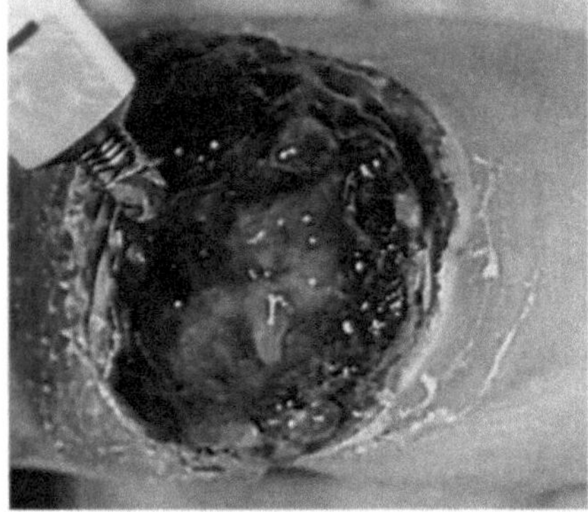

**Fig. 7.** Hydrogel

## Charcoal Dressings

**Composition – Background.** These dressings contain a layer of charcoal. This charcoal is combined with an absorbent dressing which may vary considerably in terms of its composition: cotton fibre (Carbonet), CMC (Carboflex) or a non-woven envelope. Actisorb combines silver with the charcoal.

**Mechanism of Action.** Active charcoal absorbs endo- and exotoxins and other degradation products released in situ as well as volatile amines and fatty acids responsible for the production of odours by wounds which are superinfected or colonised by anaerobic or Gram-negative bacteria (chronic wounds in the cleansing phase, cancerous wounds). In the case of Actisorb Plus 25, the micro-organisms are also inactivated in the dressing by its silver content.

**Method of Use.** These dressings are applied dry to wounds, or are sometimes moistened with physiological saline. They need to be covered with a secondary dressing. Carboflex is the most absorbent charcoal dressing, followed by Carbonet and then Actisorb. Carboflex does not adhere to a wound. When Carbonet or Actisorb are used for wounds producing little exudate, it is possible to employ a greasy interface (Jelonet, Adaptic) to prevent the dressing from adhering to the wound.

**Indications.** Charcoal dressings may be indicated as a primary or secondary dressing for wounds, which are cleansing or foul-smelling, and particularly for cancerous wounds, and because they are not exuding, cleansing or foul-smelling [18, 28], especially for malignant wounds. Because they are not occlusive, they can be used on infected wounds. Charcoal dressings are a good alternative to the use of metronidazole in the treatment of malodorous wounds [14].

**Advantages, Tolerability and Acceptability.** There are no contra-indications to the use of these dressings. Their tolerability is excellent.

**Disadvantages.** It is sometimes difficult to render these dressings conformable. Some users raise the problem of their high cost, particularly when they are used in combination with other dressings. They can often be used alone on a wound (e.g. when moistened), which may make it possible to limit the cost of each dressing without impairing patient comfort.

## Silver Dressings

**Composition and Background.** Silver sulfadiazine-based dressings have existed since 1930 in France, and are widely employed for the treatment of burns. Actisorb has been the most frequently used for several years in the treatment of chronic wounds. The more recently introduced Acticoat is used to treat acute or chronic wounds with a risk of major infection, or infected wounds.

**Forms and Products Available.** Silver sulfadiazine has been available in France since 1930 in a cream form (Flammazine, Sicazine) and more recently in the form of an impregnated lipid–colloid interface (Urgotul SSD) or in combination with hyaluronic acid (Ialuset Plus). These products are reimbursed for use by outpatients. Flammacerium combines silver sulfadiazine and cerium nitrate and is reserved for the treatment of major burns. Actisorb, already described in the section on charcoal dressings, also contains silver, but not a sulfonamide. Its cost is reimbursed. Acticoat is a nanocrystalline silver-based dressing which, when applied to a wound, releases silver ions over a prolonged period (Fig. 8). It needs to be moistened with water prior to application, and then kept moist. Of a more recent design, it is not yet reimbursed for outpatient care. Other silver-containing dressings are available in Europe or the USA: Silvercell (alginate + silver), Aquacel Ag (hydrofibre + silver), Contreet (hydrocolloid + silver) and Contreet H (foam + silver) or Advance.

**Mechanism of Action.** Silver acts as a broad-spectrum antibacterial agent. The quantity of silver released varies considerably, depending on the product (in vitro studies). Thus, the antibacterial activity of the product also varies greatly. Silver also exhibits an anti-inflammatory activity, by reducing the activity of metalloproteases. Despite its longstanding and broad areas of use, there have not as yet been any documented instances of resistance to silver ions.

**Indications.** Use of silver dressings is indicated for wounds with a risk of infection (critical colonisation) and as adjuvant treatment for certain types of infected wounds. Clinical studies are necessary to clarify these indications in acute or chronic wounds. We have already results on burns [8], donor sites [19] and leg ulcers [20].

**Comparison of Silver Dressings.** Not all silver dressings are equivalent, as has been shown by in-vitro studies which clarified some of their properties [40]. It is important to establish the quantity of silver contained in the dressing, its form (silver salt, metallic silver), whether it is released into the wound or not, at what rate it is released, for how long, what concentrations may be attained in the wound and to what depth. The correlation between these properties and clinical results concerning the prevention or treatment of infection has not yet been established.

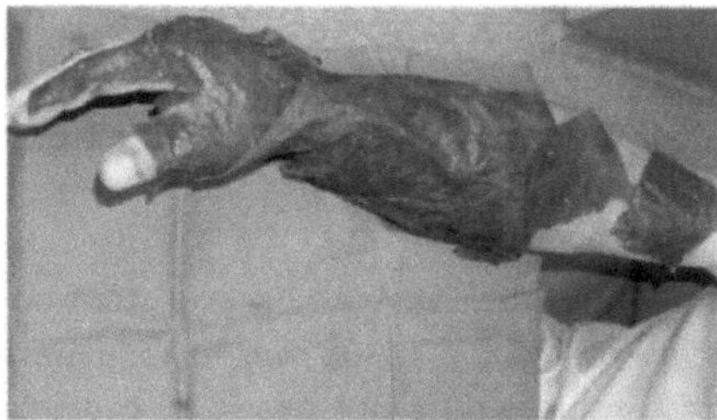

**Fig. 8.** Silver dressing Acticoat on burn

**Tolerability and Acceptability.** The use of silver dressings with silver sulfadiazine is not recommended for long time in chronic wounds by many dermatologists, because of the risks of contact eczema due to the sulfonamide or the excipient in creams when they are used on leg ulcers. However, the risk of generalised argyria is more theoretical than real. When using Flammacerium on extensive burns, a few cases of methemoglobulinemia have been reported. With silver sulfadiazine, some cases of transient and reversible leukopenia have been described in patients with burns covering more than 15% of the body, but they remain the exception.

**Disadvantages.** When using products which contain high concentrations of silver (Acticoat), a metallic-grey coloration of the wound may occur, which disappears within a few weeks.

### Impregnated Gauze "Tulles" and Interfaces

**Presentation and Composition.** Several types of "tulles" and interfaces are available. The oldest types are impregnated with antibiotics, antiseptics or corticosteroids. Their use is not without danger to the community. They may cause sensitisation to these antibiotics. By destroying the common micro-organisms which colonise slough (without preventing its healing), antiseptics select much more harmful, resistant organisms, and furthermore they may be cytotoxic in vitro to growing cells.

Other, more recently designed tulles and interfaces are impregnated with hypo-allergenic, neutral greasy substances such as vaseline or paraffin (Fig. 9). These interfaces, made of synthetic fibres have a smaller mesh and never adhere to a wound. They are sometimes coated with silicone [24, 26] or combined with CMC [25] (Fig. 10) to form a slightly absorbent gel on the surface of the wound, which facilitates painless dressing removal.

**Method of Use.** These dressings are applied directly to the wound and then covered with a secondary, absorbent dressing (gauze, pads, multi-layer dressing etc.). They need to be changed every day or every other day, depending on the stage of the wound.

**Indications.** The low absorbent potential means that their use should be reserved for little-exuding wounds (dermabrasion, wounds caused by epidermolysis bullosa, burns, superficial wounds or those undergoing epidermisation etc.). These dressings should be used during granulation and epidermisation, particularly on areas deprived of epidermis or at the ultimate phase of healing of a pressure ulcer. Finally, it is possible to place them between the foam of a VAC system and the wound, so as to render dressing changes less painful (the interface preventing granulation tissue from binding to the foam of the VAC dressing).

**Disadvantages.** The mesh of classic tulles is often quite large and granulation occurs through them, so that there is a risk that granulation tissue may be torn away and bleed when the dressing is changed. This problem does not arise with modern interfaces.

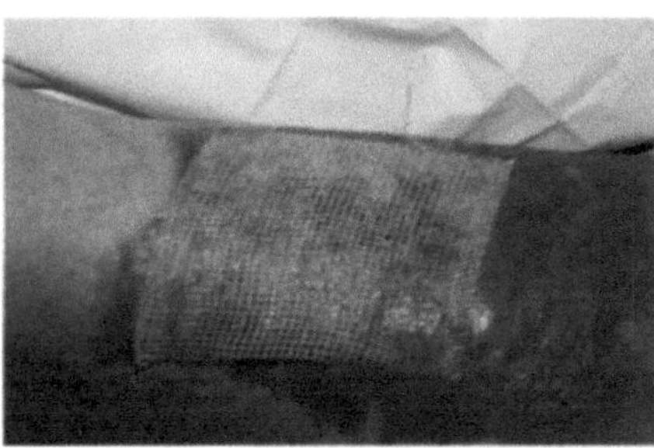

**Fig. 9.** Impregnated gauze on donor site

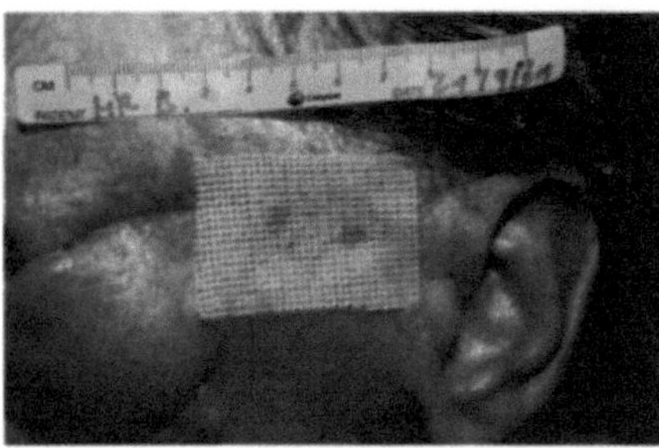

**Fig. 10.** Interface on acute wound

**Contra-Indications.** These products should not be used in the case of heavily exuding wounds.

### Hyaluronic Acid-Based Dressings

**Rationale for the Use of Hyaluronic Acid (HA) to Promote Healing.** Foetal skin heals without leaving a scar. Hyaluronic acid is present at a very high level in the dermis, but this level then declines very rapidly and the skin no longer regenerates but heals leaving a scar. Several experimental studies have demonstrated the value of HA during the different phases of healing, but in vivo, the efficacy of the product is limited by the existence of hyaluronidases.

**Presentation and Composition.** Several types of hyaluronic acid-based products are available to assist wound healing. They range from creams and impregnated gauze with hyaluronic acid, to dressings containing esterified hyaluronic acid, sometimes in combination with alginates.

**Method of Use.** Hyaluronic acid-based dressings are indicated in wounds which generally exude little. In principal, the dressing should be changed daily.

**Indications.** Hyaluronic acid-based dressings have mainly been the subject of studies in chronic wounds [33]. The tolerability of these dressings is excellent.

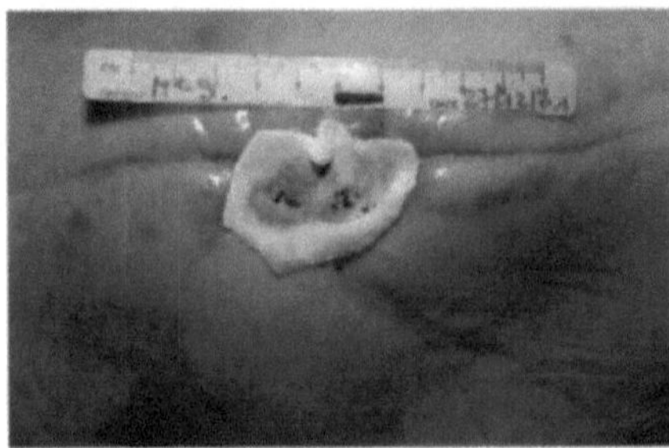

**Fig. 11.** Collagen Matrix Dressing: Promogran on acute wound

### Collagen Matrix Dressing

Promogran is a matrix combining oxidized regenerated cellulose and bovine, prion-free collagen. This collagen matrix dressing modulates and restores the balance of the environment of chronic wounds by binding and inactivating proteases and binding and protecting the growth factors naturally present in the wound (Fig. 11).

Its efficacy has been demonstrated during controlled, randomised studies as a booster to healing in cleansed leg ulcers or diabetic ulcers of the foot. The dressing is applied under an interface, directly onto the bed of the wound. It is changed daily, or less frequently. The tolerability of this product is excellent. If it is used only during the granulation phase of a wound, it can be considered as viable in terms of the time gained in healing [41, 43].

## Conclusion

The dressings and biomaterials available at present for the treatment of wounds only have little specific action on healing phenomena and on shortening the time to closure of a wound. However, they optimise natural healing in a moist environment, improve patient comfort and help nurses in the management of wounds and in allowing longer intervals between dressing changes (Tables 1 and 2).

**Table 1.** The different types of dressings available in France

| Type of dressing | Commercial products |
| --- | --- |
| Hydrocolloid | Algoplaque/Urgoderm, Askina Biofilm, Comfeel Duoderm = Granuflex, Epicol, Hydrocoll, Tegasorb, Tetracolloid |
| Foam and *super-absorbent | Askina transorbent, Allevyn, Biatain, *Cellosorb, Combi-derm, Cutinova foam, Lumiderm 6000, Lyomousse, Mepilex, Syspurderm, Tielle |
| Alginates | Algosteril, Askina Sorb, Comfeel-Seasorb, Dosastéryl, Kaltostat, Melgisorb, Sorbsan, Urgosorb |

**Table 1.** *Continued*

| Type of dressing | Commercial products |
|---|---|
| Hydrofibre | Aquacel |
| Hydrogels | Askina gel, Duoderm hydrogel, Hydrosorb, Intrasite gel, Nu-Gel, Purilon, Urgo hydrogel |
| Charcoal dressings | Actisorb Plus, Carbonet, Cardoflex, Lyomousse C |
| Silver-based dressings | Acticoat, Actisorb Plus, UrgotulS Ag, Flammazine, Cicazine, Advance, Contreet, Aquacel Ag |
| Semi-permeable films | Dermafilm, Epitect, Epiview, Hydrofilm, Mefilm, Opraflex, Opsite Flexigrid, Stéridrap, Tegaderm, Tetrafilm, Visulin |
| Non-medicinal impregnated gauze | Jelonet, Lomatuell, Unitulle, Vaselitulle |
| Interfaces, *silicone interfaces, **paraffin + CMC | Adaptic, Cutiserin, *Mépitel, **Physiotulle, **Urgotul |
| Hyaluronic acid-based dressings | Effidia, Ialuset, Hyalofill |
| Interactive dressings | Promogran |

**Table 2.** Summary of indications for different dressings and biomaterials depending on the stage and appearance of a wound

| Appearance of the wound | Therapeutic alternatives |
|---|---|
| Presence of black, dry, necrotic tissue | Hydrogel, enzymes |
| Presence of fibrin or moist necrotic tissue | Hydrocolloid, hydrogel if little exudate, alginate if heavily exuding, hydrofibre if heavily exuding, enzymes |
| Cavity wound | Alginate ribbon, hydrofibre ribbon, hydrocolloid gel, foam pad |
| Heavily exuding wound | Alginate, hydrofibre, "new-generation" hydrocolloid, foam |
| Granulating wound | Hydrocolloid, foam, hydrogel (hydrofibre alginate) |
| Superficial wound or dermabrasion, superficial burn, donor graft site | Hydrocolloid, hydrocellular or foam, hydrogel, film, tulle and interface |
| Foul-smelling wound | Charcoal dressings |
| Infected wound | Alginate, hydrofibre, charcoal dressings |

# References

1. Alm A, Hornmark AM, Fall PA (1989) Care of pressure sores: a controlled study of the use of hydrocolloid dressing compared with wet saline gauze compresses. Acta Dermatol Venereol (Stockh) 149 [Suppl]: 1–10

2. Apelqvist J, Larsson J, Stenstrom A (1990) Topical treatment of necrotic foot ulcers in diabetic patients: a comparative trial of Duoderm and MeZinc. Br J Derm 123: 787–792

3. Bale S, Baker N, Crook H, Rayman A, Rayman G, Harding KG (2001) Exploring the use of an alginate dressing for diabetic foot ulcers. J Wound Care. 10: 81–84

4. Barnett A, Berkowitz RL, Mills R, Vitnes LM (1983) Comparison of synthetic adhesive moisture vapor permeable and fine mesh gauze dressings for split skin graft donor sites. Am J Surg 145: 379–381

5. Basse P, Slim E, Lohmann M (1992) Treatment of donor sites: calcium alginate versus paraffin gauze. Acta Chir Plast 34: 92–98

6. Belmin J, Meaume S, Rabus MT, Bohbot S (2002) Sequential treatment with calcium alginate dressings and hydrocolloid dressings accelerates pressure ulcer healing in older subjects: a multicenter randomized trial of sequential versus nonsequential treatment with hydrocolloid dressings alone. J Am Geriatr Soc 50: 269–274

7. Brandrup F, Menne T, Agren M (1990) A randomized trial of two occlusive dressings in the treatment of leg ulcers. Acta Derm Venereol (Stockh) 70: 231–235

8. Caruso DM, Foster KN, Hermans MH, Rick C (2004) Aquacel Ag in the management of partial-thickness burns: results of a clinical trial. J Burn Care Rehabil 25: 89–97

9. Colin D, Kurring PA, Yvon C (1996) Managing sloughy pressure sores. J Wound Care 5: 444–446

10. Dawson C, Armstrong MWJ, Fulford SCV, Fauqi RM, Galland RB (1992) Use of calcium alginate to pack abcess cavities: a control clinical trial. J Royal Coll Surg 37: 177–179

11. Eisenberg M (1986) The effect of occlusiv dressings on reepithelialization of wounds in children with epidermolysis bullosa. J Pediatr Surg 21: 892–894

12. Freshwater MF, Su CT, Hoopes JE (1978) A comparison of polyurethane foam dressing and fine mesh gauze in the healing of donor sites. Plast Reconstr Surg 61: 275–276

13. Friedman SJ, Daniel SU (1984) Management of leg ulcers with hydrocolloid occlusive dressing. Arch Derm 120: 1329–1336

14. Hampson JP (1996) The use of metronidazole in the treatment of malodorous wounds. J Wound Care 5: 421–426

15. Handfield-Jones SE, Grattan CEH (1988) Comparison of a hydrocolloid dressing and paraffin gauze in the treatment of venous ulcers. Br J Derm 118: 425–427

16. Hermans MHE, Hermans RP (1986) Duoderm, an alternative dressing for smaller burns. Burns 12: 214–219

17. Hinman CC (1963) Effect of air exposure and occlusion on experimental human skin wound. Nature 200: 377–379

18. Holloway S, Bale S, Harding K, Robinson B, Ballard K (2002) Evaluating the effectiveness of a dressing for use in malodorous, exuding wounds. Ostomy Wound Manage 48: 22–28

19. Innes ME, Umraw N, Fish JS, Gomez M, Cartotto RC (2001) The use of silver coated dressings on donor site wounds: a prospective, controlled matched pair study. Burns 27: 621–627

20. Karlsmark T, Agerslev RH, Bendz SH, Larsen JR, Roed-Petersen J, Andersen KE (2003) Clinical performance of a new silver dressing, Contreet Foam, for chronic exuding venous leg ulcers. J Wound Care 12: 351–354

21. Lawrence JE, Blake GB (1991) A comparison of calcium alginate and scarlet red dressings in the healing of split thickness skin graft donor sites. Br J Plast Surg 44: 247–249

22. Limova M, Troyer-Caudle J (2002) Controlled, randomized clinical trial of 2 hydrocolloid dressings in the management of venous insufficiency ulcers. J Vasc Nurs 20: 22–32

23. Loiterman DA, Byers PH (1991) Effect of a hydrocellular polyurethane dressing on chronic venous ulcer healing. Wounds 3: 178–181

24. Meaume S, Van De Looverbosch D, Heyman H, Romanelli M, Ciangherotti A, Charpin S (2003)y to compare a new self-adherent soft silicone dressing with a self-adherent polymer dressing in stage II pressure ulcers. Ostomy Wound Manage. 49:44–51

25. Meaume S, Senet P, Dumas R, Carsin H, Pannier M, Bohbot S (2002)l: a novel non-adherent lipidocolloid dressing. Br J Nurs 11 [Suppl 16] S42–43, S46–50

26. Meuleneire F (2002) Using a soft silicone-coated net dressing to manage skin tears. J Wound Care 11: 365–369

27. Milburn PB, Zinger JC, Milburn MA (1989) Treatment of scleroderma skin ulcers with a hydrocolloid membrane. J Am Acad Derm (Part 1) 21: 200–204
28. Muller G, Winkler Y, Kramer A (2003) Antibacterial activity and endotoxin-binding capacity of Actisorb Silver 220. J Hosp Infect 53: 211–214
29. Neal DE, Whalley PC, Flowers MW, Wilson DH (1981) The effects of an adherent polyurethane film and conventional absorbent dressing in patients with small partial thickness burns. Br J Clin Pract 35: 254–257
30. Nemeth AJ, Eaglstein WH, Taylor JR, Peerson LJ, Falanga V (1991) Faster healing and less pain in skin biopsy site treated with occlusive dressing. Arch Derm 127: 1679–1683
31. Nielsen PG, Madsen SM, Stromberg L (1990) Treatment of chronic leg ulcers with a hydrocolloid dressing. Acta Derm Venereol (Stockh) 152 [Suppl]: 1–12
32. Oleske DM, Smith XP, White P, Pottage J, Donovan MI (1986) A randomized clinical trial of two dressing methods for treatment of low-grade pressure ulcers. JET 13: 90–98
33. Ortonne JP (1996) A controlled study of the activity of hyaluronic acid in the treatment of venous leg ulcers. J Dermatol Treat 7: 75–81
34. Phillips TJ, Kapoor V, Provan A, Ellerin T (1993) A randomized prospective study of a hydroactive dressing vs. conventional treatment after shave biopsy excision. Arch Derm 129: 859–860
35. Pometan JP, Chanut MC, Alla P (1989) Flore bactérienne et escarre. Le moniteur Hospitalier 11: 3–4
36. Porter JM (1991) A comparative investigation of reepithelialization of split skin graft donor areas after application of hydrocolloid and alginate dressings. Br. J Plast Surg 44: 333–377
37. Sayag J, Meaume S, Bohbot S (1996) Healing properties of calcium alginate dressings. J Wound Care 5: 357–362
38. Thomas DR, Goode PS, LaMaster K, Tennyson T, Parnell LK (1999) A comparison of an opaque foam dressing versus a transparent film dressing in the management of skin tears in institutionalized subjects. Ostomy Wound Manage 45: 22–24, 27–28
39. Thomas DW, Hill CM, Lewis MA, Stephens P, Walker R, Von Der Weth A (2000) Randomized clinical trial of the effect of semi-occlusive dressings on the microflora and clinical outcome of acute facial wounds. Wound Repair Regen 8: 258–263
40. Thomas S, McCubbin P (2003) An in vitro analysis of the antimicrobial properties of 10 silver-containing dressings. J Wound Care 12: 305–308
41. Veves A, Sheehan P, Pham HT (2002) A randomized, controlled trial of Promogran (a collagen/oxidized regenerated cellulose dressing) vs. standard treatment in the management of diabetic foot ulcers. Arch Surg 137: 822–827
42. Viciano V, Castera JE, Medrano J, Aguilo J, Torro J, Botella MG, Toldra N (2000) Effect of hydrocolloid dressings on healing by second intention after excision of pilonidal sinus. Eur J Surg 166: 229–232
43. Vin F, Teot L, Meaume S (2002) The healing properties of Promogran in venous leg ulcers. J Wound Care 11: 335–341
44. Vloemans AF, Soesman AM, Kreis RW, Middelkoop E (2001) A newly developed hydrofibre dressing, in the treatment of partial-thickness burns. Burns 27: 167–173
45. Von Lindern JJ, Niederhagen B, Appel T, Berge S (2002) Treatment of soft tissue defects with exposed bone in the head and face region with alginates and hydrocolloid dressings. J Oral Maxillofac Surg 60: 1126–1130
46. Winter GD (1963) Effect of air drying and dressings on the surface of wounds. Nature 197: 91–93
47. Wyatt D, Mc Gowan DN, Najarian MP (1990) Comparison of a hydrocolloid dressing and silver sulfadiazine cream in the outpatient management of second-degree burns. J Trauma 30: 857–865
48. Xakellis GC, Chrischillis EA (1992) Hydrocolloid versus saline-gauze dressings in treating pressure ulcers: a cost-effectiveness analysis. Arch Phys Med Rehab 73: 463–468
49. Zuccarelli FA (1992) A comparativ study of the hydrocellular polyurethane dressing Allevyn and the hydrocolloid dressing Duoderm in the treatment of leg ulcers. Phlebologie 45: 529–533

# Suture Materials and Techniques

U.A. Dietz, E.S. Debus, W. Hamelmann, N.G. Czeczko,
U.E. Ziegler, A. Thiede

## Introduction

A smooth healing with minimal scarring is an important goal in every wound management of the skin. Patients will judge the work of the surgeon plastically, that is on the looks of the scar; so the scar makes the reputation of the surgeon. The great variety of skin wounds calls for a differentiated approach to each one, which again is based on individual suture techniques and a multitude of available suture materials. In addition, the degree of a wound's contamination as well as a number of systemic and local factors may influence the healing process.

The healing of wounds depends on several factors, one of them being the tissue itself (pH, bacterial load, physiological stress and blood supply, the cell type responsible for the healing process and collagen metabolism). Broad scars e.g. develop especially in inadequate primary wound closure or in patients with hereditary predisposition (keloid formation in coloured patients). Some of the complications of skin sutures can be prevented by appropriated technique. The application of adequate suture materials, needles and the correct surgical technique are elementary for adequate results. In the following, suture materials and the basic principles of surgical technique in wound closure are presented.

## Suture Materials

The choice of the surgical suture material depends on a variety of factors, all of which have to be weighed up carefully. On the one hand, the choice of the suture derives from objective criteria, which are defined by the physical properties of the material as well as its biochemical attributes interacting with the body. On the other hand, subjective criteria such as handling characteristics and operative habits of the surgeon are to be considered as well.

Suture materials are discriminated according to constitutional characteristics, distinguishing parameters and handling properties. It is of value to choose the appropriate suture material in combination with an adequate needle. Constitutionally, surgical sutures are described regarding their origin (organic or synthetic), their absorbability (absorbable or non-absorbable) and regarding the structure of the material (monofilament or multifilament). Depending on their absorption and function time, absorbable sutures are divided into three main groups: ultra-short-term, short-term and medium-term absorption. The function period of an absorbable suture is the period of time in which it retains a functional tensile strength in the tissue. FT50 (function time 50%) is the period of time in which the absorbable su-

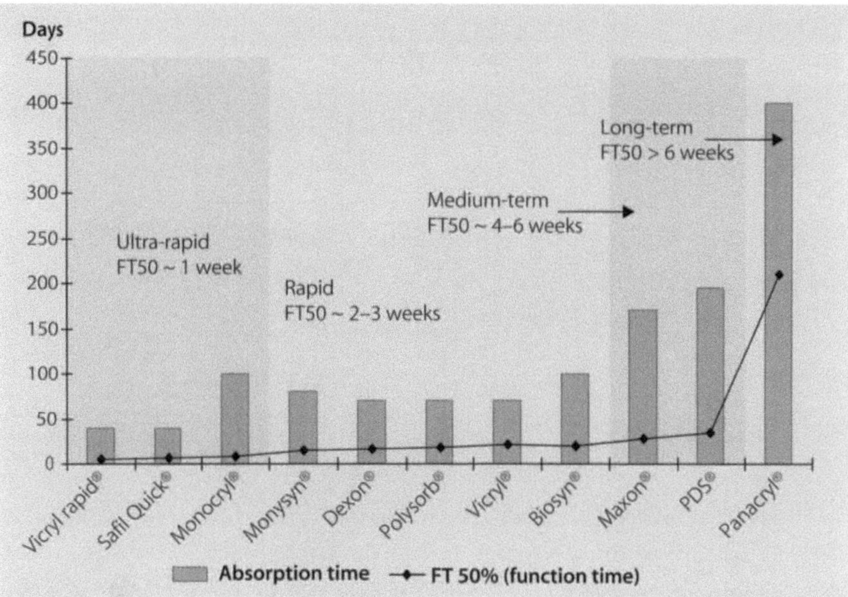


**Fig. 1.** Current absorbable suture materials with regard to their absorption and function time

ture still holds 50% of its original tensile strength. Absorption time is known as the period between the suture's implantation and its histological disappearance (complete hydrolysis) [1] (Fig. 1).

One distinguishes between monofilament sutures (homogen, unstructured and smooth surface) and multifilament sutures (multitude of single filaments). The multifilament sutures may be twisted (catgut and cotton) or braided (Vicryl, Dexon II, silk, polyester-based and polyamide-based sutures). In addition, multifilament surgical sutures can have their twisted core covered by a jacket (pseudo-monofilament); the coating has substantial influence on the function period and handling properties of the suture material [2–8] (Fig. 2). The surface of the suture material has a considerable influence on the tissue as well as on the handling. Due to their rough surface, multifilament sutures have a considerable sawing effect with pronounced tissue trauma, compared to monofilament sutures. In addition, threaded uncoated suture materials have a capillary effect (favouring bacterial and fluid transport along the thread). Multifilament sutures have a better knotting quality with better holding capacity (higher knot strength and knot security than monofilament sutures), and they are more flexible than monofilament sutures.

For a plastic skin closure, monofilament non-absorbable suture materials are used to guarantee a smooth and atraumatic passage through tissue and to prevent suture granulomas or pronounced absorption reactions. Suturing the mucous has to meet different demands: since defects of the mucosa regenerate within a few days and the mucosa is not exposed to pressure and tensile load, it is important to use suture material with a short FT50. In trauma surgery, suture material is required to have a long-lasting FT50, as several months pass until final wound stability is

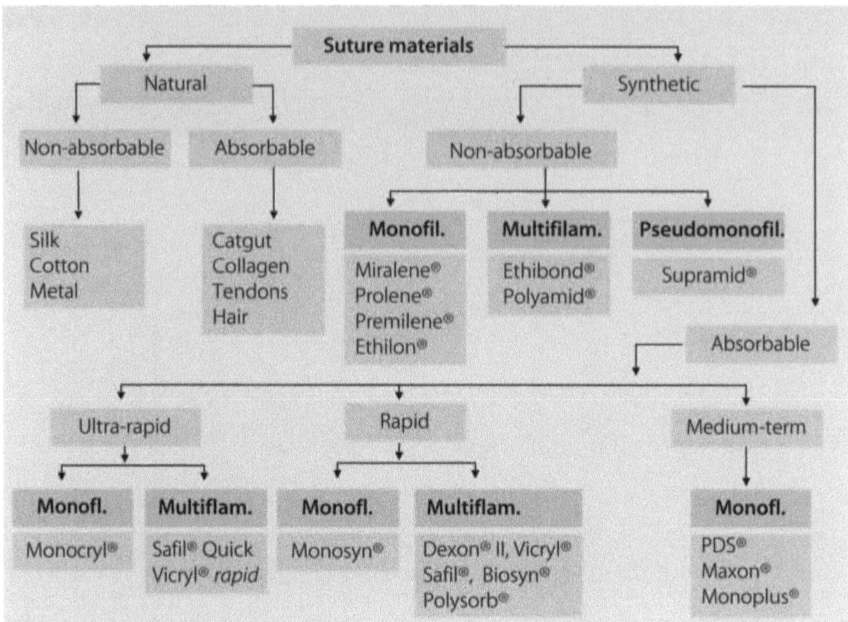

**Fig. 2.** Summary of suture materials

achieved (suture of tendons), so medium-term absorbable synthetic sutures should be used. To prevent the implantation of a persisting foreign body, absorbable sutures should be used preferentially whenever the sutures cannot be removed after the completion of the wound healing.

## Needle Configuration

A harmonic suture–needle combination and its attachment are very important. The development and conception of atraumatic sutures includes not only the properties of the thread, but also the configuration of the needle and the type of attachment to it. The attachment of the suture to the needle may have three different configurations: closed eye, French eye (split or spring) and eyeless (swaged, with the suture being bonded to the needle). The suture should be like the direct prolongation of the needle so that the tissue trauma can be optimally reduced.

The most important biomechanical attributes of surgical needles are ductility, bending resistance (elastic deformation with ultimate breaking moment) and sharpness. Needles from different companies offer an immense range of quality, which goes from breaking after a single bending stress to breaking after bending up to 27 times. These data do not depend so much on the needle configuration as on the

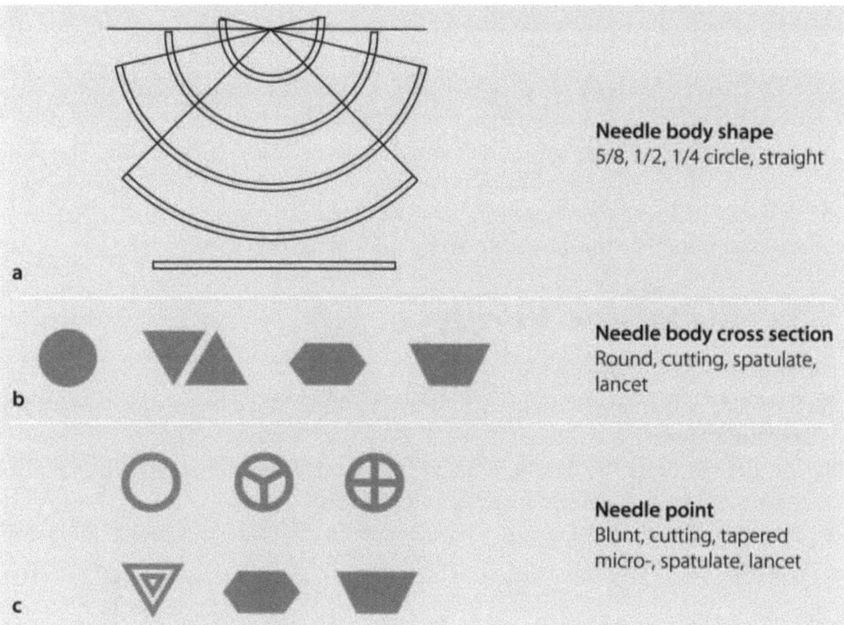



**Fig. 3.** Anatomy of surgical needles

needle's steel and size. The sharpness also depends on the needle's size and on the manufacturing process and type of the needle point: larger needles have a higher cutting power than smaller ones. Needles with cutting (sharpened point, they cut through the tissue) or tapered point (they pierce and spread the tissue) have lower tissue penetration resistance than blunt-point needles (Fig. 3).

## Suture of the Skin

### Common Guidelines

In the surgical approach to wounds, common guidelines have to be pursued. In injuries, the status of tetanus immunisation and prophylaxis with antibiotics has to be checked first. In elective procedures, the direction of the incision of the skin has to be parallel to Langer's lines (general course of bundles of connective tissue within the dermis, the so-called lines of reduced skin tension, syn. = cleavage lines). Incisions and wounds that cross these cleavage lines tend to be widened by inherent tension. In injuries an adequate debridement of the wound (Friedrich's[1] wound debridement) is necessary; highly traumatised tissue with impaired blood supply affects wound healing negatively. The wound has to be cleared from foreign bodies and cleaned with an antiseptic solution. Whenever possible, the wound should be closed primarily by suture after careful haemostasis. In special cases and for clinical control purposes (in the case of exposed fractures), wound defects can be temporarily covered with an alloplastic material and closed secondarily, after safety control and exclusion of wound infection. Wound edges have to be sutured correctly and are not allowed to be under tension; a slight eversion is desirable. The choice of adequate suture material has to be managed individually. Additional injury of the tissue by manipulation has to be avoided. The post-operative functional immobilisation can further the smooth healing in selected cases [9].

### Anatomical Basis of the Skin Layers

The skin has three main layers:
- the outer epidermis (with the stratum corneum – horn layer – and the stratum germinativum),
- the dermis (syn. = corium, with vessels, eccrine and apocrine perspiratory glands, sebaceous glands and hair follicles) and
- the subcutaneous tissue (syn. = Tela subcutanea, hypodermis), with adipose and connective tissue).

Epidermis and dermis together are called skin (syn. = cutis) (Fig. 4).

### Principles of Knotting

In describing a suture, several definitions are important. **Included layers** describe the number of anatomical layers which are included by the suture. The intracutaneous suture includes only the dermis (syn. = intradermic or corium suture), whereas the single-stitch and Donati's suture include the subcutaneous tissue in addition. **Number of rows** relates to the number of sutures that are performed one upon another; for example, an interrupted intracutaneous suture with a concomitant running intracutaneous suture (see below). **Shape of the suture** describes the geometry of the suture; the skin suture can be everted or with exact apposition of the edges. **Type of suture progression** describes if the suture is performed either in a single stitch or a continuous, running way [10].

In knotting the suture it is important to avoid too much tension on the tissue and ischemia to the tissue grasped within the loop. The key is to transfer only the minimally needed tension to the wound edges. A perfect knotting technique is indispensable. Knots can be symmetric or asymmetric. Symmetric knots (Fig. 5a) (square knot and surgeon's knot) offer a sliding-safe configuration; after knotting the first two slings, no further slippage is possible. In order to create a symmetric knot, two rules have to be noted (Livingstone's laws):
- At each step, the ears of the suture have to return to the initial position after having changed their sides in performing the anterior turn (half-knot or sling).
- In doing so, mirror-image-like movements or crossing movements have to be carried out with the surgeon's hands.
- In contrast to the symmetrical knots (Fig. 5b), the tension on the loop can be adjusted in asymmetric knots even after knotting the first two or three turns (slings) [11–14].

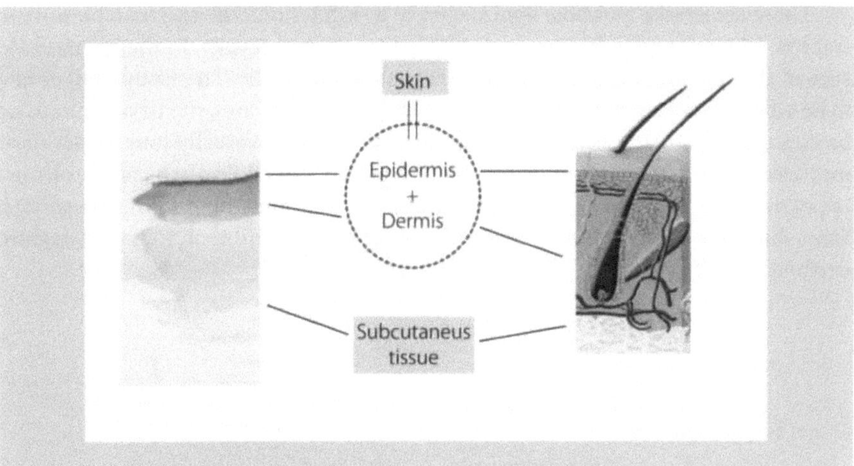



**Fig. 4.** Anatomy of the skin

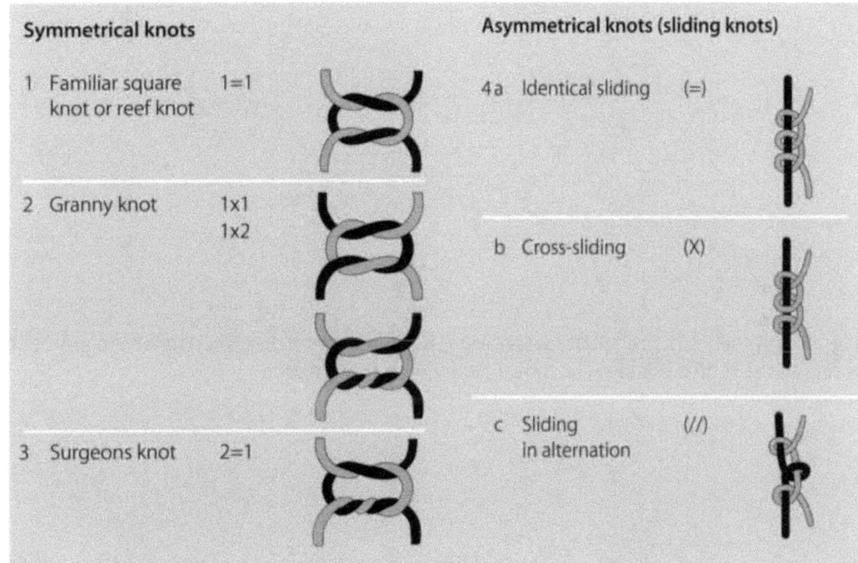



**Fig. 5.** Morphology of surgical knots

### *Principles of Suturing*

The suture of the skin should include the dermis and sometimes the subcutaneous tissue. The epidermis itself (with its stratum corneum) cannot be sutured, since needle and thread can tear through very easily (e.g. the palm of the hand and the sole of the foot).

There are several possible approaches to a skin lesion. The skin can be sutured, stapled, adapted with a zipper or glued (2-octyl-cyanoacrylat). In the primary closure of the skin, the wound edges are adapted anatomically. The wound edges have to be adapted tension-free by the suture and, in tying the knot, the tissue should not be strangulated by the suture. Leaving the sutures unnecessarily long in the tissue may cause an epithelisation of the stitch channel, which, in turn, can result in a hypertrophic scar. Scars that run parallel to the skin folds tend to disappear later. Scars that cross Langer's lines are always under tension and tend to have a negative aesthetic result.

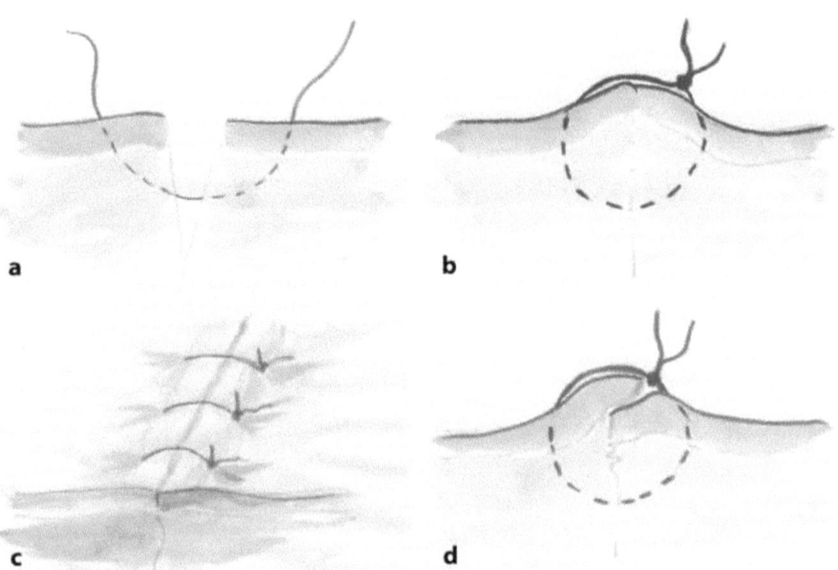

**Fig. 6a–d.** Simple stitch. **a** Stitch morphology; **b** completed stitch; **c** interrupted simple-stitch suture of the skin; **d** common technical failure with invagination

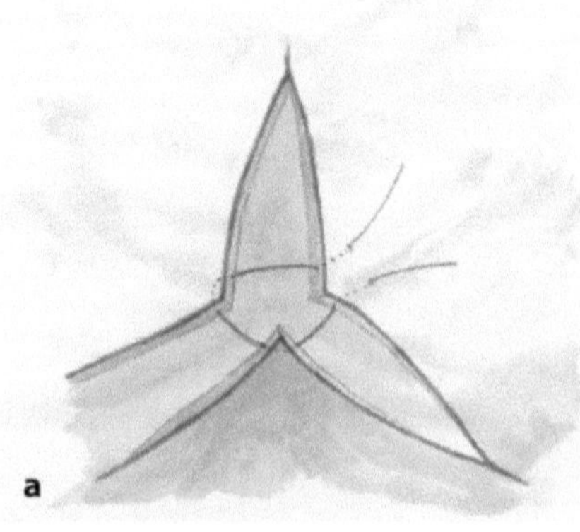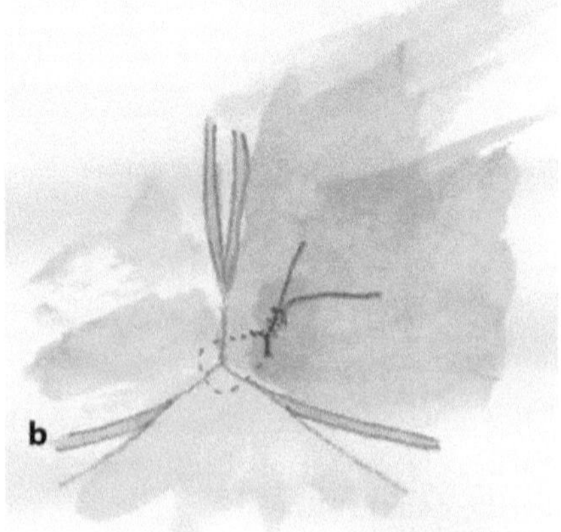

**Fig. 7a,b.** Three-point-U or corner suture. **a** Stitch path; **b** final view after tying the knot

The subcutaneous tissue is well vascularised but offers only a weak resistance for suture anchorage. It is discussed if the subcutaneous tissue should be sutured at all. Nevertheless, complications can occur by subcutaneous implantation of suture material (granuloma of the suture material or suture fistulas). A number of authors recommend the subcutaneous suture as a mechanical relief for the skin suture. The filaments are knotted with slight tension, because otherwise fat necrosis and/or sterile wound abscesses can occur. To prevent disturbances of the subcutaneous tissue wound healing, placing a suction drainage may be an efficient measure.

## Common Suture Techniques

### *Simple Stitch (syn. = Interrupted Stitch, Simple Through-and-Through Suture)*

The simple-stitch suture is recommended for most application fields. The needle should enter the epidermis at a right angle (vertical to the skin); the natural curvature of the needle should be followed by passing it through the tissue. The edges of the wound are to be seized only lightly with tweezers (to avoid additional trauma of tissue) (Fig. 6). In the case of uneven, long wound edges, symmetry can be achieved by progressively dividing the wound into half. A slight eversion is almost always favourable; inverted sutures of the skin can lead to defects and larger scars. The simple-stitch suture should not be knotted too tightly, in order to prevent strangulation and oedema of the seized tissue, which may lead to disturbances of the wound healing. Dead spaces are to be avoided in any case. In general, sutures which are placed close together and grasp less tissue lead to a good aesthetic result.

In the case of lacerated wounds, a three-point-U or a corner suture may be helpful. It corresponds to a horizontal running mattress suture with components of a common simple-stitch and an intracutaneous suture; the knot is placed away from the connecting point of the wound edges (Fig. 7).

### *Vertical Mattress Suture (syn. = Donati's[2] Suture)*

Donati's suture has a wide–wide–close–close structure, whereas the wide-through stitches seize the subcutaneous tissue and the close-through stitches seize only the dermis. Also in deeper wounds, they render a good eversion of the wound edges and a safe approximation of the depth; this prevents the formation of dead space and haematoma (Fig. 8). So the skin is adapted precisely, and by seizing the subcutaneous tissue lateral of the skin through the stitches, the tension forces are kept away from the wound edges. The knots should always be placed laterally to the wound borders. In doing so, a very good aesthetic result is achieved already after 2 weeks, but especially after 6 and 12 months [10, 16]. Also with Donati's suture, prevention of tension at the wound edges should be observed, as described above; otherwise, the advantages of the suture are lost and unnecessary rough scars develop. Donati's suture can be performed in either single-stitch or running method.

A slightly different version of Donati's suture is Allgöwer's[3] suture: The shape comprises a subcutaneous suture at one side and an intracutaneous suture (sunk), which represent a transition between Donati's suture and the intracutaneous suture (see below). Even though the aesthetic result is very good, there is the danger of not

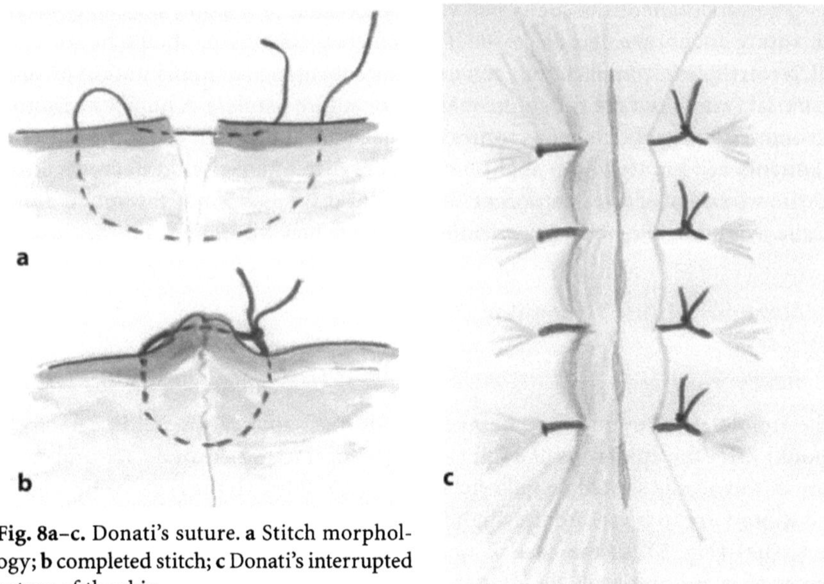

**Fig. 8a–c.** Donati's suture. **a** Stitch morphology; **b** completed stitch; **c** Donati's interrupted suture of the skin

seizing enough tissue while puncturing the layers on the "sunk" side; this is the case at the extremities, where the surgeon finds only a thin subcutaneous tissue and does not have enough draw-back possibilities with the needle in order to perform an optimal stitch.

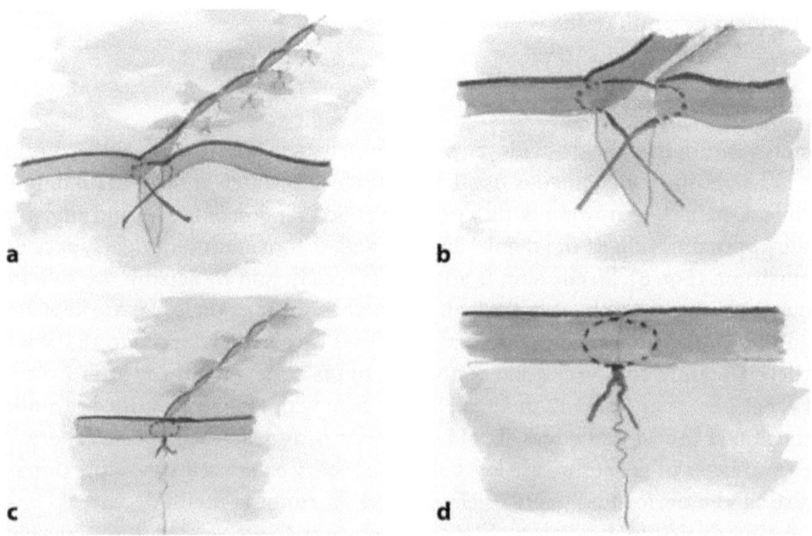

**Fig. 9a–d.** Interrupted intracutaneous suture with counter-sunk knot. **a,b** Stitch morphology; **c,d** completed stitch [note the gaping shape of the wound edges; this suture has to be complemented by an additional suture (see text)]

### Interrupted Intracutaneous Suture with Counter-Sunk Knot

It is important that the interrupted intracutaneous suture is placed perpendicular to the skin and directly underneath its surface (needle passage from the boundary between subcutaneous tissue and the dermis through the dermis, at a right angle) (Fig. 9). There should be no tension on the wound after knotting the sutures; in some cases, undermining or detaching the dermis slightly from the subcutaneous tissue may provide an improved aesthetic result. The indicated suture material for this technique is an absorbable monofilament thread. The data of a nation-wide survey in Germany shows that 47.5% of the German plastic surgeons use the interrupted intracutaneous suture with counter-sunk knot in face surgery and 86.3% use it in the area of the torso [15]. In addition to the interrupted intracutaneous suture with counter-sunk knot, a classical running intracutaneous suture, simple-stitch or horizontal mattress suture are possible, except at the nose, palpebras and ears.

### Horizontal Mattress Suture (Interrupted or Running)

The running horizontal mattress suture is a fast and sealing suture alternative. The suture is used in the area of the dorsum of the hand, after laparotomy closure or in cases of rotation flaps or secondary wound closure after vacuum-assisted therapy (Fig. 10).

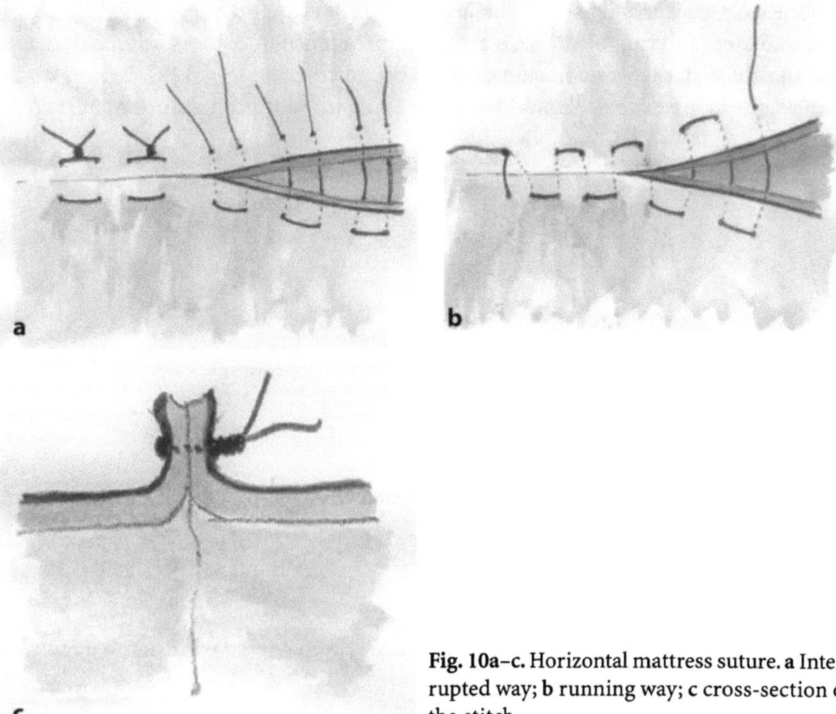

**Fig. 10a–c.** Horizontal mattress suture. **a** Interrupted way; **b** running way; **c** cross-section of the stitch

### Intracutaneous Suture (syn. = Intradermal or Subcuticular Running Suture, Halsted's[4] Suture)

The thread is pulled in meander manner through the dermis (Fig. 11a). Since the blood supply runs within the dermis, the running intracutaneous suture affects it less than single stitches do. Both ends of the filament are knotted either in the dermis (towards the subcutaneous tissue) or are fixed with adhesive tape on the surface of the skin. It is also possible to sink the ends in L-form (the sliding of the wound is prevented by redirecting the needle at a 90° angle through the skin surface) [10, 17]. Absorbable or non-absorbable monofilaments are used in the size 4/0 or 5/0 USP. Absorbable sutures are not removed and remain until their complete hydrolysis within the dermis after 90–120 days (Monocryl and Monosyn). In the case of non-absorbable sutures, these are removed after 4–7 days by the ends at the wound as well as by the loops of suture in between (Prolene, Premilene, Ethilon). Common needles for intracutaneous sutures are 3/8th circle, with cutting point. In the case of unnoticed back-suturing, the approximation of the edges may be shrunk zigzag-wise; this can be prevented by passing the needle in a symmetrical way through the dermis.

### Stapling of the Skin

Stapling of the skin for wound closure is a popular technique. The speed of the procedure and its good aesthetic result are decisive. Skin stapling promotes an anatomic approximation of the respective layers; the lateral contact between the closed staple and the skin leads to a tension relief at the site of the wound edges (Fig. 12a). Inversion and step building of the skin are the most common complications; they may lead to a delay in the wound healing and to broad scarring (Fig. 12b). To remove the staples, the same criteria should be followed as for common suture material (see below).

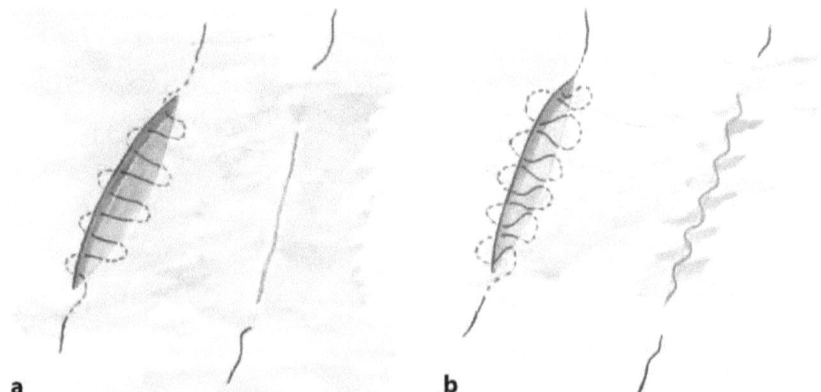

**Fig. 11a,b.** Halsted's suture. **a** Ideal stitch morphology with linear wound line; **b** unintended retrograde stitching, with contorted wound line

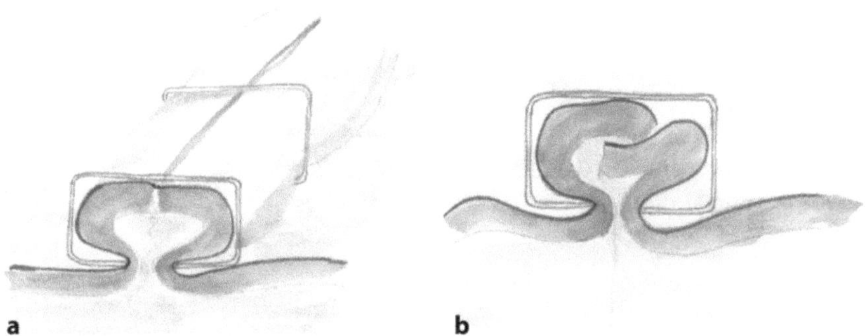



**Fig. 12a,b.** Skin stapling. **a** Anatomical adaptation of the skin with slight eversion; **b** undesirable inversion and poor edge adaptation

## Suture Removal Depending on the Anatomical Location

Removal of suture material (threads or staples) should take place as early as possible in the process of wound healing. The aim is a stress-secure linear scar with minimal tendency to developing a pronounced scarring in the follow-up. The time for removal of skin sutures varies with the different body locations. Sutures in face and neck area can already be removed after 4–5 days (SteriStrips should be applied afterwards, to prevent tension on the wound edges), on trunk and inguinal region after 8–10, on the upper extremity 10–12 and on the lower extremity after 12–14 days [15] (Fig. 13).

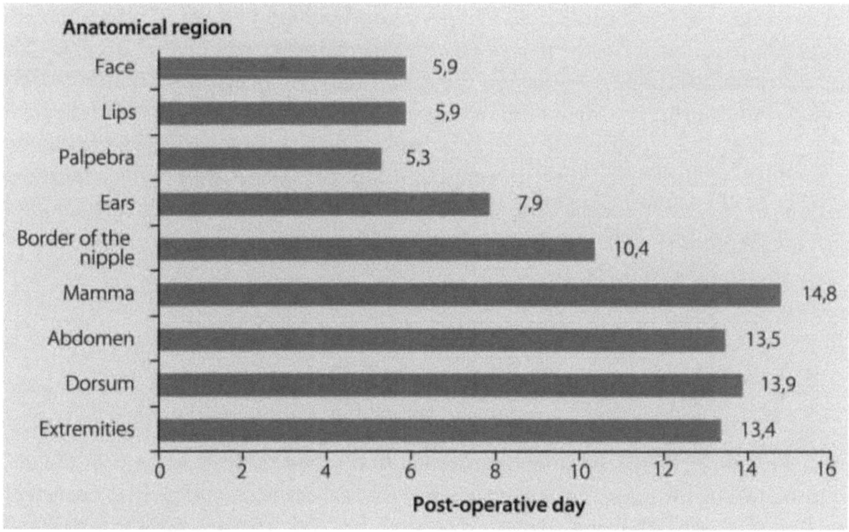



**Fig. 13.** Removal of sutures

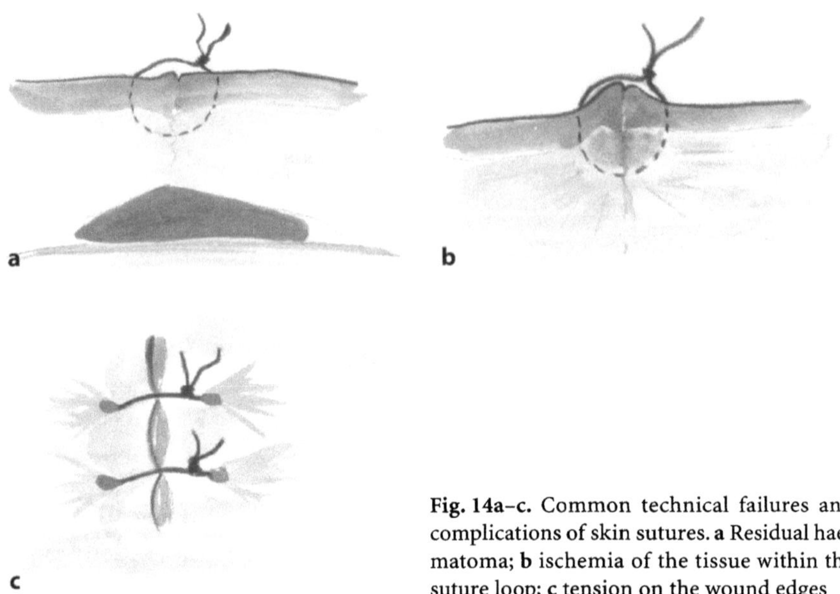

Fig. 14a–c. Common technical failures and complications of skin sutures. **a** Residual haematoma; **b** ischemia of the tissue within the suture loop; **c** tension on the wound edges

## Technical Failures and Complications of Skin Sutures

Insufficient apposition of the anatomical layers is the most common mistake in performing skin sutures. It results in delayed wound healing, dehiscence of the wound and broad scarring. Dead spaces, haematomas and tension on the wound edges are the most common sources of wound-healing complications. Reasons for haematoma may be dead spaces or insufficient haemostasis. Haematomas are a favourable culture medium for bacteria; the placement of suction drains (e.g. Redon[5] drainage) in the subcutaneous tissue may prevent the formation of a haematoma (patients with coagulation disorders). Other sources of complications may be insufficient surgical debridement, the violation of Langer's lines, poor knotting technique (loose or unintended asymmetrical knot), strangulation of the tissue in tying the knot and tension on the wound edges (Fig. 14). Last but not least, leaving dog ears can end in a bad aesthetic result.

## Suture Techniques for Fascias

A fascial suture is exposed to greater stress than other sutures. Sutures of the abdominal fascia, for example, are exposed to increased intra-abdominal pressures because of bowel distension, coughing or pressing. Tendons also have to withstand higher pressure after suturing. The healing of a fascia and a tendon requires more time than the healing of the skin or the bowel. The original tensile strength of fascias is reached after several weeks, as compared to the skin, where it is reached after the 10th post-operative day, or the bowel after 14 days. An early failure of fascial sutures (e.g. tearing out of the suture or rupture of the suture) can lead to major complications, such as hernias of the abdominal wall.

Fascias can be sutured with a running suture or in single-stitch technique. The running suture leads to an implantation of greater foreign material but has the advantage that the tension caused by the suture is divided over the total length of the wound. Functionally, this means that with increasing pressure the stress on a running suture is divided evenly and a breaking of the suture is rare; with a single stitch the pressure is transferred locally, which can result in a dehiscence. In closing the Linea alba of the abdomen, it is important to keep the proportion between the suture length and wound length of approx. 4:1 [19]. Therefore, non-absorbable sutures (Prolene) or medium-term absorbable sutures (PDS for abdominal wall and tendons) qualify for suturing fascia. However, rapid-absorbable sutures can be used for closure of muscular compartments (Dexon II, Vicryl).

## Progressive Skin Traction (syn. = Dermatotraction)

Whenever a wound or a soft-tissue defect cannot be closed primarily or secondarily, it is important to have an alternative therapy concept. This can be achieved by means of rotation flaps, by skin transplantation or progressive skin traction. Skin transplantation is discussed in a specific chapter in this book. In progressive skin traction, the chronic wound edges are brought together with intermittent tangential pull over several days, which can result in wound reduction or even in wound closure. The skin responds to the traction with distension; the plane distension of the skin's surface contributes to the stepwise reduction of the wound area. This is made possible mostly by the collagen fibres of the skin [20].

The main indication for progressive skin traction is the closure of large, primary wound defects as well as fascial incisions after decompression of compartment syndrome at the extremities [20, 21].

The procedure for progressive skin traction is as follows. The wound edges are surrounded by two silicon sticks or adapted Redon drainages. The suture at each wound edge enlaces the silicon sticks and is performed with a non-absorbable, monofile suture of the strength 1 USP (nylon or polypropylene) (Fig. 15a)[6]. The silicon sticks surrounding the wound offer an additional anchorage to the suture, reinforcing the tensile strength of the skin. The stitch technique corresponds to a Donati suture. In knotting, it is very important to do a perfect asymmetric knot (Fig. 5b) in order to allow the progressive tightening (Fig. 15b). Tightening of the wound is done meanly every 2–3 days, normally up to four times a day, in a total period of 8–12 days. In doing so, an average of 77% of all wounds can be closed completely [20].

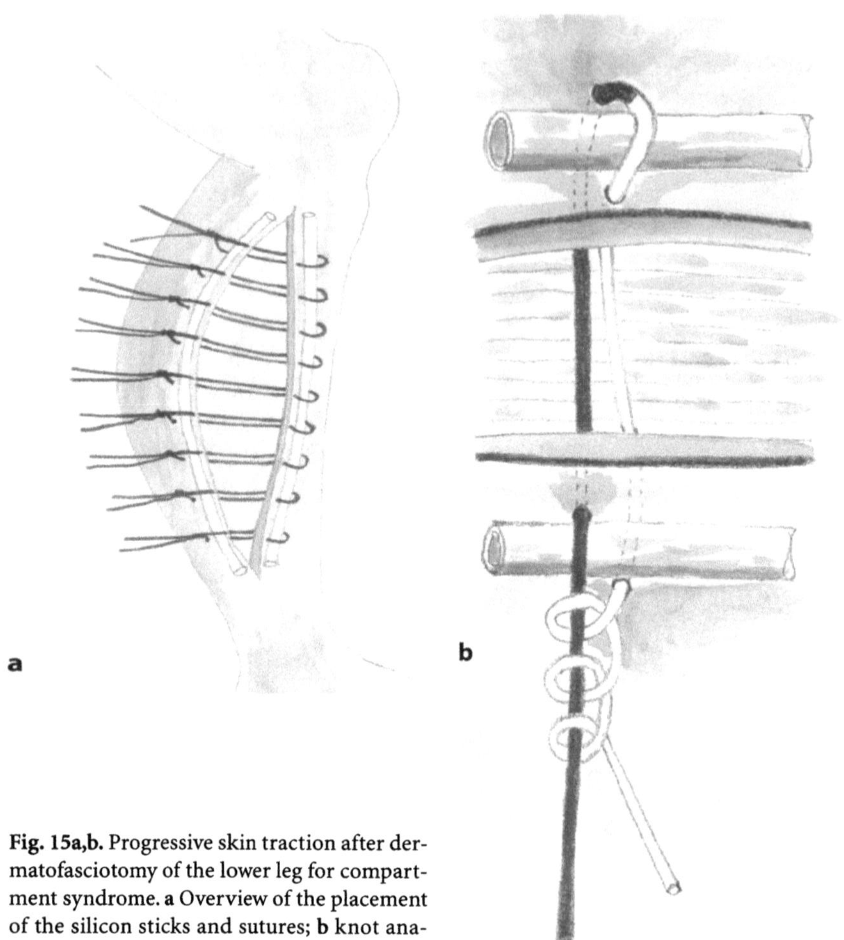

**Fig. 15a,b.** Progressive skin traction after dermatofasciotomy of the lower leg for compartment syndrome. **a** Overview of the placement of the silicon sticks and sutures; **b** knot anatomy in detail (asymmetrical knot)

## The Infected Wound

The surgical suture material may have an influence on the course of an infection. The suture's structure (monofilament or multifilament), its basic substance and its absorbability characteristics may have different behaviours in infection and interact with the course of the infection (Table 1). Also the suture technique plays an important role: both the number of suture rows as well as the layers included are correlated with different healing patterns; single-stitch sutures may be more easily drained in comparison to running sutures.

Suture material behaves differently in infected and in non-infected wounds, depending on its chemical composition; absorbable threads may lose their tensile strength prematurely, influenced by the wound's pH and type of bacterial colonisation. Last but not least, bacteria may migrate into the core of multifilament sutures

**Table 1.** Behaviour of different suture materials in infected tissue

| | Suture material | Behaviour in infected tissue |
|---|---|---|
| **Absorbable** | Dexon II®, Vicryl® | Increased absorption (depending on the type of bacteria)<br>Potentially anti-infectious activity (polyglycolic acid) |
| | PDS® | Increased absorption (depending on the type of bacteria) |
| | Maxon® | Increased absorption (depending on the type of bacteria) |
| **Non-absorbable** | Supramid® | Uninfluenced |
| | Prolene®, Premilene® | Uninfluenced |
| | Steel® | Uninfluenced |

(either by capillarity or by its own flagellum-related motility) and by being protected from the immune system, they can be responsible for late suture-related fistulas and chronic inflammatory reactions [18].

## Summary

The goal of wound management is complete healing with minimal scarring and optimal functional results. Therefore, fundamental knowledge in the field of wound conditioning and surgical techniques is indispensable. The choice of adequate suture-needle combinations, the adequate knotting technique as well as the correct application of the basic anatomic and handling knowledge are all part of the procedure towards an optimal result.

## References

1. Thiede A, Dietz UA, Debus ES (2002) Klinischer Einsatz – Nahtmaterialien. Langenbecks Arch Chir (Kongressband DGC): 276–282
2. Anderson E, Sondenaa K, Holter J (1989) A comparative study of polydioxanone (PDS) and polyglactin 910 (Vicryl) in colonic anastomosis in rats. Int J Colorectal Dis 4: 251–254
3. Anscombe AR, Hira N, Hunt B (1970) The use of a new absorbable material (PGS) in general surgery. Br J Surg 57: 917–920
4. Blomstedt B, Jacobsson S-J (1970) Experiences with Polyglactin 910 (Vicryl) in General Surgery. Acta Chir Scand 143: 259–263
5. Chu CC (1982) The effect of pH on the in vitro degradation of polyglycolide lactide copolymer absorbable sutures. J Biomed Mater Res 16: 117–124

6. Chu CC, Moncrief G (1983) An in vitro evaluation of the stability of mechanical properties of surgical suture materials in various pH conditions. Ann Surg 198: 223–228

7. Diener H (2001) Organspezifisches Resorptionsverhalten verschiedener moderner absorbierbarer Nahtmaterialien. Inauguraldissertation, Medizinische Fakultät der Julius-Maximilians-Universität Würzburg

8. Thiede A, Lünstedt B (1991) Chirurgisches Nahtmaterial – Vor- und Nachteile. In: Jahrbuch der Chirurgie. Biermann, S 243–255

9. Taylor B, Bayat A (2003) Basic plastic surgery techniques and principles: how to suture. Student BMJ 11: 182–184

10. Nockemann FP (1992) Die chirurgische Naht. Thieme, Stuttgart

11. Tera H, Åberg C (1976) Tensile strengths of twelve types of knot employed in surgery, using different suture materials. Acta Chir Scand 142: 1–7

12. Trimbos JB (1984) Securitiy of various knots commonly used in surgical practice. Obstet Gynecol 64: 274–280

13. Chu CC (1997) Classification and general characteristics of suture materials. In: Chu CC, von Fraunhofer JA, Greisler HP (eds) Wound closure biomaterials. CRC Press LLC, Boca Raton, pp 39–63

14. Thiede A, Stüwe W, Lünstedt B (1985) Vergleich von physikalischen Parametern und Handhabungseigenschaften kurzfristig und mittelfristig absorbierbarer Nahtmaterialien. Chirurg 56: 803–808

15. Ziegler UE, Dietz UA, Debus ES, Keller HP, Thiede A (2004) Nahtmaterialien und Nahttechniken in der Chirurgie. (in press)

16. Trimbos JB, Mouw R, Ranke G, Trimbos KB, Zwinderman K (2001) The Donati stitch revisited: favorable cosmetic results in a randomized clinical trial. J Surg Res 107: 131–134

17. Mohabir RC, Christensen B, Blair GK, Fitzpatrick DG (2003) Avoiding stitch abscesses in subcuticular skin closure: the L-stitch. Can J Surg 46: 223–224

18. Geiger D, Debus ES, Ziegler UE, Thiede A, Dietz UA (2003) Kapillarität von chirurgischem Nahtmaterial und fadenabhängige Bakterientranslokation: eine qualitative Untersuchung. (in press)

19. Israelsson L (1999) Bias in clinical trials: the importance of suture technique. Eur J Surg 165: 3–7

20. Böhm HJ, Jung W (2001) Hautverschlussmaßnahmen. Trauma Berufskrankh 3 [Suppl 1]: 528–531

21. Weise K, Schäffer M (2000) Behandlungsstrategien bei Wundheilungsstörungen. Unfallchirurg 103: 100–109

22. Fisher GT, Fisher JB, Stark RB (1980) Origin of the use of subcuticular sutures. Ann Plast Surg 4: 144–148

## Notes

[1] Paul Leopold Friedrich (born January 26th, 1864 in Roda, Germany, died January 15th,1916 in Königsberg). Surgeon at Greifswald and Marburg. The concept of surgical debridement of wounds was first presented at the 23rd Congress of the German Surgical Society on April 13th, 1898.

[2] Mario Donati (born February 24th, 1879 in Modena). After 1912, professor of surgical pathology in Cagliari (Italy); professor of clinical surgery at Modena (1916), Padua (1922) and Torino (1927). Founder of the Lombard Society of Surgery (1920); from 1939–1945, in exile in Switzerland. Died January 21st, 1946 in Milan.

[3] Martin Allgöwer (born 1917), former head at the University Surgical Department in Basle, Switzerland. Allgöwer M (1963) Besonderheiten der chirurgischen Weichteil-Technik bei Unterschenkelfrakturen. In: Müller ME, Allgöwer M, Willenegger H (Hrsg) Technik der Operativen Frakturbehandlung. Springer, Heidelberg, S 111–114

[4] William S. Halsted (born September 23rd,1852, died September 7th, 1922) first used the *subcuticular suture* to prevent wound infection in the cervical region in dogs (experimental parathyreoid surgery). As early as 1887, Halsted transferred this suture to patients and 1889 modified the technique in introducing the *subcuticular running suture* (Halsted WS [1889] The radical cure of groin hernia. Johns Hopkins Hospital Bulletin No. 1, p12). The credit for introducing the intradermic suture in plastic surgery belongs to John S. Davis (1919) [22].

[5] Henry Redon, craniomaxillofacial surgeon in Paris.

[6] Described by the German pioneer of plastic surgery Erich Lexer (born May 22[th], 1867 in Freiburg i. Br., Germany; died 1937) as *Zapfennaht* in his Lehrbuch der Allgemeinen Chirurgie, Ferdinand Enke, Stuttgart, 1906. Lexer studied in Würzburg, was pupil of Ernst von Bergmann and worked in Berlin, Königsberg, Freiburg and Munich.

# Surgical Incision

K. Schmidt, U.E. Ziegler

## Introduction

Surgical incision means the intentional wounding of a patient in order to treat his discomforts.

Skin incision and tissue dissection together with haemostasis and wound suture are the oldest and, as it may seem, the simplest elements of any surgical intervention [5]. At the same time, however, they are crucial elements of every surgical operation. According to Erich Lexer (1934), a wound is a more or less "gaping severance of tissue in the skin, the mucous coat or the surface of internal organs".

Technical improvement of medical devices during the past century has given a wide choice of cutting instruments to all surgeons, ranging from different types of surgical steel knives and electrosurgery to the modern standards of laser technology.

## Basic Principles of Skin Incision

Every surgical incision must be planned and performed by the surgeon, considering precisely the therapeutic aims, practicability and the functional and aesthetic results of scar formation [13]. For this reason it seems useful to develop and to stick to a standardised proceeding [3].

On the one hand, the size of the skin incision must guarantee a good visibility of all anatomic structures which are to be prepared. On the other hand, the risk of tissue hypoperfusion, consecutive skin necrosis and the size of the later scar formation increases with the size of the incision. A surgical incision must be as short as possible and as long as necessary [16].

A precise planning of the incision requires in the first place knowledge of the so-called Langer's skin lines. These lines reflect the course of the architectural axis of tension and pressure in the dermal ridge pattern. For example, they refer to the pattern of collagen and elastic fibres. The relaxed skin tension lines described first by Kraissl and later by Borges give an even better orientation (Fig. 1). Numerous named guidelines have been developed as surgeons have searched for an ideal guide for elective incisions [18]. Many surgeons prefer Langer's lines. These lines were developed by Karl Langer, an anatomy professor, from corpses in rigor mortis. However, Kraissl preferred lines running vertically to the movement of the underlying muscles. Later, Borges described relaxed skin tension lines, which follow furrows formed when the skin is relaxed and are produced by pinching the skin [2]. These lines run vertically to the tensile force vectors on the relaxed skin surface. Cutaneous and subcutaneous tissue atrophy develops parallel to these lines, contribut-

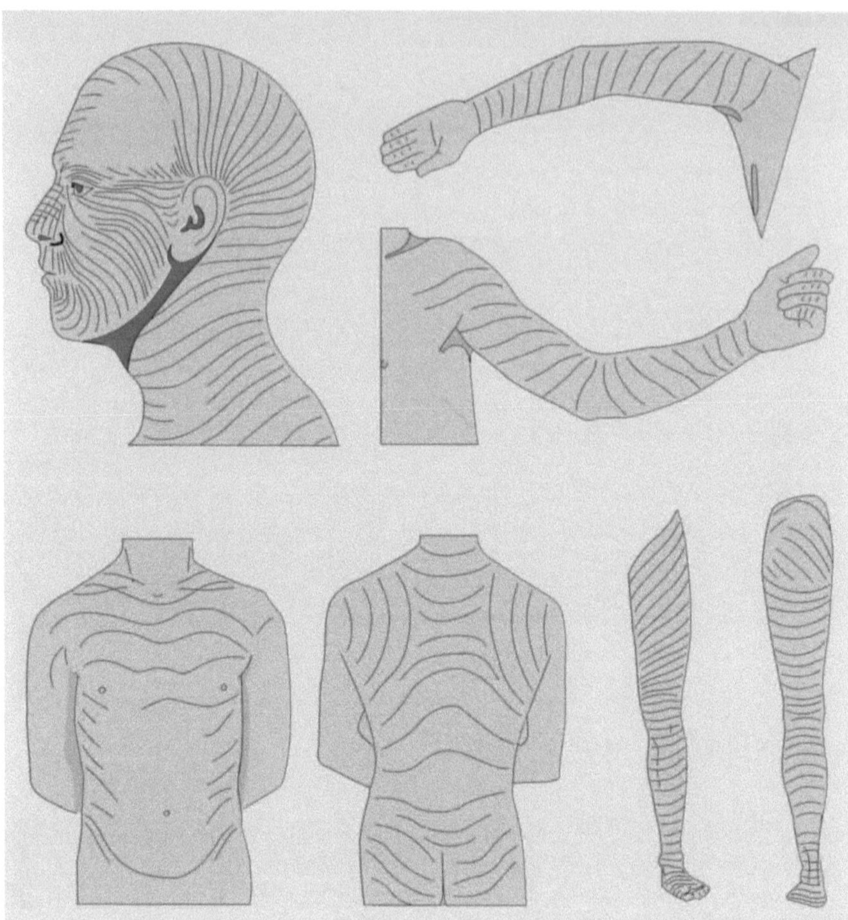

**Fig. 1.** Relaxed skin tension lines (Kraissl and Borges). (Williams et al. 1989)

ing to the formation of increased wrinkles and sagging of the skin in the life decades of the 1960s, 1970s and 1980s [1, 11, 12]. However, these are only guidelines; there are many contributors to the camouflaging of scars, including wrinkle and contour lines. Borges's and Kraissl's lines (not Langer's) may be the best guides for elective incisions of the face and body, respectively.

Incisions of the skin should be placed along or parallel to the skin tension lines whenever possible, because in terms of ideal wound healing this leads frequently to physiological scar formation with a good aesthetic and functional result without the risk of wound dehiscence or scarred contracture.

In the case of incisions in exposed regions like the face or the female breast it is recommended to conceal the scar in pre-existing wrinkles or behind the hairline (see Fig. 2 for examples) [6].

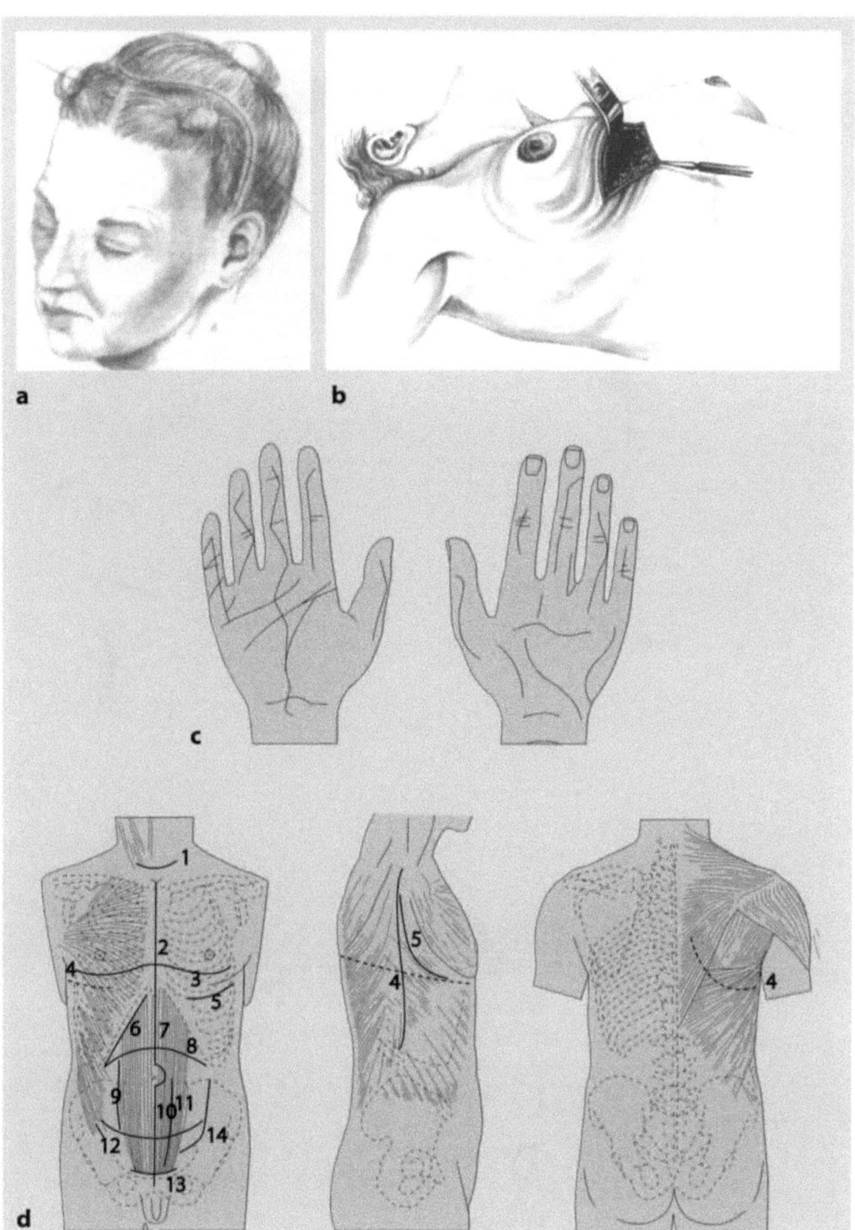

**Fig. 2a–d.** Special incision in exposed areas. **a** Incision behind the hairline, **b** in the inframammary fold, **c** hands: Brunner's incisions, **d** trunk. *1* Kocher's incision, *2* median sternotomy, *3* thoracic transversal approach, *4* dorsolateral and anterolateral thorakotomy, *5* subcostal incision, *6* epigastric median laparatomy, *7* epigastric transverse laparatomy, *8* pararectal incision, *9* median laparotomy, *10* paramedian laparatomy, *11* hypogastric transversal laparatomy, *12* gridiron (muscle splitting) incision, *13* Pfannenstiel's incision, *14* hypogastric-retroperitoneal incision

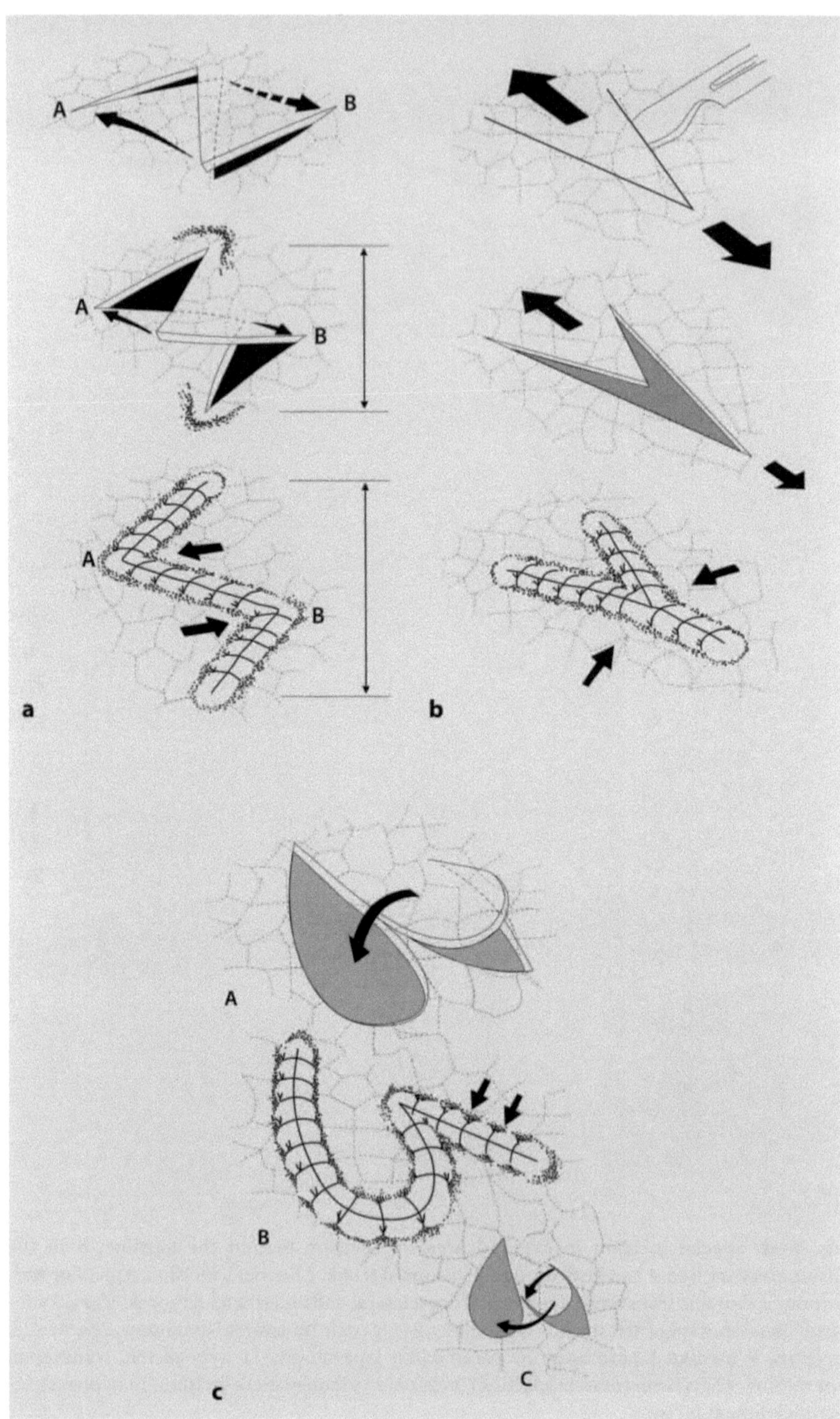



**Fig. 3. a** Z-plasty, **b** V-Y-plasty, **c** rotation-flap plasty

In any case, hand and feet incisions must be made along the lines of Brunner to prevent possible scar contraction (Fig. 2d). Abdominal incisions are closely related to the aim of the planned operation; standardised abdominal approaches were established long ago.

Special incision lines have to be respected in the case of tissue-rotation-, transposition- or interpolation flaps like the Z-plasty (useful in the management of scar contractures), multiple W-plasty (camouflage of extremely visible scars in exposed areas) or any other local flap plasties. Figure 3 shows some common examples.

## Technique of Surgical Incision

Because of the aesthetic importance of a meticulously planned and performed skin incision, it is advisable to mark each cut with a special sterile skin marker on the standing patient before the operation. In this position, the plastic constitution of the body surface becomes manifest. Examples of plastic surgery on the trunk or stoma operations show plainly the importance of this strategy.

The incision has to be strictly rectangular to the surface of the skin [14]. The total depth of the skin, i.e. both epidermis and dermis, must be cut thoroughly and at once. With this technique the occurrence of hypoperfusion at the wound edge caused by tangential slides is minimised. The suture is simplified because the incidence of skin bulging is very low. Performance of this technique is considerably simplified if the skin in the operation area is pre-stressed steady tension by an assistant [17]. The starting point of the incision should be the most difficult and problematic region, where the surgeon needs the highest precision (red margin of lip, mamilla, lacrimal papilla etc.). Whenever possible, the incision should be performed in one single lineament. If this is taken into account, the pre-operative marking will not be wiped away and the wound edges will be smooth and congruent to the opposite side (Fig. 4).

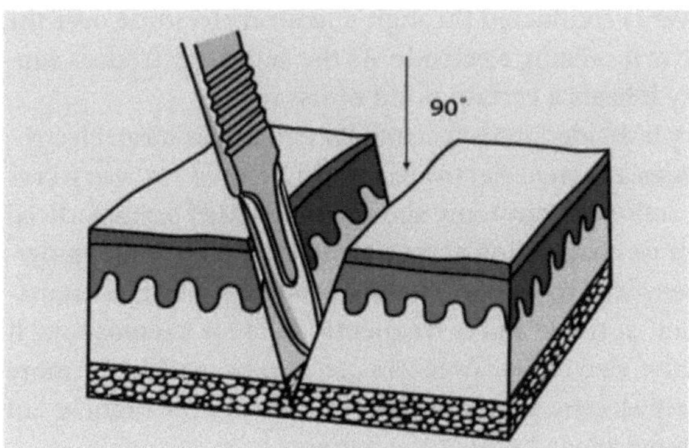


**Fig. 4.** Technique of surgical incision

Next, wound edges are elevated by subtle skin hooks in order to give the operator a better sight [10], so that he can prepare the deeper structures in the subcutaneous fat with scissors, a second so-called deep knife or by electrosurgery. No tweezers should be used for holding the skin in atraumatic skin surgery, due to the fact that tissue damage at the wound edge is caused by bruising the skin with tweezers. That might cause disturbed wound healing only in secondary intention.

It is also remarkable that thickness and structure of the skin layers vary considerably in different regions of the body [4]. The area of the upper lid shows the thinnest dermis, whereas the dorsocaudal parts of the trunk provide a thick and solid skin. The skin of the planta pedis is most complex [15]. A unique and fascinating architecture of collagen fibres is covered by a very strong dermis with a thick epithelium. For this reason, incision has to be prevented in this region. Whenever possible, incisions should be done at the dorsum pedis. If the plantar approach is not preventable, the incision at the planta pedis should be done as sparingly as possible, following the principles of Brunner's incision and the palma manum.

Because of the great variation in skin thickness and architecture, the surgeon needs to use an appropriate cutting instrument for each incision.

## Instruments for Surgical Incisions

### The Surgical Knife

Single-use scalpels have to be distinguished from scalpels with changeable blades. The most important difference is the form and size of the blade. The blade of the stitch scalpel is formed like a flat spike und used for stitch incisions. Small and bellied blades are used for incision in regions with a thin dermis or in cases of a complicated incision line (e.g. round the nipple or belly bottom). The bigger-bellied blades are useful for long-drawn-out cuts and dissection of subcutaneous fat.

### Electrosurgery

High-frequently electric power is conducted through a neutral electrode over the body of the patient to the active localizing electrode. As the active electrode is supplied with high power density it heats a certain point of tissue [8].

The field of electrosurgery is divided into electrotomy and fulguration. Electrotomy uses fine needles or lances as active electrodes. It can be used for sharp cuts with low surface coagulation action. Electrotomy should not be used for superficial incision of the epidermis, because coagulation necrosis might develop in the epidermal basal cell layers, which may lead to wound-healing problems. Electrocoagulation means electrocauterisation of tissue and is frequently used for haemostasis. It is sensible to use tweezers-active electrodes. Tweezers can also be used in the more secure bipolar technique where electric power flows only between the branches of the tweezers and not through the whole body of the patient.

## Laser Surgery

Laser (light amplification by stimulated emission of radiation) is a frequently used instrument in modern surface surgery. Argon lasers, neodym-YAG lasers, $CO_2$ lasers and colour lasers are routinely used for several indications [7].

The light of the argon laser (514–488 nm), which is an ionic gas laser, is particularly absorbed by melanin and haemoglobin. The laser light works in a depth of 1 mm. It can be increased up to 4 mm if the efficiency of the light generator is higher and if the skin surface is cooled at the same time.

Main indications are resection of haemangioma, teleangiectasia and naevi flammei. In 10–15% of all cases the major side effects are hypo- and hyper-pigmentation.

The neodym-YAG laser emits invisible light with a wavelength of 1060 nm. Its working depth is 5–6 mm. At this depth the laser light of the neodym-YAG laser generates a strong thermic tissue reaction. Indications are cavernous haemangioma, angioma of the lips or nodular parts of naevi flammei.

The $CO_2$ laser can excite the $CO_2$ molecule up to different levels of energy [9]. The most common wavelength is 10 600 nm. The light radiation is absorbed by water molecules in the tissue. The targeted tissue is vaporised except for its pigmentation. In the focused mode tissue can be dissected sharply with almost no thermal collateral damage; in the non-focused mode superficial parts of the skin are removed (e.g. laser skin resurfacing, tattoo removal).

## Reference


1. Balin AK, Klingman AM (1989) Aging and the skin. Raven Press, New York
2. Borges AF (1984) Relaxed skin tension lines (RSTL) versus other skin lines. Plast Reconstr Surg 73: 144–150
3. Brahams D (1988) Cosmetic surgery: greater duty to warn of risks. Lancet 2:1434
4. Braun-Falco O, Wolff HH, Winkelmann RK (1991) Dermatology. Springer, Berlin Heidelberg New York Tokyo
5. Dieffenbach JF (1845) Operative Chirurgie I. FA Brockhaus, Leipzig
6. Field LM (1990) Make your incision where you want your final scar to be: a surgical philosophy. J Dermatol Surg Oncol 16: 1062–1063
7. Goldman MP, Fitzpatrick RE (1994) Cutaneous laser surgery. Mosby, St. Louis
8. Goodman MM (1994) Principles of electrosurgery. Saunders, Philadelphia
9. Kirschner RA (1984) Cutaneous plastic surgery with the $CO_2$ laser. Surg Clin North Am 64: 871–883
10. Lerner SP (1985) The modified skin hook: a new instrument in cutaneous surgery. J Dermatol Surg Oncol 11: 586–588
11. Mc Carthy JG (1990) Plastic surgery. WB Saunders, Philadelphia
12. Meirson D, Goldberg LH (1993) The influence of age and patient positioning on skin lines. J Dermatol Surg Oncol 19: 39–43
13. Mustoe T et a. and the International Advisory Panel on Scar Management (2002) International clinical recommendations on scar management. Plast Reconstr Surg 110: 560–571
14. Petres J, Rompel R (1996) Operative Dermatologie. Springer, Berlin Heidelberg New York Tokyo
15. Roggero P, Blane Y, Krupp S (1993) Foot reconstruction in weight-bearing areas. Eur J Plast Surg 16: 186

16. Schumpelick V, Bleese NM, Mommsen U (1994) Chirurgie. Enke, Stuttgart
17. Wheeland RG (1994) Cutaneous surgery. Saunders, Philadelphia
18. Wilhelmi BJ, Blackwell SJ, Phillips LG (1999) Langer's lines: to use or not to use. Plast Reconstr Surg 104: 208–214
19. Williams PL, Warwick R, Dyson A, Bannister LH (1989) Gray's Anatomy. Churchill Livingstone, Edinburgh

# Skin Grafts

U.E. Ziegler, U.A. Dietz, K. Schmidt

## Introduction

Since about 2500 years skin grafting has been used in medicine, but only since the 19th century has it been established in surgery. Technical details of harvesting and the best dressing for the grafts were the greatest problems at that time. Skin from amputated parts was used to cover traumatic defects. The history of skin grafts started with Baronio in 1804 [1] who documented epidermis grafts in sheep which led to the use by surgeons at that time for coverage of granulating wounds in humans. The surgeon Jacques Louis Reverdin in Geneva (worked at Hospital Nêcker in Paris 1869) used grafts (epidermis and part of the dermis) on wounds of the forearm, and developed new techniques [10]. Today, these grafts, called Reverdin-(island) grafts, are still used in many countries as the easiest form of skin transplantation, mostly in chronic wounds. The difficult fixation of these grafts, their reduced healing potency (different thickness) and the choice of aesthetic donor sites are the greatest problems after transplantation. In 1869 Louis Xavier Ollier in Lyon transplanted epidermis and dermis in long strips (10–15 mm) and Georg David Pollock in London used this method 1 year later in an acute burn wound in an 8-year-old girl [4]. He was the first surgeon to use allografts. Girdner [5] credits himself with being the first and he believed that such grafts from a cadaver would be a permanent solution.

Pinch-grafts are single small parts of skin which are submerged in holes punched in wounds (Mangold 1895). The originator of split-thickness skin grafts (STSG) is Carls Thiersch (1874, Erlangen and Leipzig), who favoured the one-step procedure with coverage of all the defects at once [14]. His acquisition is still today standard in skin transplantations. Full-thickness skin transplantation was used by Wolfe (1875) and Krause (1893) to correct ectropion lower eyelids [7, 16].

## Skin-Graft Types

Skin grafts are a piece of skin including epidermis and parts of the dermis. They may either be full or split thickness, depending on how much dermis is included. Full-thickness skin grafts contain the entire dermis and epidermis, split-thickness skin grafts contain varying thickness of dermis and entire epidermis (Fig. 1). Depending on the thicknesses of the dermis, these grafts contain adnexal structures such as sweat glands, hair follicles, capillaries and sebaceous glands. The more dermis the graft has, the more primary is the contraction that will be experienced [11].

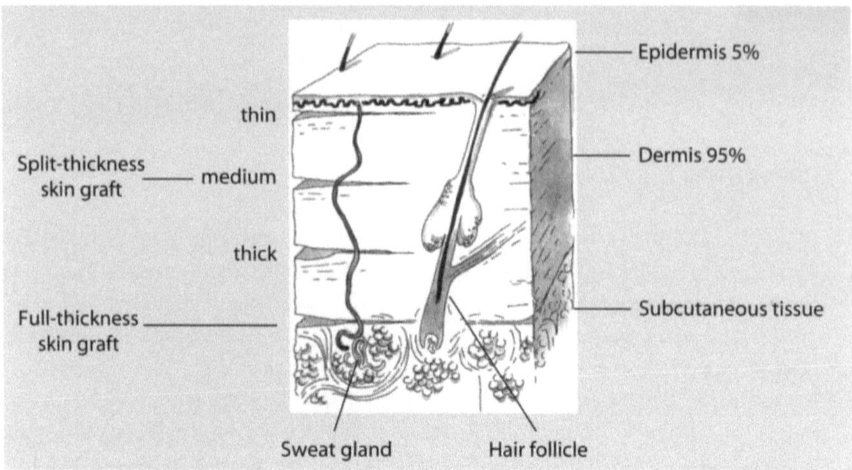


**Fig. 1.** Skin graft thickness

The skin grafts are harvested on any part of the body and can then be transplanted on wounds in order to heal in. We differentiate skin grafts into:

- epidermis skin grafts,
- thin split-thickness skin grafts (Thiersch grafts): 0.2–0.3 mm,
- medium split-thickness skin grafts (Thiersch grafts): 0.4–0.5 mm,
- thick split-thickness skin grafts (Thiersch grafts): 0.6–0.7 mm,
- full-thickness skin grafts (Wolfe-Krause grafts): 0.8–1.1 mm,
- composite grafts (e.g. skin and cartilage).

According to their origins:

- isologous (donator and recipient are identical),
- allogenic (recipient individual different but belong to the same species),
- xenogenous (donator and recipient belong to different species),
- alloplastic (skin substitute, "skin retort").

### Full-Thickness Skin Grafts (FSG)

Full-thickness skin grafts are harvested with a knife and are fixed over the index finger. All the fat has to be removed (Fig. 2). This preparation has to be done accurately to ensure good take. The same procedure is necessary with composite grafts (skin and integrated cartilage) without fat under the cartilage. Scarification is the incision made in the grafts with a sharp knife, so that blood and exudates can be caught in the dressing. The fixation of FSG is very important and has to be performed with a special tie-over bolster dressing (wound bed – skin graft – non-adherent gaze – cotton) so that no movement of the graft on the bed is possible. Immobilisation techniques (e.g. splinting of the extremities) include the use of these bolster dressings. Inspection of the grafts takes place at the end of the 5th postoperative day.

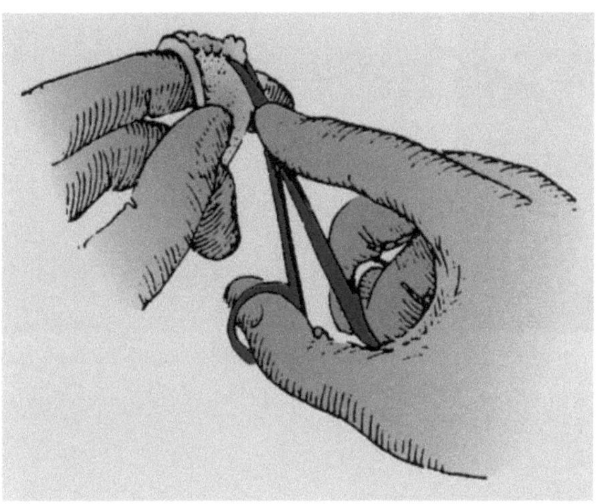

**Fig. 2.** Full-thickness skin graft is prepared before grafting. (According to [8])

Indications:
- exposed skin areas in the face (cosmetic aspect),
- where no secondary shrinking is desirable and in stressed regions (e.g. palmar aspect of hand, eyelid, joint).

Advantages:
- cosmetically favourable results if the skin is harveste near the region where it was transplanted,
- the scar in the harvest area is linear and mostly not visible,
- maximum of 10% shrinking,
- very good mechanical resistance.

Disadvantages:
- demanding on the wound bed because of the take,
- limited availability.

### Thickness Skin Graft (TSG)

The harvesting of small TSG with different thicknesses can be done with a Watson knife, Humby knife or with a de Weck dermatom. If larger grafts are necessary, pneumatic or electric (battery) dermatomes are used (Fig. 3). In areas where an irregular surface of the skin is presented (ribs, abdominal wall, buttock, thigh, back etc.) saline solution (0.9%) is injected under the skin before cutting. After grafting, the skin is not expanded, but scarification cuts are used for drainage. The dressings for the grafts can be non-adherent gaze, cotton, foamed material or compression with elastic bandages. After 5 days the dressing can be removed for the first time. Local inspection (odour, exudates etc.) is indicated in the first days.

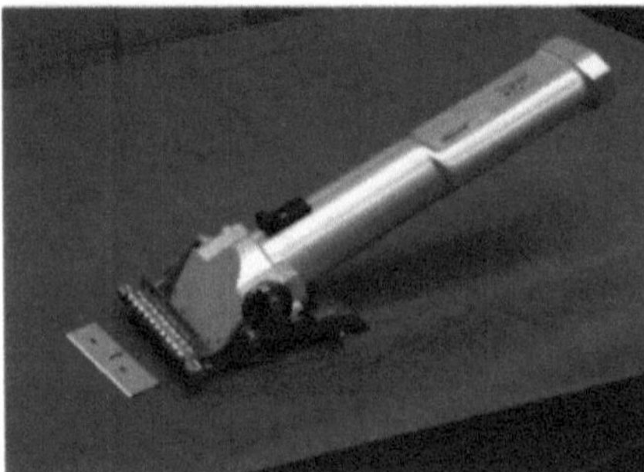

**Fig. 3.** Dermatom (battery)

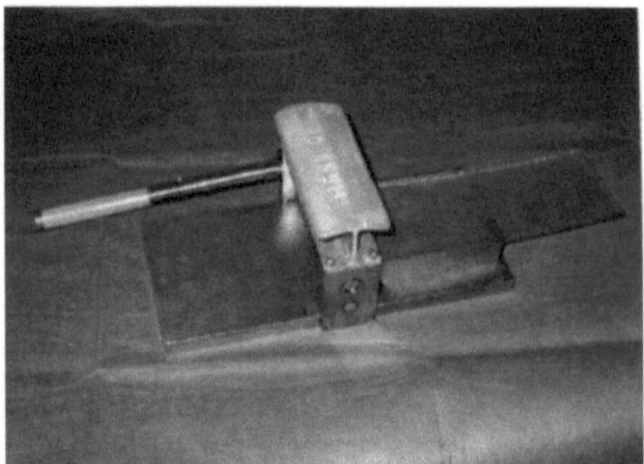

**Fig. 4.** Mesh-graft cutting machine with graft templates

Indications:
- cosmetically demanding areas where no mesh pattern is desirable (e.g. face, dorsum of the hand),
- large defects where no full-thickness skin graft or flap is possible,
- mechanical resistance areas.

Advantages:
- lots of skin is available,
- if there is good contact to the wound bed, a high take is possible.

Disadvantages:
- limited resistance,
- shrinking capacity (up to 20%),
- visible change of pigmentation,
- excessive scarring is possible.

### Split-Thickness Skin Grafts (STSG)

The harvest of split-thickness skin is done in the same way as with thickness skin grafts. Multiple mechanical incisions with the mesh-graft cutting machine (Fig. 4) result in a meshed skin graft, allowing immediate expansion of the graft. The graft templates are available in size 1:1.5 up to size 1:30, and because of the numerous holes in the grafts the drainage is quite good [13]. Different dressings are possible, non-adherent gaze, foamed material or vacuum-assisted closure techniques, for example.

Indications:
- huge defects (e.g. burns),
- chronic wounds of any type (excluding radiation ulcer),
- superinfected or exudating wounds,
- if the shrinking process is welcome (e.g. loge syndromes).

Advantages:

- best use relation between harvest and transplanted areas (burns),
- less demanding on the wound bed,
- very good drainage because of the grafts,
- mostly high take.

Disadvantages:

- mesh pattern is visible,
- shrinking up to 30%, with functional problems and contractions.

## Skin-Graft Donor Sites

The donor-site epidermis regenerates from the immigration of epidermal cells' origin in the hair follicle shafts and adnexal structures left in the dermis. The dermis itself never regenerates. FSG donor sites are closed by primary sutures. An elegant method is the pre-expanded skin before harvesting FSG or for composite grafts. The donor site can also be closed primarily. SPSG harvest only a part of the dermis, so the original donor site can be used again for subsequent SPSG harvest (mostly after 10 days, depending on the harvest area). Dressings for the donor sites are nonadherent gauze and cotton (mostly painful); hydropolymere, polyurethane foil dressings or perforated silicone sheets are better (Fig. 5). Fibrin glue seams a good alternative procedure to increase the take [8].

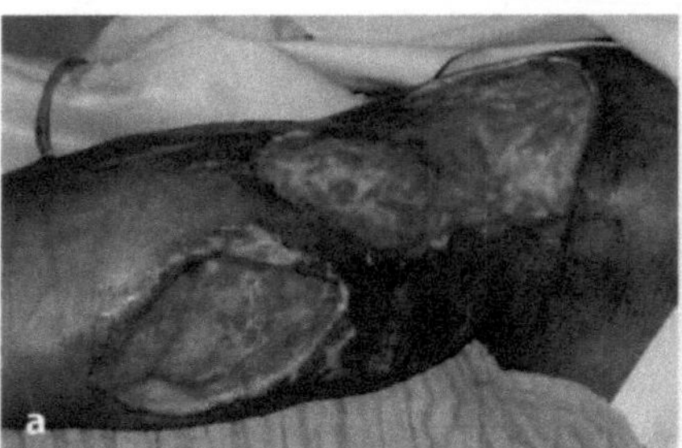
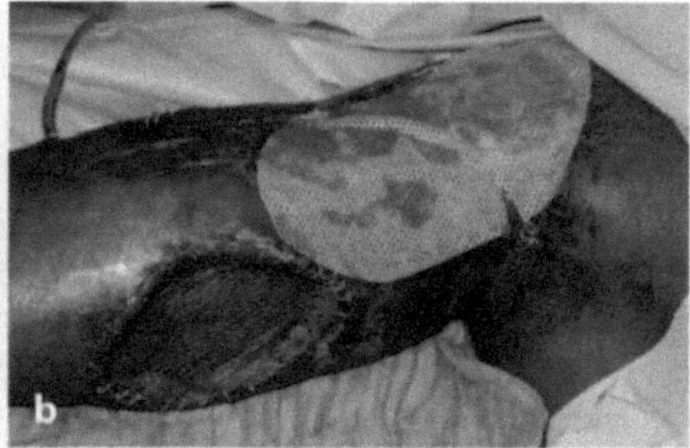
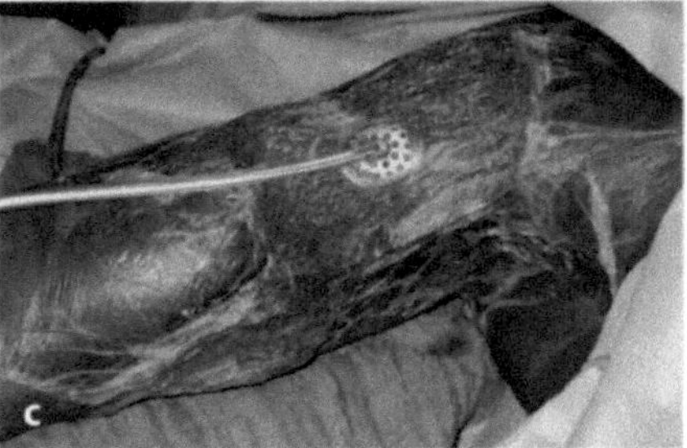

**Fig. 5. a** Defect of lower extremity. **b** Transplanted split-thickness skin graft (ratio 1:1.5), fixed with stables and covered with a perforated silicon sheet. **c** Applied vacuum-assisted closure technique with polyurethane foam

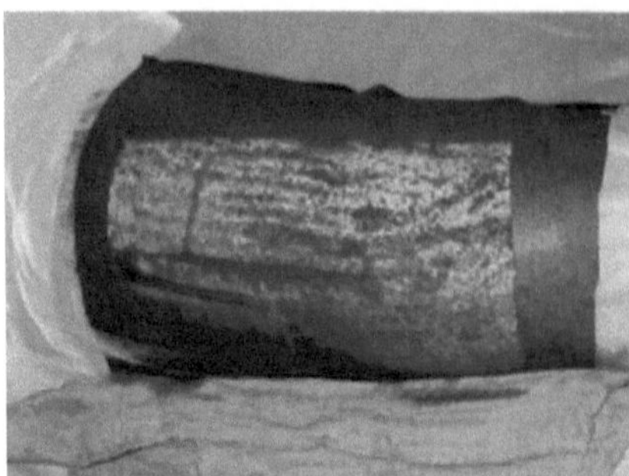

**Fig. 6.** Donor site

Skin grafts can be taken from anywhere in the body (Fig. 6). Colour texture, thickness of the dermis, vascularity and donor-site morbidity vary considerably. The best area for harvesting SPSG is the lateral lower leg area, in children the back of the head. FSG can be taken from the groin, but the upper eyelid skin can also be used, as it provides a small amount of very thin skin. Skin grafts taken from the superior or inferior area of the clavicles provide a superior colour match for defects in the face. Retro-auricular areas are also available.

## Skin Graft Healing Process

Skin grafts heal in with three different phases [6]. The first is the plasmatic-inhibition or avascular phase, the second is an inosculatory phase and in the third phase the graft is revascularised through the "kissing" capillaries.

If the skin grafts are transplanted on the wound bed, they look pale, and fibrins to adhere them [3]. Fibrinolytic activity is usually not seen in acute wounds. In the first hours (48–72 h) the grafts live from the plasmatic inhibition (from diffusion), depending on the thickness of the grafts (0.2–0.3 mm = 72 h, 0.4–1.1 mm = 48 h) and the recipient bed. In the first hours the grafts swell with water (oedema) up to 40% of their original weight and blood vessels are spastic. Superficial blood vessels from the wound bed grow in the grafts (starting 4 h after transplantation) and after 24 h find a connection to the degenerated graft vessels (capillary alignment, second phase). This is the reason why in the first 48 h no movement or force is allowed on the transplanted grafts. The blood vessels penetrate in the dermis vertically, which is the most important procedure for the take. The grafts start living from the circulated blood, and the revascularisation goes on for up to 14 days after grafting, depending on the thickness of the skin (third phase).

Because the full-thickness skin grafts are thicker, a survival of the graft is more precarious, demanding a well-vascularised bed [2]. The elevated weight of the skin grafts persists up to 5 days and the skin colour becomes more red. After this time it is no longer possible to shift the grafts from the wound bed. Close contact between graft and wound bed is essential. Haematomas or seromas under the skin grafts will compromise the healing process. Immobilisation in the first days is absolutely necessary for the take of the grafts.

The recipient wound bed has to be prepared (wound-bed preparation) in order to optimise the take of the skin grafts. The wound bed requires a well-vascularised area, and grafts will fail on exposed bones, cartilage or tendon (without periostium, perichondrium or peritendon). Quality of the wound bed, quality of the skin graft and quality of the operation technique are the guarantees for successful healing. Infection (especially with *Pseudomonias aeruginosa*), necroses and elevated exudates reject skin grafts [15]. Wound-bed preparation controls these three major topics.

## Special Skin Grafts

Skin with hair in it can be transplanted. This is necessary in reconstruction of e.g. eyebrows (after burns). In the haired temporo-occipital area full-thickness skin grafts can be harvested and the defect is closed by primary sutures. The incisions for same way as in the original. It is difficult to calculate the result concerning hair density and growth.

In special situations (e.g. major amputations) living skin can be harvested for delayed transplantation of rest defects in the same patient. In these cases split-thickness skin grafts can put in Ringer's solution gauze in the refrigerator at +4 to +6 °C. The grafts can be transplanted after 10 to 14 days, but the best time is within the first 7 days after harvesting.

## Skin and Skin-Replacement Procedures in Chronic Wounds

There is a large demand for skin substitutes for the coverage of chronic wounds. Due to intensive and local wound treatment, impaired dermal and epidermal repair still remains a major problem. Known treatments such as SPSG, Reverdin and pinch grafts make adequate and solid wound closure possible. However, in such procedures the take rate of grafting often fails. Graft healing can be increased with a combined mesh graft (1:1.5 meshed, 0.2 mm thick) and vacuum-sealing technique (50–125 mmHg).

Controlled and comparative studies concerning the healing rate of split-thickness skin grafts do not exist sufficiently. The clinical work shows that this type of defect coverage with autologous skin (epidermis and part of dermis) has a high take rate, using a simple and standardised procedure. The healing rate of SPSG should be at least 90% in chronic wounds (opinion of the authors), in order to prevent an early re-occurence of the ulcer. The grafts have to lie horizontally to the extremities, preventing scarring, and the meshed skin has to lie really tight. Comparative studies on skin-replacement material, like autologous outer root cell sheaths, show a healing rate of little over 40% in SPSG, which seems very low to us [9]. The autologous outer root cells (keratinocytes) are comparable, with shortly under 40%, but still at a very low rate. Our own experience with autologous keratinocytes in fibrin glue confirms the low healing rate [12]. Epidermis- and dermis-replacement procedures will be available with improved application and will be more reliable in the near future. It appears that dermis equivalents (bovine or equine) can result in better scars after grafting.

## References


1. Baronio G (1804) Degli Innesti Animali. Stamperia e Fonderia del Genio, Milan
2. Birch J, Branemark PI (1969) The vascularization of a free full thickness skin graft. I. A vital microscopic study. Scand J Plast Reconstr Surg 3: 1–10
3. Burleson R, Euseman B (1973) Nature of the bond, between partial thickness skin and wound granulation. Am Surg 177: 181
4. Freshwater MF, Krizek TJ (1978) Georg David Pollock and the development of skin grafting. Ann Plast Surg 1: 96–100
5. Girdner JH (1881) Skin-grafting with grafts taken from the dead subject. Med Rec 20: 119–120
6. Haller JA. Billingsham RE (1967) Studies of the origin of vascular in free skin grafts. Ann Surg 166: 896.
7. Krause F (1893) Über die Transplantation großer ungestielter Hautlappen. Verh Dtsch Ges Chir 22: 46
8. Krupp S (1989) In: Gosepath J (ed) Aktuelle Methoden der Gewebeklebung im Kopf-Hals-Bereich. Urban & Schwarzenberg, München.
9. Nielsen PG, Madsen SM, Stromberg L (1990) Treatment of chronic leg ulcers with a hydrocolloid dressing. Acta Derm Venereol (Stockh):152 [Suppl]: 1–12
10. Reverdin JL (1872) De la greffe épidermique. Arch Gen De Med 19: 276, 55, 703
11. Rudolph R (1964) Inhibition of myofibroblasts by sham skin grafts. Plast Reconstr Surg 63: 473
12. Stark GB, Kaiser HW, Kopp J, Spilker G et al. (1992) Kultiverte autologe Keratinozyten in einer Fibrin-Matrix zur Deckung von Brandwunden. 30th Annual Meeting of the German Society for Plastic and Reconstructive Surgery. Berlin, 8.–10. Okt. 1992
13. Tanner JC, Vandeput J, Olley JF (1964) The mesh skin graft. Plast Reconstr Surg 34: 287
14. Thiersch C (1874) Über die feineren anatomischen Veränderungen bei Aufheilung von Haut auf Granulationen. Verh Dtsch Ger Chir 3: 69
15. Vogt PM, Andree C et al. (1995) Dry, moist and wet skin wound repair. Ann Plast Surg 34: 493
16. Wolfe JR (1875) A new method for performing plastic operations. Br Med J 2: 360

# Local and Regional Flaps

O. Heymans, N. Verhelle

## Introduction

Due to major advances in local wound care, superficial or small-sized wounds can be managed by secondary healing. However, more complex defects necessitate other treatment options because secondary healing will not provide an adequate and stable scar. Some of these more complex defects consist frequently in bone, tendinous or articular exposure, and delaying their coverage can be disastrous. The deep structures will be longer exposed to bacterial contamination, inducing infection and necrosis. In these cases, therefore, wound coverage has to be achieved by other techniques.

Several diseases such as diabetes, atherosclerosis, renal failure or connective disorders induce wounds that are very difficult to manage in a proper way. The systemic disturbances impair the normal healing process and more extensive wound coverage procedures such as flaps have to be performed. However, these diseases which caused the primary wound can also interfere with the healing process after soft-tissue coverage.

A wide range of techniques, including skin grafts, local, regional or free flaps, are available to cover these more difficult wounds. With these tools, healing can be obtained in very complex wounds providing optimal and stable coverage. The key point, however, is to distinguish as soon as possible the wounds where spontaneous healing will be unlikely and thus other surgical techniques have to be applied. Once this selection has been established, the right surgical technique for that specific wound has to be chosen.

## Surgical Techniques

### Skin Graft

Skin can be harvested as a split thickness skin graft (STSG) or a full-thickness skin graft (FTSG). Once harvested, it is applied onto the defect, whereas the donor site will heal spontaneously (STSG) or will be closed primarily (FTSG). In both situations, the graft will stick to the wound (graft take, due to the angiogenic process which provides a vascular supply to the transplanted skin). This means that the graft take is directly linked to the quality of the recipient site. Optimal recipient site quality implies a well-vascularised wound bed containing healthy granulating tissue. Once the graft has been applied to this optimal recipient site, wound coverage can be achieved, although local factors such as mechanical stress, haematomas or infection may lead to partial failure. Due to their poor protective characteristics, skin grafts are not indicated in demanding areas such as in pressure sores or on weight-bearing areas. Moreover, they cannot be used on bone, tendons or hardware due to the quality of the recipient site.

## Flaps

Contrary to a skin graft, flaps carry their own vascularisation to ensure survival and adequate healing on the recipient site. Since they do not rely on the revascularisation by the recipient site, the wound bed quality is not of prime interest although a proper debridement has to be performed before transfer. On the other hand, this vascular autonomy allows the use of large and thick tissular volume which cannot be provided by simple skin grafts.

Flaps can be divided roughly into local flaps, pedicled flaps and free flaps. Local flaps can be either skin flaps or fasciocutaneous flaps. The skin flaps are supplied by a non-individualised vascular network arising from muscle perforators, giving them the name of random flaps. They consist of skin and subcutaneous fat. However, fasciocutaneous flaps include also the underlying fascia containing a supplementary vascular supply. Pedicled flaps are supplied by a well-individualised vascular pedicle which enters into the flap. Free flaps correspond to one or more tissues with their own vascular pedicle which has been divided and needs a microvascular procedure to revascularise the flap on the recipient site.

### Local Flaps

Since the vascular supply of these flaps is random, flap size and proportions are of major importance. Although the old surgical law on local flaps states that "flaps are safe when their width is equal to their length", it differs in each anatomical area. In the head and neck for example, the flap length can be five times more than the width, due to the extremely well-supplied environment. The general rule nowadays for most other parts of the body is that the width/length ratio should be 1:2 or 1:2.5.

The principles of local flap coverage are based on tissue redistribution. The flap is moved into the defect by means of rotating or transposing or sliding while the defect created by flap harvesting is closed primarily or by simple tissue mobilisation.

In this type of coverage, due to its vascular basis, the distal part of the flap has the poorest vascular supply. Hence, ischemic events occurring at this level can cause partial necrosis. Unfortunately, frequently these distal parts are located on the crucial part of the defect that has to be covered (bare bone, for example).

Successful use of these flaps depends on the location and size of the defect, the vascularisation and the trophic qualities of the region, the soft-tissue redundancy and the thickness needed. Although in the head and neck area small- to medium-sized defects are frequently covered by these local flaps, they have only limited clinical value in the limbs and especially in the lower extremity. Indeed, the vascular conditions present in the head and neck area allow excellent viability and reliability of local flaps. Moreover, the good colour match and the unique facial skin quality make these local flaps a workhorse in the head and neck area. In the lower leg, however, these flaps have almost no clinical value due to the sometimes poor vascular conditions, the traumatic origin of the wounds, the poor pliability of these flaps and horrible donor sites. However, scar contracture caused by prolonged secondary healing and burns can be treated by local flap such as z plasties. In these cases, two triangular local flaps are turned to increase the scar length and break the scar contracture. This procedure can be performed safely, even in lower legs, due to the well-designed flap proportions.

### Pedicled Flaps

As mentioned before, these flaps are based on an individualised arterio-venous pedicle. Mobility and ability to reach the recipient site are obtained after proper dissection of the flap and the pedicle. The donor site can be closed primarily or can be skin-grafted if necessary. Within this large group of flaps, several different types of tissues can be transferred (cutaneous, muscular, fascial etc.) and the physiological principle can be very variable (perforator flap, neurocutaneous flap, axial flap etc.). In spite of these physiological and anatomical differences, all these flaps have a well-described vascular territory based on the angiosome and venosome concept. Due to this concept, their maximal size [1] is well determined, and harvesting can be performed as a pedicled flap or as a free flap. A huge number of pedicled flaps have been described to cover defects located all over the body. It is therefore impossible to discuss them all. Since the lower leg often presents with different kinds of wounds (arterial, venous, diabetic, traumatic etc.), we will focus this chapter on this area.

The **anterolateral thigh flap** [2] is based on the descending branch of the circumflex lateral femoral artery and vein. It can be used as a pedicled flap proximally based and will reach the groin. When it has been harvested as a distally based flap, defects around the knee can be covered. The **gastrocnemius flap**, nourished by the sural artery and vein, both branches from the popliteal vessels, can be used to cover up defects from the anterior part of the knee down to the first third of the lower leg [3]. Harvesting this muscle results, however, in a certain functional and cosmetic impairment and, moreover, the size of defects that can be covered is limited. The **soleus muscle** can be harvested to cover defects over the middle one-third of the lower leg. It is nourished by branches from the fibular artery and has the same limitations: donor site morbidity (loss of the deep venous pump) and a limited size. The **anteromedial adiposo-fascial flap** [4] can cover defects from the knee down to the heel. It is nourished by perforators from the posterior tibial artery as well as by the saphenous pedicle. However, its use is limited to cover defects up to 30 to 40 cm$^2$.

The **sural neurocutaneous flap** [5] is a distally based flap which is supplied by a distal peroneal perforator giving a perineural arterial network. This is a fasciocutaneous flap harvested on the proximal posterior calf region. The pedicle, which consists of the lesser saphenous vein and nerve surrounded by the fine arterial network, is long and makes it possible to reach the distal third of the leg, the heel and the ankle. The **supramalleolar flap** is a thin fasciocutaneous flap harvested on the lateral malleolar area, on a short retrograde pedicle. As the sural neurocutaneous flap, the donor site cannot be closed primarily and needs a skin graft.

Several flaps on the foot have been described. However, due to their poor reliability and often horrible donor sites, they have lost their popularity and are only rarely used [6]. The **medial plantar flap** is supplied by the medial plantar vessels ending the posterior tibial vessels. The harvested tissues correspond to the soft tissue of the plantar sole. Although the donor site has to be grafted, the main advantage of this flap is that thick, protective and sensate coverage can be transferred to the weight-bearing area of the foot.

### Free Flaps

Free tissue transfer corresponds to the transfer of tissue-based on an arterio-venous pedicle, needing arterial and venous micro-anastomosis to recipient vessels in order to re-establish blood supply to the flap. The microsurgical anatomosis remains one of the most important steps during this procedure. These sutures are frequently performed on vessels with diameters from 1–3 mm.

Because the major vessels in the lower leg should be spared whenever possible, most sutures in lower leg reconstructions are performed in a termino-lateral fashion for the artery, and termino-terminal for the vein [7]. While this nourishing pedicle is, in the first days after transfer, the only blood supply to the flap, perfect permeable microsutures are essential for flap survival. It is generally accepted that the microsutures are most at risk for thrombosis during the first 2 days, after which endothelialisation of the anastomosis has occurred. This nearly constitutes an "all or nothing phenomenon", which can lead to a total necrosis necessitating a new coverage procedure.

By converting the pedicled flap into a free flap, there will be no limit any more in the range of motion. Indeed, any kind of tissue, based on a pedicle, can be transferred to any other part of the body. Moreover, not only one single type of tissue (cutaneous, muscular, osseous) can be harvested to transfer. Compound tissue transfers (musculo-cutaneous, osteo-cutaneous etc.) can be performed safely as long as the angiosome/venosome concept has been respected.

### Different Types of Free Flaps

The choice of free **muscular** flaps depends essentially on the amount of tissue needed and the desired pedicle length [8]. Indeed, muscles like the latissimus dorsi, serratus anterior and gracilis provide different characteristics; they all give low donor-site morbidity. The **rectus-abdominis** muscle has been a workhorse for a long time, but nowadays it has been abandoned by many surgeons because of its important donor-site morbidity (abdominal weakness). All muscle flaps are frequently harvested as pure muscle flaps and will be skin-grafted in order to enhance the cosmetic result of the reconstruction and to limit donor-site morbidity. The **latissimus-dorsi** muscle is able to cover large areas, which makes it unique. It has a long pedicle with large diameter vessels (1.5–2.5 mm, thoraco-dorsal vessels). The **serratus anterior** muscle (two or three inferior digitations) has the same pedicle as the latissimus dorsi but its volume is much smaller. The **gracilis** muscle is also a relatively small muscle with a shorter pedicle (6–8 mm, art. circumflexa femoris med.) with a smaller diameter (1–1.2 mm).

If a free **fascio-cutaneous** flap is required, the radial forearm flap, nourished by the radial artery, remains one of the most popular flaps in Western countries. It is a very reliable and thin flap, supplied with a long, large calibre pedicle [9]. If harvested as a fascio-cutaneous flap, then the donor site has to be covered with a skin graft, often resulting in an unsightly scar. Mainly for this reason, we nowadays tend to harvest it as a pure fascial flap that will be grafted once applied to the receptor site. The donor site can be closed primarily without impairing the cosmetic and functional result of the reconstruction. Some other examples of pure fascial flaps that can be harvested are the fascia temporalis (superficial temporal vessels), the fascia of the serratus anterior or the fascia of the antero-lateral thigh.

Whenever **bone** is needed as a free flap, the fibular flap remains the workhorse. It is harvested on the fibular artery and can provide a long segment of bone. Together with the bone, fascio-cutaneous or muscular tissue (M. soleus) can be harvested on the same pedicle [10]. This arsenal of about ten flaps allows us to perform most of our microsurgical reconstructive procedures.

## Indications and Reconstructive Ladder

When spontaneous healing is not able to provide a good qualitative result (aesthetic results, with a stable scar and good protective properties) or if primary healing is not expected in the first weeks, a surgical option has to be considered. The reconstructive ladder helps to select the right surgical option for a defect. It advises the use of skin graft prior to a local flap, prior to a pedicled flap, and only as a last resort should free flaps be used. In fact, it recommends the use of the simpler method to solve, with a maximal quality, the presenting wound.

Basic rules for procedure selection are quite simple: skin grafts are contraindicated for bone, tendinous or hardware coverage or in regions which undergo a lot of mechanical stress. Moreover, it requires healthy or granulating tissue as a recipient site. Local flaps can be performed for superficial wounds if their vascularisation and mobilisation can be considered as reliable, for example, in the head and neck region or on the proximal part of the limbs. Pedicled flaps have to be preferred to free flaps if their harvesting does not induce excessive morbidity and if they are able to cover and fill out the entire defect. If not, free flaps are indicated.

Usually it is quite obvious which coverage procedure has to be selected, except when a choice has to be made between a pedicled or a free flap. Although free flaps have become the first choice for reconstructive procedures in the lower leg since the popularisation of microsurgery, local flaps can still be indicated in selected cases [11]. In some clinical circumstances short operative times are preferred, high risks for microvascular procedures are present or minimal donor-site morbidity is a must, so pedicled flaps can provide an alternative for free-tissue transfer.

The use of pedicled muscle flaps such as the gastrocnemius and the soleus has proved to be valuable in the management of soft-tissue defects over the tibia. However, due to local contusion of the soft tissues after trauma, local muscle flaps are not always perfectly healthy and will not have the trophic qualities of a free flap. Moreover, there will be local devascularisation subsequent to the removal of the flap and the tissue defect will often be covered with the least vascularised distal part of the muscle flap.

Pedicled fascial and fasciocutaneous flaps have regained popularity recently and can provide an excellent alternative for coverage of lower leg defects, even when (fractured) bone has to be covered. However, they have limited reach and can be unreliable, especially if the area around the wound has been traumatised or is chronically scarred. Moreover, they leave often ugly donor site scars due to the need of skin grafting. In contrast to other pedicled fasciocutaneous flaps, the medial adiposofascial (maf) flap has some advantages:

- no major vessel has to be sacrificed,
- the flap is reliable even in traumatised areas,
- no skin is harvested, leaving minimal donor site scarring,
- due to its dual vascularisation, well-vascularised tissue can be harvested to cover a defect up to 40 cm$^2$.

Although the Gillies' concept "replace tissue with like tissue" remains one of the key stones in plastic surgery, a grafted muscle flap can replace a loss of fascio-cutaneous tissue [12]. Due to the lack of available local fascio-cutaneous tissue and the often subcutaneous position of bony structures, especially in limbs, free muscle flaps became in the 1980s the workhorse of soft-tissue coverage. A huge amount of work has been published by pioneers as Mathes and co-workers [13, 14], stating that muscle is more resistant to infections than any other tissue. Since exposed bone, and especially osteomyelitis cases even after debridement, were considered as infected structures, bone coverage became a matter of course in literature. Recent clinical work, however, indicates that also non-muscular tissue can be successfully transferred to cover bone defects after aggressive debridement. Moreover, muscle harvesting can induce a certain morbidity of the donor site and may induce some aesthetic disadvantages on the recipient site. Due to these findings, several authors continued to search for better solutions as thin fascio-cutaneous free flaps, in order to avoid complications in simple soft-tissue losses [15]. In all these studies, aggressive debridement of bone and adjacent soft tissue, removing all infected, non-viable or fibrotic skin and soft tissue, is performed to reduce bacterial colonisation. Subsequently, all dead space has to be filled out during the soft-tissue coverage procedure to prevent fluid collections which may cause bacterial colonisation and infection. Moreover, these collections will also prevent optimal tissue contact between the flap and surrounding tissues, thereby impairing the optimal collaboration in terms of cicatrisation and angiogenesis.

# References


1. Taylor GI, Palmer JH (1987) The vascular territories (angiosomes) of the body: experimental study and clinical applications. Br J Plast Surg 40: 113–141
2. Wei FC, Jain V, Celik N, Chen HC, Chuang DCC, Lin CH (2002) Have we found an ideal soft tissue flap? An experience with 672 anterolateral thigh flaps. Plast Reconstr Surg 109: 2219–2230
3. McCraw JB, Fishman JH, Sharzer LA (1978) The versatile gastrocnemius myocutaneous flap. Plast Reconstr Surg 62: 15–23
4. Heymans O, Verhelle N, Peters S, Nélissen X, Oelbrandt B (2002) Use of the medial adiposofascial flap of the leg for coverage of full thickness burns exposing the tibial crest. Burns 28: 674–678
5. Hollier L, Sharma S, Babigumira E, Klebuc M (2002) Versatility of the sural fasciocutaneous flap in the coverage of lower extremity wounds. Plast Reconstr Surg 110: 1673–1679
6. Attinger CE, Ducic I, Zelen C (2000) The use of local muscle flaps in foot and ankle reconstruction. Clin Podiatr Med Surg 17: 681–711
7. Wells MD, Bowen CV, Manktelow RT (1996) Lower extremity free flaps: a review. CJS 39: 233–239
8. Godina M (1986) Early microsurgical reconstruction of complex trauma. Plast Reconstr Surg 78: 285–292
9. Musharafieh R, Atiyeh B, Macari G, Haider R (2001) Radial forearm fasciocutaneous free tissue transfer in ankle and foot reconstruction: review of 17 cases. J Reconstr Microsurg 17: 147–150
10. Pelissier P, Casoli V, Demiri E, Martin D, Baudet J (2000) Soleus-Fibula free transfer in lower limb reconstruction. Plast Reconstr Surg 105: 567–573
11. Hallock GG (2000) Utility of both muscle and fascia flaps in severe lower extremity trauma. J Trauma 48: 913–917
12. Nahai F, Mathes SJ (1981) Aesthetic aspects of reconstructive microsurgery of the lower extremity. Clin Plast Surg 8: 369–372
13. Mathes SJ, Alpert BS, Chang N (1982) Use of the muscle flap in chronic osteomyelitis: experimental and clinical correlation. Plast Reconstr Surg 69: 815–828
14. Chang N, Mathes SJ (1982) Comparison of the effect of bacterial inoculation in musculocutaneous and random-pattern flaps. Plast Reconstr Surg 70: 1–9
15. Weinzweig N, Davies BW (1998) Foot and ankle reconstruction using the radial forearm flap: a review of 25 cases. Plast Reconstr Surg 102: 1999–2005

# Free Flaps: Interests and Limits

L. Téot

## Introduction

Free flaps were introduced three decades ago after the pioneering works of Cheng, who reimplanted a thumb, realizing for the first time a microsuture on vessels whose diameter did not exceed 1 mm. The flap technique, pediculising a skin area on its vessels, was initially proposed by McGregor in 1972 with the groin flap, and by Orticochea with the combined musculo-cutaneous gracilis flap. Since then, many surgical techniques have been proposed, based on important anatomical studies on the microvascularisation of new skin or composite flaps.

During more than 20 years, these techniques have made it possible to save limbs from amputation, to cover exposed noble structures and to offer reconstructive strategies in most of the situations where reconstructive surgery was needed. Some indications of free flaps are now in balance with more recent techniques based on a step-by-step approach.

## Principles

Microsurgical flaps offer a one-time procedure in which wound-bed preparation and coverage are done in the same surgical sequence. The flap is harvested at the donor-site area, then revascularised using microsurgical techniques on the vessels located close to the recipient site.

Several principles were adopted in the 1980s concerning the characteristics of ideal flaps like a constant anatomy, an easy harvesting procedure and an aesthetic adaptation between the donor and the recipient sites. Over the years, ideas and new concepts emerged, some of them still remaining active after two decades, others being progressively abandoned.

Some flaps, including richly vascularised structures like aponeurosis or muscles, are supposed to help the revascularisation process on the recipient site. This fact was demonstrated in the 1980s by several experimental works.

Prefabrication can help to design exceptional flaps not found in the normal human anatomy but suitable for a specific purpose. The combination of skin expansion and microsurgically transplanted vascular carriers is the basic principle of this procedure.

In the past decade, fasciocutaneous flaps branched on perforator vessels were developed, and the concept of composite flaps was examined in discussions concerning the benefits/risks of these techniques.

In fact, gaining good functional results justifies in most of the cases any deficit in aesthetic sequellae. Thus, indications followed these principles and microsurgical techniques have gained precedence in most reconstructive strategies in cancerology, hand surgery, oral and maxillofacial surgery, digestive surgery, amputation stump coverage and extensive burn-scar resurfacing.

## Different Types of Flaps

Historically, Manchot in 1889, Spalteholz in 1893 and Salmon in 1936 were the first anatomists interested in arterial and venous vascularisation of skin and muscles. Microsurgery started in fact after the pioneer works of Cheng and the first publication by McGregor of the groin flap. Extensive anatomical works were developed during the 1970s, providing each month a new flap in the catalogue. Complexity in harvesting increased, adding to pure skin flaps the possibility of using muscle, bone and fascias; in fact, a large panel of solutions adapted to the necessities of the recipient site and the strategy proposed by the surgical team. Microsurgery is a technique allowing transfer in another location of a piece of tissue that could not rotate or advance to cover a determined area.

Different classifications concerning anatomical structures and vascularisation patterns were successively proposed.

### Skin

Nakayama in 1986 defined four types of vascular compartments reaching the skin and proposed a classification in four groups: skin flaps corresponding to randomly vascularised flaps, fascio-cutaneous flaps, divided by the author into six types following the arterial pattern (I to VI), adipo-fascial flaps, septo-cutaneous flaps and musculo-cutaneous flaps.

Many authors presented the results of their research, so by and by a complete catalogue of flaps was established. Variations in thickness of the skin and of the subcutaneous tissue and colour matching between donor and recipient sites were evaluated.

### Skin and Muscles

The subsequent works of Saijo in 1988 defined three types of musculo-cutanous perforators, allowing three groups of flaps to be distinguished: cutaneous, septo-cutaneous and musculo-cutaneous.

## Muscles

Muscle vascularisation interested several authors, the first being Mathes and Na-hai in 1980 and 1981 [1]. They classified muscle vascularisation into five types, depending on the vascular anatomy. Type 1 are muscles presenting one single vascular pedicle (tensor fascia lata). In type 2, like the gracilis muscle, one dominant pedicle and several accessory pedicles are present. In type 3, two dominant pedicles come from different arteries (gluteus maximus, rectus abdominis). In type 4, several segmental pedicles are present as in the sartorius muscle. In type 5, one dominant pedicle and several secondary segmental pedicles are present as in the latissimus dorsi (Fig. 1).

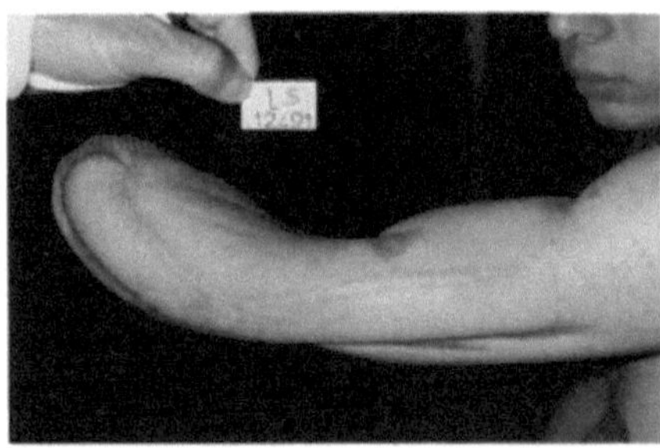

**Fig. 1.** Double composite latissimus dorsi-parascapular flap (one pedicled, the other microsurgically revascularised) in a large electrical burn of the upper limb

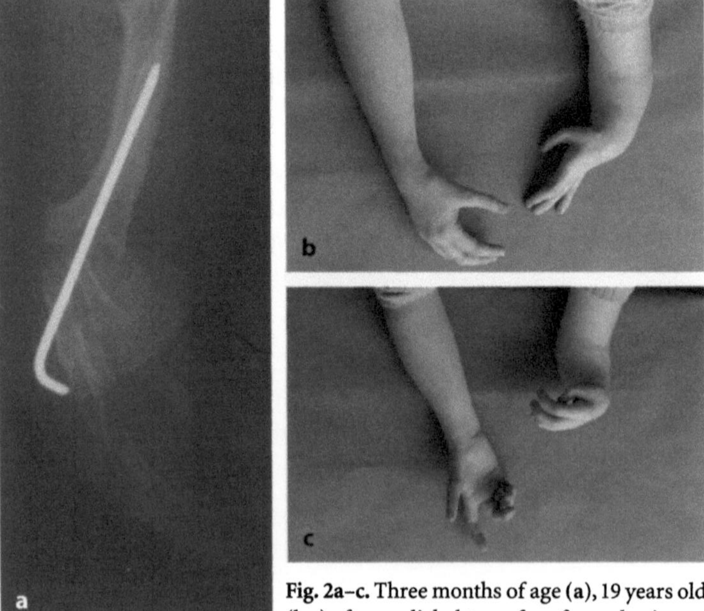

**Fig. 2a–c.** Three months of age (a), 19 years old (b,c) after pedicled transfer of apophysis

In 1984, Cormack and Lamberty added a classification concerning the fascio-cutaneous flaps in four different types (A, B, C, D). Type A corresponds to several longitudinal fascio-cutaneous arterioles (gastrocnemius), type B to the parascapular muscle, one large dominant fascio-cutaneous pedicleand type C presents a vascular lamina as in the antebrachial flap, which can be transferred as an island flap alternatively with an anterograde or a posterograde flow. Type D is a variation of type C: septal branches providing several structures in the same composite flap.

In 1994, Taylor proposed a simplification of this classification. Microsurgical transfers of muscles are usually proposed in acute wounds to cover large defects like exposed fractures of the tibial area, and, more recently, in revascularisation of devascularised feet. In this last case, the pedicled muscle was transposed at the distal end of a vascular prosthesis or venous grafts in a revascularisation process, in order to enhance the microcirculation distally. Some successes have been described.

### Bone

Many authors have tried to define the bone vasculature, and the different components (diaphyseal, epiphyseal, cortico-medullary systems) were described after the pioneer works of Gilbert et al. [2] concerning the thumb and the fibula. Other authors described the vascular systems of bones like the scapula, the iliac crest or the upper fibular epiphysis (Fig. 2).

### Epiploon and Jejunum

The vascularisation of epiploon and jejunum was re-examined in the light of the new microsurgical possibilities. Selective procedures were developed by surgeons interested in reconstructive digestive surgery, specifically on oesophageal reconstruction after carcinologic resections. Epiploon was also proposed in the treatment of defects of the anterior thoracic area.

By the right choice of flap, vascularisation opened new possibilities of using a flap without microsurgical techniques. Reverse flaps, branched on perforators distally located along a structure (skin or fascia, or muscle) were developed and presented alternatives to previous techniques or to microsurgery.

Venous flaps were used in difficult situations where arteries could not be used for any reason. The results of these venous-based flaps were fair, a certain number of thrombotic complications being reported. New possibilities like VAC for controlling venous engorgement can improve the results of these procedures.

Perforator flaps have been more recently proposed as a consequence of the anatomical work on cadavers. Composite flaps using fascia and a defined piece of skin were successfully proposed either as local flaps or transplanted microsurgically.

The advantages of free flaps are numerous. The skill necessary to perform microsurgery depends on the quality of the training of the surgeon or the team. Once this initial step is overcome, the choice of the technique depends on the compatibility between donor and recipient areas. Colour, type of tissue transplanted, quality of the function restored and usefulness of the technique have to be anticipated. When no better solution exists, microsurgery will offer a real ability to bring locally a new suppleness, fitting functionally to the recipient site and piece of tissue. The rate of failure is less than 5% and the overall rate of complications less than 10%. The fact of having a one-step procedure is an advantage, and cases where a function is re-established immediately after surgery arouse enthusiasm.

In most cases, the limited iatrogenicity is an important factor in the success of this technique. In the three decades since microsurgery started, guidelines for good practices have been developed and training includes the necessity of respecting the donor site area as far as possible.

Microsurgery can be practised even on older people, particularly on diabetic patients, where good results of covering techniques using flaps were described.

Revascularisation of lost digits or segments of limbs is still a real challenge, and clinical reports of success are numerous. Globally, reimplantation is useful depending on the age of the patient and his capacity for re-innervation (higher age means more sources of late complications). Re-innervation and revascularisation of partially traumatised digits, hands or wrists are good indications for microsurgery.

Prefabrication was proposed recently as a new possibility for creating flaps not existent in the normal anatomy. The angiogenesis offered by skin expansion, combined to a transfer of a vascular carrier just above the expander can create new vessels and link them with the carrier. Expansion of arterial and venous territories is one of the most striking events observed when using this technique. Thus, new areas and new possibilities of developing extra-large flaps are proposed. In exceptional situations, this technique can be very useful (Fig. 3).

Recently, vascularised homotransplantations were proposed by some authors in order to replace a missing limb, especially after trauma. In unilateral or bilateral amputations of the upper limbs, the results were amplified by an intense mediatisation. Apart from the spectacular sight offered by an apparently miraculous recovery, the inconveniences are numerous. The necessity of being submitted to the permanent use of immunosuppressive drugs, the risk of failure even after a long period of time, the relatively poor functional results and the lack of donors limit extension of the technique. The National Ethical Committee recently refused in France to grant authorisation for facial homotransplantation.

Limits of the free-flap techniques are linked to the difficulty of integration of the different vascular anatomies, the experience of the surgeon considering a specific flap and the rate of complications.

Colour matching is also a problem, and imposing a piece of light or brown tissue in the middle of a leg in a young teenager will cause aesthetic problems. Make-up can help and, if there is no other sequella, can be a temporary solution.

The "cake" scar induced by the flap and causing trouble in lymphatic circulation is sometimes encountered in not expanded skin flaps when the subcutaneous tissue is not submitted to pressure by previous transfer. The lack of lymphatic connections prevents a normal drainage, ending in a cake flap difficult to compress or to drain. This complication shows the limits of the technique.

The discrepancy in volume between donor and recipient sites obliges repetitive defatting surgical procedures in the following months or years. These procedures imply new hospitalisations, jeopardising the results and creating new opportunities for complications.

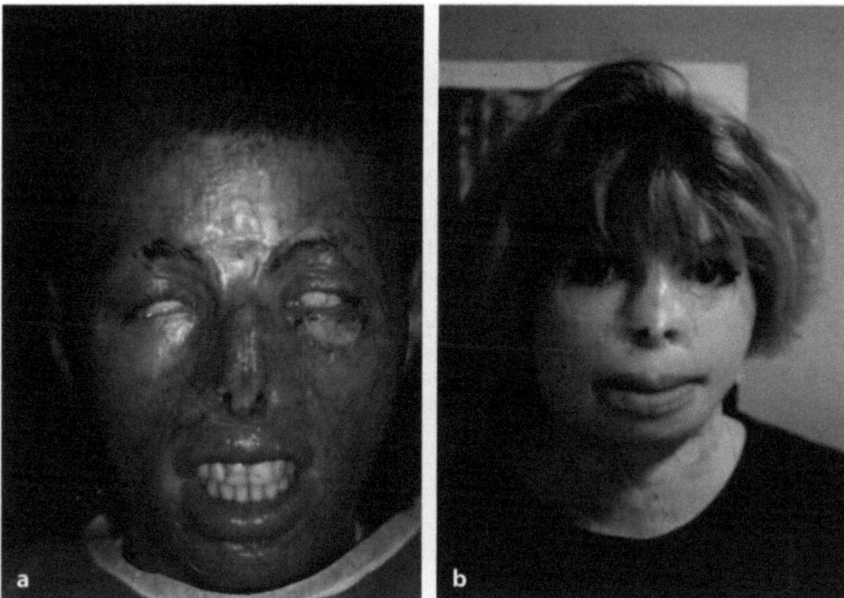

**Fig. 3a,b.** Prefabrication of facial flap to resurface a scar face after third-degree burns: before (a) and after (b)

Suppression of the donor site area is seldom described as a complication, but remains a problem in some cases. Suppression of one of the two main axes of vascularisation in the upper distal limb has been the subject of several reports emphasising the variable collaterality of the supplying vessels.

## Conclusion

Microsurgery in wounds remains a fantastic possibility to solve the covering problem in one single procedure. This technique is demanding in terms of skill, experience and team approach. In well-trained hands, the results approximate 90% uncomplicated procedures.

In the new area of wound healing microsurgical techniques are integrated in the sequential approach and it is the responsibility of the surgeon to use an adapted solution when needed. Examples of this type of combination of techniques (e.g. a microvascularised fascia covered with a dermal substitute) are progressively appearing in the literature, as well as new gene therapies applied to cells being transferred with their vessels.

New technologies will profit from the experience of microsurgical techniques already developed.

## References

1. Mathes SJ, Nahai F (1979) Clinical atlas of muscles and musculocutaneous flaps. CV Mosby, London
2. Gilbert A, Teot L (1982) The free scapular flap. Plast Reconstr Surg 69: 601–604
3. Wood M, Gilbert A (1997) Microvascular bone reconstruction. Martin Dunitz, London
4. Brunelli G (1988) Textbook of microsurgery. Masson, Paris
5. Teot L, Bosse JP, Mouffarege R, Papillon J, Beauregard G (1981) The scapular crest bone graft. Int J Microsurg 4: 1–10
6. Teot L, Gilbert A, Bosse JP, Tremblay GR (1985) Pedicled iliac crest epiphysis transplantation. Clin Orthop Rel Res 180: 286–296
7. Teot L, Bosse JP, Souyris F (1992) Pedicle scapular apophysis transplantation in congenital limb malformations. Ann Plast Surg 29: 332–340
8. Dupoirieux L, Teot L, Jammet P, Souyris F (1994) The role of microsurgery in salvage operations for cranio-cerebral gun shot wounds. J Craniomaxillofac Surg 22: 81–85
9. Teot L (1997) Prefabrication of combined scapula flaps for microsurgical reconstruction in oro-maxillofacial defects: a new technique. J Craniomaxillofac Surg 3: 174
10. Teot L, Giovannini UM, Colonna MR (1999) Use of free scapular crest flap in pediatric epiphyseal reconstructive procedures. Clin Orthop Rel Res 365: 211–220
11. Teot L, Otman S, Giovannini UM, Cherenfant E (2000) Prefabricated vascularised supraclavicular flaps. Lancet 355: 1695–1696
12. Fauré P, Canovas F, Bonnel F, Téot L, Quatra F, Giovannini UM, Colonna MR (2001) Free osteocutaneous scapular apophysis flap for reconstruction of the lateral malleolus. Ann Plast Surg 47: 328–331
13. Giovannini UM, Téot L (2002) Aesthetic complex reconstruction of the lower leg: application of a dermal substitute (Integra) to an adipofascial flap. Br J Plast Surg 109: 1747

# 21

# Post-Operative Management of Skin Graft and Flap

O. HEYMANS, N. VERHELLE

## Introduction

Even though precision and careful execution are essential during the operative procedure, an optimal result is achievable only with an optimal post-operative care. Obviously, skin grafts, flaps and free flaps follow this basic rule. In this field, as in many others, an optimal result implies functional and cosmetic concerns. Hence, the major interest seems to be the operative procedure itself. The post-operative period starts at the time of the dressing and is finished when the obtained result is stable and acceptable. So this post-operative period will be divided into early and late post-operative. Whereas the importance of the immediate post-operative care is usually well known, the late post-operative period can also be important to obtain the final result.

## Skin Graft

### Immediate Post-Operative Period

After graft inset, it is very important to pay special attention to the factors and complications that can contribute to the survival of the skin graft. Particular attention should thus be paid to ensure:

- careful haemostasis and avoiding haematomas and fluid collections between the graft and the recipient site and thus minimizing the infection risk,
- adequate postoperative graft immobilisation.

### Careful Haemostasis and Preventing Haematomas

#### Peri-Operative

Since the percentage of graft take depends on the extent and speed at which vascular perfusion is restored to the graft, a close contact has to be insured. Clots will isolate the undersurface of the graft from the recipient site so that neovascularisation will not take place, leading to graft take failure. During the operative procedure, a complete debridement of the wound has to be performed, removing all dead tissue to avoid bacterial contamination. By this debridement, a new well-vascularised bed should be obtained in a chronic wound as well as in acute burns. However, careful haemostasis should be performed and some additional surgical techniques can be used to prevent accumulation of blood. By meshing the grafts, multiple small slits can be made prior to transplantation, allowing adequate blood drainage through the interstices. On the other hand, in meshed grafts, there is a considerable surface area that must heal by secondary intention, decreasing the cosmetic result. These grafts will be used to cover large areas with minimal morbidity, but they cannot be applied to cover functionally important or visible regions such as the hands and the face.

### Dressing

A light pressure dressing on the grafts is of major importance. Indeed, adequate compression crushes the opened small vessels, which will reduce the post-operative bleeding. On the other hand, excessive pressure (exceeding 30 mmHg) on a fresh graft may also cause it to die. A light compression can be obtained by a three-layer dressing. A Vaseline gauze is placed on the skin graft, while the second layer consists in a tie-over which is stapled to the edges of the graft. The third compressive layer consists of simple gauzes. Although these three-layer dressings will not be able to prevent arterial bleeding, they will minimise the overall haematoma risk very efficiently.

### Post-Operative

Since blood accumulation under the graft has to be avoided, a decrease of the venous pressure is of prime interest. Adequate limb compression by any kind of bandages combined with limb elevation will reduce the venous pressure, decreasing the bleeding risk and post-operative swelling. In difficult cases, we advise bed rest with proper elevation of the operated limb until skin graft take has been established (i.e. post-operative day 5 to 7).

Unfortunately, primary contraction of the graft, probably due to recoil of the dermal elastic fibres, and skin graft shrinkage (secondary contraction) will already start early after transfer to the recipient site. This wound contraction can be clinically useful in selected areas in order to reduce the wound surface, but in functional areas such as hands or articulations it should be minimal. To control the degree of contraction, the thickness and proportion of the dermis in the graft is of major importance: full-thickness grafts will prevent wound contraction better than split-thickness grafts. Compression garments, immobilisation and splinting of the grafted "functional" areas of the structures can also help to exercise some control over the degree of graft contraction.

### Adequate Post-Operative Graft Immobilisation

Since close contact between the graft bed and the graft is required for optimal graft take, a light compressive dressing should be applied as described above. However, frequently the skin is placed on a muscle surface after debridement. To allow optimal vascular ingrowth in these cases, the total immobilisation of the underlying muscular structure is essential. Otherwise, new-formed vessels will be squeezed and disrupted, decreasing the graft take. Even if all efforts have been made to prevent post-operative bleeding, it will occur at a minimal level. This blood accumulation, however, will pass into the Vaseline gauze without crust formation between the graft and the gauze. This allows an easy removal of the dressing after 5 to 7 days, thus avoiding traumatic forces onto the newly taken graft. Moreover, some blood or exudate can be absorbed by the tie-over.

### Late Post-Operative Period

This period starts after the blood flow has been restored in the transferred graft (on post-operative day 5 or 6) and will last until the complete stabilisation of the healing process. Although a proper vascular system can be re-established within the graft somewhere between the fifth and sixth post-operative day, resulting in excellent graft take, there are some conditions under which grafts will heal by secondary intention. In meshed grafts, for example, secondary healing will occur at the interstices of the meshed graft, or even in non-meshed grafts secondary healing can occur in the areas between applied grafts. During this period it is thus mandatory to continue a moist environment by applying dressings.

### Sun Prevention

As for every scar, during the early post-operative period, sun exposure can be deleterious. As prescribed in simple linear scars, sun exposure has to be avoided until the pink graft colour has faded to a basically normal skin tone. Otherwise, the hyperpigmentation state of the graft, following the cutaneous grafting, will be prolonged or might be permanent.

### Substitution of the Hydratation Process

Normal skin benefits from a complex mechanism, including neural, humoral and hormonal factors, regulating the hydratation process. These different controls are decreased after transplantation since especially in split skin grafts no sweat glands or sebaceous glands will be transplanted. These grafts will appear typically dry and brittle after take, which has to be prevented by applying fatty creams to avoid hyperkeratosis.

### Physical Therapy and Prevention of Hypertrophic Scars

During graft healing, wound contraction occurs, leading to tight and immobile areas often with distortion of the surrounding normal tissue. Although this phenomenon is less important in full-thickness grafts, it may cause contractures around flexion areas or other functional zones such as articulations. It is therefore essential to exercise some control on the degree of wound contracture in the grafted zones for aesthetic and functional reasons. Manual massages, mobilisation and LPG® can help the surgeon to control this problem.

Prevention of hypertrophic scars is also essential. Although the previously cited methods reduce the occurrence of hypertrophic scars, several other treatments have to be addressed. Compression of the grafted area, 23 h/24 h for a long period (1 to 1½ year) remains very important in terms of prevention and treatment. Constant pressure on scar formation, nowadays mostly in combination with silicone gel, makes a softer and thinner scar, and should be applied for the total period of scar maturation. The mode of action of silicone gel is thought to be physical, chemical or a combination of both. Whenever scar contractures are encountered, this conservative treatment may soften the contractures, but due to the localisation of these contractures, this technique is often inadequate. In web space contractures, for example, additional physical therapy such as manual therapy, mobilisation and LPG has to be started in combination with the compression therapy. In selected cases, intralesional injection of steroids can be performed to retard the excessive collagen deposition. Drawbacks to this technique are possible local hypopigmentation, skin atrophy and teleangiectasia.

If these therapies remain unsuccessful, surgical correction of the contracture has to be considered.

## Flaps

As mentioned before, flaps correspond to a unit of vascularised tissue that can be used for many purposes. Island flaps or pedicled flaps remain attached by their vascular pedicle while free flaps need a microvascular anastomosis after transfer.

As in the skin-graft post-operative care, the post-operative evolution can be divided into two periods: the immediate post-operative and the late post-operative period. Although some differences exist between free and pedicled flaps during the early post-operative period, the general principles remain similar.

### Early Post-Operative Period

#### Vascular Survey

In free flap transfer, the microvascular permeability remains the key point during this early post-operative period. Indeed, survival of the transferred tissue is totally dependent on the vascular inflow. Unfortunately, processes of vasospasm and thrombosis exist and can sometimes be controlled by pharmacologic agents. Post-operative surveillance is thus fundamental. This surveillance will consist of clinical assessment of skin colour, temperature and capillary refill in combination with Doppler examination of the nutrient pedicle. A pale coloration combined with an absence of capillary refill and Doppler tone will suggest an arterial occlusion and no bleeding will occur after perforating the flap with a needle. On the other hand, when the flap becomes bluish and swollen, a venous occlusion can be suspected even when a good arterial Doppler tone can be heard. In these cases, needle puncture will usually produce an abundant bleeding of dark blood.

Laser-Doppler, transcutaneous oxymetry, microdyalisis or thermography can be applied, but are expensive and not superior to the clinical expertise. Although there is no microsurgical procedure during the transfer of pedicled flaps, post-operative monitoring can provide some useful information under certain conditions after these flap transfers.

### Revision

Whenever the decision is made to revise a flap, it will be based on the argument of the vascular survey. Indeed, suspicion of an arterial or venous problem requires immediate revision in order to restore the in- or outflow as soon as possible. Causes of arterial or venous problems are numerous but the result is quite similar: microvascular thrombosis, which has to be corrected as soon as possible to avoid ischemia-reperfusion injury and especially flap necrosis.

During revision, the cause of the flap failure has to be established (compression due to a haematoma, poor suture quality, pedicle torsion etc.). Once the cause has been found, correcting the problem can often salvage the failing flap although a thrombectomy and new microvascular anastomosis has to be performed. Unfortunately, due to thrombosis and vascular distension, the endothelium and subendothelium of the vessel walls can be permanently disturbed, causing recurrent microsuture thrombosis. In these cases, an anti-thrombotic therapy (heparin or low molecular weight heparin therapeutic dose) is frequently started in order to reduce the thrombotic risk.

Depending on the experience of the observer, the devices to monitor the blood flow, the skills of the nursing team and the availability of OR facility, the revision can be performed quickly. It is obvious that the time before revision is essential concerning the prognosis. Depending on the staff skills (surgeon, anaesthetist, nurses) and the patient's profile, the revision rate varies from 2 to 20%. Although these revisions need an important infrastructure and maximal expertise, they will be successful in only 50 to 60% of the cases.

### Postural Requirements

Since tissue viability is highly dependent on the inflow, postural considerations are important. Declivity improves the flap inflow whereas proclivity improves venous drainage. However, under normal conditions the patient is positioned in a strictly prone position. On the other hand, compression to the flap or to the pedicle is absolutely forbidden. This means that the position of the patient in his bed should be checked regularly.

### Anti-Thrombotic Therapy

As mentioned above, vascular and microvascular surgery is classically associated with a marked risk of thrombus formation. These thrombi can develop in the arterial or venous anastomotic site, due to many technical or pathologic events. Although technical errors cannot be corrected by pharmacologic agents, an anti-thrombotic prevention is usually prescribed.

Unfortunately, in literature only few reports can be found on experiments in humans dealing with anti-thrombotic therapy. Many trials have indeed been performed on animals but in humans there is still a lack of standardisation. So, the applied post-operative anti-thrombotic therapy is mainly empiric or has a purely theoretical basis. Plasmatic expanders (pentastarch, dextran etc.), heparins, low molecular weight heparin, Buflomedil, aspirin, NSAID etc., correspond to this large armentarium. Despite the low haemorrhagic risk, aspirin combined with pentastarch and low molecular weight heparin seems to be becoming standard therapy.

### Dressing

Whenever a skin flap or composite flap with a skin pedicle is used, wound healing will occur uneventfully. However, care must be taken to avoid any compression of the dressing onto the flap or near to the pedicle to avoid any circular compression. In muscle flaps, skin grafting can be delayed for several days to allow the formation of granulation tissue and to make the early follow-up easier (colour, bleeding of the muscle flap). During this period, a Vaseline dressing is recommended in order to avoid any superficial desiccation, which may induce necrosis and difficult clinical assessment.

## Late Post-Operative Period

The critical period for thrombus formation in the anastomosis is in the first 3 to 5 days. After this critical period, other events such as pedicle compression or section of the pedicle can still occur. Whenever flap coverage is performed, the main goal is to obtain good healing of the flap edges and excellent graft take on, for example, muscular flaps. However, oedema is usually an important factor affecting the post-operative period, and can negatively interfere with the flap survival. Finally, the mechanical properties of the transferred tissues together with their complete anaesthesia make post-operative care and protection essential to obtain a stable result.

### Graft Take and Healing

Since flaps are vital tissues with adequate vascularisation, normal healing and good graft take are expected. However, in some situations, delayed healing can occur. It is a basic principle and technique to harvest a piece of tissue which corresponds to the angiosome of a certain pedicle. In this way, the harvested tissue will be well vascularised up to the edges of the flap. However, atheromatosis, diabetes and other comorbidities can decrease the flap size which normally corresponds to the angiosome.

In pedicled flaps, the distal flap tissue is often located where the defect closure is essential. Unfortunately, the viability of this distal flap tissue is less reliable, especially when important tension is used to close the defect. This is one of the main reasons why distal necrosis or poor graft take is encountered in areas where coverage is essential. Although in free flap surgery distal necrosis may occur, it is a situation which is less frequent.

In chronic wounds, flap coverage is often required. Well-vascularised tissues are thus brought into a damaged area. However, imbalance between the vascular status of both tissues (donor and recipient site) may cause healing problems. In these situations, non-union of the flap edges frequently occurs, which can be treated by leaving the stitches for a long time and by prolonged secondary healing. However, these situations should be avoided and, whenever possible, a well-vascularised recipient bed should be obtained after debridement.

### Oedema

Although the flap size is selected to fit perfectly into the defect, post-operative swelling of the flap occurs and may cause important problems. Oedema of a flap placed on a heel, for example, causes functional disturbances in terms of gait rehabilitation and for footwear. In other sites, flap oedema may cause serious aesthetic problems.

Salmi described the evolution of oedema after transfer. Flap oedema starts immediately after flap transfer and will be at its maximum after 3 months. After the third post-operative month, the volume of the flap will decrease until the ninth post-operative month, but it will never reach a volume similar to that obtained right after flap inset. Discussion has been going on for years to explain the cause of this oedema which can be vascular, lymphatic, a result of an ischemia-reperfusion injury or the inflammatory phenomenon following any kind of surgery.

It is probable that whenever a flap is isolated on its pedicle and an adventitectomy has been performed, a sympathetic blockage is induced, resulting in an intra-flap vasodilatation. This increases the flap inflow and will have an immediate effect on the venous network, which will dilate thanks to its important capacity.

During flap harvesting, pedicular dissection disrupts the lymphatic vessels. Moreover, when a flap is isolated, the lymphatic channels going to the neighbouring tissues will also be disrupted. It is obvious that during the immediate post-operative period, there is no lymphatic return. However, the lymphangiogenitic process will start immediately after transfer, creating new lymphatic vessels merging with the lymphatics located in the neighbouring tissues. A lymphoscintigram, realised several days after transfer, already shows an efficient lymphatic uptake.

The ischemia-reperfusion injury is a well-known problem encountered when a perfusion is re-installed after a prolonged time of warm ischemia. This phenomenon is likely to occur after 3 h of warm ischemia and induces tissue necrosis and major oedema. Although under normal conditions the ischemic time is no longer than 60 min, this phenomenon can develop after difficult anastomosis or later after thrombotic occlusion of the microsurgical anastomosis.

### Post-Operative Oedema Management

Due to the induced denervation, the transferred tissue will atrophy, especially when the transferred and denervated tissue is muscular. Transferred tissue can be hard, needing manoeuvres to make it more supple and help the lymphatic drainage. So, when a complete healing has been obtained, physical therapy will be started, including mobilisation, massage, lymphatic drainage and LPG. As prescribed after skin grafting, customised compressive garments can be applied. This treatment improves the flap contour and flap integration.

### Flap Inflow

Depending on the location, external compression will be applied to the flap. This is, for example, obvious for flaps transferred to the plantar surface. However, also flaps transferred to the ankle region can be compressed by footwear or external compression can be induced by wearing a bra after breast reconstruction. Immediately after transfer, the flap viability is directly dependent on its pedicle inflow. Thus, any compression to this pedicle may cause ischemia and may put this flap in danger. All previous examples illustrate this concept. However, during the healing process, new capillaries (angiogenic process) sprout from the surrounding tissues into the flap, establishing a dual inflow to the flap. The extent of this phenomenon depends on many factors such as the area of contact between tissues, the type of transferred tissue, the type of surrounding tissue etc. Thanks to the dual inflow, the flap will become less dependent on the pedicle and less vulnerable to mechanical stress such as compression. For these reasons, compression garments are not applied during the early post-operative period.

Even if direct vascular compression is avoided, mechanical stress to the flap can cause ulcerations or other wounds. The risk for these injuries is directly linked to the hyposensitivity of the transferred tissues. Indeed, it is rare that flaps are sensate. Much has been written in the literature on this type of prevention but discussion still persists and it seems to be highly dependent on individual configuration of the reconstructed area. For example, after flap coverage of a sacral pressure sore, the flaps should be protected by reposition of the patient every 2 h, whereas the flap on a reconstructed heel reconstruction should be protected with special footwear and protective soles.

# 22

# Dermabrasion and Management of Donor Sites

K.N. Dolynchuk

## Introduction

Since the 1940s dermabrasion has been used the world over for various pathological conditions as well as cosmetic rhytid removal by dermatologists and plastic surgeons [1]. However, since the 1980s the risk of blood-borne pathogens has reduced the popularity of dermabrasion. Since then, a resurgence in the approach to skin pathology has appeared anew with the advent of microdermabrasion and ancillary techniques such as laser ablation [1–3]. This chapter will highlight the clinical aspects of the dermabrasion techniques and management of the acute wounds resulting from them. Since skin graft donor sites are similar in nature to dermablated wounds, they are covered here as well. The surgical techniques for each will be discussed.

## Clinical Aspects

Indications for dermabrasion include acne scarring, actinic keratosis, seborrheic keratosis, acne rosacea, rhinophyma, traumatic and decorative tattoos, Hailey–Hailey disease, Darier's disease, tylosis, keratoderma, rhytids and nitrogen mustard exposure. The techniques employed vary according to the location of the lesion and the degree of depth required. The use of refrigerants has been shown to be helpful by allowing better depth of ablation as well as pain relief. However, these agents are dangerous as well as toxic to the ozone.

Dermaplaning is essentially the tangential excision of skin with a dermatome. It can be useful over large areas of skin involvement, such as acne on the back. It is recommended that tumescent solutions should be used to minimise pain and bleeding. The amount of infiltration is sufficient to palpably distend the skin. Blood loss would be expected to be similar to harvesting a split-thickness skin graft, that is, 45 cc per 46 cm$^2$ or less with the use of tumescence.

Microdermabrasion has been studied as a less invasive approach to rejuvenation of facial skin; since the dermis is not entered, there is less risk of blood splatter. However, there is clinical improvement of fine rhytids by a reparative mechanism in the dermis and the epidermis [4]. Patients may require multiple sessions and active acne is a relative contra-indication.

Resurfacing lasers such as carbon dioxide ($CO_2$) and erbium yttrium aluminum garnet (er:YAG) have been a valuable adjunct for many of the same indications as dermabrasion. Since the early 1980s the er:YAG laser has been gradually gaining in popularity over $CO_2$ laser resurfacing since it is able to ablate as deeply without the complications or delayed healing seen with $CO_2$. The ability to contract the dermis 16% at 16 weeks is equivalent to $CO_2$ as well [5]. However, no randomised control trials exist to support the use of er:YAG over $CO_2$ in acne scar management [6]. These lasers are also indicated in verrucous hamartoma, extensive benign superficial dermo-epidermal lesions, and they are particularly indicated in extensive diffuse lesions or when potential HIV contamination is an issue [7].

The acute wound created by dermabrasion and ablative lasers heals by epithelialisation. The mechanism involves cell-cycle changes in the perifollicular stem cells and epithelial cells along the wound margin, leading to migration from appendageal structures and the wound edge by epiboly. The $\alpha$ 9 integrins are involved as well as syndecan-1 in mediating cellular proliferation in wounded epithelial tissue [8].

The differences in amino propepeptide containing collagen type I (pN-I collagen) and that of type-III collagen (pN-III collagen) are consistent in amount and duration with that of any fibroblastic response to injury in the dermis. The levels of TGF $\beta$ are also in keeping with normal fibroplasia [9].

The time to complete epithelialisation will depend on the depth of the injury and the conditions in the wound. The average time for healing in a dermabraded wound is 2 weeks, with that of $CO_2$ and er:YAG 5–10 days, respectively. The use of *cis*-retinoic acid has been suggested to increase the rate of healing in dermabrasion injury but this does not appear to be beneficial in normal patients. Donor-site wounds are usually altered somewhat in terms of skin texture, as are deep dermabrasion results (Fig. 1).

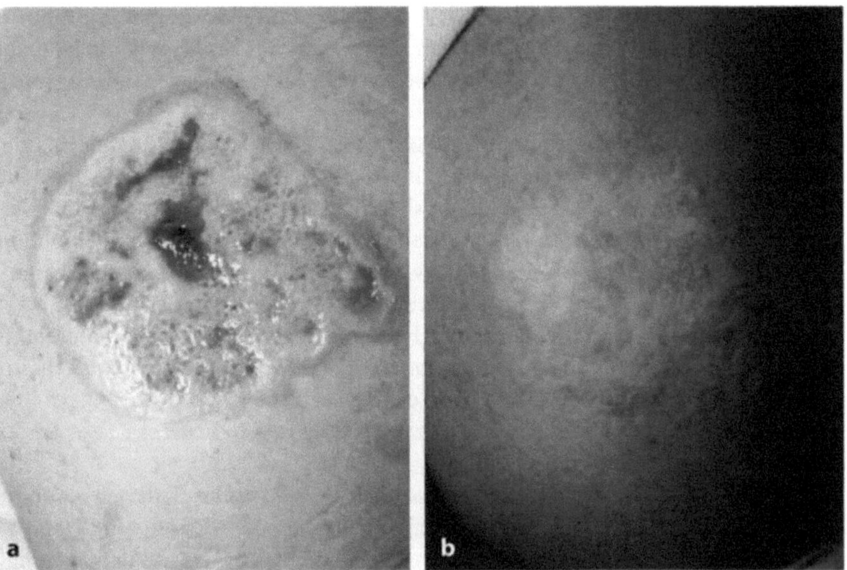

**Fig. 1a,b.** Intra-operative (a) and 6 weeks post-operative (b) tattoo removal: results after dermabrasion

## Surgical Aspects

The safe use of ablative techniques requires a thorough understanding of the technique and its potential complications in order to avert problems. This starts with proper patient selection, as Fitzpatrick types V and VI are contra-indicated for use of dermabrasion and $CO_2$ ablation techniques [10]. However, even darkly pigmented patients can be treated safely with er:YAG laser at shallow depths. True keloid formers are not recommended for dermablation. Alt describes several aids to the safe use of dermabrasion. Use of Turkish towels for retraction and special refrigerant handling are of questionable benefit, because few people use cooling since it is environmentally hazardous, and any woven dressing near the tip of the dermabrader can easily get wrapped in it and spun around dangerously. If possible, scar revision should be carried out before dermabrasion, either by subcision or by actual excision and closure techniques [1]. Control of acniform lesions pre-operatively is desirable. The need to discontinue Accutane at least 6 months before the operation will reduce hypertrophic scarring. The patient should be informed of the potential risk of hyperpigmentation, and solar avoidance is advised. The possibility of hypopigmentation at deeper levels is also a risk and difficult to treat if it occurs. Herpes simplex type I and Herpes zoster need to be prophylaxed with the use of antiviral medication such as famcyclovir, 250 mg po BID starting the night before surgery until the wound is closed [11]. Antibiotics are seldom necessary with the use of moisture-retentive dressings such as film dressings, e.g. Omiderm and Tegaderm, or hydrogel dressings, e.g. Fexzan or Vigilon [12]. However, triple antibiotic ointment has been shown to be the best choice if infection supervenes [13]. Awareness of unusual infections is also necessary [11]. Pain is difficult to control with dermabrasion, although tumescent techniques and topical EMLA are helpful [14]. Carbon dioxide and er:YAG laser ablation can be done with topical anaesthetic and/or nerve block, as well as conscious sedation. Eye protection is mandatory with both techniques. Desiccation of the wound will lead to delayed healing and possible scarring as well as infection. The use of moisture-retentive dressing for the first 2–3 days followed by topical Elta or Aquafor will prevent this sequela. Though no proven technique exists, it is known that skin heals faster in a moist environment [15]. The redness that persists after the treatment varies with the technique used. Dermabrasion is usually the worst, being 3–6 months. $CO_2$ is prolonged in terms of erythema as well. Er:YAG, on the other hand, remains visibly red for a period of 3–6 weeks. Use of a camouflage mineral-based cover can be helpful during this early phase of recovery.

The techniques used are published widely in the literature. However, a brief description is offered here. Dermabrasion is conducted with a wire brush, fraise burr or diamond wheel attached to a variable-speed hand engine. The skin may be turgid with tumescent-anaesthetic fluid containing 1:1 million epinephrine to reduce bleeding and pain. The area to be treated is firmly stabilised and care taken not to avulse the skin by abrading toward the thinner, more mobile, skin edge. The bleeding encountered may be reduced with metal shields and care in avoiding splatter into the air is taken by adjusting the speed of the bur. The depth of ablation is sometimes gauged by application of gentian violet or methylene blue to the skin. Its removal indicates the uniform depth of ablation but penetration into the papillary dermis is noted by the presence of punctate bleeding. The wound is compressed briefly and dressings applied. Dermaplaning is carried out with a deratome, either hand-held or power-driven, by removing successive thin layers of skin from the affected area. The results are similar, but finer control is maintained with the burr.

The use of laser ablation is usually carried out with either a free-hand technique for small lesions or a computer-generated scanner to treat larger areas. Skin preparation may be with topical anaesthetic or nerve blocks; general anaesthesia may also be required as with dermabrasion.

Successive passes of the $CO_2$ laser result in a chamois appearance to the skin, indicating that the mid reticular dermis has been entered. The depth of ablation is not as obvious with er:YAG. However, the new lasers allow the operator to set the depth that a single pass will achieve. The usual initial pass is through the epidermis and the subsequent one or two passes are into the dermis to varied depth, depending on the desired outcome; the deeper the penetration the greater the bleeding. Therefore, the ability to use a long pulse duration at an alternating frequency with the ablating pulse will reduce this problem. The result is a clean wound surface and a limited thermal gradient, unlike that seen with $CO_2$ lasers [16].

Dressings are as individual as the operator, though certain points are deemed desirable for optimal healing. In the case of donor sites, tulle dressings and dry castings with scarlet red not only heal more slowly, the pain is also greater as compared to moist dressings. The haemostatic absorbent contact layer used commonly is an alginate, such as Kaltostat or Aquacel. This is covered with film or semi-occlusive dressings such as Opsite or Biocclusive. Donor-site dressings do not need to be removed for 7 to 10 days.

In the case of laser peels, the wound is less exudative but the face is contoured and more difficult to dress. The careful application of hydrogel sheets or silicone sealants such as Diamond Seal will often be used in the first few days, followed by frequent washing, with application of a rich emollient such as Crisco, Eucerin or Elta afterwards until healing. The exclusive use of emollients can be used in an open fashion as well. The patient needs to participate in the management, and this requires selection as opposed to the closed technique, which may be easier for the patient. However, dressing-related problems have been described, such as infection and pattern formation on the skin [17].

## Conclusion

The use of dermabrasion has been in and out of favour over the years. However, it provides an inexpensive alternative to ablation or dermopathology, which respond to these techniques. The clinical example shown of a tattoo removal using dermabrasion in Fig. 1 demonstrates its effect. The time to healing and attendant pain, swelling and redness have been reduced somewhat by the use of lasers, of which er:YAG is currently the gold standard.

## References

1. Alt T (1987) Technical aids for dermabrasion. J Dermatol Surg Oncol 13: 638–648
2. Kitzmiller W et al. (2000) A controlled evaluation of dermabrasion versus $CO_2$ laser resurfacing for the treatment of perioral wrinkles. Plast Reconstr Surg 106: 1366–1372
3. Kwon S, Kye Y (2000) Treatment of scars with a pulsed Er:YAG laser. J Cutan Laser Ther 2: 27–31
4. Freedman B, Rueda-Pedraza E, Waddall S (2001) The epidermal and dermal changes associated with dermabrasion. Dermatol Surg 27: 1033–1004
5. Fleming D (1999) Controversies in skin resurfacing: the role of erbium. J Cutan Laser Ther 1: 15–21
6. Jordan R et al. (2001) Laser resurfacing for facial acne scars. Cochrane Database Syst Rev 1: CD001866
7. Mazer J (2002) Indications for medical lasers in dermatology. Presse Med 9: 223–231
8. Stepp M et al. (2002) Defects in keratinocyte activation during wound healing in the syndecan-1-deficient mouse. J Cell Science 1: 4517–4531
9. Nelson B et al. (1996) A comparison of wire brush and diamond fraise superficial dermabrasion for photoaged skin: a clinical, immunohistologic, and biochemical study. J Am Acad Dermatol 34: 235–243
10. Seckel B (1996) Aesthetic laser surgery. Little and Brown, Boston, p 162
11. Garman M, Orengo I (2003) Unusual infectious complications of dermatologic procedures. Dermatol Clin 21: 321–325
12. Smith R (1997) Dermabrasion: is it an option? Aust Fam Physician 26: 1041–1044
13. Berger R et al. (2000) A newly formulated topical triple-antibiotic ointment minimizes scarring. Cutis 65: 401–404
14. Goodman G (1994) Dermabrasion using tumescent technique. J Dermatol Surg Oncol 20: 802–807
15. Ryan TJ (1990) Wound healing and current dermatologic dressings. Leg Ulcers 4: 21–29
16. Koch R (1999) Laser resurfacing of the periorbital region. Facial Plast Surg 15: 263–270
17. Weinstein C (2000) Postoperative laser care. Clin Plast Surg 27: 251–262

# V  Specific Wound Problems



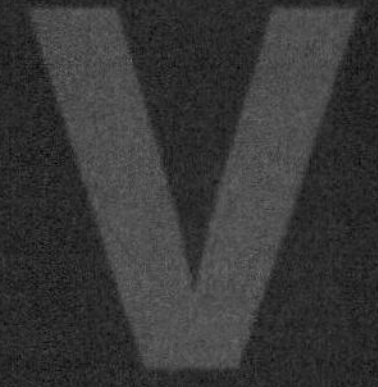

G. Pivato, A. Gilbert

## Introduction

Tissue defect has always been a challenge for the reconstructive surgeon. The first systematic procedure using a flap for repairing a mutilated nose in an adult female is attributed to Suœruta, who lived in the 6th or 7th century B.C. [1]. More recently, the Italian surgeon Gaspare Tagliacozzi described a delayed flap taken from the arm and also used for reconstruction of the nose [2]. After that, few clinical applications were described until 20 years ago; however, we may be astonished by the discrepancy between the incredible sum of knowledge available in the early 20th century and the applications that have been performed.

## History

We believe that three concomitant axes of development can be considered from historical points of view.

**The Empirical Development of Surgical Concepts.** Many of the now familiar concepts of reconstructive surgery were already known a long time ago and have been rediscovered only recently. To our knowledge, the first true axial pattern cutaneous flap was performed in 1862 by John Wood [3], who treated a severe burn deformity of the hand with a flap that based the superficial epigastric vessels: he called it the groin flap. There is no doubt that Wood's groin flap significantly predates that described by Shaw and Payne, also based on the superficial epigastric vessels. It also corresponds to the axial pattern flap which was introduced by McGregor and Jackson in 1972 [4].

In 1892, three decades after the first groin flap, the Italian surgeon Igino Tansini [5] covered a radical removal of a breast cancer by a dorsal skin flap, whose pedicle was based in the armpit; however, the flap did not survive completely, but with his studies he established the fundamental notion of the pedicled muscle flap and the myocutaneous flap with corresponding overlying skin territory. Unfortunately, Tansini's procedure of radical mastectomy was swiftly supplanted by Halsted's technique. The latissimus dorsi flap was abandoned and forgotten for many years before being rediscovered in 1986 by Olivari [6] and Quillien [7].

At the beginning of the 20th century and even later, the method used by all surgeons in elevating skin flaps followed the dogma of the never-to-be-exceeded length/breadth ratio of 1:1. The Dutch surgeon Esser felt that the notion of including a band of skin as large as possible in the pedicle of a flap was wrong. He first introduced the concept of "island flap" [8]: With his method, he elevated flaps where the skin had been completely removed around the pedicle. In this way, Esser presented the concept of pedicled flaps long before modern authors such as Littler [9] and Moberg [10].

**Anatomical Knowledge.** Concerning the anatomical knowledge about blood supply to the skin, the earliest study of value is that of Carl Manchot from Hamburg. He gives a detailed description of the deep cutaneous arteries and their emergence from the underlying muscles [11]. However, he does not accord importance to the small but continuous vessels which arise from the main arteries and directly supply the skin. The definitive work on the cutaneous arteries was done by the French anatomist and surgeon Michel Salmon in 1936 [12]. The work of Salmon was complete and innovative, and is still valid; today it represents a mine of information, and several authors have thought of new flaps as a result of reading it.

**The Technical Achievement of Vascular Anastomoses and the Use of Binocular Microscopes.** Recent advances in reconstructive surgery would not have been possible without the ability to suture vessels and to perform microsurgical anastomoses under the microscope. The earliest and most fundamental work was probably done by Alexis Carrel in 1902 [13], in which he described experimental studies of vascular end-to-end anastomoses. He also worked with Charles Guthrie to perform organ transplants in animals. The other basic advance was the introduction of the operative microscope by the Swedish surgeon Carl Nylen in 1921 [14].

## Application

This historical review of the pioneers demonstrates that at the beginning of the 1920s all the concepts, anatomical knowledge and technical abilities were sufficiently established to make flap surgery and even the free vascular flap possible as we know it now. So why has it been necessary to wait more than 30 years, and 50 years in some fields, to see the true development of surgical procedures? We believe that the principal obstacle to development was the dogma of the never-to-be-exceeded length/breadth ratio of 1:1.

Undoubtedly, microsurgery, and especially microvascular surgery, have been the catalyst for the explosive development of modern reconstructive surgery. All researches and clinical applications were dramatically stimulated by the publication of the work of Jacobson and Suarez on the anastomoses of 1-mm blood vessel in 1960 [15]; in 1960 Buncke reported the successful replantation of amputated rabbit ears [16]; in 1962 Malt achieved the world's first arm replantation (without a microscope) [17], in 1965 Tamai performed the first microsurgical replantation of a completely amputated thumb and in 1969 Cobbett reported first hallux-to-thumb transfer [18]. Microvascular surgery also enabled free tissue transfer in experimental research and the first clinical applications were carried out at almost the same time.

The early 1970s saw the fusion of the concept of the flap, the technical possibility of using the operative microscope for microvascular surgery and the anatomical knowledge necessary for the procedures. It became increasingly clear that all tissues could be transferred with their blood supply. In the later 1970s, events accelerated. Olivari rediscovered the latissimus dorsi flap in 1976 [19]. In the same year, Baudet proposed the term musculocutaneous flap, and in 1979 Mathes and Nahai established a systematic and still valid classification of muscle vascularisation [20].

Three major advances took place in the early 1980s: a Chinese military surgeon, Yang Kuofan, demonstrated the possibility of elevating a skin flap based on a main artery which is not the vascular artery of the flap (the radial forearm flap) [21]; in 1981, Ponten demonstrated empirically the survival of a pedicled flap taken from the leg with a length/breadth ratio of 4:1 when the skin is elevated with the subcutaneous tissue on the fascia en bloc [22]; in 1982, Chinese authors took a new step in proposing the distally based pedicled island flap, which seemed extravagant, as it defied Harvey's law for the venous return.

All these new discoveries stimulated in the 1980s the interest in anatomy in order to find new applications and undescribed flaps. Today, clinical research is oriented towards compound transfers and prefabricated microsurgical tissue units. Decades after the first free revascularised skin flap, we believe that the solutions provided by reconstructive surgery are limited only by the imagination of the surgeon.

## Vascular Anatomy

### Skin Vascularisation

In terms of the descriptive vascular cutaneous anatomy, Salmon [12] distinguished between direct and indirect arteries. This distinction is still valid.

Direct arteries are destined directly for the skin, they arise from the deep tissues and pass through the fascia. They can be classified into two groups according to their size, their length and their direction: namely, arteries with a long course and septal arteries. **Long-course arteries** perforate the aponeurosis obliquely and then follow a pathway in the depths of the subcutaneous tissue. These arteries are of limited number at the level of the extremities and are of significant size (between 1 and 2 mm at their origin). Included in the long-course arteries are those neurocutaneous arteries that accompany superficial sensory nerves. **Septal arteries** are branches of an axial artery. They course in a septum situated generally between two muscles and run perpendicular to the principal artery in the skin. After they have perforated the aponeurosis, they run in a tortuous manner, with anastomoses linking them in the immediate subaponeurotic plane. These anastomoses constitute an extremely important axial plexiform network when the aponeurosis is included in the elevation. These anastomotic curls or ringlets give birth to branches that comprise a second plexiform network in the plane of the subcutaneous tissue where the terminal arterials of the skin are borne [23]. Additional indirect vascularisation is provided by the arterials of muscular origin that traverse the aponeurosis and are distributed to the skin. There exists then a correlation between the type of cutaneous vascularisation and the method of vascularisation of flaps. The long-course arteries are the basis of those flaps with axial vascularisation, of which an example is the groin flap. Septal vascularisation constitutes the foundation of septocutaneous flaps. This term implies that it is necessary to include the septum containing the vascular axis during the elevation of these flaps. Finally, indirect vascularisation of muscular origin is the basis for musculocutaneous flaps, a fact known for a long time [24, 25]. This kind of vascularisation is provided by the arteries of muscular origin that traverse the fascia and are distributed to the skin.

### Skin Territory and the Territory of Flaps

It is remarkable that the same cutaneous territory can give rise to the description of three flaps with different modes of vascularisation. In effect, at the level of the limbs, certain privileged sites are nourished by all three types of cutaneous vascularisation described above, with, in addition, multiple anastomoses between these three systems. Once the vascularisation of a flap has been determined, the extent of its territory is difficult to determine precisely. An anatomical territory can be marked out by following for as long as possible the vascular axis of the flap, but this method is only valuable for those flaps with axial vascularisation. The cutaneous territory of an artery under physiological conditions is surely smaller than the anatomical territory: the existence of peripheral pressure due to neighbouring arteries in effect limits the cutaneous territory of the artery of the flap. This, then, is a dynamic territory. In reality, the surgical territory of a flap is wider than the corresponding anatomic or dynamic territories of the nutrient artery. There is thus a potential territory which is the result of a combination of two factors: first, the basic geometry which is derived from the blood flow in the flap, including suppression due to peripheral pressure; and second, an element of territorial extension made possible by anastomoses that do not offer resistance to the vascular supply obtained from the main flap pedicle. It is possible to obtain a good appreciation of the territorial potential of an artery by injection of coloured materials in the fresh cadaver.

## Classification

In considering the above factors, a flap can be defined according to three criteria: vascular anatomy, method of utilisation and component tissues.

### Vascular Anatomy

According to the mode of vascularisation, we have seen that we can distinguish:
- the **axial pattern** flap,
- the flap with **connective tissue,**
- the **neurocutaneous** flap, which can be considered as an axial pattern flap,
- the **musculocutaneous** flap.

The distinction is of paramount importance because the same skin territory can be raised using different modes of vascularisation.

### Utilisation

In terms of utilisation, three types of flap should be distinguished:
- the **free** flap requires microsurgical anastomoses for its revascularisation. It can depend on all three modes of vascularisation;
- the **peninsular** flap is characterised by the maintenance of a cutaneous hinge proximally or distally. It can be utilised as a rotation flap, and its possibilities for coverage are limited;
- the **island** flap is characterised by a vascular pedicle whose length confers to the flap an arc of rotation which defines its possibilities. Most island flaps are typically vascularised by the septal mode.

### Component Tissues

The final criterion characterising a flap concerns its component tissues. The recognised existence of different modes of vascularisation permits isolation of the following flaps:
- the **fascial** flap, including the deep fascia and a thin layer of subcutaneous tissue to protect the immediate suprafascial plexiform network;
- the **subcutaneous** flap, which is dissected at a subdermal and suprafascial level. This shows an axial pattern vascularisation;
- the **cutaneous** flap, the plane of dissection of which lies over the superficial surface of the fascia or of the muscular aponeurosis;
- the **fasciocutaneous** flap, elevated en bloc with the skin, the subcutaneous tissue and the deep fascia.

In conclusion, all skin flaps can thus be defined according to their method of utilisation, their modes of vascularisation and their component tissues. The most important notion is that the same cutaneous artery can give birth to many radically different types of flap.

## The Main Pedicled Flaps for the Upper Limb

### Scapular and Parascapular Flaps

Dos Santos reported a detailed anatomical study of the circumflex scapular artery and its branches in 1980 [26]. Gilbert in 1982 [27] first described the clinical use of scapular flap, while Nassif [28], also in 1982, first reported on the clinical use of the parascapular flap.

The region of scapula is an interesting skin-flap donor site. The blood supply is reliable, the quality of skin is resistant, but the flaps are not sensory. Initially used as free flaps, the scapular and parascapular flaps have gained indications as island flaps in reconstruction of the axilla.

**Indications.** Free-flap indications are for regions where very resistant skin is needed. A very large flap can be raised by including the two flaps in the same design; however, the donor site should be grafted.

Other compound flaps are possible, associating a scapular or parascapular flap with latissimus dorsi. A parascapular flap can also be associated with a bone segment from the rim of the scapula.

Pedicled island flaps: the scapular and parascapular flaps are now routinely used in the reconstruction of the axilla following release of a contracture (Fig. 1).

**Vascular Supply.** The flaps are entirely supplied by the cutaneous branch of the circumflex scapular artery. This artery arises from the subscapular artery and passes between teres major and teres minor on the axillary border of the scapula. Here, it divides into two cutaneous branches, namely the scapular artery, which runs horizontally, and the parascapular artery, which runs longitudinally. A small ascending branch has recently been described [29]. The parascapular artery is the larger of the two and also the more constant. Both arteries are accompanied by venae comitantes. The flaps can be raised, using either of the two arteries as a base, either singly or together. The position of the vascular pedicle can be identified by use of the simple formula:

$$D = \frac{L - 2}{2}$$

where D is the distance between the spine of the scapula and the pedicle and L is the distance from the spine of the scapula to the inferior angle of this bone, both measurements being expressed in centimetres [29, 30].

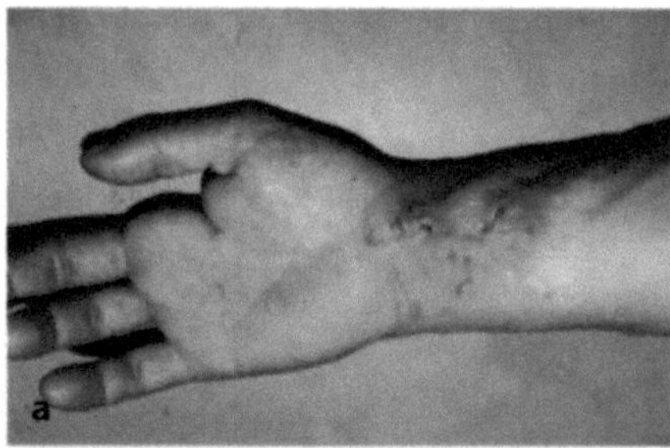

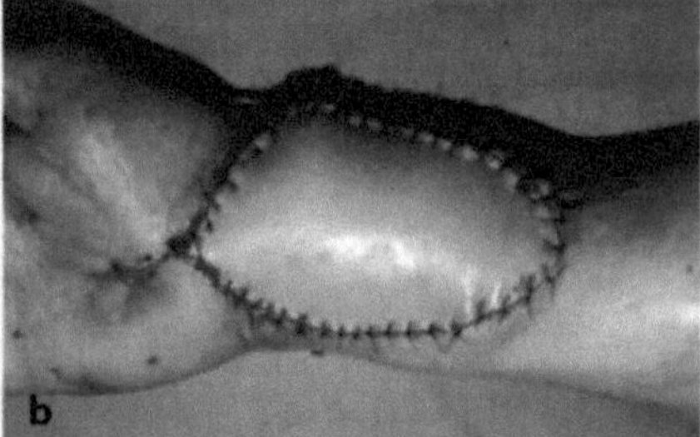

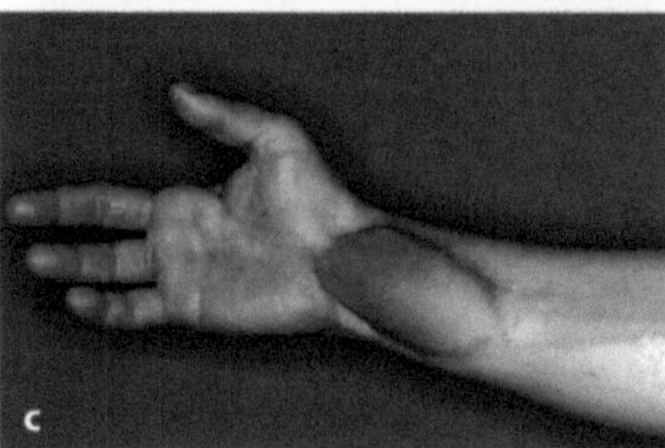

**Fig. 1. a** Amputation of index and crush injury of median nerve. **b** Covering with a free scapular flap. **c** Result after 6 months

**Operative Procedures.** The patient is placed either prone or in midlateral position. The position of the cutaneous branch of the circumflex scapular artery is localised as described above. The parascapular and scapular branches are dissected and ellipsoid flaps are marked on the skin. The flap is raised, commencing distally, but the deep fascia covering the underlying muscles is left intact. The main vascular pedicle should be mobilised with the intermuscular septum. Several muscular branches must be ligated when a long pedicle is needed. The flap can now be moved to the axilla to cover defects following the release of scar contractures.

### Latissimus Dorsi Flap

The latissimus dorsi myocutaneous flap was first described in 1896 by Igino Tansini [5], who used this flap for breast reconstruction after radical mastectomy. In 1978, Maxwell reported the successful transfer of a free latissimus dorsi flap for reconstruction of a scalp defect [31]. This flap is probably the most often employed and the most reliable flap in the whole body. It has many indications, as it can be used as a free or pedicled flap, as a covering procedure or as a functional transfer. The functional deficit associated with its elevation is negligible.

**Indications.** As a proximally based flap it is used to cover defects over the shoulder girdle and the upper arm, including the posterior aspect of the elbow, and the anterior chest, including the clavicle, as well as for restoration of elbow flexion in the paralysed upper limb. The proximal insertion of the muscle should be transferred to the coracoid process. The free transfer flap is used for covering large defects of the limbs.

The main indications for the distally based flap are defects of the posterior trunk (Fig. 2).

**Vascular and Nerve Supply.** The vascular pedicle arises from the thoracodorsal vessels. The subscapular artery divides into the circumflex scapular and thoracodorsal arteries (in the former, the diameter is 3–4 mm to 3–12 mm; in the latter, the diameter is 1.5–3 mm to 1.5–4 mm). Before entering latissimus dorsi, the thoracodorsal artery supplies one or two small branches to teres major and at least one main branch to serratus anterior. The motor nerve arises from the posterior cord and enters latissimus dorsi with the vascular pedicle 10 cm distal to the axillary vessels. In the muscle, the vascular pedicle in most cases (94%) divides into two branches, a horizontal and an oblique branch, each supplying a distinct segment of muscle. Numerous intramuscular anastomoses link the two systems. Latissimus dorsi also receives blood supply from the intercostal artery at the point of its insertion into the spine. The muscle can be distally based on three of these pedicles for covering a defect of the lower back. The skin overlying the muscle can be raised in its entirety with complete confidence. The largest flap reported is 35×20 cm [32].

**Operative Procedure.** The patient lies in midlateral position. The upper limb is inclu-ded in the operative field and supported throughout to avoid traction being applied to the brachial plexus.

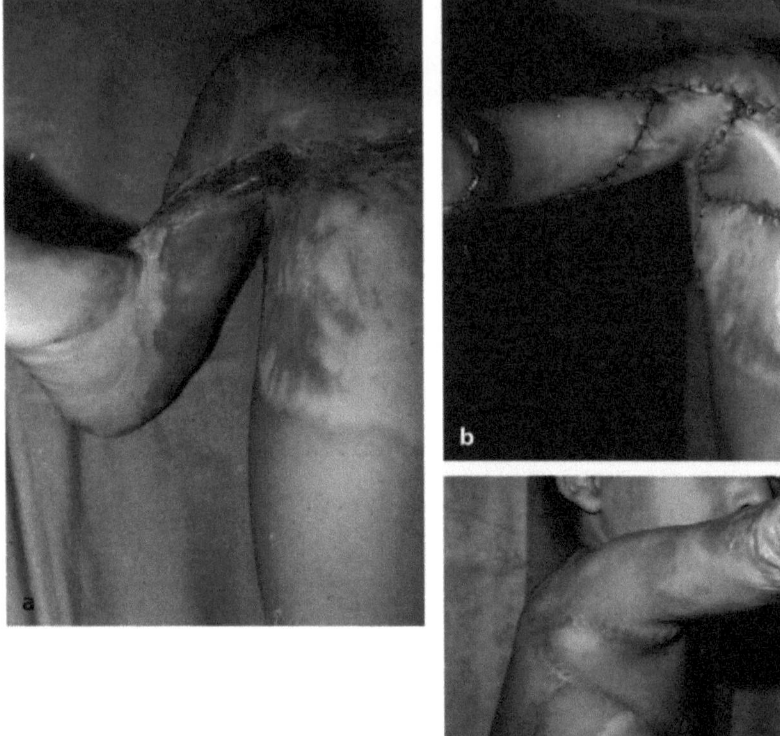

**Fig. 2. a** Sequelae of burns with significant scar contracture. **b** A latissimus dorsi flap with cutaneous palette. **c** Result after 4 months

A longitudinal incision is made from the axilla to the posterior iliac crest. The eventual desired skin paddle should be marked out and its margin incised. By anterior dissection the lateral border of the muscle is exposed. The spinal origin of the muscle is demonstrated by reflection of the posterior skin flap.

The key point of the technique is to dissect the anterior border, which should be slightly retracted in order to expose the vascular distribution. When the muscle is used as a rotation flap, the pedicle does not need to be dissected, but the thoracic branches of the thoracodorsal vessels should be ligated and divided to allow mobilisation of the muscle. When a free flap is raised, it seems to be better to retain the distal insertion of the muscle until the pedicle is carefully dissected; then the muscle is released from its spinal origin and from the iliac crest, beginning the dissection distally and working proximally. The scapular attachments are divided. Care should be taken to ligate the small vessels lying deep to teres major. The segmental vascular intramuscular division allows the surgeon to split the muscle and to raise the medial portion only.

### Lateral Arm Flap

In 1982 R.Y. Song reported his anatomical study on lateral arm flap and its clinical application [33]. This flap could be taken from the posterolateral aspect of the upper arm between the deltoid insertion and the elbow.

**Indications.** This kind of flap can be used as a local flap to cover defects over the shoulder and elbow and it may have either a proximal or a distal pedicle. With a proximal pedicle, the flap can reach to the coracoid area or the axilla. With a distally based pedicle, the flap is an excellent procedure to resurface the anterior or the posterior aspect of the elbow.

**Vascular and Nerve Supply.** The flap is based on the posterior radial collateral artery (PRCA) with 1.5–2 mm in diameter, a direct extension of the profunda brachii artery, which arises from the brachial artery. Venous drainage of the flap is provided by two concomitant veins, with a mean diameter of 2.5 mm [33]. From the insertion of deltoid muscle, the length of pedicle is 7–8 cm, and could be 9–13 cm if an extended approach for the pedicle of the flap is performed. The posterior cutaneous nerve of the arm and forearm arises from the radial nerve accompanying vessels to innervate the skin of the distal part of the lateral upper arm and the skin of the posterolateral forearm. The distal lateral humerus receives some periosteal blood supply from the terminal periosteal branches of the PRCA and this allows the creation of a vascularised bone segment of approximately 1×10 cm extended from the deltoid insertion to the lateral humeral metaphysic. The presence of many fasciocutaneous perforators arising from the PRCA allows for the possibility of a free fascial flap when a thick or bulky flap is undesirable for reconstruction.

**Operative Procedure.** Flap markings are initiated by drawing a line from the acromion over the deltoid insertion to the lateral epicondyle which delineates the lateral intramuscular septum and the closely associated PRCA. A flap is then designed with the above line as the central axis. Concerning its size, in cadaver study it was between 8×10 cm and 15×14 cm and can be extended for 3–4 cm distal to the lateral epicondyle. The maximum size in clinical application was 24×6 cm.

The lateral arm flap, as a pedicled flap, could effectively facilitate release of either an anterior or posterior axillary fold contracture; or, when oriented transversely, could release an antecubital contracture, based either proximally or distally. Elevated in its fasciocutaneous form, without isolation of the pedicle, it could be used to reconstruct soft-tissue defects of the contralateral hand as a two-stage procedure if microvascular capabilities were not available.

### Posterior Interosseous Flap

In 1986, Zancolli et al. described a dorsal forearm island flap based on the posterior interosseous artery which was first published in Spanish. In 1988, his work was published in English [34]. In 1986, Penteado et al. also reported on an anatomic study on the fasciocutaneous flap of the posterior interosseous artery and its clinical application [35].

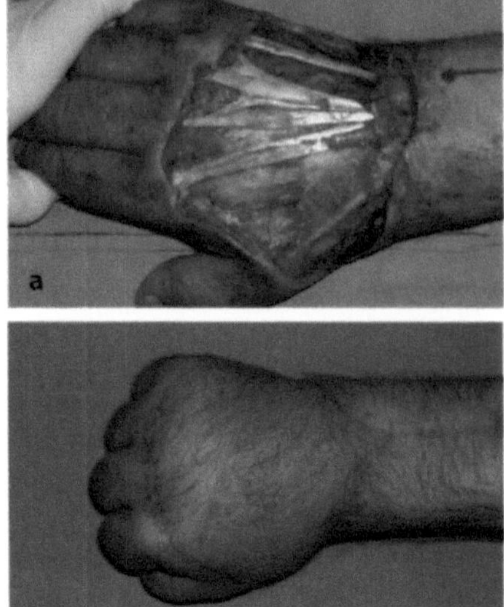

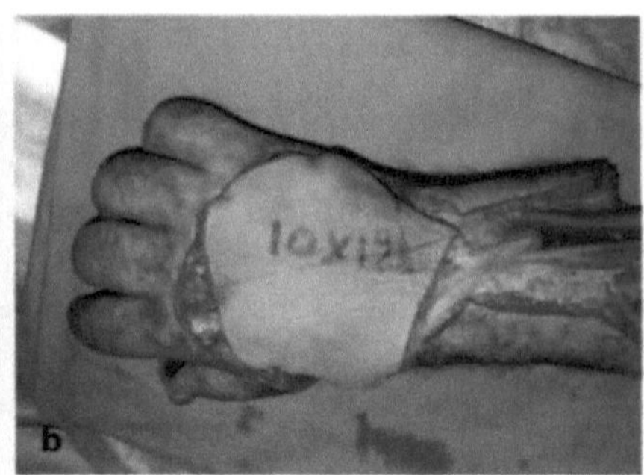

**Fig. 3. a** Loss of substance of the dorsum of the hand with tendons exposure. **b** Covering of the dorsum of the hand with a posterior interosseous flap. **c** Cosmetic and functional result after 6 months

**Indications.** The flap is used most frequently with a distal pedicle to cover soft-tissue defects on the dorsum of the hand. Areas which can be covered by this flap depend on the size of the flap and the length of the pedicle: the bigger the flap, the shorter the pedicle. When a flap of moderate size (5×4 cm) is raised, the pedicle will allow reaching the first web space and the whole of the dorsal and palmar aspect of the hand (Fig. 3).

**Vascular Supply.** The common interosseous artery arises from the ulnar artery at the level of the radial tuberosity and divides into the posterior and anterior interosseous arteries. The posterior interosseous artery runs deep to supinator and enters the posterior compartment of the forearm. The surface marker of its point of entry is the junction of the middle and proximal thirds of a line drawn from the lateral epicondyle to the distal radioulnar joint. The artery is accompanied by the posterior interosseous nerve, which soon divides into sensory and motor branches. A small sensory branch and two venae comitantes accompany the artery as far as the wrist. The pedicle enters the septum between extensor digiti minimi and extensor carpi ulnaris. Along its course, the posterior interosseous artery gives off several cutaneous arteries (between 7 and 14). The largest of these arteries is proximal. At the wrist, the artery anastomosis with the perforating branch of the anterior interosseous artery, the dorsal carpal arch and the vascular plexus surrounds the ulnar head.

Considering the vascular pedicle, the posterior interosseous artery has an average external calibre of 1.6 (0.9–2.7) mm and the average length is 7.1 with the range 5.8–8.3 cm (based on the dorsal transverse anastomotic branch and a segment of posterior interosseous artery) to 15 cm (based on the posterior interosseous artery and the most proximal relevant septocutaneous perforator) [35, 36].

The flap can reach the dorsal aspect of the hand, including the first web space. The dorsal aspect of the proximal phalanx can also be covered.

**Operative Procedure.** The elbow is flexed to a right angle and the lateral epicondyle and distal radioulnar joint are marked on the skin. The line which joins these two points is the axis of the flap. The vascular pedicle is located just distal to the junction of the middle and proximal thirds of this line. If a small flap is required, the flap should be raised predominantly distal to the vascular pedicle. A huge flap can be raised, extending as far proximally as the elbow. Theoretically, it is possible to raise all the dorsal skin of the forearm on this vascular pedicle. When the flap is raised with a distal pedicle, the pedicle is dissected on the distal radioulnar joint and the flap is rotated around this point to its desired position. An incision is made on the posterolateral border of the flap and is extended distally as far as the distal radioulnar joint in order to expose the vascular pedicle. The intermuscular septum is defined by identification of the septal arteries that pass through the deep fascia to the skin. The fascia is incised on both sides of the septum. Extensor carpi ulnaris is retracted towards the ulna, and extensor digiti quinti and extensor indicis proprius are retracted to the radial side. This allows exposure of the posterior interosseous artery distal to the flap. The flap is then raised with the deep fascia, beginning the dissection on the radial side. The septum between extensor digitorum communis and extensor digiti quinti should be divided. One must take care not to divide the intermuscular septum, between extensor digiti quinti and extensor carpi ulnaris, which contains the skin arterioles. The plane of the dissection is defined between the two above muscles, and extensor digiti quinti is gently retracted. Proximally, the artery must be dissected from the posterior interosseous nerve, which lies on its lateral side. Optical magnification and microsurgical instruments should be used at this stage. Sometimes the motor nerve to extensor carpi ulnaris runs superficial to the artery, which should be ligated distal to this important motor nerve. The ligature of the posterior interosseous artery should be performed just proximal to the first arteriole to the flap. The medial border of the flap overlying extensor carpi ulnaris is then incised and the pedicle within the septum is dissected from the ulnar shaft. The distal vascular anastomotic arch is also released from the interosseous membrane. The ligature of the ramus perforans of the anterior interosseous artery allows the pivot point of the pedicle to be placed more distally on the vascular network of the wrist. This procedure increases the arc of rotation of the pedicle. The flap can now be mobilised to reach the dorsal aspect of the hand, including the first web space. The dorsal aspect of the proximal phalanx can be covered. The donor site can be covered by an immediate split-thickness skin graft when a primary suture is not possible.

### Radial Flap

Also called forearm flap or Chinese flap, it was first described by G.F. Yang in 1978 as a free flap in the Chinese Medical Journal; in 1981, and later, R.Y. Song reported this flap in a western journal.

When this flap appeared in the 1980s, it undoubtedly opened a new chapter in reconstructive surgery. Three main concepts were raised by the Chinese flap:

1. A new mode of vascularisation of flap. The forearm flap was not an axial pattern flap because the pedicle did not belong to the skin territory. This type is now called a flap with meso (loose connective tissue), as the flap is nourished by small arteries in a very thin membrane which links the vascular axis and the flap.
2. A very wide range of applications, as the flaps could be used in any way, pedicled or free.
3. Most surprisingly, the possibility of using this flap with an arteriole retrograde flow.

The forearm flap is a versatile and reliable fasciocutaneous flap raised on the anterior aspect of the forearm.

**Indications.** The proximally based pedicle island flap can be used for soft-tissue defect repair of the elbow. The distally based pedicled island flap is used for repairing defects of the hand and digits. The free flap has many applications in head and neck surgery, urology and limb reconstructive surgery. In a complex defect, the radial artery can be utilised for repairing a main vascular axis. A composite transfer can be raised, including a piece of bone from the radius, tendons, nerves and even brachioradialis.

**Vascular and Nerve Supply.** The flap is supplied by the radial artery, from which many small arteries arise perforating the anterior brachial fascia. These small vessels are more abundant in the distal third of the forearm than in the proximal third; the skin is also supplied by the arterioles arising from the underlying brachioradialis muscle. A systematic description of the precise blood supply cannot be given as the number of arterioles is variable. Nonetheless, three main branches are constant [37]:

1. A proximal branch which arises near the origin of the radial artery, or sometimes from the anterior recurrent radial artery, and which can be considered as a long-course artery. It supplies a rather long skin territory located on the anterolateral aspect of the proximal half of the forearm.
2. A mid-course branch which arises 7–8 cm proximal to the styloid process of the radius.
3. A distal branch which arises 2 cm proximal to the styloid process, runs beneath pronator quadratus and supplies the metaphyseal region of the radius, which can be included in the transfer.

Venous return is ensured by the venae comitantes which have a diameter of more than 1 mm close to the elbow, and by the superficial venous network of the forearm [37]. In the case of a distally based island pedicled flap it is not necessary to include a superficial vein.

Sensibility is mainly supplied by the anterior cutaneous nerve of the forearm, but the discriminative sensibility is poor and the forearm free flap cannot be considered a true neurovascular flap.

Theoretically, all the skin of the forearm can be raised on the radial artery. In practice, however, the limits of the flap are the border of the ulna, medially, and the midline of the dorsal aspect of the forearm, laterally, including the volar skin [38, 39].

**Operative Procedure.** The patient is placed supine with the arm abducted on a hand table. Allen's test should be performed before surgical procedure to assess the viability of the ulnar artery. The flap is marked on the skin approximately over the middle third of the anterior aspect of the forearm. The length of pedicle needed to allow the flap to cover the defect is estimated. Two pivot points can be defined for the pedicle. When the defect is located on the dorsum of the hand, the pivot point is at the base of the thenar eminence just proximal to the division of the radial artery. When a longer pedicle is needed, the pivot point is at the apex of the first web, which implies the inclusion of the deep branch of the radial artery in the pedicle and passing the pedicle and the flap under the tendons of the thumb. Distally to the flap, the incision is made over the radial vascular axis to expose the pedicle. Proximally to the flap, a short incision allows the control of the radial artery. The superficial veins which cross the flap are ligated. Dissection is begun on the ulnar side, including the fascia until it reaches the lateral border of the flexor carpi radialis. The muscle and its tendon are then retracted ulnar-wards to deepen the dissection in order to spare attachments of the meso and the radial artery to the flap. On the radial side, the flap is released from the underlying brachioradialis muscle. Care should be taken with the sensory branch of the radial nerve. On the medial border of brachioradialis the dissection is deepened to pass beneath the radial artery. The radial artery and venae comitantes are then clamped. The tourniquet is released to verify the vascularisation of the flap and the hand. The tourniquet is then re-inflated and the vascular axis is divided proximal to the flap. The flap and its vascular axis are progressively released from the underlying flexor muscles. Diathermy should be applied to the numerous small arteries to the muscles. The flap and the pedicle have been completely released as far as the base of the thenar eminence. The flap reaches the first phalanx of the fingers but cannot cover the distal end of the digits. In order to increase the length of the pedicle, an incision is made over the snuffbox as far as the apex of the first web. The deep branch of the radial artery is identified and released from the floor of the snuffbox as far as the apex of the first web, where it plunges between the two heads of the first interosseous muscle. Ligation of the superficial branch is necessary. Sometimes, ligation of the branch to the carpus and the first dorsal intermetacarpal artery is needed. Care should be taken with the branches of the radial nerve. The tendons of abductor pollicis longus and extensor brevis are isolated and their sheath is slightly released from the styloid process of the radius to allow the passage of the flap. The flap and the pedicle are also passed beneath extensor pollicis longus. The provided arc of rotation allows the flap to cover the extremities of the digits. The donor site is covered by a split-thickness skin graft after the tendons of flexor carpi radialis and brachioradialis are brought together. A cast immobilisation is required to obtain graft healing.

### Dorsal Ulnar Artery Flap

This flap was first described by Beker and Gilbert in 1992 [40]. The dorsal ulnar artery flap is a fasciocutaneous flap raised on the ulnar side of the wrist and forearm. Its axial pattern vascularisation is based on a cutaneous branch of the ulnar artery.

**Indications.** The flap is chiefly used to resurface defects over the anterior aspect of the wrist, especially when well-vascularised tissue is needed to cover the median nerve, which may be surrounded by dense scar tissue following previous injury or surgery. In these indications, it may be preferable, if the skin is of suitable quality, to use a fascial flap, which can be wrapped around the nerve in order to protect and supply it. The distal ulnar artery flap can also be used to reach the dorsal aspect of the wrist and hand. The small length of pedicle, constituted by the origin of the cutaneous branch, limits the arc of rotation of the flap.

**Vascular Supply.** The main trunk of the pedicle is called the ulnodorsal artery, which arises from the ulnar artery at a distance of 2–5 cm proximal to the pisiform. The artery passes beneath flexor carpi ulnaris and divides into three branches:
1. The proximal branch supplies the distal portion of flexor carpi ulnaris.
2. The middle branch is devoted to the skin and divides into two small arterioles which pass through the fascia. The ascending one runs between the ulna and the flexor carpi ulnaris and supplies the skin of the medial side of the lower forearm. The descending one accompanies the dorsal branch of the ulnar nerve and gives off several arterioles to the skin.
3. The distal branch is devoted to the pisiform and constitutes the pedicle of the vascularised pisiform transfer to replace the lunate.

The flap can extend over the whole distal half of the forearm. It averages 20 cm in length and 9 cm in breadth. The pedicle is the common trunk. The length of the pedicle is no more than 3 cm. The ulna constitutes the median axis of the flap.

**Operative Procedure.** The flap could be taken as fascial or fasciocutaneous flap. It is outlined on the medial side of the forearm and wrist. The landmark of the emergence of the pedicle is included in the design. After cutaneous incision, the pisiform is identified. The pedicle emerges between 2 and 5 cm from the pisiform. The flap is released on its radial side. It is progressively retracted, exposing the underlying flexor carpi ulnaris muscle. The emergence of the pedicle has been identified; the flap is released on its medial side. A distal hinge can be maintained. A simple rotation of the flap permits the coverage of the midpalm of the hand.

### Groin Flap

N.H. Antia in 1971 first reported on the direct transfer of a large area (13×9 cm) of skin and subcutaneous tissue in the lower abdominal wall by direct vascular anastomoses of the superficial epigastric vessels to the facial area for facial soft tissue reconstruction [41]. I.A. McGregor in 1972 first reported on the groin flap as a pedicled flap based on superficial circumflex iliac vessels [42]. Latter, in 1973, R.K. Daniel first successfully reported on transfer of groin flap as a free flap for his clinical application [43]. The groin flap has been one of the main advances in reconstructive surgery and should be considered as a milestone, particularly in hand surgery. It has been practically abandoned as a free flap because of the variation in diameter of the vascular pedicle and the thickness of subcutaneous tissue in some patients. However, many indications for this flap remain, as it is very reliable as a pedicled flap to cover defects involving the hand in emergencies. The groin flap must be considered a basic procedure for all surgeons.

**Indications.** The pedicled flap is used for treatment of soft-tissue defects of the upper limb involving the elbow, the forearm and the hand. It can also be used for local treatment of soft-tissue defects resulting from a trochanteric pressure sore when no other procedure is available.

The main advantage of the free flap is that there is very little cosmetic prejudice at the donor site.

**Vascular Supply.** The groin flap is supplied by the superficial circumflex iliac artery accompanied by venae comitantes. This artery is a long-course artery, which defines the groin flap as an axial pattern flap. The vessel arises from the femoral artery about 2 cm distal to the inguinal ligament. It pierces the fascia on the medial border of sartorius and then courses obliquely in the subcutaneous tissue and curls around the iliac crest. It passes about 2.5 cm distal to the anterior superior iliac spine. Beyond this landmark, the artery is well defined for 5–6 cm and then divides off in small branches.

**Operative Procedures.** The design of the flap is an ellipse, the long axis of which is the presumed course of the artery. The landmarks are the femoral artery, the inguinal ligament and the anterior superior iliac spine and sartorius. In the lateral part (distal portion of the flap), the elevation is very quick and easy and should not include the aponeurosis of the muscles, which are attached deeply by fibrous septa. The lateral border of sartorius must be cautiously identified. The elevation can stop at this level. If a long pedicle is needed, the dissection is continued. The aponeurosis of sartorius is incised to be included in the flap. Thus it protects the origin of the vascular pedicle. The dissection can be continued until the origin of the artery. It usually gives a branch to sartorius. The origin of the vein is located more medially on the femoral vein.

## Other Flaps

### Posterior Arm Flap

A. Masquelet in 1985 reported on his anatomical study on posterior arm flap and its clinical use [44, 45]. The flap is taken by the posterior aspect of the arm. It could be composed by skin, subcutaneous tissue and fascia. It is based on an unnamed artery with 1.0–2.5 mm in diameter, which is from the humeral artery or the deep humeral artery or directly from the axillary artery. The length of pedicle is on average 6.2 mm. It could be used as a free flap to cover defects of soft tissues (wrist, hand etc.), or as an island flap to cover the defects of axilla.

### Radial Recurrent Fasciocutaneous Flap

Y. Maruyama in 1986 first reported on its clinical application and later published a detailed anatomical study on this flap [46, 47]. The donor site is the lateral aspect of the upper limb; it is possible to use skin, subcutaneous tissue and fascia. It is vascularised by radial recurrent artery or arterial arcade of radial recurrent artery of 2.6 mm in diameter. Both as an island flap and as a free flap it could be used to cover defects of soft tissue of the elbow.

### Ulnar Artery Forearm Flap

M.J. Lovie in 1982 first used this flap as a free flap and in 1984 published his clinical experience [48]. The donor site is almost the entire aspect of the forearm up to the ulnar border. It is based on the ulnar artery and can be assessed in different composition using skin, subcutaneous tissue, fascia with or without nerve (medial cutaneous nerve and the motor branch to FCU), tendon (FCU, PL) or bone (ulna). As a free flap it can cover many defects of composite tissues; as a distal-based island flap it could be used to cover defects of composite tissues on the hand.

### Brachioradialis Myocutaneous Flap

A. Gilbert first used this flap as an island flap [49]. The flap is taken by the posterolateral lower half of the upper and the lateral upper third of the forearm. It can be used only as a muscular flap or with skin; it is nourished by radial recurrent artery or radial artery. As a proximal-based island flap, it can cover defects of soft tissue of elbow; as a distal-based island flap it can reach the hand.

### Pronator Quadratus Muscle Flap

A.L. Dellon in 1984 first used this flap as an island flap [50]. The donor site is the volar aspect of the distal forearm; the muscle could be taken also with the bone to reconstruct the bony defects of the wrist when it is taken as a distal-based island flap. The artery that nourishes the flap is the anterior interosseous artery.

**Indications.** Replacement of tissue loss necessitates a graduated response depending upon the importance of the lost tissue, its location and the deep structures that are exposed. This section covers the indications for pedicled flaps of the upper extremity according to the location of tissue loss. It is assumed that other conditions which both necessitate and permit a flap are fulfilled.

Formerly, when a skin graft was insufficient or likely to be unsuccessful, the treatment for tissue loss was to utilise random cutaneous flaps elevated from the abdomen, the thorax or the contralateral extremity. These techniques, besides their inherent limitations of mobilisation in awkward position and the multiplicity of surgical procedures, were frequently the source of complications caused by infection and maceration. Great progress resulted from the introduction of the inguinal or groin flap. This technique provided and still provides immense surgical service, particularly for distal injuries of the upper extremity. It nonetheless has the inconvenience that it requires a second stage for flap separation.

Microsurgery liberated these flaps from the demand to maintain their nourishing pedicles intact and offered possibilities that have been exploited in order to accomplish reconstruction in one step. Another benefit has been revascularisation of the recipient site through the use of vascular transfers. As with any new technique, considerable excesses have been committed in the past 10 years regarding the indications for free transfer of tissue.

Microvascular free-tissue transfer techniques served to introduce the present era because the anatomical investigations conducted in parallel with widespread clinical applications of free-tissue transfer made apparent the technical possibility of providing tissue covered by means of local or regional flaps. Thus, in their search for new free flaps, surgeons and anatomists discovered that the vascular anatomy suggests that most tissue losses at the level of the extremities may be covered with a cutaneous flap or neighbouring muscular flap.

The problem is different for the upper compared with the lower extremity. In the lower extremity, numerous muscular flaps can be elevated without important functional detriment. In contrast, in the upper extremity, very few muscles can be sacrificed that will not alter function. The latissimus dorsi and the brachioradialis are two exceptions. Cutaneous arterialised flaps still find their best indications in the upper extremity even though these indications have been considerably reduced in number during the past few years. There are still also good indications for free-flap transfers to the upper extremities: for example, reconstruction of a missing digit calls for transfer of the toe, either complete or partial.

The inguinal flap remains an alternative procedure to many local or regional flaps and this is mentioned as appropriate. The local and regional flaps are described hierarchically according to their location.

## Tissue Losses from the Shoulder

Three regions must be distinguished in the shoulder: the shoulder stump, which corresponds to the region of the deltoid muscle and includes the area over the humeral articulation and the superior part of the humerus, and the preclavicular and axillary regions.

### Shoulder Stump and Preclavicular Region

Large tissue losses in the preclavicular region and the shoulder contour are the incontestable domain of the latissimus dorsi muscle or musculocutaneous flap. The pedicle, which is located deeply under the protection of the scapula, is generally intact even in severe injuries. The arc of rotation of this muscle permits easy coverage of anterior tissue losses: the flap reaches just to the sternoclavicular articulation.

Sectioning of the humeral insertion of the muscle increases the arc of rotation. When there is complex loss of tissue that includes bony and soft tissue, for example after a gunshot injury, reconstruction of both these elements can be accomplished in one stage by elevation of the latissimus dorsi with one or two ribs, usually the posterior curvature of the ninth or tenth rib, to reconstruct the humerus or to ensure bone continuity while an arthrodesis is accomplished.

Tissue loss that is localised or of a limited size requires an important sacrifice if the latissimus dorsi muscle is used; even though the functional impairment is minimal. In such cases, a cutaneous flap is preferable. The anterior and lateral surfaces of the shoulder may be covered with a lateral upper-arm flap, while the posterior surface can be covered by a scapular or parascapular flap turned through 90°–180° on its pedicle.

### Axilla

The axilla is limited by two pillars, anterior and posterior, and represented by the border of the latissimus dorsi posteriorly and the pectoralis major in front. It includes the lateral thoracic region immediately adjacent to the breast under the border of pectoralis major muscle. Reconstruction of the axilla is indicated for sequelae of burns with significant scar contracture and for resurfacing of cutaneous lesions secondary to post-surgical radiation.

Use of the latissimus dorsi in the first case represents two important sacrifices even if only a portion of the muscle is utilised: the excess of tissue here causes obliteration of the axilla. In the second case, the reliability of the muscular pedicle could be in question after surgical removal of lymph nodes and then radiation. Thus, the latissimus dorsi is less indicated for reconstruction of the axilla.

Instead, three cutaneous flaps may be utilised: the scapular flap, the parascapular flap and the posterior brachial or upper-arm flap. They offer a cutaneous surface that is supple and thin. Our preference is the parascapular flap, for which closure of the donor site is easier than for the scapular flap. The posterior brachial flap is an excellent alternative to the parascapular flap. Its cutaneous cover is thinner and its arc of rotation permits coverage of the lateral thoracic areas adjacent to the axilla.

## Tissue Losses from the Arm and Hand

The latissimus dorsi is indicated for elective coverage of tissue loss from the arm. It can be utilised with or without a cutaneous portion. Its greatest indication is when it is required to treat simultaneously a significant tissue loss and a deficit of elbow flexion. The arc of rotation of the muscle permits coverage of all the surfaces of the arm just to and including the elbow. Certain compound fractures of the elbow that ascend towards the humerus can also justify elevation of the latissimus dorsi.

### The Elbow Region

Until quite recently the elbow region was the most difficult to cover. Numerous periarticular flaps are now available which simplify this problem. It is proper to distinguish four surfaces in the elbow region.

**Anterior Surface.** The anterior surface of the elbow is the typical area for burn scar contracture which, after release, leaves a significant cutaneous deficit, usually with exposure of the tendons, the neurovascular bundles and occasionally even of the articular surfaces, when an anterior capsuleotomy is necessary. The choice of flaps thus depends essentially on the scale of the tissue loss. The brachioradialis muscle is convenient for tissue loss which is deep but limited in width. The flap of the anterior lateral surface of the forearm, utilised as a long, narrow (peninsular) flap with a proximal pedicle, is indicated in cases where the contracture includes the medial part of the elbow. In our opinion, when tissue loss is significant, this is an indication for the external brachial flap as an island flap with a reverse pedicle based on the posterior radial collateral vessels. Occasionally, a tissue bridge can be retained medially, which converts this flap into a peninsular flap with a distal base. This technical variation offers rapid and reliable execution but limits the available surface area of the flap.

**Lateral Surface.** Only infrequently is flap coverage necessary for tissue loss from the lateral surface of the elbow: the muscle based in the epicondyle, the triceps and the brachialis usually provide sufficient granulation tissue for a split-thickness skin graft. Three flaps may be utilised in this region: the flap from the anterolateral surface of the forearm, the lateral brachial flap and the radial arm flap.

The flap from the anterolateral surface of the forearm permits coverage from the epicondylar region just to and including the olecranon. This flap is useful for small tissue losses which expose both the epicondyle and olecranon and which do not justify the use of the other two flaps.

Elevation of the flap to cover the lateral surface of the elbow is difficult. It should be considered in cases where the anastomotic plexus between the posterior radial collateral artery and the recurrent posterior interosseous is compromised. It is then necessary to elevate the lateral brachial flap as a reverse pedicled island flap, based on the anterior radial collateral artery, in which separation of the radial nerve is difficult in the external bicipital groove.

A third solution is offered by radial arm flap of the forearm as a direct pedicled island flap based on the radial artery. The importance of the tissue loss must justify the elevation of this or any similar flap.

**Medial Surface.** The medial surface is the most difficult region of elbow to cover. The most frequent situation is that of ulceration of the medial epicondyle, particularly in quadriplegic patients. The flexor carpi ulnaris muscle mobilised on its superior pedicle is a good means of covering this region if this muscle is already paralysed, as is typically the case in tetraplegic patients. Sacrifice of an active muscle is not warranted. A flap from the anterolateral surface of the forearm with a wide subcutaneous pedicle that supports a distal cutaneous paddle is probably an interesting solution but we do not have any experience of it. It should not be forgotten that, in a number of cases, the simple technique of resection of the epitrochlea constitutes a satisfactory approach. Utilisation of the Chinese flap with a direct pedicle is difficult to envisage except in the case of a large tissue loss or where it is required to resurface an unstable cutaneous zone, for example prior to repair of the ulnar nerve.

**Olecranon.** The olecranon is an equally difficult region to cover. Decubitus ulcers and unstable scars furnish the usual indications for coverage by a flap. Small losses of tissue less than 4 cm in diameter can be treated by a posterior interosseous flap with a direct pedicle elevated from the dorsal surface of the inferior one-third of the forearm. A lateral brachial island flap with a reversed pedicle is an interesting alternative. Its advantage is that it does not leave a scar on the forearm. Large tissue losses justify, as for other regions of the elbow, a Chinese flap with a direct pedicle.

### The Wrist Region

Essential zones to cover in the wrist are the dorsal surface and in particular the palmar surface. The recently developed medial ulnar flap and posterior interosseous flap have taken the place of other distant tissue-transfer techniques, either free or pedicled.

**Posterior Surface.** The indications for flap coverage of the posterior surface of the wrist are infrequent. They include extension contractures of the wrist and rarely flexion contractures, and post-traumatic loss of tissue treated on an emergency basis or subsequently when it is required to provide a supple and protective covering prior to extensor tendon reconstruction. A third indication might be loss of dorsal skin after extensive dorsal synovectomy in a patient with rheumatoid arthritis. The medial ulnar flap is indicated for tissue losses of limited dimensions situated in the proximal portion of the wrist. In effect, the pedicle limits the utilisation of this flap.

Other tissue losses, in particular secondary to an extensor carpi ulnaris loss, are indications for a posterior interosseous flap. The choice of this flap to cover a loss secondary to trauma is delicate: in such cases, in effect, the distal anastomoses of the posterior interosseous artery may be destroyed or thrombosed. It is then necessary to have available either the Chinese flap with a reverse pedicle or the groin flap. This last procedure is our preference because it is reliable and permits preservation of the capital flap of the upper extremity.

**Palmar Surface.** The indications for a local regional flap in the palmar surface of the wrist are rare and are principally flexion contractures and tissue losses which are limited in nature and which follow skin avulsions. Another indication is after recurrent carpal tunnel syndrome, where the objective is simultaneous to provide cover and vascularised protection for the median nerve. Grave sequelae that result from complex lacerations of the wrist in which there is only cutaneous covering of poor quality adherent to the bone, with a complete interruption of all of the underlying structures, are an indication for a free flap. The ideal flap in such cases is the Chinese flap elevated from the contralateral arm. It permits simultaneously cutaneous covering and restoration of the vascular axis to the hand. Reconstructive surgery will thus be possible under ideal conditions. Major losses of tissue that involve only the cutaneous covering are an indication for the posterior interosseous flap. Limited contractions and tissue needs for recurrent carpal tunnel cases can be resolved by a medial ulnar flap.

To provide protective tissue, it is possible to use either the flexor carpi ulnaris subcutaneous tissue flap (including fascia and fatty tissue) or a posterior interosseous flap that is purely fascial to avoid the unaesthetic swelling that occurs with a fasciocutaneous flap. Small losses of tissue at the distal aspect of the wrist at the junction with the palm can be treated by a muscular flap of the abductor of the fifth finger. This area is difficult to reach with the flexor carpi ulnaris flap, and the use of the posterior interosseous flap in our opinion represents a sacrifice that is too major.

**Medial and Lateral Surface.** The medial surface of the wrist can be covered by a posterior interosseous flap provided that the posterior interosseous artery is intact. Complex trauma with open fractures of the lower portion of the ulna generally precludes this technique. These cases call for the use of a distant pedicled flap such as the groin flap or a free flap. Coverage of the lateral surface of the wrist is an uncommon indication but responds well to the posterior interosseous flap.

### The Hand

It is not the purpose of this section to discuss all of the indications that arise from tissue loss in the hand. It is sufficient to discuss several regions of particular interest that can be covered by the flaps which have been described earlier.

**Dorsal Surface of the Hand.** Indications for covering the dorsal surface of the hand, previously the exclusive domain of the inguinal flap, were altered by the development of flaps elevated from the forearm. The tissue losses are generally secondary to direct trauma or scars that result from the extravasation of chemotherapeutic agents. The posterior interosseous flap is here in competition with the Chinese flap. If the tissue loss is centred on the dorsal surface, we prefer the posterior interosseous flap because its elevation is less detrimental than the Chinese flap. Further, if there is a bony defect associated with a metacarpal loss, a composite posterior interosseous flap may be elevated to include a portion of ulna. This technique is particularly indicated for complex tissue losses from the medial surface of the hand or within the elective territories of the posterior interosseous flap.

When the tissue loss occurs on the distal half of the dorsal surface of the hand and projects onto the metacarpophalangeal joints of the first phalanx, it is preferable to use the Chinese flap, in which the arc of rotation is more distal than that of the posterior interosseous flap. This remark concerning the suppleness of the two flaps is equally pertinent to tissue losses in the transverse axis situated in the distal half of the dorsal surface of the hand. The Chinese flap falls naturally into place, whereas the posterior interosseous flap pedicle must be sent in order to position the flap and this represents a risk to the variability of the flap.

**First Commissure.** Indications for a flap are frequent after the release of contractions of the first commissure which are secondary to trauma, vascular causes or burns. The posterior interosseous flap finds an elective indication here because the length of the pedicle permits coverage of both sides (palmar and dorsal) of the first commissure. Extension of the flap along the palmar side requires the wrist to be placed in extension which must be maintained for 10 days post-operatively. The palmar flap described by Vasconez is indicated for small tissue losses where a simple skin graft or a z plasty is not sufficient.

**Palmar Surface of the Hand.** The palmar surface of the hand only exceptionally requires coverage by a flap except in cases of scar contracture secondary to burns that were initially maltreated, where the scar release exposes tendons and neurovascular components. The Chinese flap and the posterior interosseous flap are frequently in competition in such cases. Without doubt, cutaneous dehiscence secondary to local necrosis along the surgical incision occurs between the thenar and hypothenar areas. The thickness of the fatty tissue in the proximal zone of the palm does not facilitate granulation. Limited tissue losses are thus best treated by use of the adductor muscle of the fifth finger mobilised on a proximal pedicle.

## References


1. Sùsruta (Bhishagratna KL) (1844) An English translation of the Susruta Samhita based on original Sanskrit text. Bose, Calcutta, p 107
2. Tagliacozzi G (1597) De curtorum chirurgia per insitionem. Bindoni, Venice
3. Wood J (1863) Care of extreme deformity of the neck and forearm from the cicatrices of a burn, cured by extension, excision and transplantation of skin adjacent and remote. Med Chirurg Trans 46: 149
4. McGregor IA, Jackson IT (1972) The groin flap. Br J Plast Surg 25: 3
5. Tansini I (1896) Nuovo processo per l'amputazione della mammella per cancer. Reforma Medica 12: 3
6. Olivari N (1976) The latissimus dorsi flap. Br J Plast Surg 29: 126
7. Quillen CG, Shearin JL, Georgiade NG (1978) Use of the latissimus dorsi myocutaneous island flap for the reconstruction of the head and neck area. Plast Reconstr Surg 62: 113
8. Esser JFS (1917) Island flaps. Med J New York 106: 205
9. Littler (1953) The neurovascular pedicle method of digital transposition for reconstruction of the hand. Plast Reconstr Surg 12: 303
10. Moberg E (1955) Discussion of D Brooks: The place of nerve grafting in orthopaedic surgery. Annual Meeting of the American Orthopedic Association, June 1954. J Bone Joint Surg 37A: 305
11. Manchot C (1889) Die Hautarterien des menschlichen Körpers. Leipzig (Translated as The cutaneous arteries of the human body. Springer, New York, 1983)
12. Salmon M (1936) Les artères de la peau. Masson, Paris
13. Carrel A (1902) La technique des anastomoses vasculaires et la transplantation des viscères. Lyon Med 98: 589
14. Nyelen CO (1954) The microscope in aural surgery, its first use and later development. Acta Otolaryngol 116 [Suppl]: 226
15. Jacobson JH, Suarez EL (1960) Microsurgery in anastomoses of small vessels. Surg Forum 11: 243
16. Buncke HJ, Schulz WP (1966) Total ear reimplantation in the rabbit utilizing microminiature vascular anastomoses. Br J Plast Surg 19: 15
17. Malt RA, McKhann CF (1964) Replantation of severed arm. JAMA 189: 716
18. Cobbett JR (1969) Free digital transfer. Report of a case of transfer of a great toe to replace an amputated thumb. J Bone Joint Surg 51B: 677
19. Olivari N (1976) The latissimus dorsi flap. Br J Plast Surg 29: 126
20. Mathes S, Nahai F (1979) Clinical atlas of muscle and musculocutaneous flaps. Mosby, Saint Louis
21. Yang K, Chen B, Gao Y (1981) Free transfer of forearm flaps. Report of 56 cases. Nat Med J China 61: 139
22. Ponten B (1981) The fascio-cutaneous flap: its use in soft tissue defects of the lower leg. Br J Plast Surg 34: 215

23. Guneder R, Montandon D, Marty F et al. (1986) The subcutaneous tissue flap and the misconception on fasciocutaneous flap. Scand J Plast Reconstr Surg 20: 61–65

24. Ger R (1971) The technique of muscle transposition in the operative treatment of traumatic and ulcerative lesions of the leg. J Trauma 11: 502–510

25. MacCraw J, Dibbell DG, Carraway JH (1977) Clinical definition of independent myocutaneous territories. Plast Reconstr Surg 60: 341

26. Dos Santos LF (1980) Retalho scapular: Um novo retalho livre microcirùrgico. Rev Bras Cir 70: 133

27. Gilbert A, Teot L (1982) The free scapular flap. Plast Reconstr Surg 69: 601–604

28. Nassif TM, Vidal L, Bovet JL et al. (1982) The parascapular flap: a new cutaneous microsurgical free flap. Plast Reconstr Surg 69: 591–600

29. Dos Santos LF (1984) The vascular anatomy and dissection of the free scapular flap. Plast Reconstr Surg 73: 599–603

30. Nassif TM, Rocha JR, Bijos PB et al. (1988) Retalhos livres cutaneos. In: Melega JM, Zanini SA, Psillakis JM (eds) Cirurgia plàstica reparadora e estética. Medsi, Rio de Janeiro, pp 921–930

31. Maxwell GP, Manson PN, Hoopes JE (1978) A free latissimus dorsi myocutaneous flap. Plast Reconstr Surg 62: 462–466

32. Maxwell GP, Manson PN, Hoopes JE (1979) Experience with 13 free latissimus dorsi myocutaneous flaps. Plast Reconstr Surg 64: 1–8

33. Song RY, Song YG, Yu YS et al. (1982) The upper arm free flap. Clin Plast Surg 9: 27–35

34. Zancolli EA, Angrigiani C (1988) Posterior interosseous island forearm flap. J Hand Surg 13B: 130–135

35. Penteado CV, Masquelet AC, Chevrel JP (1986) The anatomic basis of the fasciocutaneous flap of the posterior interosseous artery. Surg Radiol Anat 8: 209–215

36. Masquelet AC, Penteado CV (1987) Le lambeau interosseux postérieur. Ann Chir Main 6: 131–139

37. Timmons MJ (1986) The vascular basis of the radial forearm flap. Plast Reconstr Surg 77: 80–92

38. Foucher G, Van Genechten F, Merle M et al. (1984) A compound radial artery forearm flap in hand surgery. An original modification of the Chinese forearm flap. Br J Plast Surg 37: 139–148

39. Song R, Gao Y, Song Y et al. (1982) The forearm flap. Clin Plast Surg 9: 21–26

40. Becker C, Gilbert A (1992) The dorsal ulnary artery flap. In: Gilbert A, Masquelet AC, Hentz RV (eds) Pedicle flaps of the upper limb. Martin Dunitz, London, p 129

41. Antia NH, Buch VI (1971) Transfer of an abdominal dermo-fat graft by direct anastomoses of blood vessels. Br J Plast Surg 24: 15–19

42. McGregor IA, Jackson IT (1972) Groin flap. Br J Plast Surg 25: 3–16

43. Daniel RK, Taylor GI (1973) Distant transfer of an island flap by microvascular anastomoses. Plast Reconstr Surg 52: 111–117

44. Rinaldi S (1985) Le lambeau brachial posterieur. Mém Lab Anat Fac Med, Paris, p 54

45. Rinaldi S, Masquelet AC (1985) Anatomical basis of the posterior brachial skin flap. Anat Clin 7: 155–160

46. Maruyama Y, Takeuchi S (1986) The radial recurrent fasciocutaneous flap: reverse upper arm flap. Br J Plast Surg 39: 458–461

47. Hayashi A, Maruyama Y (1990) Anatomical study of the recurrent flaps of the upper arm. Br J Plast Surg 43: 300–306

48. Lovie MJ, Duncan GM, Glasson DW (1984) The ulnar artery forearm free flap. Br J Plast Surg 37: 486–492

49. Gilbert A, Restrepo J (1980) The brachio-radialis muscle: anatomy and use as a muscular rotation flap. Ann Chir Plast 25: 72–75

50. Dellon A, Mackinnon SE (1984) The pronator quadratus muscle flap. J Hand Surg 9A: 423–427

# 24 Loss of Soft Tissue in Lower Limbs

N. PALLUA, A. HEITLAND

## Introduction

The expertise of plastic surgery in lower-extremity reconstruction is established in the field of many vascular, surgical, oncologic and orthopaedic defects. A very important indication is the acute reconstruction of the lower extremities in emergency cases. These demand a high knowledge of anatomy, of local and free flap operative techniques and a well-defined algorithm of therapy methods to save the injured limb. The aims of lower extremity reconstruction are a stable, closed wound, enhanced bone healing, restored ambulation, pleasing aesthetic appearance and ultimately the functional restoration of the saved limb.

## Epidemiology

Historically, military injuries were the main cause of lower-extremity trauma. This changed in the past century to a higher incidence of high-energy injuries in car and train accidents.

There has been a steady decline in motor vehicle-related injuries since 1960 in the USA, which actually showed an increase of killed persons of 1.5% to 42 815 and a decrease of injured persons of –3.5% to 2 926 000 in 2002 [1]. Similar trends are reported from Europe with 40 812 persons killed and 1 295 600 injured persons in car accidents [2]. Especially in older people aged 65 years and more the risk of lower-extremity fractures is increasing [3].

## Pathology

These high-energy injuries create a wound that initially appears small, but which is in reality wider and deeper. The zone of injury of these wounds becomes larger due to the onset of the inflammatory response of the contused tissue. This leads to a high rate of microvascular thrombosis caused by an increased friability of the vessels and perivascular scar formation [4]. Serial debridements are necessary and the soft-tissue coverage in high-energy injuries has to be postponed.

## General Principles of Soft-Tissue Coverage

The goal of reconstruction in cases of soft-tissue loss in the lower extremity is an early wound closure. Cannon and Constable [5] postulated that "the restoration of an intact cutaneous covering is the primary surgical requisite following trauma of the lower extremity because deep healing can be no better than the surface covering". Quick wound closure requires consideration of the following facts: the amount of injured tissue, the size of the defect, the patient's condition in an emergency case, the operative risk and the functional and aesthetic outcome of the reconstruction.

The existing ladder of soft-tissue reconstruction management consists of primary closure, skin grafts, pedicled and free flaps.

Basic indications for salvage of a severely damaged limb are:

- any limb in a child,
- limbs with intact sensitivity in adults,
- limb trauma with a nerve injury allowing a return of at least partial function within a reasonable period.

Age should not be a contra-indication for the salvage of a complex injury in the elderly if meticulous peri- and post-operative monitoring is possible. Goldberg et al. [6] proved that microvascular reconstruction in the elderly can be performed in a safe and successful way.

The basic principles of wound treatment also apply to open wounds of the lower limbs. Devitalised and contaminated tissue has to be debrided, the wound has to be explored, damaged structures repaired and the defect covered with soft tissue.

The indications for free tissue transfer to cover defects of the distal lower extremities are:

- defects exposing the Achilles tendon,
- exposed fractures,
- open joints,
- compromise of the distal arterial flow,
- exposed bypass grafts.

The aims of free-tissue transfer are an early definitive wound healing and restoration of function, salvage of impending amputations, functional stumps for prosthetic reconstruction and, finally, good aesthetic results [7].

## Surgical Planning

The necessity for an angiogram is still subject to debate. Sometimes a Doppler can give enough information about a possible discontinuity of the vessels. Therefore, there is no absolute need for an angiogram in young patients. In mature patients we suggest debridement, followed by an angiography and, when necessary, free-flap coverage within 72 h.

## Microsurgical Principles

According to microsurgical principles, the recipient site has to be chosen outside the zone of injury. Sometimes this requires a second incision to prepare the recipient vessels or to interpose the distance with a venous graft. The pedicle of the standard free latissimus-dorsi flap or serratus flap is usually long enough and therefore there is rarely a need for vessel grafts.

Another important point is the exact planning of the flap dimensions. First, the recipient site is prepared and secondly the donor site. When available, the work can be done by two teams simultaneously. The flap should be inserted first, then the venous end-to-end anastomosis and finally the arterial end-to-side anastomosis should be performed. Post-operatively, the leg has to be elevated, the foot dorsiflexed and the flap clinically monitored.

A considerable problem in an acute injury to the lower extremities is venous hypertension. In free flaps an anastomosis is preferably performed to the deep veins as long as they are undamaged. However, when the deep vein system is damaged, an anastomosis to the deep and also the superficial veins (the greater saphenous vein) has to be performed. This is because spasms are common in superficial veins.

## Timing of the Lower-Extremity Coverage

An exact timing of the lower-extremity coverage depends on a variety of factors: the amount of damaged tissue, the type of concomitant fracture, the involved functional structures, the bacterial contamination and the patient's condition. Nevertheless, there is still a controversy concerning the exact timing of soft-tissue coverage.

The studies of Byrd et al. [8, 9] showed that early aggressive wound debridement and soft-tissue coverage with a free flap within 5 days had a positive effect on post-operative infection, flap take and the rate of bony non-union and osteomyelitis. Godina [10] proved the importance of early aggressive wound debridement and soft-tissue coverage within 72 h in open fractures. His study demonstrated that the rate of flap take is higher, the infection rate lower and the period of hospitalisation shorter in the group with early soft-tissue coverage.

These studies showed the benefit of an early microsurgical flap transplantation which then led to the first case of an immediate free flap coverage by Lister and Schecker [11], who defined the so-called emergency free flap as a flap transplantation at the end of primary debridement or within 24 h after the injury. The great advantages of an emergency free flap have been demonstrated by Arnez [4], who proved that the infection and revision rate were lower and consequently the hospitalisation period and costs were lower and the bone healing time shorter. It is well known that the flap survival in chronic wounds is generally lower because of contamination, infection, injured lymphatics, injured veins, tissue oedema, perivascular fibrosis and valvular incompetence. Nevertheless, in high-velocity accidents the rules of early wound coverage have to be weighed against the needs of serial wound debridements. Yaremchuk [12] had good results with free flap transfer between the 7th and 14th day after injury and several debridements.

The timing of the microsurgical tissue transplantation has to be tailored to the patient's status, the injury mechanism and the condition of the wound. Ideally, the defect should be covered on the 3rd to 4th post-traumatic day with the exemption of an emergency flap in a young patient with clean wounds and a well-defined injury zone.

## Surgical Principles

In an emergency case, the findings of the wound exploration determine the immediate repair of functional structures, the methods of possible fixation, the need to open compartments, the timing and the type of coverage of the defect. Figure 1 gives an overview of the multiple operative procedures and serves as a decision-making aid.

In general, all functional structures have to be repaired with special attention to nerve injuries. Sensitivity in the sole of the foot is the key to a functional or nonfunctional extremity. Unfortunately, high-velocity injuries to the lower extremity tend to occur more proximal than in upper-extremity injuries. In a case of any suspected nerve damage, the nerve has to be explored to rule out a transsection with the differential diagnosis of a compartment syndrome. Uncontaminated sharply transsected nerves need immediate repair within 72 h whereas contaminated or tractioned nerves require secondary reconstruction. In the case of a distal injury and loss of the distal nerve stump, a neurotisation [13] helps to reconstruct a neuromuscular union. Then the proximal nerve stump is dissected and transposed into the muscle belly.

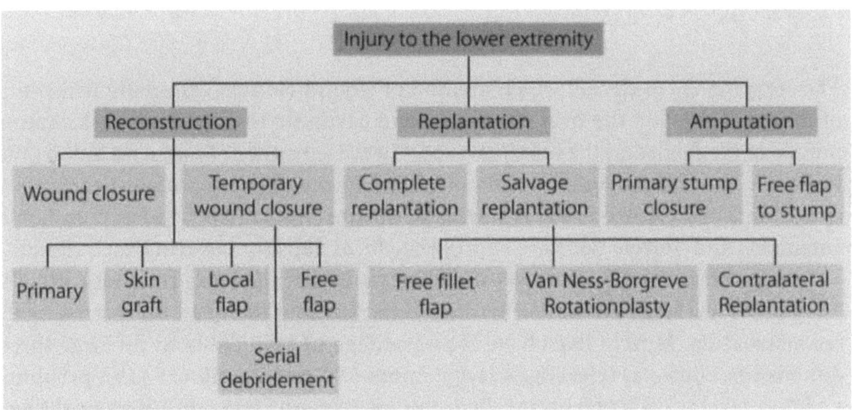


**Fig. 1.** Algorithm for the operative care of acute lower-extremity traumas

Open joint injuries should be covered within 72 h and will not lead to infection if irrigated and covered with sufficient soft tissue. Small bone defects up to 6 cm in size can be reconstructed with non-vascularised grafts. Non-vascularised bone grafts require a clean wound ground, small defect size and sufficient soft-tissue coverage. An immediate coverage with a free flap is possible, but most of the time the infected wound ground has to be cleaned and a two-stage procedure of free-flap coverage with delayed cancellous bone grafting is chosen. After an interval of at least 6 weeks the secondary bone transplant is performed.

In cases of bone gaps larger than 6 cm the defect can be closed with vascularised bone transplants such as a contralateral free fibula bone graft. Alternative techniques are the synostosis of the fibula and the tibia, the Papineau technique or the Ilizarov distraction. In the Papineau procedure the bone is debrided and stabilised. After the formation of granulation tissue the wound bed is filled with cortical bone from the iliac crest and covered with a moist dressing for 3 days. After several dressing changes the free cortical bone grafts are vascularised and the wound can be closed with a skin graft.

In cases of acute trauma to the lower extremities the risk of a compartment syndrome is often underestimated. Blick et al. [14] estimated the incidence of a possible compartment syndrome to be 9.1% in 198 acute open fractures of the tibia. Symptoms of compartment syndrome in a massive trauma to the leg are tingling, pain, painful passive extension of the involved muscle or a deficit of sensitivity. The actual tissue compartment pressure can be measured with a fine needle catheter. Compartment pressure levels up to 30 mmHg should raise concern, and pressures between 35 and 40 mmHg are an indication for a fasciotomy. Furthermore, a compartment fasciotomy is recommended whenever there is a circulatory interruption of a lower extremity, a clinical suspicion of reduced neurological function or compartments with verified pressure elevation. A devascularised lower extremity requires a four-compartment fasciotomy in any case.

## Recommended Flaps in Relation to the Anatomical Injury Level

The surgeon has to decide which method of wound closure, especially which type of flap, will provide the best functional and aesthetic result. In general, exposed muscle of the thigh and the proximal aspect of the leg can be closed with a skin graft. Defects in the exposed anterior tibia and distal aspect of the leg, weight-bearing foot, open joints and exposed neurovascular structures need a flap closure. Both fasciocutaneous and muscle flaps are appropriate local flaps for covering such defects.

Fasciocutaneous flaps are more useful in low-velocity and non-traumatic wounds. They provide a large amount of tissue with or without the need for microsurgical reconstruction. Muscle flaps have the advantage of being able to fill large three-dimensional defects, releasing a large amount of growth factors [15], providing a higher level of vascularisation than fasciocutaneous flaps and thus enabling a better wound healing with higher antibiotic delivery and collagen deposition.

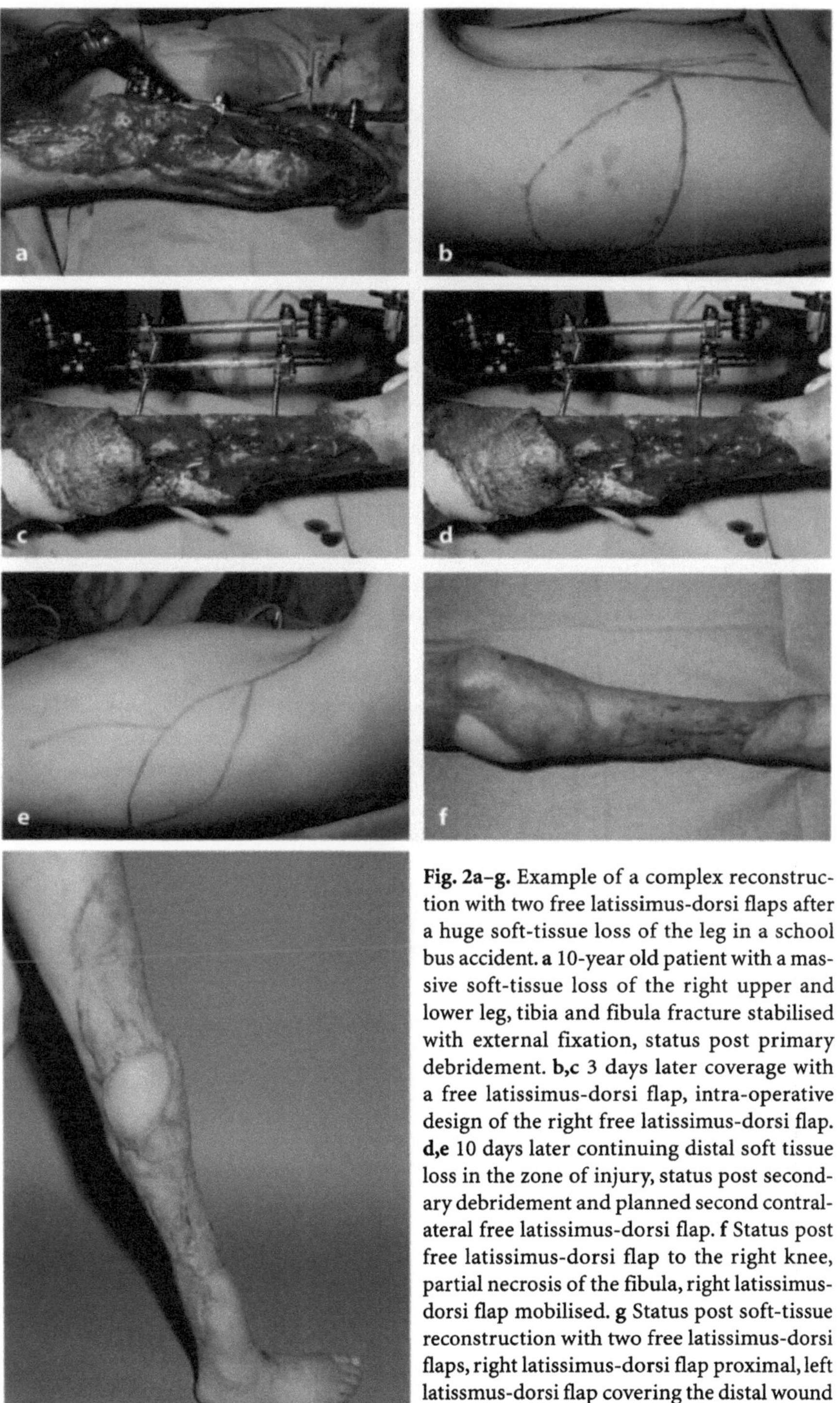

**Fig. 2a–g.** Example of a complex reconstruction with two free latissimus-dorsi flaps after a huge soft-tissue loss of the leg in a school bus accident. **a** 10-year old patient with a massive soft-tissue loss of the right upper and lower leg, tibia and fibula fracture stabilised with external fixation, status post primary debridement. **b,c** 3 days later coverage with a free latissimus-dorsi flap, intra-operative design of the right free latissimus-dorsi flap. **d,e** 10 days later continuing distal soft tissue loss in the zone of injury, status post secondary debridement and planned second contralateral free latissimus-dorsi flap. **f** Status post free latissimus-dorsi flap to the right knee, partial necrosis of the fibula, right latissimus-dorsi flap mobilised. **g** Status post soft-tissue reconstruction with two free latissimus-dorsi flaps, right latissimus-dorsi flap proximal, left latissmus-dorsi flap covering the distal wound field

The advantages of distant tissue transplantation with free flaps include the transfer of a large amount of tissue in a one-stage procedure, without the need for long periods of immobilisation. Our favourite free flaps are the latissimus dorsi, the gracilis or the serratus anterior muscle flap, with possible additional skin grafts. One of the few indications for a cross-leg flap would be in a child, who could tolerate the knee flexion without subsequent joint stiffness and contracture, if free flaps are not possible.

The following is a summary of the recommended flaps in relation to the anatomical injury level.

In the **thigh**, reconstruction consists of

- local rotation or advancement flaps of the thigh muscles, i.e. gracilis, vastus lateralis and tensor fascia lata flap (with or without skin grafts)
- fasciocutaneous flaps, i.e. medial thigh-, lateral posterior thigh-, anterolateral thigh and mediolateral thigh flap,
- more distant flaps, i.e. rectus abdominis flap.

A common method is to divide the lower leg into thirds, covering the upper third with a pedicled gastrocnemius flap, the intermediate third with a pedicled soleus flap and the lower third with a free flap. However, this procedure has to be adjusted to provide the best functional and aesthetic results and not just the easiest procedure.

In the **knee** and **proximal tibia area** the medial or lateral gastrocnemius flap are the first choices. Alternatively, adequate soft-tissue coverage is possible with either the fasciocutaneous saphenous flap or the distally based vastus lateralis flap with a high risk of necrosis. However, larger soft-tissue defects will need a free-flap coverage.

In the **midtibial region** the soleus flap or the anterior tibial muscle turnover flap are recommended.

The difficult area of the **ankle** and **distal tibia** can be covered by a dorsalis pedis flap, an extensor brevis muscle flap or a sural neurocutaneous flap. The **weight-bearing heel** and **midplantar region** require neurosensory reconstruction with the instep flap.

Figure 2 gives an example of a complex reconstruction with two free latissimus dorsi flaps after a large soft-tissue loss in the leg.

## New Trends

Recently, there have been several new trends in tissue reconstruction. The concept of free perforator flaps reduced the morbidity of the harvesting defect to a minimum. The perforating vessels are dissected through the muscle. Figure 3 shows the free DIEP (deep inferior epigastric artery perforator) flap. This provides an optimal harvest-site defect without damaging the muscle fibres, but demands a longer preparation time of the pedicle. Several cases have been reported in the literature [16], but this technique of closing wounds of the lower extremity is still not completely established and needs further clinical experience. Also, cases using the artificial dermis Integra™ have been reported, but are limited to smaller wounds which require only dermal and epidermal reconstruction.

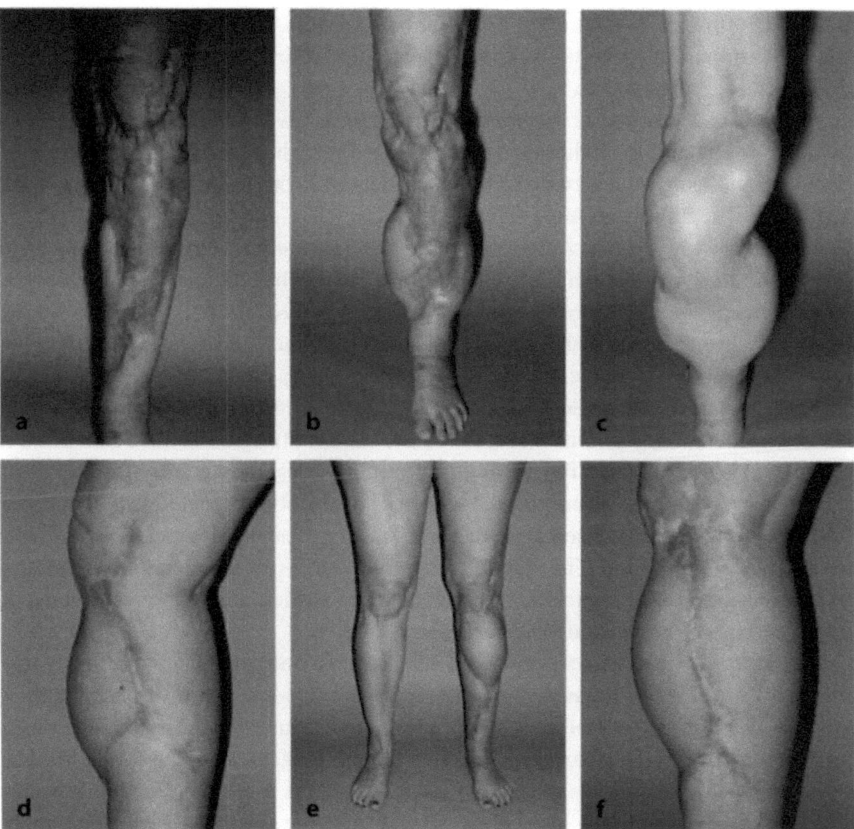

**Fig. 3a–f.** New trends. Example of secondary soft-tissue coverage with multiple expanders and free DIEP (deep inferior epigastric artery perforator) flap. **a,b** Status post motorbike accident with 3° open tibia and patella fracture left leg, extremely painful tibia. **c,d** Status post 4 expander implantation and tissue expansion **e,f** 6 months status post free DIEP flap, planned flap thinning by liposuction

## Replantation

A completely amputated lower extremity is a very demanding situation which needs a careful decision between replantation, salvage replantation or amputation. Historically, the first successful replantation of a completely amputated arm was described in 1962 by Malt [17].

The following principles have to be considered in an attempt to replant a lower limb. The tolerated ischemia time of muscle is 4–6 h. Surface cooling of a large extremity is not effective because it does not cool the core of the extremity. The most vulnerable parts are the muscles. Ischemia time can be reduced by a temporary shunt if the time limit is too short for the reconstruction order given below.

The ideal indication for a replantation is a clean amputation at a single level without crush or avulsion injuries and an ischemic time less than 6 h. A wider zone of injury increases the amount of reconstruction. Especially extensive muscle or nerve injuries have a poor functional outcome. The recommended maximum of bone shortening is 8–10 cm [18] unless both extremities are amputated. In general, the indication for a replantation should be handled more liberally in young patients and bilateral amputations.

Contra-indications for replantation are a poor level of health, multi-level injuries to joints and an ischemic time of more than 6 h. After all, the principle life before limb has to rule. Crushed compartments and extensive bone injuries make a successful replantation more difficult.

The following surgical order of replantation is widely accepted. The zone of injury has to be debrided including all avascular parts other than large pieces of bone which can survive on periosteal vascularisation. The procedure is performed in the following chronological order: bone fixation, arterial and venous anastomosis, nerve repair, soft-tissue coverage.

In debridement a muscle-unit concept should be followed. By not cutting through the muscle, bleeding is minimised. However, muscle stumps should be retained in order to cover vital structures. For better functional results it is important to minimise bone shortening. Some gait disturbances cannot be corrected by pelvic tilt or heel lift and will need subsequent bone lengthening. The use of arterial, venous and nerval grafts is justified. The standard external fixation is less stable than internal fixation and does not compress the bone endings sufficiently. The disadvantage of internal fixation is reduced vascularisation.

Replants of the lower extremity can survive with only one reconstructed artery. It is recommended to harvest vein grafts from the opposite leg. If necessary, nerve grafts should be performed only under ideal conditions with clean wounds, sharp transsection and without any tension on the nerve (Fig. 4). In above-knee amputations a proper fascicular coaptation of the sciatic nerve is very important to regain a neurosensory functional lower extremity. Middle-leg amputations require repair of the sural nerve, distal leg amputations require superficial peroneal nerve repair. Foot amputations require tibial nerve repair or repair of the medial plantar, lateral plantar and the medial calcaneal nerve. The neurovascular structures should be covered with adequate soft tissue. Fasciotomy has to be done routinely after a revascularisation to prevent compartment syndrome.

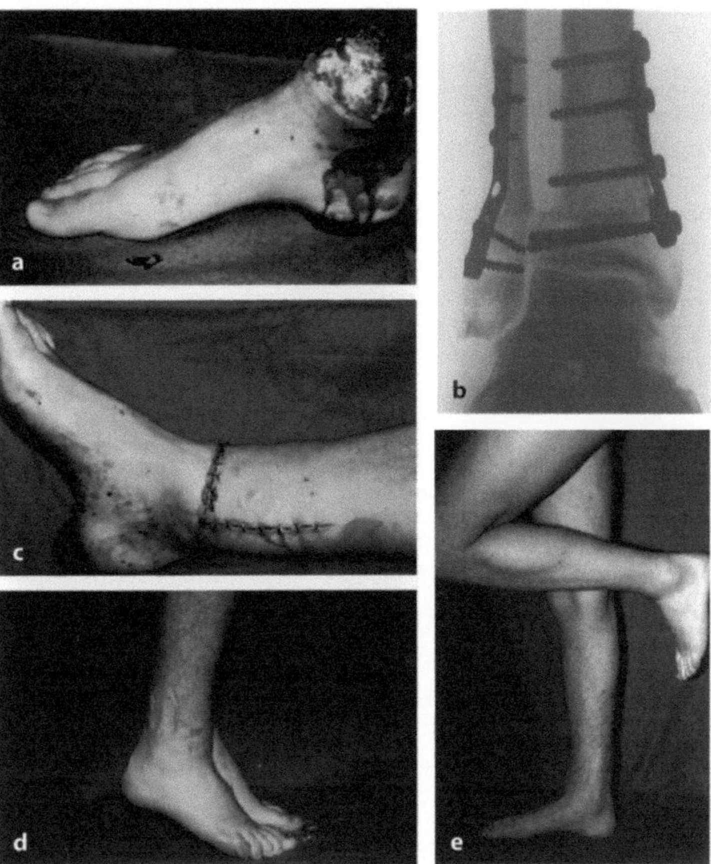

Fig. 4. **a** Example of a traumatic right foot amputation. **b,c** Status after successful replatation and osteosynthesis. **d,e** Full functional rehabilitation. Patient is able to stand on one foot (**e**), on his toes (**d**) and his heels. (The author would like to thank Prof. Berger for kindly providing him with these pictures of a patient taken during their shared, very productive years in Hannover)

## Salvage Replantation

Salvage replantation involves using nerve, skin or bone grafts from the amputated part. Portions of the foot can be used as a free muscle- or fillet flap to cover the proximal stump and allow retention of bone length. A heel pad over the distal stump can be re-innervated and allows for neurosensory stump reconstruction.

Rare procedures include the use of the contralateral foot in a bilateral amputation for a heterotopic replantation.

Another possibility to create a functional and sensory stump is the Van Ness-Borgreve-rotation plasty [19, 20]. After resection of the "zone of injury" of the injured part, the tibia is rotated 180°. This procedure enables a sensitive stump.

## Principles of Amputation

The principles of amputation should provide a reliable stump. The best function can be achieved with a below-the-knee amputation. The preservation of the knee simplifies rehabilitation, the more distal the better. Above-knee amputations should be performed at the mid-thigh region, whereas below-knee amputations should be performed 12 cm below the knee. In an above-knee amputation a patello-femoral fusion can provide bone to tendon anchorage.

## References


1. Administration N.H.T.S (2003) Motor Vehicle Traffic Crash Fatality and Injury Estimates for 2002. United States Department of Transportation, National Highway Traffic Safety Administration
2. Federation E.U.R. (2003) Transport Statistics 2003. Statistic 6.1. European Commission EUROSTAT
3. Moran SG et al. (2003) Relationship between age and lower extremity fractures in frontal motor vehicle collisions. J Trauma 54: 261–265
4. Arnez ZM (1991) Immediate reconstruction of the lower extremity – an update. Clin Plast Surg 18: 449–457
5. Cannon B, Furlaw L, Hayburst JW, McCarthy JG, McGraw JB (1977) Reconstructive surgery of the lower extremity. In: Converse JM (ed) Reconstructive plastic surgery, 2nd edn. W.B. Saunders, Philapdelphia
6. Goldberg JA, Alpert BS, Lienaweaver WC (1991) Microvascular reconstruction of the lower extremity in the elderly. Clin Plast Surg 18: 459
7. Khouri RK, Shaw WW (1989) Reconstruction of the lower extremity with microvascular free flaps: a 10-year experience with 304 consecutive cases. J Trauma 29: 1086–1094
8. Byrd HS, Cierny G III, Tebetts JB (1981) The management of open tibial fractures with associated soft-tissue loss: external pin fixation with early flap coverage. Plast Reconstr Surg 68: 73
9. Byrd HS, Spicer TE, Cierny GD (1985) Management of open tibial fractures. Plast Reconstr Surg 76: 719
10. Godina M (1986) Early microsurgical reconstruction of complex trauma of the extremities. Plast Reconstr Surg 78: 285
11. Lister G, Scheker L (1988) Emergency free flaps to the upper extremity. J Hand Surg (Am) 13: 22
12. Yaremchuk MJ, Brumback RF, Manson PN (1987) Acute and definitive management of traumatic osteocutaneous defects of the lower extremity. Plast Reconstr Surg 80: 1
13. Wigand ME, Naumann WH, Thormann J (1976) Microsurgical nerve implantation for rehabilitation of atrophied and transplanted muscles. In: Koos W, Böck FW, Spetzler R (eds) Clinical microsurgery. Thieme, Stuttgart, p 271–273
14. Blick SS, Brumback RJ, Poka A, Brugess AR, Ebraheim NA (1986) Compartment syndrome in open tibial fractures. J Bone Joint Surg 68 A: 1348
15. Pallua N, Ulrich D (2003) Expression of basic fibroblast growth factor and transforming growth factor-Beta 1 in patients with fasciocutaneous and muscle flaps. Plast Reconstr Surg 111: 79–82; discussion 83–84
16. Blondeel PN et al. (2003) Soft tissue reconstruction with the superior gluteal artery perforator flap. Clin Plast Surg 30: 371–382
17. Malt RA (1964) Replantation of severed arms. JAMA 189: 716
18. Chen ZW, Zeng BF (1983) Replantation of the lower extremity. Clin Plast Surg 10: 103–113
19. Veenstra KM et al. (2000) Quality of life in survivors with a Van Ness-Borggreve rotation plasty after bone tumour resection. J Surg Oncol 73: 192–197
20. Heise U, Minet-Sommer S (1993) [The Borggreve rotation plasty. A surgical method in therapy of malignant bone tumors and functional results]. Z Orthop Ihre Grenzgeb 131: 452–460

# Vacuum-Assisted Closure: Orthopaedic Applications

D. Laverty, L.X. Webb

## Introduction

Vacuum-assisted wound closure (VAC) was introduced in the early 1990s by Argenta and Morykwas [1] and was initially called the decubivac, because it was developed for the management of large, infected, chronic wounds in debilitated patients. The indications for its use rapidly expanded. Around the same time, trials were underway by Fleischmann in Europe utilising a similar technique for the treatment of open fractures and infection [2, 3]. Essentially, negative pressure is used to exert a "pull" on the tissue of a wound cavity. This mechanically induced negative pressure removes fluid from the extravascular space, improves circulation in oedematous tissue by lowering capillary afterload and enhances the proliferation of reparative granulation tissue by virtue of the ilyzarovian [45] effect on surface reparative tissues.

## Basic Science

Wounds heal by progressing through phases. After the initial injuring mechanism, an inflammatory response is brought about characterised by an array of vascular, cellular and humoral events. The traumatised tissue causes a release of vasoactive substances which, in turn, causes the capillaries to allow for the leaking of plasma proteins, followed by fluid moving from the intravascular compartment to the extravascular tissue space. The process also triggers white cell migration and enzymatic action on dead cells which, in turn, increases the osmotic load in the tissue space. This is followed by the further release of fluid from the intravascular space into the extravascular tissue space with elevation of tissue pressure and increased capillary afterload. This results in a slowing of capillary flow, decreased oxygen exchange at the tissue level and the potential for further cellular necrosis, establishing a positive feedback loop on this destructive process. Once this inflammatory course and sequential events have run their course, and the necrosis is cleared, this phase gives way to a reparative phase, marked by heightened angiogenesis, granulation, collagen production and re-epithelialisation.

The positive effects of subatmospheric pressure on a wound bed are many. First, the technique acts to pull fluid from the interstitial space, thereby lowering the capillary afterload in the zone of stasis [1]. Evacuation of this fluid removes the embarrassment to the venular side of the microcirculation, enhancing flow and the delivery of oxygen and glucose to and the removal of waste products from the affected tissues. Inhibitory factors that suppress the formation of fibroblasts, keratinocytes and vascular endothelial cells are removed with this fluid as well [1, 4–9]. Secondly, there is a notable increase in blood flow in the tissues of the wound. In a study by Morykwas et al. [10], paired wounds were created equidistant from the dorsal midline in 20-kg pigs. Continuous laser-Doppler needle probes were inserted adjacent to the wound, and subatmospheric pressure applied in 25-mmHg increments (range 0 to 400 mmHg) for 15-min intervals. Intermittent applications of negative pressure (on for 1 to 10 min, off for 1 to 5 min) as well as continuous settings were studied. Peak increases in blood flow (four times baseline) were noted at 125 mmHg below ambient pressure in the intermittent mode (optimum cycle of 5 min on, 2 min off). Combined, these factors may account for the successful prevention of the progression of partial-thickness burns in an animal model [11]. As well, these mechanisms most likely play a role in preventing ulceration after injection of doxorubicin in a swine model [12].

Next, it has been shown that VAC treatment lowers bacterial counts present on wound surfaces. Prior studies have proven that bacterial colonisation hampers wound healing [13–15]. Use of VAC therapy has been studied in a swine model to assess the rate of bacterial clearance [10]. Matched wounds were created and infected with *Staphylococcus aureus* and *Staphylococcus epidermidus*. One wound received treatment with subatmospheric pressure (–125 mmHg), and the other saline-soaked gauze for a paired control. Punch biopsies of each wound were performed at 24-h intervals for 2 weeks. Quantitative bacterial counts remained below $10^5$ organisms/g tissue for all VAC-treated wounds. Control wound bacterial levels remained high, above $10^5$/g tissue, until day 11 (peak count occurred at day 5).

Granulation tissue formation was studied in five animals using subatmospheric pressure. Paired wounds were created, one receiving VAC therapy and the other control wound managed with saline-moistened gauze dressings. The mean increase in the rate of granulation tissue formation for saline-moistened dressing-treated wounds was $63.3 \pm 26.1\%$; in wounds treated with intermittent VAC therapy the granulation tissue response was $103.4 \pm 35.3\%$ [10].

Flap survival was evaluated using dorsally based flaps. Four groups were created:
1. pre-operative and post-operative exposure to negative pressure,
2. only pre-operative exposure to negative pressure,
3. only post-operative exposure to negative pressure,
4. no exposure to negative pressure (control group).

Groups 1 and 2 were exposed to subatmospheric pressure of 125 mmHg continuously for 4 days prior to surgery. Groups 1 and 3 had continuous negative pressure for 72 h after surgery. A percent of flap survival was calculated, with the viable surface areas of each flap expressed as a percentage of the entire flap surface area. Group 1 had the greatest survival (72.2%), followed by the flaps treated only postoperatively (group 3: 67.4%). Flaps with only pre-operative exposure (group 2) had 64.8% survival, while flaps in control group 4 had the lowest survival at 51.2%. The difference between groups 1 and 4 was statistically significant ($p < 0.01$) [11].

Laboratory data have shown the VAC system to be an effective adjunct in treating soft-tissue wounds. By reducing oedema, promoting blood flow, enhancing granulation tissue formation and reducing bacterial counts, VAC therapy positively affects a myriad of wounds on an accelerated timetable.

In utilising the system for the management of the fasciotomy wounds in the setting of acute crural compartment syndrome, Chang et al. [27] showed a more rapid and complete resolution of the oedema in the muscle bed as evidenced by a quicker time to healing (stable definitive closure or coverage) in those wounds managed with a vacuum vs. those managed with conventional dressings.

## Application of the VAC System

Several essential elements make up the VAC system. A sterile reticulated polyurethane foam sponge is cut to conform to the surface of the wound and is then placed onto the wound bed, making contact with the entire wound surface. A plastic sheet with adhesive on one side is then placed over the sponge with enough overlap of the surrounding skin to provide an airtight seal (recommended around 5 cm). Once this closed system is created, a 2-cm opening is made in the drape over the sponge; this allows for application of the adherent track pad and egress tubing that will connect with the vacuum pump and reservoir. The settings for the vacuum pump are adjustable for either continuous (most common) or intermittent operation at negative pressures of 50–200 mmHg (the most common setting is continuous at negative 125 mmHg).

Obtaining a seal can be difficult in some orthopaedic wounds. Proximity of moist skin (burn patients) or external fixation pins can prove to be challenging. Sterile hydrocolloid gel (e.g. Duoderm, Convatec, Princeton, NJ, USA) helps provide a secure seal when applied circumferentially to these areas, as well as around the external fixation pin about an inch above the skin. In areas where an intact skin bridge is present between open wounds, Adaptec (Johnson and Johnson, Arlington, TX, USA) can be placed over the intact skin and a connecting sponge conformed between the two wounds to provide continuity of the vacuum system. Elderly patients with thin skin or patients on steroids may need any skin areas exposed to negative pressure protected with Adaptec; skin grafts bolstered using the VAC technique may also benefit from an intervening layer of Adaptec, as would exposed nerves and tendons in the wound bed.

Direct contact of the sponge on blood vessels should probably be avoided, lest there be any tearing of the vessel at the time of changing of the sponge.

Sponge changes most commonly occur at 48-h intervals. This can be done as a bedside procedure if the wound tissue is limited and mature. The authors have used 1% plain lidocaine inserted into the sponge after the vacuum has been turned off as a "topical" means of alleviating patient discomfort. These sponge changes are done as a clean (not sterile) procedure, with normal blood and body fluid precautions. Some patients with extensive, semi-acute wounds may require general anaesthesia in an operating room; this is often done in concordance with other procedures such as fracture stabilisation or surgical debridement with irrigation.

Fluid volumes can be substantial in the first 24 to 48 h, not uncommonly a range of 100–1000 ml. Much of this depends on the size of the wound, location and general health status of the patient. In patients with generalised or local oedema (low protein levels, congestive heart failure etc.), more fluid is produced as the vacuum pulls third-spaced fluid from the wound. These patients may need careful monitoring of their haemodynamic status in an ICU. Anticoagulated patients should have drainage observed at regular intervals; any excessive blood loss is an indication to inspect the wound for bleeding sources and to potentially discontinue VAC therapy. Direct placement of the sponge on any exposed blood vessels should be avoided, lest these be torn at the time of sponge removal or exchange (tissue ingrowth into the sponge can be vigorous).

The VAC technique has been used on debilitated patients without adverse impact on electrolyte balance, kidney or liver function, or other vital systems. Most cases do not require special systemic or laboratory monitoring.

## Indications

Wounds treated with vacuum-assisted closure can be grouped into 11 basic descriptive categories [16] as listed below.
1. Wounds with a split-thickness skin graft
2. Previously infected, clean wounds (after debridement)
3. Open-fracture wounds
4. Acute soft-tissue wounds (low energy; exposed bone, joint, tendon, hardware)
5. Fasciotomy wounds after compartment syndrome
6. Chronic wounds (>3 months duration)
7. Difficult to close surgical wounds
8. High-energy injuries involving bone, joints
9. Irritated external fixation pin sites
10. Surgical wounds prone to weep
11. Severe traumatic degloving injuries (Morel-Lavallee lesion)

The standard pressure setting for wound types 1–8 is –125 mmHg, with sponge changes every 48 h. For wound types 2, 3, 4, 6 and 8, application of the VAC technique is only appropriate after complete removal of all devitalised and necrotic tissue (i.e. a complete debridement). This often means that severely contaminated acute wounds may need a second look operative debridement to ensure confidence that the wound has been cleared of all devitalised tissue and potential contaminants.

Wounds of type 9 require a lower pressure setting, generally –50 mmHg. The sponge is placed at the base of the external fixator pin and can be changed about once per week.

VAC therapy for wound type 10 (surgical wounds prone to drainage beyond post-operative day 2) has proven useful. The typical setting is –50 mmHg, although –75 mmHg has been used with precautions to avoid skin irritation (usually a small piece of Adaptec is used as an intermediary between the sponge and the skin).

The type-11 wound is a recent addition to the potential uses for VAC therapy.

## Specific Techniques

### Split-Thickness Skin Graft

Many orthopaedic traumatologists perform split-thickness skin grafting as a part of soft-tissue management for open fractures and degloving injuries. With the advent of VAC therapy, wounds that may have required a rotational flap or free-tissue transfer are now amenable to final coverage with a skin graft. The recipient bed created in orthopaedic wounds is often complex, with a highly irregular surface geometry, exudative surface and location of the body subjected to repeated motion. All of these factors tend to limit the intimate contact required for a skin graft to survive and adhere to the granulating recipient bed.

The classic method of securing skin grafts has been with tie-over bolsters. Cotton balls soaked in a modified Bunnell's solution (acetic acid and glycerine) are used as a dressing material, and firmly held in place by multiple over-lying sutures. While this method may work well on flat, motionless surfaces, it has proven to be cumbersome with many orthopaedic wounds. Other methods have been utilised, including fibrin glue, splints made from silicones, foams and self-adherent wraps.

VAC therapy addresses many of the difficulties encountered with split-thickness skin grafting in complex orthopaedic wounds. Using this technique, pressure is uniformly distributed to the wound, promoting continuous contact between graft and host regardless of recipient bed surface geometry. Any exudative fluid that may accumulate is immediately evacuated, limiting the chance of infection. Minor amounts of motion are accommodated for by the pliability of the sponge.

Schneider et al. [17] describe the technique and results. Standard skin graft harvest is performed, and the graft is meshed 1:1 or 1.5:1 to limit potential fluid accumulation beneath the graft. Absorbable sutures or staples are then used to secure the graft, and a VAC foam dressing is cut to contour the defect. A porous monolayer barrier of Adaptec (Johnson and Johnson, Arlington, TX), Xeroform (Kendall, Mansfield, Mass.) or Vaseline gauze (Sherwood Medical, Markham, Ontario, Canada) is placed between the sponge and graft to limit adherence of the sponge. Standard adhesive application is then performed.

Figure 1a–c represents this technique in a degloving injury of the leg associated with a mid-shaft tibia fracture. Excellent graft take was accomplished with uneventful healing.

Continuous negative pressure is then applied at 125 mmHg, leaving it in place for 3–4 days. Patients are allowed to participate in limited therapy as long as the device is in place. It is critical to carefully remove the foam dressing and barrier after

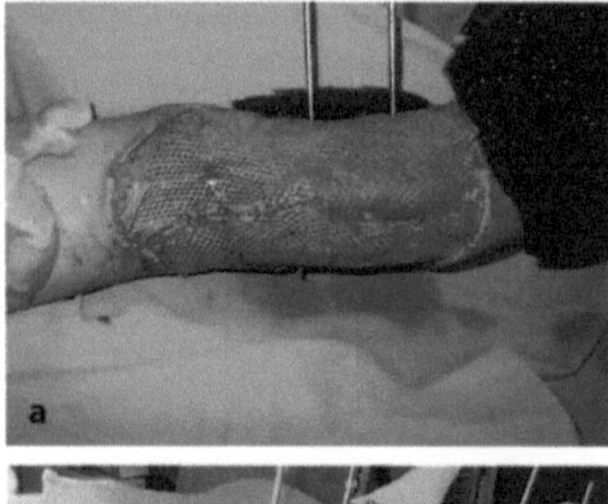
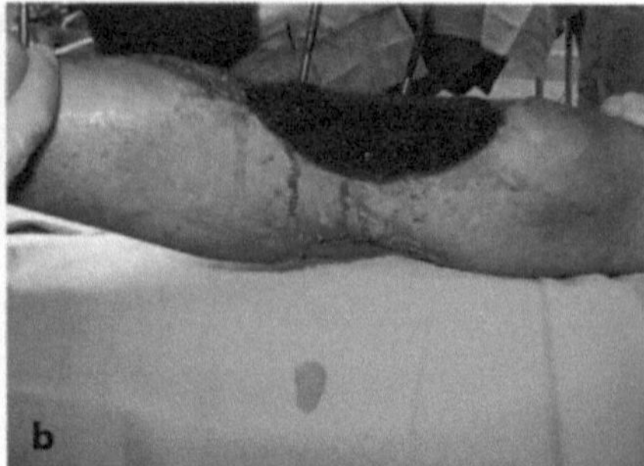
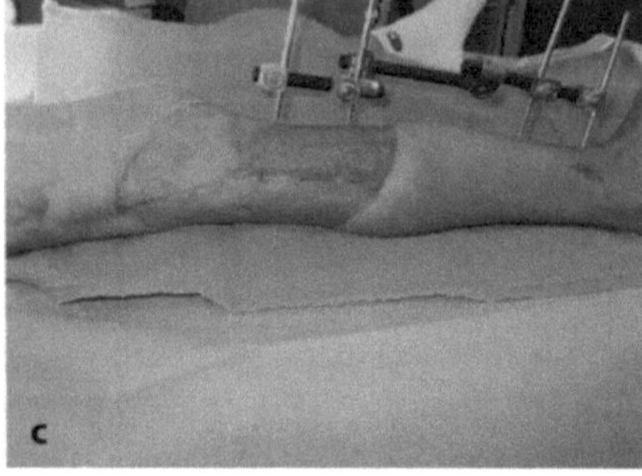

**Fig. 1a–c.** Split-thickness skin graft in a degloving injury of the leg associated with a mid-shaft tibia fracture

release of the negative pressure; potential for shearing and graft dislodgement is possible. If granulation tissue buds have protruded through the graft, they will usually be rapidly replaced (72 h) by a layer of epithelium even with the graft once the negative pressure is removed.

Over 100 acute wounds, chronic wounds and burns in patients aged 2 months to 97 years were reviewed utilizing this method [17]. Grafts were applied to all regions of the body (feet, lower extremities, perineum, genitalia, trunk, hands, face and scalp). No grafts were lost due to intervening fluid collections. A complete take was evident in all but two grafts (both in grossly contaminated chronic wounds), and patients tolerated the procedure well. In another study, Blackburn et al. [18] had 95% graft survival. Use of portable VAC units has been studied as a method of dressing skin grafts on the lower extremities [19]. Excellent results were obtained in all patients evaluated.

Application of VAC therapy to split-thickness skin grafts covering complex orthopaedic wounds has proven to be effective, easy to use and well tolerated by patients. Fewer secondary procedures may be needed, decreasing hospital stay and cost.

### Previously Infected Clean Wounds (After Debridement)

The application of VAC therapy does not substitute for sound surgical principles. The ultimate success of treatment may be defined as the transition of a traumatic wound to stable wound closure or coverage. When confronted with an infected

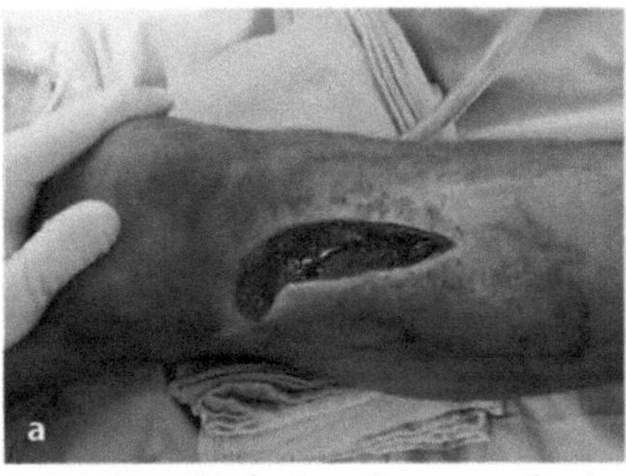
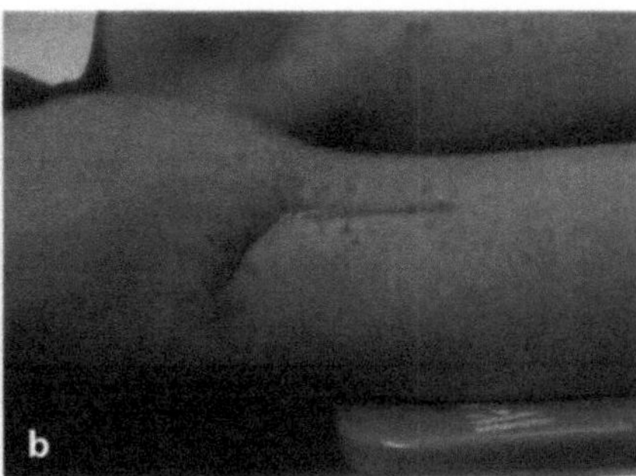

**Fig. 2. a** Wound infection after open reduction internal fixation of a lateral tibial plateau fracture; **b** result after VAC therapy

wound bed, the primary goal remains debridement of all contaminated or devitalised tissue. If orthopaedic implants, such as plates and screws, are part of the wound, they will often need removal. When there is a small area of exposed bone and/or implant at the base of a well-vascularised wound, VAC treatment may encourage the overgrowth of clean, healthy granulation tissue amenable to simple closure methods, such as split-thickness skin grafting. Using the VAC techniques as described by Fleischmann et al. [3], larger areas of exposed or infected hardware may be treated.

In a study by DeFranzo et al., VAC therapy was used in 75 lower-extremity wounds with exposed bone, tendon or hardware [20]. Continuous subatmospheric pressure (125 mmHg) was applied at the wound site, and dressings were changed every 48 h. Tissue oedema was greatly reduced, with a decrease in leg circumference and size of the wound. Granulation tissue formed profusely, covering bone and hardware. Successful coverage, as defined by primary closure, split-thickness skin graft or regional flap was obtained in 71 of 75 wounds, stable at 6 months to 6 years.

Sixteen patients who developed an infected soft-tissue defect with exposed bone and/or implants after stabilisation of lower-extremity fractures were followed with VAC therapy [21]. Deep wound infection was diagnosed at an average of 4 weeks following initial surgical intervention (average 1–6 weeks). Initial irrigation and debridement was performed, with administration of intravenous antibiotics. Wet to dry gauze dressing changes were instituted for the first 48 h, at which time patients were returned to the operation room for repeat irrigation and debridement, with application of VAC therapy. Fourteen patients responded favourably to VAC therapy, with a mean time to healing of 16 days (range 7–28), and an average of 3.7 applications. All exposed bone and/or implants were covered in these 14 patients. Wound coverage was achieved by secondary intention in two patients, and split-thickness skin grafting in 12. All fractures healed in an expected amount of time.

Figure 2a is a wound that became infected after open reduction internal fixation of a lateral tibial plateau fracture. The wound was irrigated and debrided. VAC therapy was utilised to assist with bacterial clearance and granulation tissue formation. Subsequent delayed primary closure was successful, as seen in Fig. 2b.

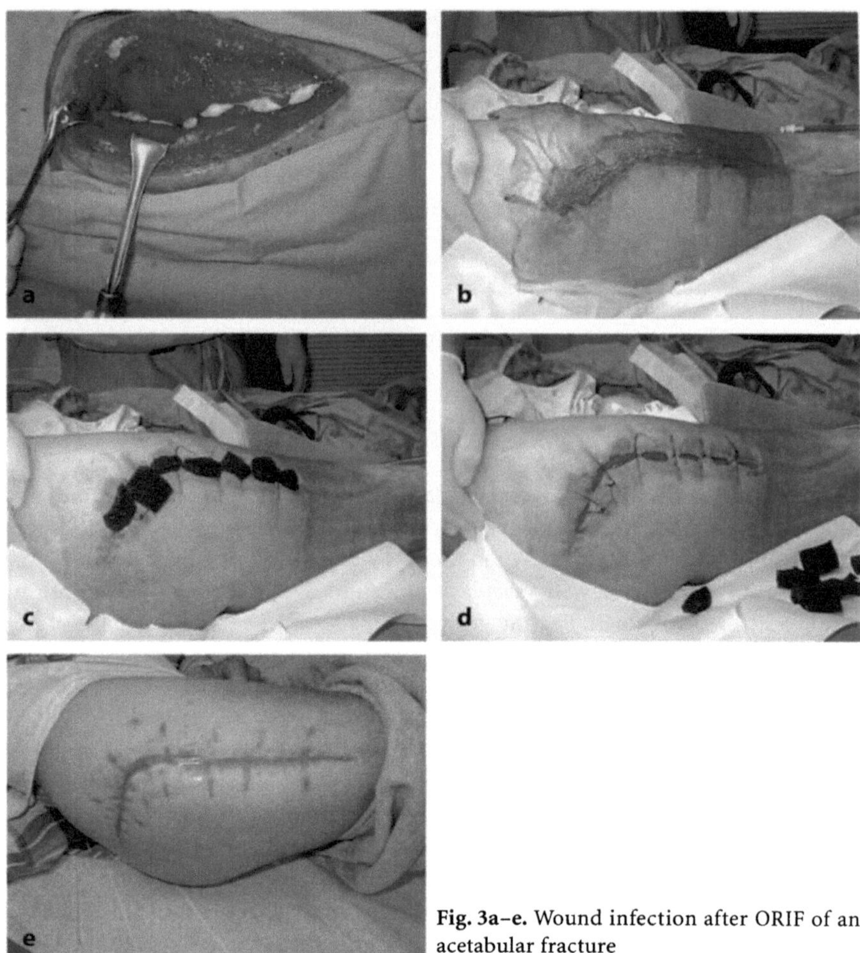

**Fig. 3a–e.** Wound infection after ORIF of an acetabular fracture

Figure 3 a–e represents a surgical wound infection after ORIF of an acetabular fracture. Initial management included irrigation and debridement. Antibiotic beads were temporarily placed in the wound. VAC therapy was used to promote granulation and assist in obtaining a delayed primary closure. Infection-free wound healing was obtained.

Benefits of closed-system VAC therapy in the treatment of infected wounds include the ability to inspect and characterise the effluent, a decrease in the number of dressing changes, and limited possibility of cross-contamination between wounds. The algorithm used in treating orthopaedic wound infections has changed over time. With the advent of antibiotics, specialised techniques such as the bead pouch and hyperbaric oxygen, and improved results with free-tissue transfer, fewer infected limbs require amputation. Thorough irrigation and debridement remain the critical steps to bring about a stable wound bed, free of devitalised tissue and contamination. VAC therapy has proven to be an effective adjunct in promoting granulation, improving vascularity and lowering bacterial counts at these compromised sites, making the ultimate treatment more effective.

### Open Fractures

Open fractures encompass a wide variety of injuries, from low-energy, inside-out skin lacerations to high-energy, limb-threatening injuries with significant bone and soft-tissue damage. Numerous classification systems have come about in an effort to categorise these injuries. Perhaps the most widely used is that of Gustilo and Anderson [22], which sorts open fractures based on the degree of soft-tissue injury and contamination.

Typically, the grade-I injury is caused by a low-energy mechanism, where the bone pierces the skin from inside outward, producing a skin laceration measuring less than 1 cm. These wounds are clean, with relatively little associated soft-tissue injury, and have relatively simple fracture patterns. Unless the fracture occurs in a highly contaminated environment, such as a barnyard, bacterial colonisation is low.

Type-II injuries are characterised by a wound measuring greater than 1 cm, with moderate soft-tissue damage. This is generally an outside-to-inside mechanism, with fairly simple fracture patterns, moderate comminution and little stripping of the soft tissues from bone.

Type-III injuries are divided into subtypes A, B and C. All have wounds resulting from an outside-to-inside mechanism. These injuries have more extensive muscle devitalisation and soft-tissue stripping from the bone. Grade-IIIA injuries are the least severe, where coverage of the bone is possible without free-tissue transfer or rotational flap coverage. Grade-IIIB injuries require soft-tissue reconstructive procedures, often in the form of a free-tissue transfer, while IIIC injuries require a vascular repair to effect survival of the distal portion of the limb.

VAC therapy does not alter the initial treatment of open fractures. Orthopaedic surgical principles of antibiotic and tetanus prophylaxis, early, thorough surgical debridement and acute stabilisation of open fractures, whether by internal or external fixation, still apply. Often, there is a need for multiple repeat debridements during the course of treatment. At issue is how to manage these wounds while the patient is awaiting further debridement or operative closure.

Many techniques have been applied, including simple packing of open fracture wounds, performing serial wet-to-dry dressing changes and, more recently, insertion of antibiotic-impregnated polymethylmethacrylate beads, the so-called bead-pouch procedure as described by Seligson [23]. The advantage of simple packing and dressing changes is their relative ease of application, availability of materials and familiarity for nursing staff. However, the wound remains unsealed and open, potentially leading to secondary contamination (especially in the ICU setting). The bead-pouch technique seals the wound while providing a high local concentration of antibiotic. While this technique appears promising, toxicity to osteoblasts and the generation of selective pressure toward antibiotic-resistant organisms is generated; further study is needed.

Surgeons who take care of high-energy open fractures have come to recognise the fact that even after a thorough initial debridement, in which all contamination and devitalised tissue has been removed, there is an extension of the initial zone of injury. Similar to thermal injuries, a zone of primary injury exists, with obviously necrotic tissue, surrounded by a zone of borderline tissue, which at the initial debridement appears viable, but over time may become necrotic. It is in this borderline zone, or zone of stasis, where the inflammatory cascade is present in response to the initial injury. This cascade evolves over the course of the following hours and days, releasing inflammatory mediators and oxygen-free radicals. Interstitial soft-tissue oedema ensues, with ultimate inclusion in the circulation to the tissue, thus leading to an extension of the initial primary zone of injury, manifested by more necrotic tissue present at repeat debridements.

We have used the VAC system in open fractures to limit this secondary necrosis. Utilising subatmospheric pressure, interstitial oedema is reduced in the zone of stasis and increased blood flow is thereby encouraged. There is often little necrotic tissue present at repeat debridements. The VAC offers a closed, negative pressure environment with little chance for contamination from nosocomial pathogens. Nursing requirements have proven to be few, and patients tolerate the procedure well.

Our current protocol calls for use of the Versajet®, a device based on the Bernoulli principle, to perform our initial debridement, with subsequent fracture stabilization [46]. In patients with functioning clotting parameters and no exposed neurovascular structures, the VAC sponge is applied to the open wound in the standard fashion. We use a setting of –125 mmHg. Grade-II and -III wounds are brought back to the operating room between 24 to 48 h for repeat irrigation and debridement. At this time, a determination is made regarding the possibility of primary closure versus alternative techniques. With the efficacy of VAC treatment in promoting healthy granulation tissue over limited areas of exposed bone and hardware, a longer duration of VAC therapy may be warranted, perhaps averting the need for free-tissue transfer.

### Acute Soft-Tissue Wounds

VAC treatment has found a role in acute soft-tissue wounds with exposed tendon, bone or joints. Regardless of the area, similar principles to the management of open fractures apply – adequate, thorough initial debridement, with removal of all contaminated and devitalised tissue is the goal. VAC therapy is subsequently initiated at a pressure of –125 mmHg, and continued for 24 to 48 h. Patients are then returned to the operating room for repeat irrigation and debridement. Soft-tissue coverage procedures may be appropriate at that time. Wounds showing a positive granulation response but determined not amenable to closure or coverage may have VAC therapy extended for an indeterminant amount of time. It is advised to provide a barrier between the sponge and nearby neurovascular structures, most commonly petrolatum-impregnated gauze. Healing by secondary intention is possible, with ultimate granulation and epithelialisation. Similarly to the mechanism proposed for open fracture management, VAC treatment may help limit extension of the primary zone of injury, maximising the preservation of host tissue.

In a prospective study evaluating the efficacy of VAC treatment for acute soft-tissue defects, 12 patients were followed until closure [20]. All wounds were located on the lower extremity, with a mean size of 12 cm². Standard irrigation and debridement were performed, as well as administration of intravenous antibiotics. Continuous VAC therapy was utilised for an average of 2 weeks (range 0 to 5). All patients healed uneventfully, with three closures via secondary intention and nine skin grafts. Patients underwent an average of six VAC changes (range 3–8), with a mean duration to healing of 16 days (range 10–27). No clinical signs of infection were evident at the time of definitive closure.

Degloving injuries to the hand and foot have been treated successfully with VAC therapy. In a small case series, DeFranzo et al. [25] reported on one severely degloved hand and one degloved foot. Both had greater than 95% take of the full-thickness injuries, with no complications. In a similar report by Josty et al. [26], greater than 95% take of full-thickness, defatted skin graft was seen in a degloving injury to the foot.

VAC therapy is a useful tool in the treatment of acute soft-tissue wounds. Excellent results can be expected, maximising the retention of host tissue, limiting infection, and aiding in viable soft-tissue coverage.

## Fasciotomy Wounds

Many orthopaedic patients require fasciotomy, most often after treatment of lower-extremity compartment syndrome. These wounds require serial dressing changes and debridement, with ultimate skin closure primarily or via split-thickness skin graft. There is often an extension of non-viable tissue found between the first and subsequent debridements, potentially compromising function of the limb. Significant oedema is common.

VAC therapy applied to these wounds minimises soft-tissue oedema and preserves the maximum amount of viable muscle. A retrospective analysis of simple saline dressings compared to VAC treatment demonstrated several advantages of the VAC technique. Earlier definitive closure/coverage was obtained in the VAC group, with the VAC group having a higher percentage of primary closure as opposed to skin grafting for wound coverage [27]. Application of subatmospheric pressure to fasciotomy wounds is now the standard of care at our institution.

Figure 4a–g represents a case of VAC therapy after crural fasciotomy for compartment syndrome. A two-incision technique was utilised. Primary closure of the lateral wound was obtained, and only a small skin graft was required on the medial sided wound.

## Chronic Wounds

Chronic, non-healing wounds prove to be a difficult challenge for both patients and treating physicians. Definitions may vary, but any wound that has been open for longer than 1 week and shows no progression towards healing can be considered chronic [1]. Examples include pressure ulcers, venous stasis ulcers, radiation ulcers, vasculitic and diabetic ulcers, as well as prolonged wound dehiscence.

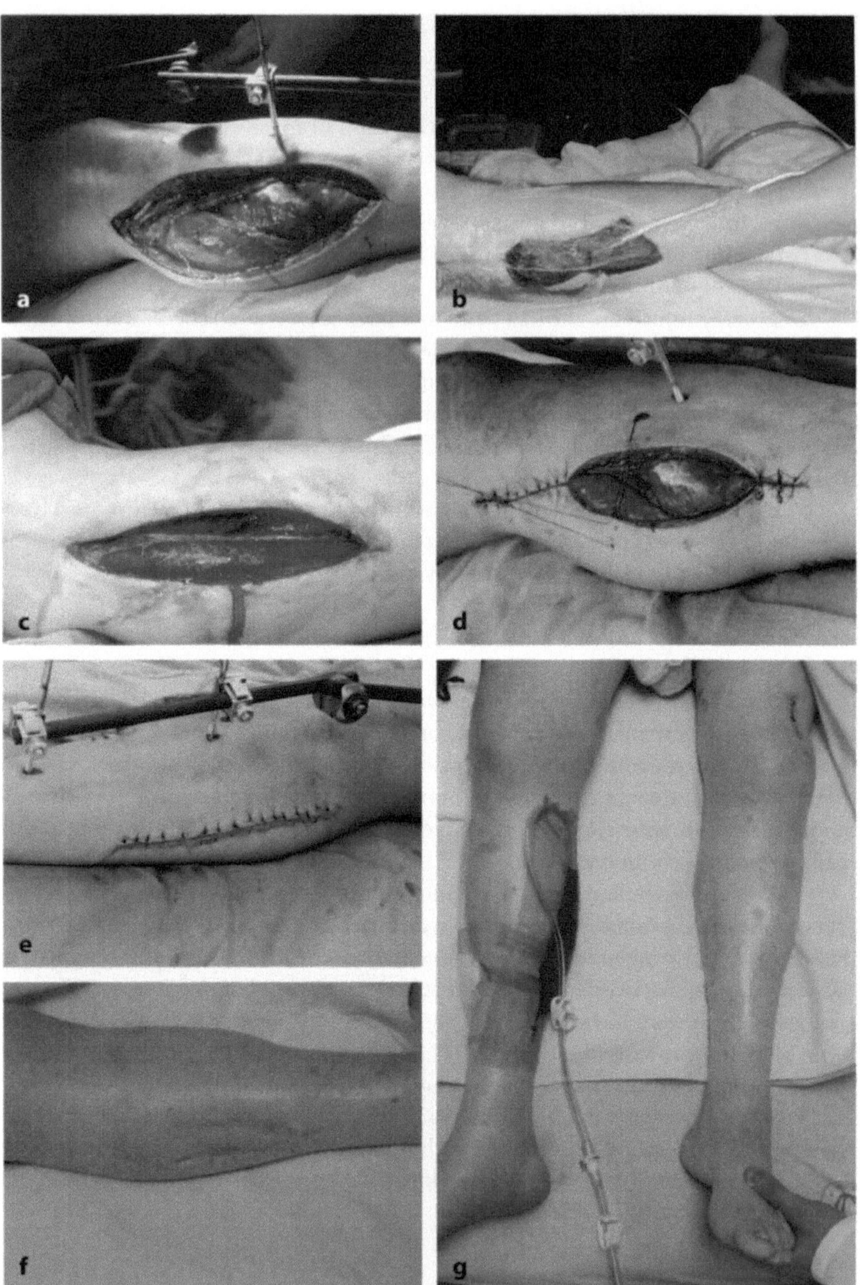

**Fig. 4a–g.** Case of VAC therapy after crural fasciotomy for compartment syndrome

Paramount to successful wound closure is adequate initial debridement of all non-viable tissue. Once haemostasis is obtained, the stage is set for application of VAC therapy. In an evaluation of 175 wounds treated, 171 responded favourably to subatmospheric pressure. In this series, continuous VAC therapy was applied for the first 48 h, followed by intermittent therapy (5 min on, 2 min off), with dressing changes taking place every 48 h. Simple debridement or hydrotherapy was performed at the time of dressing change. All wounds were treated to completion, with end points being delayed primary closure, skin grafting or local flap coverage. Large volumes of oedema fluid, up to 1000 ml, were removed during the initial application. Most notably, tissues that were indurated and firm became much more pliable over the course of treatment [1].

Diabetic foot wounds continue to burden the health-care system in terms of utilisation and morbidity for patients. Approximately 300 000 admissions are made for diabetic foot infections yearly in the United States, leading to 92 000 amputations in the diabetic population [28]. In a randomised prospective study evaluating the efficacy of VAC therapy versus conventional moist dressings in the treatment of large diabetic foot wounds, VAC dressings decreased wound volume and depth significantly more than moist gauze dressings (59 vs. 0% and 49 vs. 8%, respectively). VAC-treated wounds had a decrease in all dimensions, while wound width and length increased with moist gauze dressings [29]. In a similar study, McCallon et al. [30] randomised ten patients to receive either negative pressure wound therapy or saline-gauze dressing. They observed complete healing with VAC therapy occurred more rapidly (22 vs. 42 days), and wound dimensions decreased more rapidly in the VAC group.

From its initial use to more recent studies, VAC therapy has proven to be safe and effective in treating chronic wounds. Patients benefit from more rapid wound healing, preservation of host tissue and ultimately quicker return to function.

## Difficult-to-Close Surgical Wounds

Orthopaedic wounds in which primary closure is desired but not possible may be successfully treated with VAC therapy and delayed primary closure. This includes some fasciotomy wounds in the upper and lower extremities, surgical incisions made in areas of swollen soft tissues, as well as others. In situations where primary suturing leads to strangulation and necrosis of the skin, a loose closure is made with the VAC sponge filling the dead space of the wound. Subatmospheric pressure of 125 mmHg is applied, promoting the removal of oedema and the re-establishment of tissue elasticity with re-approximation of wound edges. After a period of 24 to 48 h, the wound is re-assessed for suitability of a primary closure. If only a tight closure is possible, VAC therapy is continued with either a gradual closure by "dynamic" wound-edge reapproximation or skin grafting at the next operative procedure.

## High-Energy Soft-Tissue Wounds

Herscovici et al. [31] evaluated the efficacy of VAC therapy in the management of high-energy soft-tissue injuries. Twenty-one patients requiring soft-tissue procedures beyond split-thickness skin grafting were treated using the VAC device. The primary indication for treatment was an attempt to avoid local or free-tissue transfer. Wounds averaged 4.1 sponge changes (range 2–16), with 77% performed at bedside. Duration of treatment averaged 19.3 days (range 5–84). Twelve wounds (57%) avoided the need for further treatment. Five additional wounds required split-thickness skin grafting only; free tissue transfer was necessary in nine wounds (43%). Only two soft-tissue complications were encountered, neither related to the use of the VAC. Average cost of treatment was calculated at $ 100.– per day, similar to wet-to-dry gauze dressing changes ($ 100.– per day). The average surgical fee for free-tissue transfer cited in their study was $ 6000.–.

The patient in Fig. 5a–i sustained a close-range, high-energy shotgun wound to the left arm. Significant bone and soft-tissue damage resulted. Serial irrigation and debridements were performed, with VAC therapy between surgeries. The wound was infection-free with exuberant granulation tissue, allowing an allograft reconstruction, flap coverage and skin grafting to be performed. Uneventful healing ensued with a stable soft tissue envelope.

### Irritated External Fixation Pins

External fixators are often used to treat fractures of the pelvis and extremities in polytraumatised patients. While this method of treatment continues to evolve and gain popularity, pin-track irritation and infection remain problematic. Prolonged drainage, erythema and pain may arise in areas of exuberant tissue (obesity) and excess motion, potentially limiting the duration for which an external fixator can be left in place. Although some authors with extensive experience using this method of treatment approach the irritated pin as merely an "obstacle" [43], others view it as more troublesome and remove the external fixator pin at the first sign of trouble.

We have adopted a method of treating external fixation pin sites that includes VAC therapy. In areas of potential irritation (pelvis, thigh, proximal tibia, humerus, others), pins are inserted in the standard fashion. Tension-free closure is performed on incisions used for insertion. A VAC sponge is then fashioned to fit around the pin, with adjacent pins connected by a bridging sponge. The intervening skin can be bridged with Adaptec (Johnson and Johnson, Arlington, TX). A sterile hydrocolloid gel helps provide a secure seal when applied circumferentially around the pin, about 1 inch above the skin. The area is sealed, and negative pressure applied at a setting of –50 to –75 mmHg. This dressing can be left in place for as long as necessary, with less frequent changing (once a week), due to the low pressure and minimal likelihood of native skin irritation. With time, VAC therapy may be discontinued once the pin site is clean and dry.

In areas where irritation and superficial cellulites are evident, appropriate local wound care with debridement of excess scab is performed, proper oral antibiotics are begun and VAC therapy as described above is initiated. Pin sites are re-evaluated in 48 to 72 h, with therapy continued until pin sites are dry and infection-free. This technique is not used in grossly infected, loose pins, which should be removed.

### Surgical Wounds Prone to Weep

Numerous orthopaedic surgical wounds have a tendency to weep. Patients with significant oedema, obesity and protein malnutrition are at risk for incisional drainage. These wounds often exhibit a delayed healing response, and are at risk for development of nosocomial infection. An estimated 10% of patients undergoing elective hip

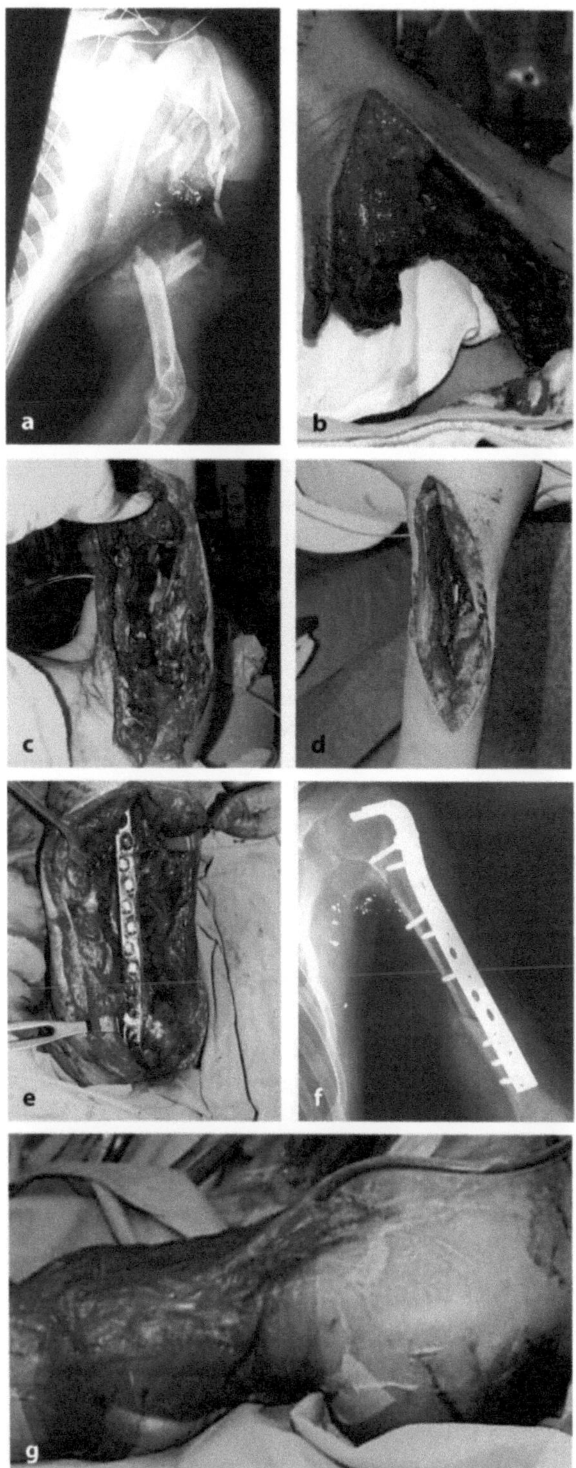

**Fig. 5a–g.** High-energy shot-gun wound. (See text)

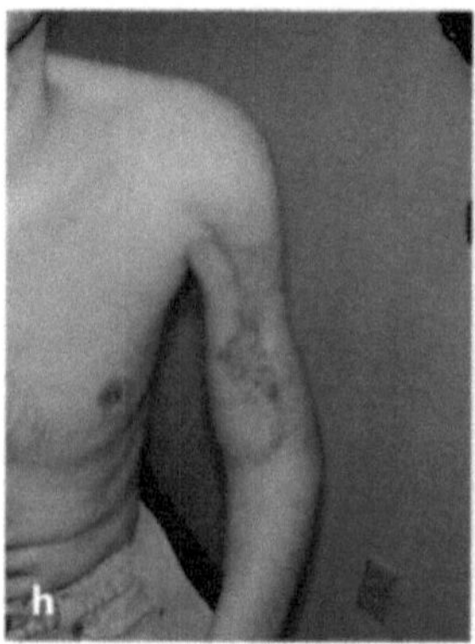
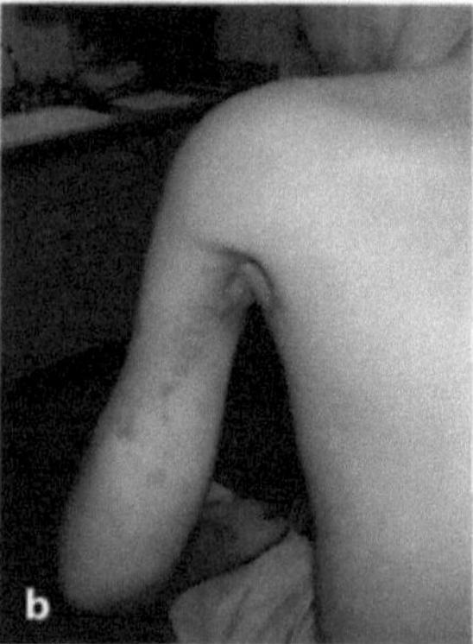

Fig. 5h,i. High-energy shot-gun wound. (See text)

and knee surgery have wound drainage to the extent that requires continued surgical dressing beyond the second post-operative day. These wounds have been shown to heal better when the seroma is drained [32]. Successful outcome is deemed the transition to a clean, dry wound free of infection.

In our experience with 56 such wounds, 54 were transitioned to clean, dry wounds that underwent uneventful healing with just one 24-h application. The remaining two wounds required two or more applications. This has prompted the routine use of low-pressure VAC treatment (–50 to –75 mmHg) to wounds with a tendency to weep, or wounds in need of isolation (anticipated prolonged ICU stay). Often, a protective layer of Adaptec (Johnson and Johnson, Arlington, TX), is applied between the closed wound and sponge. We have not experienced any deleterious outcomes utilising this technique, and have adopted it as a routine dressing in ilio-inguinal and Kocher–Langenbeck approaches to the acetabulum, as well as in most patients returning to the ICU after extensive surgery.

### Treatment of Morel-Lavallee Lesions

In the middle of the 19th century, Morel-Lavallee described a closed degloving injury [33]; Letournel and Judet later referred to degloving injuries over the region of the greater trochanter as a Morel-Lavallee lesion [34]. These injuries are the result of a shearing mechanism in which the skin and subcutaneous tissue separates from the underlying fascia, creating a cavity that is filled with haematoma and a mixture of viable and non-viable fat [35]. Presence of a soft, contused, fluctuant area is the hallmark physical exam finding. In a review of 16 cases, Hudson et al. [35] reported that diagnosis was initially missed in one-third of the cases. Necrosis of the overlying skin may occur as a result of the direct trauma and ischemia that develops secondary to swelling [35, 36].

Routt et al. [37] emphasised that flap survival may be jeopardised by operating through these areas. They also cautioned against the use of external fixation pins in these areas due to the risk of contamination. Helfet and Schmelling [38] advocated the evacuation of these lesions prior to extensile or posterior approaches for acetabular fractures. Other methods have included aspiration, injection of sclerosing agents such as tetracycline, deep fascial fenestration, compression dressings and prolonged surgical drainage [35, 36, 39–41].

In a review of 24 patients sustaining closed internal degloving injuries, Hak et al. [42] reported a 46% incidence of positive wound cultures at the time of initial debridement. All wounds except one were treated with debridement and gauze dressing changes. Fifteen patients healed by secondary intention, while five had a delayed primary closure; one patient required a posterior thigh flap. Three patients subsequently developed a deep bone infection, owing to the troublesome nature of these lesions.

We have utilised VAC treatment as a way of dealing with these wounds. Our current protocol is similar to that described by Hak et al. [42]; surgical debridement is performed first, with fracture stabilisation as necessary. Bony coverage is obtained by closure of viable deep fascia. However, instead of transitioning to gauze dressing changes, a VAC sponge is placed in the open wound with contiguous radiating 1-inch-wide "arms", arranged like the spokes of a wheel, in the zone of degloving at a pressure of –125 mmHg. The wound is revisited every 48 h for assessment of flap viability, need for debridement and VAC dressing change. When the healing response is deemed adequate, the sponge spokes are progressively shortened to promote full wound granulation, and closure is performed via primary or secondary intention as necessary.

In a preliminary review of this technique, we have had no deep or superficial infections, and all wounds have healed without flap coverage.

## Results

Perhaps the most important point in discussing results of VAC therapy is the emphasis on adequate surgical debridement accompanying the initiating therapy. This method of treatment does not remove infected, necrotic, devitalised tissue, but rather serves to thwart the development of (for lack of better terminology) the secondary soft-tissue compartment syndrome or impairment of the microcirculation in the zone of stasis due to heightened capillary afterload. In addition to this, and as shown in the previously presented cases, the institution of VAC treatment has been successful in accelerating wound healing and promoting wound granulation. In a number of cases, VAC therapy has either circumvented the need for or enhanced the success of flap coverage of a wound [20]. These early results are very encouraging, and inspire longer follow-up and new applications in orthopaedic wound management.

## Complications

There have been few complications reported with use of the VAC technique. The most common is a rash on the skin resulting from direct contact with the sponge; this generally resolves within 24 h without specific intervention. In a series of 270 patients, 2.2% developed a rash, with resolution within 48 hours in all cases [16]. The rash was not associated with itching or pain. Care should be taken to confine the sponge to the wound and avoid overlap onto normal skin. If this is not possible, a setting of –50 mmHg can be used, with a layer of Adaptec (Johnson and Johnson, Arlington, TX) between the sponge and skin.

If the sponge is left deep in a wound for more than 48 h, it can be difficult to extract due to the overgrowth of exuberant granulation tissue. Once the sponge is removed, minor bleeding may occur; this can easily be controlled with direct pressure. In a case report soon to be published (White et al.: Vacuum assisted closure complicated by erosion and haemorrhage of anterior tibial artery – a case report. Journal of Trauma), bleeding secondary to arterial "erosion" during VAC therapy is reported. This emphasises the need to take special precautions, such as a protective layer between the sponge and vessels, when applying negative-pressure therapy in these areas.

## Contra-Indications

Few contra-indications exist; first and foremost, VAC technique should not be used on wounds that are grossly infected or inadequately debrided with eschar present. If a patient has thin skin (elderly patients, long-term steroid use), shearing avulsion may occur during sponge exchange as the adherent drape is lifted from the skin. VAC technique is therefore not recommended in patients who are mechanically intolerant to the procedure, as well as in those with an allergy to the adhesives or the polyurethane sponge used in the technique.

Caution must be exercised when using subatmospheric pressure on wounds in anti-coagulated and bleeding patients; while this is not an absolute contra-indication, close observation is required. When applying the sponge near blood vessels and nerves, a protective layer of overlying fascia, tissue or Adaptec (Johnson and Johnson, Arlington, TX) should be placed. Pressures may be reduced to –50 mmHg as well, and careful monitoring is required.

The effects of VAC therapy on neoplasm are unknown; if malignancy is present in the wound, the VAC should not be used. In cases of osteomyelitis, definitive treatment with VAC is not indicated. However, after appropriate surgical debridement and antibiotic treatment, VAC therapy may be beneficial is reducing oedema and promoting healing of sinus tracts.

## Discussion

As discussed earlier in the chapter, wounds heal by progressing through phases. After the injuring mechanism, an inflammatory response is initiated, triggering numerous vascular, cellular and humoral events. There is an outpouring of tissue fluid, with associated swelling and vascular compromise. Over time, this phase gives way to a reparative phase, with concordant angiogenesis, granulation, collagen production and re-epithelialisation.

Critical in understanding the efficacy of VAC treatment is the concept of soft-tissue compartment syndrome. We propose this entity exists as a sequel to any major wound in the zone of stasis. This is the volume of tissue which immediately surrounds the area of direct wound trauma and is characterised by the outpouring of oedema due to the release of vasoactive mediators involved in the inflammatory cascade. Theoretically, the oedema accumulates in the extra-vascular space and causes a reduction of venular volume and a heightening of capillary afterload. This, in turn, causes an impairment of microcirculation and a decreased exchange of $O_2$, glucose, $CO_2$ and waste products. This is the basis for further necrosis of tissue in the zone of stasis and the cascading necrosis of tissue evident to the surgeon at the time of a 48-h second-look debridement procedure. The use of a VAC during this period acts to clear the oedema, thereby minimising the venular embarrassment and microcirculatory impairment. For want of a better analogy, therefore, the VAC acts as the microcirculatory fasciotomy for the microcirculatory compartment syndrome which develops in the zone of stasis.

It has been shown that bacterial colonisation hampers wound healing [13–15]; the effect of lowering wound bacterial counts [10] may give VAC therapy an advantage over other methods in the treatment of contaminated wounds or those with a history of infection. The mechanism for this may reside in the avoidance of micro-tissue necrosis as it otherwise eventuates in a microcompartment syndrome. Theoretically, the level of tissue necrosis is minimised if negative pressure is utilised early, for the reasons that were just discussed.

VAC appears to have some distinct advantages over traditional wound closure methods. A closed system is created, limiting the chance of contamination (particularly in the hospital setting where resistant organisms predominate). Wound fluid is evacuated, bacterial counts are lowered and granulation tissue is formed. Cost analysis in the outpatient setting has shown an advantage with VAC therapy over conventional management with dressing changes [44]. Wound fluid is collected on a continuous basis during therapy, providing a valuable research tool. While the clinical benefits of VAC treatment need to be further scrutinised with well-controlled prospective studies, early results have proven its usefulness as an adjunct to wound healing.

## References


1. Argenta LC, Morykwas MJ (1997) Vacuum-assisted closure: a new method for wound control and treatment: clinical experience. Ann Plast Surg 38: 563–576
2. Fleischmann W, Lang E, Russ M (1997) Treatment of infection by vacuum sealing. Unfallchirurg 100: 301–304
3. Fleischmann W, Strecker W, Bombelli M, Kinzl L (1993) Vacuum sealing as treatment of soft tissue damage in open fractures [German]. Unfallchirurg 96: 488–492
4. Baynham SA, Kohlman P, Katner HP (1999) Treating stage IV pressure ulcers with negative pressure therapy: a case report. Ostomy Wound Manage 45: 28–35
5. Grinnell F, Ho CH, Wysocki A (1992) Degeneration of fibronectin and vitreonectin in chronic wound fluid. Analysis by cell blotting, immunoblotting, and cell adhesion assays. J Invest Dermatol 98: 410–416
6. Bucalo B, Eaglstein WH, Falanga V (1993) Inhibition of cell proliferation by chronic wound fluid. Wound Rep Regen 1: 181–186
7. Falanga V (1992) Growth factor and chronic wounds: the need to understand the microenvironment. J Dermatol 19: 667–672
8. Wysocki AB, Grinnell F (1993) Fibronectin profiles in normal and chronic wound fluid. Lab Invest 63: 825–831
9. Wysocki AB, Staiano-Coico L, Grinnell F (1993) Wound fluid from chronic leg ulcers contains elevated levels of metalloproteinases MMP-2 and MMP-9. J Invest Dermatol 101: 64–68
10. Morykwas MJ, Argenta LC, Shelton-Brown EI, McGuirt W (1997) Vacuum-assisted closure: a new method for wound control and treatment: animal studies and basic foundation. Ann Plast Surg 38: 553–562
11. Morykwas MJ, David LR, Schneider AM, Whang C, Jennings DA, Canty C, Parker D, White WL, Argenta LC (1999) Use of subatmospheric pressure to prevent progression of partial-thickness burns in a swine model. J Burn Care Rehabil 20: 15–21
12. Morykwas MJ, Kennedy A, Argenta JP, Argenta LC (1999) Use of subatmospheric pressure to prevent doxorubicin extravasation ulcers in a swine model. J Surg Oncol 72: 14–17
13. Hunt TK (1988) The physiology of wound healing. Ann Emerg Med 17: 1265–1273
14. Seiler WO, Stahelin HB, Sonnabend W (1979) Effect of aerobic and anaerobic germs on the healing of decubitus ulcers [German]. Schweiz Med Wochenschr 109: 1594–1599
15. Daltrey DC, Rhodes B, Chattwood JG (1981) Investigation into the microbial flora of healing and non-healing decubitus ulcers. J Clin Pathol 34: 701–705
16. Webb LX, Schmidt U (2001) Wound management with vacuum therapy [German]. Unfallchirurg 104: 918–926
17. Schneider AM, Morykwas MJ, Argenta LC (1998) A new and reliable method of securing skin grafts to the difficult recipient bed. Plast Reconstr Surg 102: 1195–1198
18. Blackburn JH 2nd, Boemi L, Hall WW, Jeffords K, Hauck RM, Banducci DR, Graham WP 3rd (1998) Negative-pressure dressings as a bolster for skin grafts. Ann Plast Surg 40: 453–457
19. Sposato G, Molea G, Di Caprio G, Scioli M, La Rusca I, Ziccardi P (2001) Ambulant vacuum-assisted closure of skin-graft dressing in the lower limbs using a portable mini-VAC device. Br J Plast Surg 54: 235–237
20. DeFranzo AJ, Argenta LC, Marks MW, Molnar JA, David LR, Webb LX, Ward WG, Teasdall RG (2001) The use of vacuum-assisted closure therapy for the treatment of lower-extremity wounds with exposed bone. Plast Reconstr Surg 108: 1184–1191
21. Mullner T, Mrkonjic L, Kwasny O, Vecsei V (1997) The use of negative pressure to promote the healing of tissue defects: a clinical trial using the vacuum sealing technique. Br J Plast Surg 50: 194–199
22. Gustilo RB, Anderson JT (1976) Prevention of infection in the treatment of one thousand and twenty-five open fractures of long bones: retrospective and prospective analyses. J Bone Joint Surg Am 58: 453–458
23. Seligson D (1984) Antibiotic-impregnated beads in orthopedic infectious problems. J Ky Med Assoc 82: 25–29
25. DeFranzo AJ, Marks MW, Argenta LC, Genecov DG (1999) Vacuum-assisted closure for the treatment of degloving injuries. Plast Reconstr Surg 104: 2145–2148
26. Josty IC, Ramaswamy R, Laing JH (2001) Vacuum assisted closure: an alternative strategy in the management of degloving injuries of the foot. Br J Plast Surg 54: 363–365

27. Chang D, Castle J, Webb LX (2001) Abstract: Vacuum assisted closure for fasciotomy wounds after compartment syndrome of the leg. Orthopaedic Trauma Association Final Program, 17th Annual Meeting. Orthopaedic Trauma Association, Rosemont, IL, p 57

28. Bloomgarden ZT (2001) American diabetes association 60th scientific sessions, 2000: the diabetic foot. Diabetes Care 24: 946–951

29. Eginton MT, Brown KR, Seabrook GR, Towne JB, Cambria RA (2003) A prospective randomized evaluation of negative-pressure wound dressings for diabetic foot wounds. Ann Vasc Surg 17: 645-649

30. McCallon SK, Knoght CA, Valiulus JP (2000) Vacuum-assisted closure versus saline-moistened gauze in the healing of postoperative diabetic foot wounds. Ostomy Wound Management 46: 28–34

31. Herscovici D Jr, Sanders RW, Scaduto JM, Infante A, DiPasquale T (2003) Vacuum-assisted wound closure (VAC therapy) for the management of patients with high-energy soft tissue injuries. J Orthop Trauma 17: 683–688

32. Varley GW, Milner SA (1995) Wound drains in proximal femoral fracture surgery: a randomized prospective trial of 177 patients. J R Coll Surg Edinb 40: 416–418

33. Morel-Lavallee VAF (1863) Decollements traumatiques de la peau et des couches sous-jacentes. Arch Gen Med 1: 20–38, 172–200, 300–332

34. Letournel E, Judet R (1993) Fractures of the Acetabulum, 2nd edn. Springer, Berlin Heidelberg New York Tokyo

35. Hudson DA, Knottenbelt JD, Krige JEJ (1992) Closed degloving injuries: results following conservative surgery. Plast Reconstr Surg 89: 853–855

36. Kottmeier SA, Wilson SC, Born CT, Hanks GA, Innacone WM, DeLong WG (1996) Surgical management of soft tissue lesions associated with pelvic ring injury. Clin Ortho Relat Res 359: 446–453

37. Routt MCL Jr, Simonian PT, Ballmer F (1995) A rational approach to pelvic trauma: resuscitation and early definitive stabilization. Clin Orthop 318: 61–74

38. Helfet DL, Schmeling GJ (1995) Complications. In: Title M (ed) Fractures of the pelvis and acetabulum, 2nd edn. Williams and Wilkins, Baltimore, pp 451–467

39. Letts RM (1986) Degloving injuries in children. J Pediatr Orthop 6: 93–97

40. Kudsk KA, Sheldon GF, Walton RL (1981) Degloving injuries of the extremities and torso. J Trauma 21: 835–839

41. Matta J (1992) Surgical treatment of acetabular fractures. In: Browner BD, Jupiter JB, Levine AM, Trafton PG (eds) Skeletal trauma. WB Saunders, Philadelphia, PA, pp 899–922

42. Hak DJ, Olson SA, Matta JM (1997) Diagnosis and management of closed internal degloving injuries associated with pelvic and acetabular fractures: the Morel-Lavallee lesion. J Trauma 42: 1046–1051

43. Paley D (1990) Problems, obstacles, and complications of limb lengthening by the Ilizarov technique. Clin Orthop (250): 81–104. Review

44. Philbeck TE Jr, Whittington KT, Millsap MH, Briones RB, Wight DG, Schroeder WJ (1999) The clinical and cost effectiveness of externally applied negative pressure wound therapy in the treatment of wounds in home healthcare Medicare patients. Ostomy Wound Manage 45: 41–50

45. Ilizarov GA, Lediaev VI, Shitin VP (1969) The course of compact bone reparative regeneration in distraction osteosynthesis under different conditions of bone fragment fixation (experimental study) [Russian]. Eksp Khir Anesteziol 14: 3–12

46. Webb LX (2004) Management of High Energy Soft-Tissue Trauma in Orthopaedics. ICL 104, March 10, 2004, AAOS San Francisco, CA

R.E. HORCH

## Introduction

Osteomyelitis is an acute or chronic inflammatory process of the bone and its structures secondary to infection with pyogenic organisms. The term osteomyelitis has become more or less restricted to the haematogenous type and has lately been replaced by the term osteitis, because not only the osteomyelon is affected but always all elements of the bone are involved. It is a very expensive disease for patient and society because of the involved costs of diagnosis, inpatient and outpatient treatment, rehabilitation, lost productivity and sequelae [1]. Bone and joint infections are difficult to cure [2]. This difficulty is related to the presence of bacteria adherent to dead bone and foreign material in many cases and also to drug resistance and limited distribution of antibiotics into infected bone.

## Pathophysiology of Osteomyelitis and Associated Factors

Infections associated with osteomyelitis arise either from direct inoculation, extension from a contiguous site (exogenous form) during trauma or surgery, or haematogenous spread (endogenous form) caused by the seeding of bacteria within the bone from a remote source. Children's rapidly growing and well-vascularised metaphysis of the growing bones are primarily afflicted by this condition with a prevalence of 1 per 5000 children in the US per year.

Prior to the availability of antibiotics, mortality from haematogenous osteoarticular infection approached 20% and morbidity 45–50% but decreased considerably in developed countries after the introduction of surgical drainage and antibiotic therapy after 1944 [2]. Severe illness due to sepsis from osteomyelitis has become more seldom, while the number of patients presenting with a mild or subacute form has increased.

Clinical manifestations of direct inoculation osteomyelitis are more localised than those of haematogenous osteomyelitis and tend to involve multiple organisms. Direct osteomyelitis generally is more localised, with prominent signs and symptoms. Although a variety of numerous different bacteria can infect the wounds, the most common bacteria are *Staphylococcus aureus*, *Staphylococcus epidermidis* and *Pseudomonas aeruginosa*.

Osteomyelitis may be localised or may spread through the periosteum, cortex, marrow and cancellous tissue. Based on the age of the patient and the mechanism of the infection, the bacterial pathogen may vary. The number of bacteriae, their resistance and virulence, as well as the general immunocompetence of the patient and the local tissue milieu, are responsible for the clinical manifestation. Compromised patients have decreased healing potential when compared to uncompromised patients. Compromised healing conditions include major associated diseases or conditions such as diabetes mellitus, malignancy, chronic alcoholism, use of steroids, drug addiction, poor nutrition, extensive scarring or nicotine abuse. Diabetic patients are concerned with osteomyelitic foot complications when a peripheral neuropathy is present.

Application of implants enhances the infect susceptibility of bones. Osteomyelitis secondary to peripheral vascular disease is a special entity. Although often listed as an aetiology, peripheral vascular disease is actually rather a predisposing factor than a true cause of infection.

By definition, any bone infection lasting for more than 6 weeks is termed a chronic osteomyelitis. Chronic osteomyelitis persists or recurs, regardless of its initial cause and/or mechanism and despite aggressive intervention.

## Clinical Features

Haematogenous long-bone osteomyelitis is rare and characterised by the typical signs of fatigue after an abrupt onset of high fever with malaise, restriction of movement and local signs like erythema, oedema and tenderness/swelling of the surrounding tissues.

Post-traumatic osteitis can be distinguished into an acute early onset type starting immediately or within a few days after the trauma.

On the other hand, a chronic osteomyelitis is classically characterised by a non-healing ulcer, chronic fatigue, malaise, and sinus tract drainage. The incidence of post-traumatic osteitis after open fractures ranges generally between 5 and 10% and may reach up to 30% in open fractures of the distal lower leg.

One of the most common classification systems is the Cierny-Mader classification, which is based on the anatomy of the bone infection and the physiology of the host [3]. The Cierny-Mader staging allows stratification of long-bone osteomyelitis and the development of comprehensive treatment guidelines for each stage. In long-standing osteomyelitis wounds a carcinoma has to be ruled out by histology, especially when after a clinically quiet period of many years the fistula relapses.

## Diagnosis

### Laboratory Findings

In acute haematogenous osteomyelitis a typical leftward shift with increased polymorphonuclear leukocyte counts in the WBC (white blood cell count) is seen, whereas in chronic osteomyelitis the WBC count may be elevated but is frequently normal. The C-reactive protein level is usually elevated and non-specific; it may be more useful than the erythrocyte sedimentation rate. The erythrocyte sedimentation rate is usually elevated (90%); this finding is clinically non-specific [5].

With osteomyelitis, culture or aspiration findings in samples of the infected site in osteomyelitis are normal in 25% of cases. Blood-culture results are positive in only 50% of patients with haematogenous osteomyelitis.

### Imaging

Virtually all radiological imaging techniques from conventional radiographs to MRI or CT scans can contribute to identify osteomyelitis, depending on the individual case and stage of disease.

**X-ray** evidence of acute osteomyelitis first is suggested by overlying soft-tissue oedema at some 3–5 days after infection; however, bony changes are not evident for 14–21 days. They initially manifest as periosteal elevation followed by cortical or medullary lucencies. Approximately 40–50% focal bone loss is necessary to cause detectable lucency on plain films. X-ray investigations have a poor specifity but are comparably inexpensive, easily available and therefore the first imaging method of choice.

The **MRI** is excellent in the early detection and surgical localisation of osteomyelitis. Studies have shown its superiority compared with plain radiography, CT scan and radionuclide scanning in selected anatomic locations. The sensitivity ranges from 90–100%. However, it is expensive.

A three-phase **radionuclide bone scan** with technetium 99 m is probably the initial imaging modality of choice, but offers a poor specifity with falsely negative results in infection, false-positive findings in infarction and tumour. It may well be performed in the first week. In special circumstances, additional information can be obtained from further scanning with leukocytes labelled with gallium 67 and/or indium 111.

**CT scans** have a good specifity in the first 2 weeks and can depict abnormal calcification, ossification and intracortical abnormalities. They are probably most useful in the evaluation of spinal vertebral lesions. These images, when used alone or in combination for timed sequential images, can be highly sensitive, specific and accurate [6]. They can be useful in surgical planning.

## Therapy

The management of osteomyelitis is based on an understanding of the disease process and the underlying bone pathology. In the acute condition, it is important to prevent progression to a chronic form, to prevent exacerbation of the infection, to restore normal anatomy and function and to minimise complications such as joint destruction, bony deformity and overgrowth, and amyloidosis or limb loss due to sepsis. Treatment should be initiated the moment osteomyelitis is suspected [2].

Hence, haematogenous osteomyelitis is intravenously treated with high doses of appropriate antibiotics according to the microbial strains. In early stages, high dose antibiotics together with abscess drainage may lead to definitive cure; but as soon as necrosis or extended empyema is present, surgical debridement is indicated.

One of the major achievements in treating patients at high risk for osteomyelitis is the early defect coverage of open comminuted fractures within the first 5 to 7 days after the injury [15]. If the viability of the injured zone is questionable, repeated surgicalk debridements and temporary coverage with a vacuum device have been shown to be efficient tools until a definitive coverage can be performed. This helps to prevent post-traumatic osteitis.

**Radical aggressive surgical procedures** and antibiotics are the mainstays of treatment. Since no wound can properly heal unless it is clean, healthy and free of infection, a thorough surgical debridement is of paramount importance in achieving this goal. It is the quickest and most efficient way of getting the wound ready for healing. The ultimate goal is to excise all unhealthy and non-viable tissue until the wound edges and base consist of only normal and healthy tissue. Necrotic bone forms a nidus for persistent infection and is therefore debrided until there is punctuate bleeding from the Haversian canals that indicate bone viability [4]. Once the surgical debridement is completed, the principles of treatment include dead-space management, soft-tissue coverage, minimally invasive bone stabilisation if needed and delayed bone grafting if necessary.

Special problems such as the presence of **hardware** must be handled appropriately. It is sometimes difficult to determine if hardware has to be removed. Microorganisms exist in the glycocalix, which is a biofilm or slime that adheres to metal, dead bone and tissue, and protects bacteria from antibiotics and host defence mechanisms. It is speculated that bacterial drug resistance increases in parallel with the increased biofilm formation. Therefore, in our experience removal of all metallic implants is suggested whenever possible. Only in selected cases if no alternative stabilisation of the bone after debridement can be achieved, may internal exposed hardware be left in place while infection is controlled with antimicrobials and the fracture heals. Adequate debridement frequently leads to inadequate fixation or bone defects. These problems can be addressed with sophisticated techniques such as external fixation devices, Ilizarov frames and bone transport. Infected pseudarthrosis with segmental osseous defects may also be treated by debridement and microvascular bone transfers. Vascular bone transfers in the case of bone defects more than 3 cm in length can be placed after 1 month of inactive sepsis.

Since soft-tissue problems frequently occur in cases of osteomyelitis as a result of previous surgeries, radiation injury or trauma, an interdisciplinary approach of orthopaedic or trauma surgeons together with plastic surgeons and, if necessary, vascular surgeons or interventional radiologists is the key to achieve stable wound coverage and healing.

A **two-staged procedure** with radical debridement, implantation of antibiotic beads or a variety of resorbable antibiotic carriers until sufficient eradication of the microbial load is established and wound-bed preparation has been sufficiently achieved, is followed by soft-tissue coverage and later by cancellous bone grafting if necessary. The continuous **vacuum sealing** of such wounds (continuous vacuum-

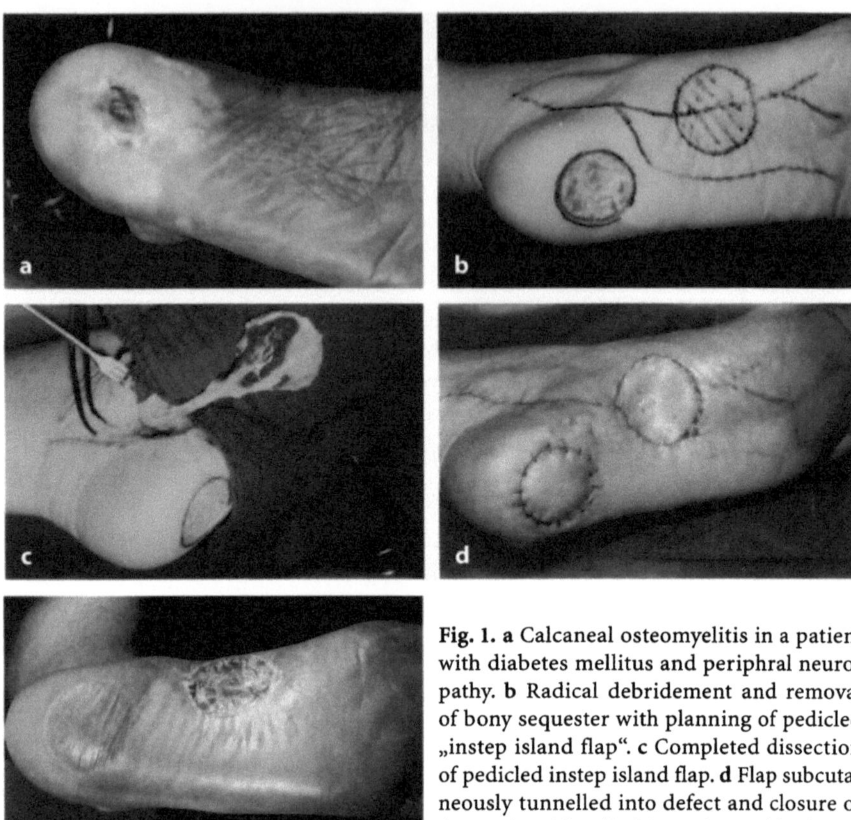

**Fig. 1. a** Calcaneal osteomyelitis in a patient with diabetes mellitus and periphral neuropathy. **b** Radical debridement and removal of bony sequester with planning of pedicled „instep island flap". **c** Completed dissection of pedicled instep island flap. **d** Flap subcutaneously tunnelled into defect and closure of donor site with split skin graft. **e** Stable closure in weight-bearing heel zone

assisted closure systems, VAC) has been shown to be a very efficient means to eliminate exudation and haematoma after radical surgical debridement, to induce neovascularisation, and to prepare the recipient site for flap transfer [13, 16].

The choice of appropriate defect coverage after the debridement adheres to the principles of a so-called reconstructive ladder. This means that surgeons must determine the ideal method for each scenario and try to keep the donor-site morbidity as minimal as possible, at the same time achieving satisfactory wound closure and restoring functional integrity in the least time and with the least resultant morbidity. In the schema of a reconstructive ladder each procedure is generally more complex and requires more expertise. Methods to consider are skin grafts, random (local) pattern flaps, axial pattern flaps and **microvascular free flaps.** The latter may range from free transplants consisting of one tissue up to composite flaps with skin, muscle, bone, fascia and tendons. Another step within this escalation of complexity is the advent of specially designed prefabricated flaps to meet all the requirements needed in the recipient area [13]. Presently, this involves the transfer of tissue from one part of the body to reconstruct another with the goal of over-all improvement. Disadvantages lie in the long operating time and the considerable expertise

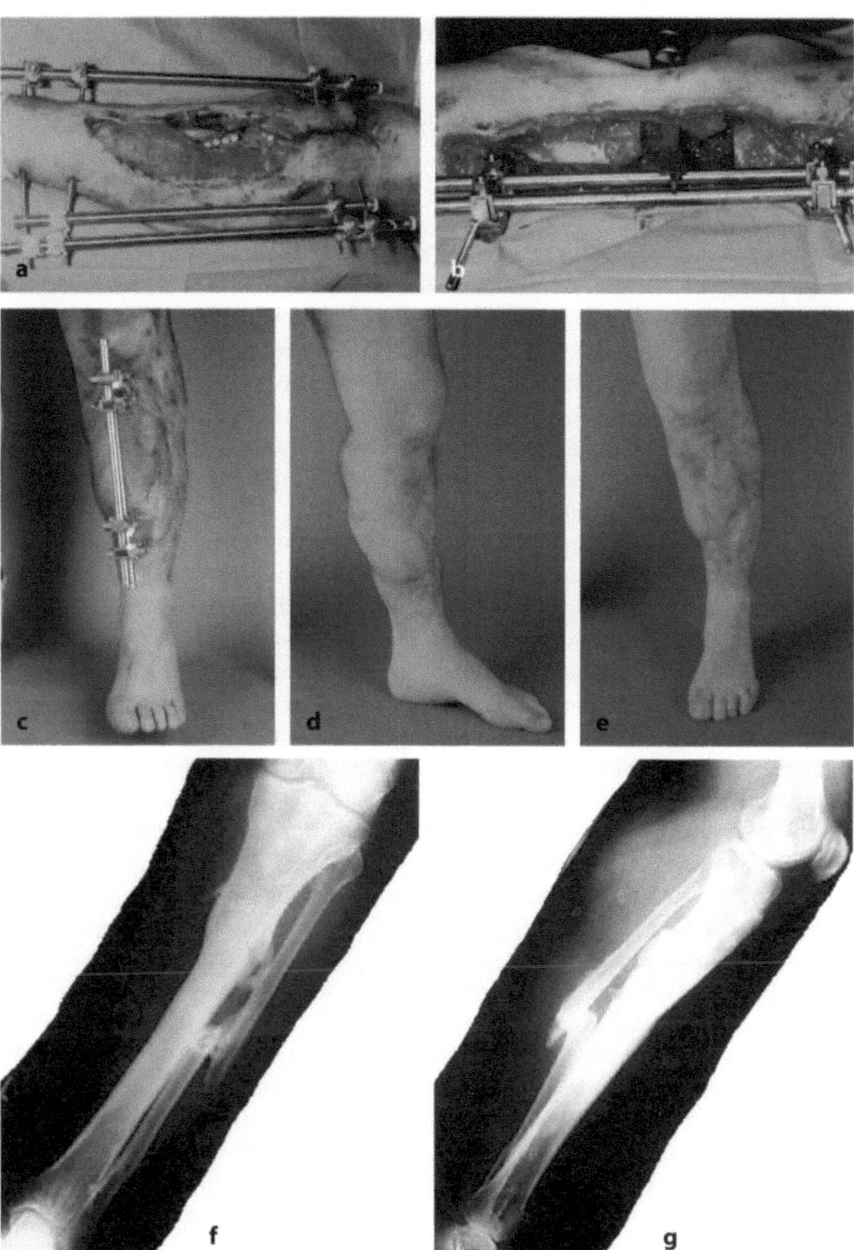

**Fig. 2a–d.** 36-year old patient with severely comminuted open fracture of the lower leg 12 and a half weeks after a motorcycle accident; sepsis and osteomyelitis had been previously addressed with debridement and antibiotic bead implantation into the bone cavity (**a**); radical surgical debridement with resection of non-vital tibial bone (**b**) and defect coverage with microsurgical latissimus dorsi flap harvested with two separate skin paddles to close anterior and posterior defect (**c**). Stable wound coverage after bone lengthening with Ilizarov procedure for now more than 10 years (**d,e** lateral and frontal aspect), and healed bone after bone lengthening by secondary distraction osteogenesis (**f,g**). ([16], with kind permission of mhp Verlag, Wiesbaden)

needed to perform the delicate operation. Post-operative flap monitoring requires intensive care and experienced nursing to identify signs of flap failure or vascular compromise. This may require additional trips to the operating room for anastomosis revision to restore blood flow to the flap. Fortunately, flap failure is becoming increasingly rare; as the procedures have evolved over the past two decades, flap success can be seen in up to 95% of patients [14].

Each technique provides advantages and disadvantages which must be weighed in the decision-making process. As a rule, the most easily accomplished and least costly procedure, not just in terms of money, but in discomfort to the patient, should be selected.

One of the most problematic soft-tissue problems to deal with is the zone of the **distal lower leg** and the ankle and heel region. Split-thickness skin grafting, lateral calcaneal artery-island flap, lateral supramalleolar flap and numerous flaps from the plantar aspects of the foot may be considered to deal with bony heel and ankle defects (Fig. 1). In most cases, however, a muscle flap is the adequate solution to fill the cavity with sufficient blood supply (Fig. 2).

One of our working horses to fill the debrided osseous cavity in the lower leg and to provide ample soft tissue cover to large defects of uniform depth is the rectus abdominis-muscle free flap with skin graft [7–11]. The paired rectus abdominis muscles arise from the pubic tubercle and insert into the costal cartilages of the fifth, sixth and seventh ribs. Entering along the lateral border of the muscle near its inferior aspect, the deep inferior epigastric artery is the dominant blood supply. It originates from the medial aspect of the external iliac artery and is usually accompanied by two large venae comitantes. It courses along the posterior aspect of the muscle and arborises to connect with the deep superior epigastric artery by means of a plexus of periumbilical choke vessels [12]. The rectus muscle can be harvested either as a segmental flap or more often as a full muscle flap, depending on the amount of muscle needed (Fig. 3). The origin of the muscle is divided after identification of the deep inferior epigastric vessels. Following transfer and microscopic anastomosis to the recipient site in either an end-to-end or end-to-side fashion with the recipient vessels always out of the zone of injury, the anterior rectus sheath is repaired without prosthetic reinforcement.

In all cases where two similarly sized venae comitantes accompany the deep inferior epigastric artery, we anastomose both veins to recipient veins in the leg. The muscle is then properly contoured, inset and covered with a meshed spilt-skin graft. For ease of post-operative monitoring, we leave a small skin paddle on the muscle, which is removed after 5 to 7 days. The rectus muscle flap looks quite bulky immediately after its transfer, but with time, atrophy of the muscle produces a good contour to such reconstructions [8, 12].

One more typical entity in chronic osteomyelitis is the long-standing decubital ulcer. The treatment adheres to the above-mentioned principles of radical debridement and soft-tissue cover. However, despite improvements in surgical repair of pressure sores (recurrence rates greater than 80% are reported), we escalate our surgical armamentarium from axial fasciocutaneous flaps to myocutaneous flaps in order to keep further options open to deal with the relapse or secondary sore (Fig. 4). In the literature, the results achieved with musculocutaneous flaps were

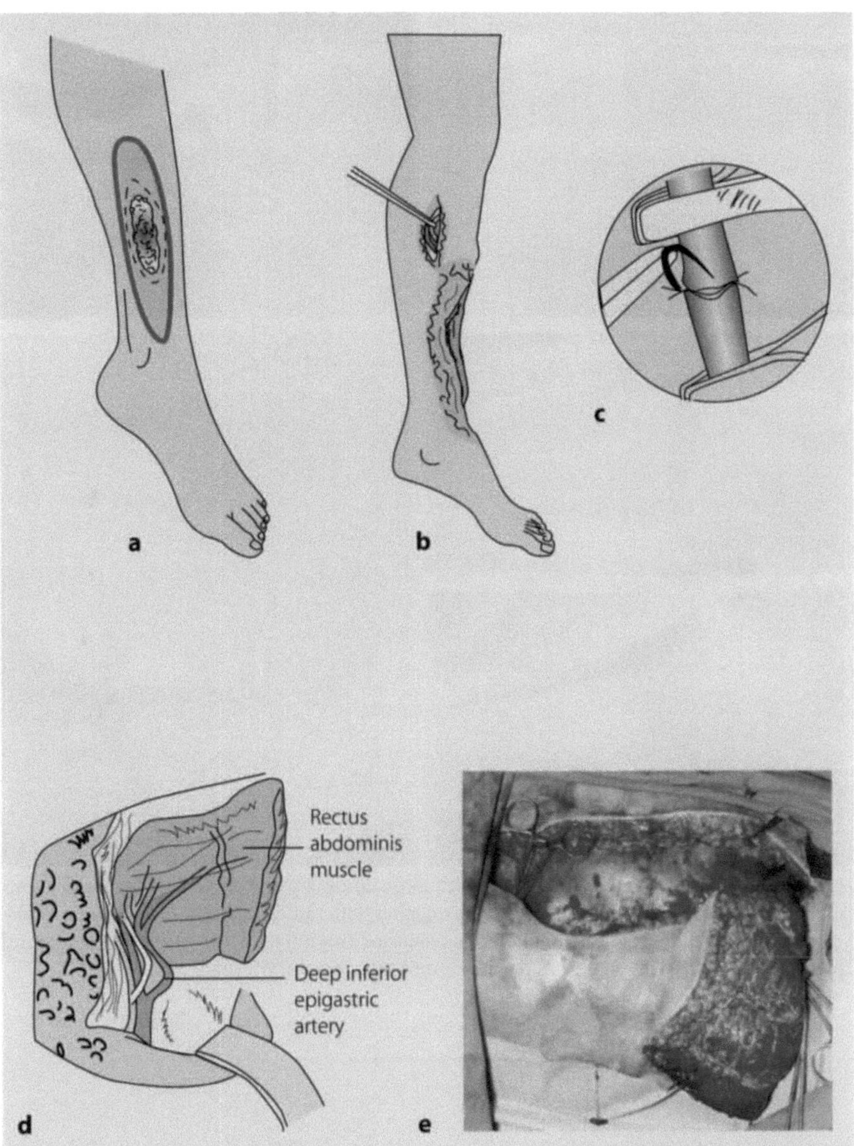



**Fig. 3. a** Schematic drawing of rectus abdominis muscle flap harvest for free-flap transfer with deep inferior epigastric vessels dissected from their origin of the iliac vessels. **b** Dissection of the recipient vessels at the lower leg outside the zone of injury after radical debridement of the infected tibial parts with thorough removal of all sequesters. **c** Microsurgical anastomosis of flap vessels to recipient vessels. **d** Scheme of free rectus muscle dissection. **e** Clinical aspect of completely dissected rectus muscle with „monitor" skin paddle

comparable to those reached by closure with cutaneous flaps. In these patients free flaps are seldom indicated and local axial pattern type flaps will suffice to stable coverage.

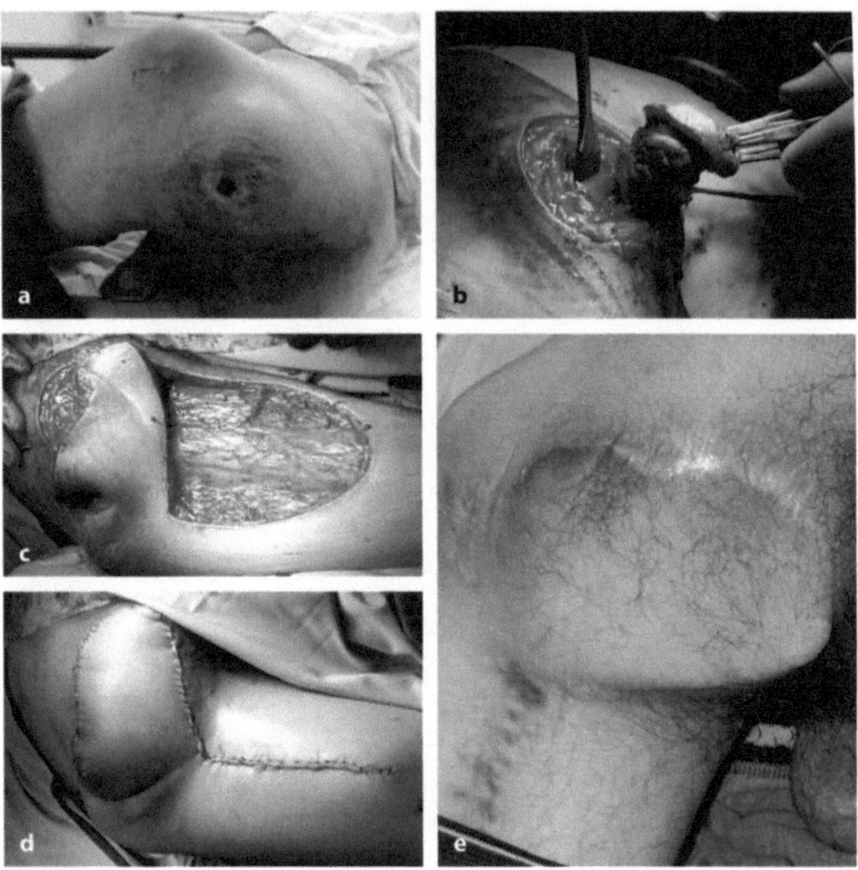

**Fig. 4. a** 23-year old paraplegic patient with longstanding decubital ulcer and ischial osteo-myelitis. **b** Removal of afflicted ischial bone together with radical surgical debridement of ulcer. **c,d** Defect coverage with fasciocutaneous posterior thigh flap. **e** Stable healing at 6 months post-operatively. ([16], with kind permission of mhp Verlag, Wiesbaden)

## Conclusion

Osteomyelitis still remains a challenge for surgery. The mainstay of osteomyelitis therapy is radical surgical debridement followed by sufficient soft-tissue coverage and accompanied by antibiotic therapy. The choice of an antibiotic therapy is guided by the bone biopsy or debridement culture results. Osteomyelitis is the typical challenge to an interdisciplinary team approach involving orthopaedic or trauma surgeons, plastic surgeons and vascular surgeons followed by specialised physio-therapists to achieve an optimal treatment outcome. The choice of the reconstructive procedure is characterised by numerous developments and advances in reconstructive options available today. With experience and proper training, the reconstructive surgeon is likely to choose the better if not the best alternative with the others as "lifeboats" if the original idea fails; if the initial plan does not work, then go to the next plan. With careful documentation and evaluation of the methods chosen to date, we as a society should expect continual improvement and nothing less in order to promote the care of patients with such severe problems as osteomyelitis.

## References


1. Eisenberg JM, Kitz DS (1986) Savings from outpatient antibiotic therapy for osteomyelitis. Economic analysis of a therapeutic strategy. JAMA 255: 1584
2. Moon MS, Moon JL (2000) Editorial management of osteomyelitis. J Orthop Surg 8: VII–X
3. Cierny G, Mader JT (1984) Adult chronic osteomyelitis. Orthopedics 7: 1557–1564
4. Levin LS, Heitmann C (2003) Lower extremity reconstruction. Sem Plast Surg 17: 69–81
5. King RD (2002) Osteomyelitis. http://www.emedicine.com/emerg/topic349.htm
6. Blum R, Wilkins R (2002) Osteomyelitis. Limb Preservation 9: 1–2
7. Horch RE, Meyer-Marcotty M, Stark GB (1998) Preexpansion of the tensor fasciae latae for free-flap transfer. Plast Reconstr Surg 102: 1188–1192
8. Horch RE, Stark GB (1999) The rectus abdominis free flap as an emergency procedure in extensive upper extremity soft-tissue defects. Plast Reconstr Surg 103: 1421–1427
9. Horch RE, Stark GB (1994) Prosthetic vascular graft infection defect covering with delayed vertical rectus abdominis muscular flap (VRAM) and rectus femoris flap. Vasa 23: 52–56
10. Walgenbach KJ, Voigt M, Andree C, Stark GB, Horch RE (2001) Management of hypovascularized wounds not responding to conventional therapy by means of free muscle transplantation. Vasa 30: 206–211
11. Walgenbach KJ, Horch R, Voigt M, Andree C, Tanczos E, Stark GB (1999) Free microsurgical flap-plasty in reconstructive therapy of diabetic foot ulcer. Zentralbl Chir 124 [Suppl 1]: 40–44
12. Reath DB, Taylor JW (1991) The segmental rectus abdominis free flap for ankle and foot reconstruction. Plast Reconstr Surg 88: 824–828
13. Schipper J, Ridder GJ, Maier W, Horch RE (2003) The preconditioning and prelamination of pedicled and free microvascular anastomised flaps with the technique of vacuum assisted closure. Laryngorhinootologie 82: 421–427
14. Fee TE, Spillert LJ (1997) Reconstructive principles. J Duval County Med Soc, www.dcmsonline.org
15. Gustilo RB, Anderson JT (1976) Prevention of infection in the treatment of one thousand and twenty-five open fractures of long bones: retrospective and prospective analysis. J Bone Joint Surg Am 58: 453–458
16. Loos B, Jeschke MG, Kopp J, Lang W, Horch RE (2003) Modern plastic surgical concepts to reconstruct chronic wounds. ZfW J Wound Healing 8: 186–193

# Principles of Surgical Management of War Wounds

S. MEINERS, H. GERNGROSS, C. WILLY

## Introduction

Military surgeons must decide how best to apply evolving civilian trauma management techniques to the difficult logistic environment of recent and future wars. This usually requires compromise of the new clinical methods as practiced in civilian trauma surgery for use in the theatre of war. In the fast-moving, far-forward, austere military environment, it is quite likely that the surgeon will not have the luxury of being able to perform topical and definitive surgery on every casualty. In addition to the problems of dispersed operations, highly mobile front lines, extended lines of logistics and delayed and inadequate evacuation, the surgeon is likely to be called upon to treat soldiers, as well as civilians, with a requirement to offer immediate care that is far removed from his/her own speciality. It is necessary to underline that up to 60% of the wounded persons are civilians (~10% children) [1, 2]. Thus, only 7% of the patients with hand grenade injuries sustained their wounds in battle; 50% were women, children or older men [3]. In this situation, the surgeon is required to perform life-saving operations and achieve both pathophysiological and biomechanical stability so that the patient can be transported. Our objective is to present the principles of modern surgery of war wounds against this background. This requires the discussion of the injury pattern, the known guidelines of wound treatment and some modern aspects.

## Injury Patterns

The majority of war wounds are caused by anti-personnel fragments from munitions such as mortars and bomblets. Modern munitions aim to incapacitate soldiers with multiple wounds from very small fragments of low available kinetic energy. Many of these fragments may be stopped by helmets and body armour, and this has led to a predominance of multiple wounds to the face, neck, pelvis, groin and limbs in those casualties requiring surgery [4, 5]. The patterns of injuries sustained on the modern battlefield are likely to be changed by the type of engagement and modern protective equipment. Thus, the rate of penetrating injuries due to bullets or fragments will depend on the nature of the battle, with blunt injury and burns likely to comprise a significant part of the injuries. The changing scope of modern military operations, in which urban and guerrilla warfare predominate, provides an opportunity to make new observations and develop new strategies in the treatment of wounded patients. For example, the incidence of injuries to the lower extremities is high in modern warfare [1]. This knowledge explains why, for instance, 80% of all life-threatening injuries in the US soldiers in Iraq 2003/2004 were wounds to the extremities. Among non-fatal injuries, head and torso wounds were almost non-existent. The injury pattern shows the following distribution [1, 4–10]:

- 20% traumatic brain injuries (TBI),
- 13% eye injuries,
- 10–15% chest injuries, abdominal trauma,
- 60–70% limb injuries (vessel injuries!),
- 80–90% soft-tissue trauma.

Whereas penetrating trauma dominates in most cases of war injuries, injuries caused by accidents (road accidents, sports accidents etc.) are mostly characterised by blunt trauma mechanisms which show the typical injury pattern as published, for example, by the trauma registry of the German Society of Traumatology [11–13]:

- 60% traumatic brain injuries (TBI),
- 60% chest injuries,
- 25% abdominal trauma,
- 40% limb injuries,
- 1–5% soft-tissue trauma.

## Injury Mechanisms

### Penetrating Trauma

Ballistic wounds are produced by penetrating missiles (bullets, metallic fragments from bombs, shells, rockets and grenades). These missiles cause injury by transferring their energy to the body, which results in laceration, contusion and disruption of tissue. Penetrating wounds are the most prevalent types of injury, followed by lacerations, open fractures and closed fractures. The most frequent anatomical regions sustaining penetrating injuries are the leg, head, hand, and arm [5].

#### Gunshot Injuries

Ballistics may be defined as the movement of a projectile. An understanding of ballistics is essential for the correct identification and treatment of wounds and fractures resulting from gunshots. Ballistics can be broken down into three components:

1. Interior ballistics – occurrences within the gun barrel (firing).
2. Exterior ballistics – the property of the missile while in flight.
3. Terminal ballistics – the effect in the target until the missile is at rest.

**Interior ballistics** relates to the type of weapon, the length of the gun barrel, the diameter, weight and composition of the projectile, and the type and amount of gunpowder used to discharge the missile. All these factors are involved in setting the missile in motion, and therefore they determine the maximum velocity of the missile as it leaves the gun barrel.

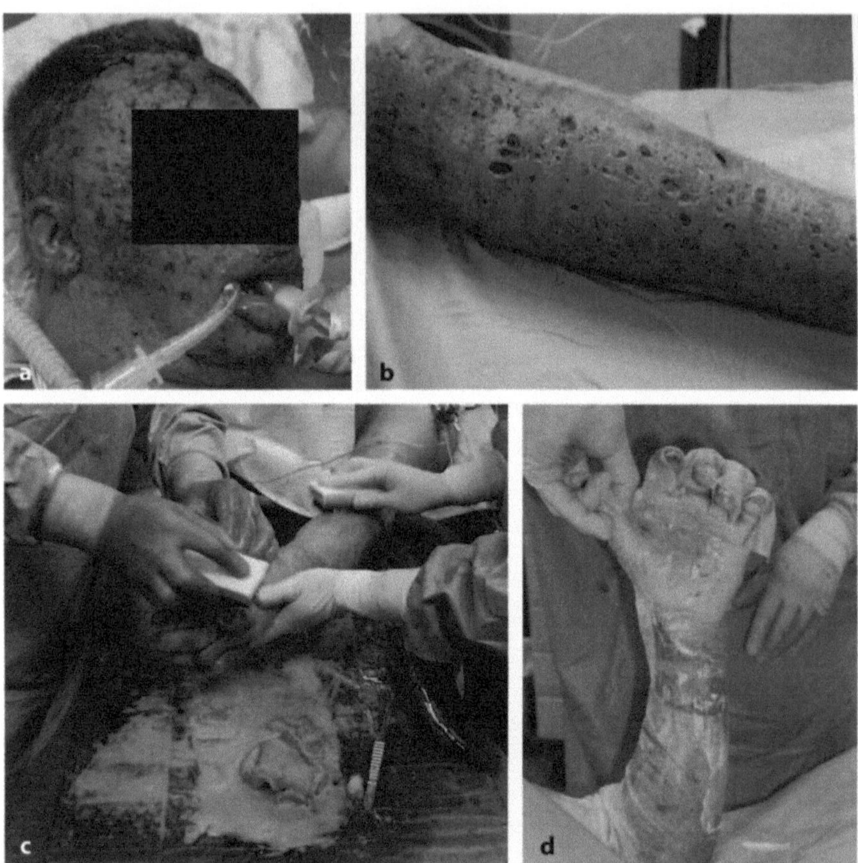

**Fig. 1. a,b** Multiple superficial and deep skin lesions due to hundreds of small pieces of glass and metal in face and upper limb. Fragments tend to be small and numerous and are fairly regular in shape to ensure adequate range and consistent performance. Terror attack June 2003 Kabul/Afghanistan. Therapy at lower arm: brushing and bandages (**c**) with sulfadiazine-silver-creme (**d**)

**Exterior ballistics** relates to the distance of discharge and the behaviour of the missile in flight. Since the missile begins to slow down when it leaves the gun barrel, the distance the missile travels will have a significant effect on the impact velocity and the amount of remaining energy. This affects the type and severity of the wound.

**Terminal or wound ballistics** describes the effect of the missile as it releases energy on its path through the tissues.

### Injuries by Metallic Fragments

Fragments are the most common wounding agents in war, accounting for between 44 and 92% of all surgical cases (in civilian practice, bullets are the predominant penetrating missiles) [5]. Fragments from military anti-personnel munitions tend

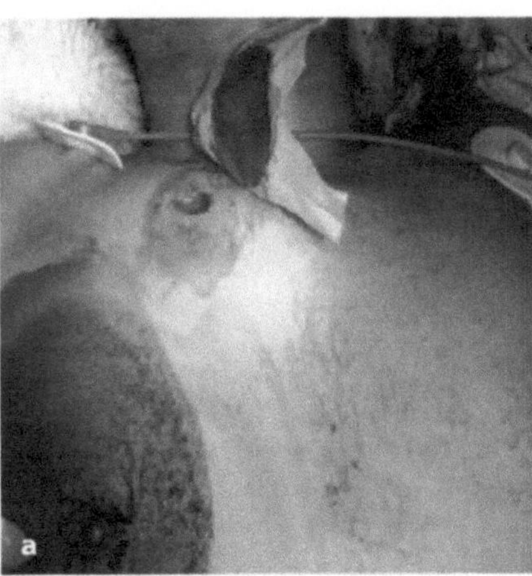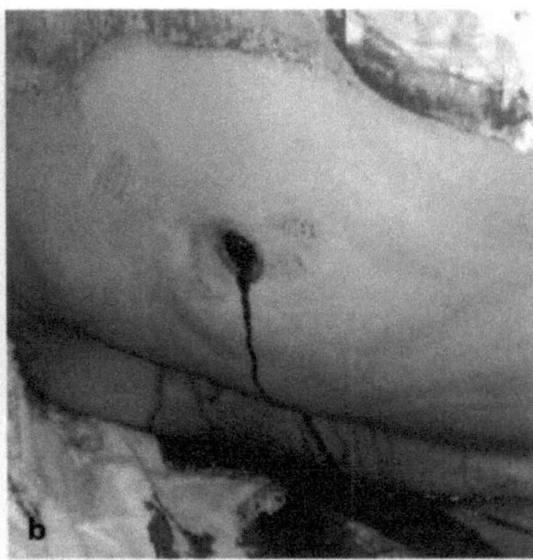

**Fig. 2a,b.** Penetrating thoracic gunshot wound (low-energy transfer injury; Prizren/Kosovo 2000). **a** Entry wound parasternal, infraclavicular. **b** Exit wound on the back medial of the scapula. Therapy: first, „only" chest tube drainage, then, due to haemorrhagic shock, thoracotomy and non-anatomical lung resection

to be small and numerous and are fairly regular in shape to ensure adequate range and consistent performance (Fig. 1). Thus, wound tracks produced by fragments have a consistent pattern. Most military anti-personnel fragments have a slight penetrating power and limited effective range.

### Energy Transfer, Wound Track and Cavitation Effect

The amount of damage caused is related to the amount of energy that the missile transfers to the tissues. Injuries can broadly be classified into low-energy-transfer and high-energy-transfer injuries. The greatest amount of tissue damage is caused by high-energy transfer, which is related to the retardation of the missile. Retardation depends upon missile factors such as shape, stability and composition, as well as tissue factors such as density and elasticity. When a projectile hits the body, it produces a wound track. Low-energy-transfer wounds (bullet velocity: ~200–400 m/s) are characterised by the injury being confined to the wound track. The principal injury results from a simple cutting mechanism, and the severity depends on the nature of the tissue penetrated (Fig. 2). In high-energy-transfer wounds (bullet velocity: >600–800 m/s) the missile lacerates the tissue and creates a surrounding zone of pressure and shock waves. As the tissue is pushed away from the passing projectile, a temporary cavity is formed. This cavity may be up to 40 times the diameter of the bullet. After passage of the projectile, the walls of the permanent cavity are temporarily stretched radially outward. The maximum lateral tissue displacement delineates the temporary cavity. Any damage resulting from temporary cavitation is due to stretching of the tissue. Resistance or vulnerability to stretch damage depends mostly on tissue elasticity. The same stretch that causes only moderate contusion and minor functional changes in relatively elastic skeletal muscle can cause devastating disruption of the liver. Analysing the size of gunshot wounds in over

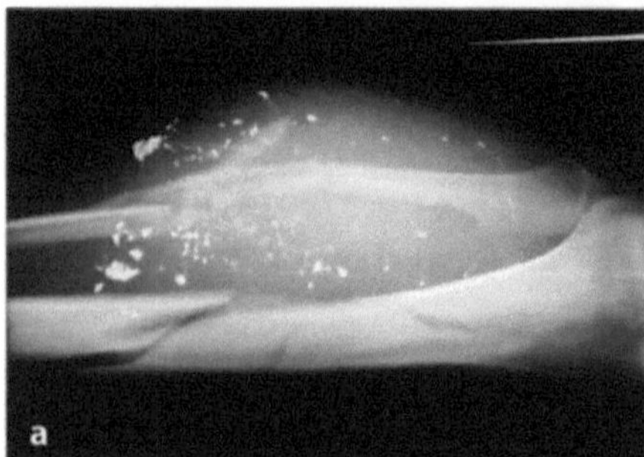
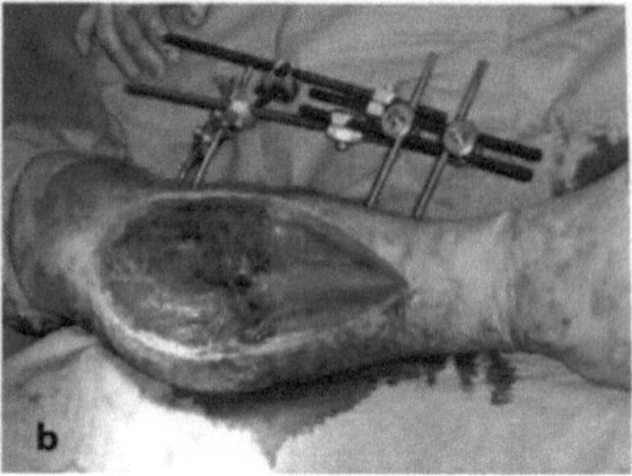


**Fig. 3. a** Gunshot wound of the lower limb (high-energy transfer injury; Prizren/Kosovo 2000) (*left*). Destruction of the nervus peronaeus communis, arteria fibularis (*right*). **b** Therapy: ligation of the artery, fasciotomy, external fixation, vacuum sealing therapy (not demonstrated)

5000 patients, Coupland demonstrated that about 50% of the wounds without fragmentation of bullets were large wounds. In the case of fragmentation of the bullets, the rate of wounds with a clinically detectable cavity increases to over 70%. Nevertheless, most large wounds do not contain bullet fragments. Thus, fragmentation of bullets is neither a necessary nor sufficient cause of large wounds, and surgeons should not diagnose extensive tissue damage because of the presence of fragments on the radiograph [15].

The result of temporary displacement of tissue is analogous to a localised area of blunt trauma surrounding the permanent cavity left by the projectile's passage. In the case of bone fractures, fragments can also act as secondary missiles. Nerves and blood vessels near the bullet track can also be damaged because of the cavitation effect (Fig. 3). In addition, indirect injuries can occur. For example, the spinal cord may be involved when the wound track comes close to the vertebral column, or a long bone may fracture in a limb even if it is not hit by the missile itself.

### Clinical Presentation of Penetrating Injury

Most wounds resulting from a penetrating injury are extensive and very deep. The risk of underestimating the extent of a war wound is high, because cavitation effects result in significant damage, often far greater than expected after visual inspection of the entry or exit wound. In about 60% of the cases, a larger-exit-than-entry wound is evidence of the devastating potential of increases in velocity. The larger-exit wound, when present, is caused by projectile yaw, by projectile fragmentation or as a result of multiple secondary bone fragment projectile. Projectile yaw represents a deviation of the longitudinal axis of the bullet from its line of flight. All war wounds are contaminated to various degrees by bacteria from clothing, skin, fragments, bullets and the external environment (e.g. mud and earth). Contaminants can enter the wound track from both entry and exit wounds. The contamination of low-energy-transfer wounds is limited to the wound track itself, whereas, with high-energy-transfer wounds, it spreads beyond the boundaries of the temporary cavity. In patients with multiple wounds, the largest one may not be the most important. Small-entry wounds from bullets can be associated with extensive internal damage. Gas in the tissue (X-ray: soft-tissue emphysema) is not pathognomonic of gas gangrene or infections by gas-producing organisms. In cases of traumatic amputation by mines, air as well as debris and other foreign bodies may be blown into the intermuscular compartments of the leg, and gunshot wounds are often accompanied by intramuscular localised air; this is sucked in as a consequence of the negative pressures occurring in the process of cavitation [16].

To score these wounds, Coupland developed the Red Cross classification of war wounds – the E.X.C.F.V.M. scoring system [17]. The wound score is based on the skin wounds and the presence of a cavity, fracture, vital injury or metallic bodies in the wound. All wounds scored in this way can be graded according to severity and typed according to structures injured. However, along with some other authors, we believe that the Red Cross wound classification is valuable in assessing a wound as part of a secondary survey, but that this wound score has little part to play in triage. It may help in the decision on the management of individual wounds in clinical practice and is useful for recording the nature of wounds for future analysis and in military surgical research [18].

### Blast Injuries

Explosions inflict injury in a number of ways. It is likely to coexist with missile injuries, blunt trauma, burns and other injuries. Primary blast injury is due solely to the direct effect of the pressure wave on the body. Secondary blast injury results from penetrating or non-penetrating damage caused by ordinance projectiles or secondary missiles, which are energised by the explosion and strike the victim. Tertiary blast injury results from whole-body displacement and subsequent traumatic impact with environmental objects. Tertiary effects generally result from the bulk flow of gases away from an explosion and occur when the individual is in very close proximity to the explosion. Primary blast injury is seen almost exclusively in gas-containing organs: the ear and the respiratory and gastrointestinal tracts.

Of the three organ systems, the **ear** is the most sensitive, but injury to the **lung** is the cause of the greatest morbidity and mortality. Primary blast injury of the lung presents a clinical picture similar to that of pulmonary contusion from blunt chest trauma, but without rib fractures or chest wall injury. The manifestations of "blast lung" may develop over the course of 24–48 h and may have the appearance of a local or diffuse infiltrate.

The **gastrointestinal tract** may be damaged wherever there are collections of gas. Injury to the gut is particularly severe in underwater blasts. While hollow visceral injury is also present in airblast, it is generally overshadowed by the more dramatic presentation of air emboli or acute respiratory insufficiency (brain vessels, coronary arteries). The colon is the hollow viscus that is most commonly disrupted. Gastric injuries are usually less common and less severe. Rarely, one encounters rupture of the spleen or liver in the absence of superimposed blunt abdominal trauma. Pathologically, injuries to the bowel range from subserosal or intramural haemorrhage to frank rupture.

## Treatment of Warfare Injuries

The aim of surgical treatment of war wounds is to save the life and the limb, to prepare for evacuation and to prevent serious sepsis by primary wound excision. The wound closure can be carried out later, after 4 or 5 days, in a second step.

### Basic Principles of Surgical Wound Management

The basic surgical procedures are haemostasis and debridement. The first operation should be performed as soon as possible after wounding to prevent the establishment of an infection. Patients suffering from blast injury should be managed in the same way as those with blunt trauma.

#### Haemostasis

Haemostasis is best achieved by ligation with absorbable material, diathermy or application of pressure with a compress or dressing. During the major amputation of a limb, double ligation of large vessels is indicated. Very rarely, adequate haemostasis cannot be achieved because of difficulty of access. This is the only indication for packing a wound or using a tourniquet.

#### Debridement

The tissue is a potential culture medium and therefore forbearance in removing dead and contaminated tissue and foreign matter is the principal cause of wound infection. The initial surgical treatment of war wounds is the most essential [16]. As part of the excision, all dead and contaminated tissue, mud, earth, clothing and loose bullets and fragments which are embedded in tissue have to be removed completely ("the best antibiotic is a good wound excision"). Prolonged surgery to locate bullets and fragments that have come to rest in undamaged tissue is unnecessary and dangerous; they should be removed later if symptoms subsequently occur. If necessary, a decompressive fasciotomy is indicated for limb wounds (any injury of a leg may be complicated by a compartment syndrome!). Furthermore, there must be no hesitation to make extensive incisions to see what needs to be done. The extent of damaged tissue should not be underestimated – often, it is much greater than anticipated. At the end, the wound must be washed out generously with saline. Repaired vessels should not be left exposed but require covering with viable muscle and may require a muscle flap. Nerves exposed after wound excision can be left without soft-tissue cover until delayed closure. Certain small and uncomplicated fragment wounds can initially be treated without surgery [3]. Small-fragment wounds affecting only the skin and muscle can be managed non-operatively with antibiotics and dressings [19, 20]. Even after efficient debridement, a tetanus prophylaxis is additionally required (unless this has already been done).

Animal experiments in pigs demonstrated the importance of early debridement. Cultures from tissue judged viable and left in the wound indicated contamination in 25% of the wounds when debridement was performed within 1 h (no antibiotic prophylaxis). A surgical delay of 6 h resulted in a rate of contamination of 37% and an infection in 11%, while a delay of 12 h resulted in an infection in 60% [21]. The authors' conclusion is that wound infection can be overcome by adequate surgical treatment within 6 h but will be out of control after a 12-h delay.

### Antibiotics

The analysis of the development of infections in war wounds showed an overall infection rate of over 20%, but varied with the type of injury [22]. Three risk factors were found to be associated with infection regardless of the number of injuries:

- penetrating abdominal wounds involving the colon,
- fractures involving the femur,
- burns involving more than 25% of body surface.

The most common bacteria are *Clostridium welchii* (causes gas gangrene), *Staphylococcus aureus, Streptococcus pyogenes, Pseudomonas aeruginosas* and *E. coli* [23, 24].

Antibiotics have to be only an adjunct to – and not a substitute for – surgery. They should be used early on in the treatment for maximum effect and should be discontinued as quickly as possible (after 5–7 days) to prevent the emergence of resistant strains of bacteria. Animal experiments in pigs demonstrated the importance of the early start of antibiotic prophylaxis. An intramuscular antibiotic regimen, commenced 1 h after wounding, could prevent infection in penetrating soft-tissue missile wounds for up to 3 days. A delay of 6 h renders treatment ineffective [25]. Therefore, timely and prophylactic prescription of a broad-spectrum antibiotic with a long half-life has great importance in the treatment of war wounds [26, 27]. All patients with abdominal wounds and suspected peritoneal perforation should receive metronidazole in addition to penicillin or a second-generation cephalosporin. Nevertheless, the incidence of wound infection in recent military conflicts strongly suggests that infection in open war wounds occurs with relative frequency despite strict adherence to the principles of surgical debridement and the administration of prophylactic antibiotics. Further research leading to improved methods for the prevention of wound sepsis is warranted in order to reduce the incidence of wound infections in the future [28].

### Temporary Closure and Delayed Definitive Closure

All war wounds of the face, scalp, neck, buccal mucosa, dura, peritoneum, pleura and synovium of joints should be closed primarily. All other wounds have to be regarded as contaminated and must be left open or must be dealt with using temporary closure techniques. The reasons for leaving wounds open are:

- to permit unrestricted swelling of tissues next to the wound, thereby allowing decompression and avoiding ischaemia,
- to admit exudation of serum,
- to avoid the formation of an anaerobic environment,
- (as a precautionary measure) to ensure that no residual, incompletely excised dead and contaminated tissue is enclosed.

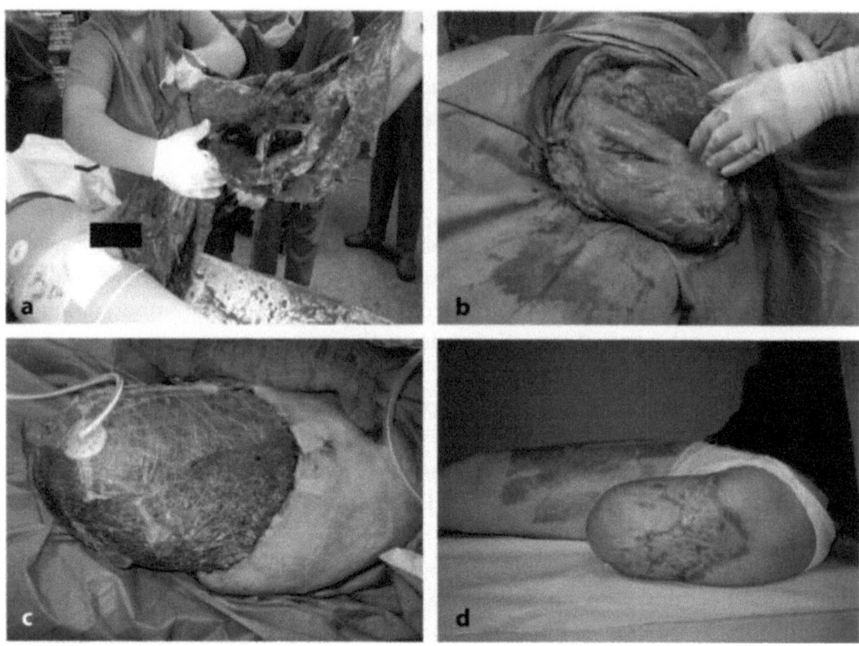

**Fig. 4a–d.** Roll-over trauma resulting in traumatic amputation left leg. **a** Severe bony and soft tissue injury. **b** After debridement. **c** Vacuum sealing therapy to close the wound. **d** After mesh-graft transplantation and vacuum-sealing therapy to fix the skin graft (6 weeks after trauma)

Alternatively, the vacuum-sealing technique is a new, simple-to-use procedure for temporary closure after the resection of dead and contaminated tissue (Fig. 4). Vacuum sealing can also be used for closing fasciotomy wounds.

The prevailing adequate time for wound closure is between 4 and 6 days after primary surgery treatment. Post-traumatic swelling has decreased by then, and the early process of wound healing is under way. Tissues left open for longer are indurated and inelastic, making the adaptation of wounds difficult. On the other hand, closing the wound is only indicated when it is clean. Direct suture and skin grafting are the most frequently employed methods of restoring integrity of skin cover. The decision to revert to healing by second intention should be well considered. In certain cases, reconstructive procedures such as muscle flaps etc. are indicated.

Nevertheless, it is noteworthy that some authors advocate proper primary reconstructive treatment of wounds aimed at early flap closure. Reconstructive surgery can be used within a framework of management of war wounds by basic principles. It is divided into three groups:

- primary (emergency) reconstruction, performed as part of initial surgery and as a life-saving procedure,
- delayed primary (essential) reconstruction, performed at the time of delayed closure,
- elective or non-essential reconstruction.

All surgeons involved with the early management of war wounds should be prepared to perform primary and delayed primary reconstruction [29]. This type of management can result in a significantly shorter hospitalisation and leads to a more effective rehabilitation and recovery of patients [30, 31]. It was shown that one-stage reconstruction with free composite flaps provides a reliable treatment solution with a good functional outcome even in patients with osteocutaneous defects [32].

## Specific Treatment of War Wounds

### Chest Wounds

The widespread use of modern body armour has reduced mortality from injuries to the chest. The incidence of penetrating wounds of the thorax in military conflicts ranges from 10–15%. After identification (X-ray), most life-threatening thoracic injuries (80–90%) can be simply and immediately treated by fitting a chest tube for drainage. Injuries to the chest wall, thoracic viscera, pericardial tamponade or persistent intra-thoracic bleeding over 300 ml/h must be treated by thoracotomy (see Fig. 2).

If thoracotomy is performed to control ongoing intrapleural bleeding, the operation consists of suturing the lung wounds, electrocautery haemostasis and drainage of the pleural cavity. Resection of the lung by lobectomy or pneumonectomy is performed less frequently. Patients with gunshot wounds to the chest (see Fig. 2) with normal vital signs, physical examinations and normal X-rays can be reasonably treated as outpatients after 4 h of observation, at the physician's discretion [33]. Minimally invasive videothoracoscopy to perform surgical manipulations of the thorax wall, the pleural cavity, the lung and the mediastinum could be a modern option in military conflicts but, unlike in civilian trauma surgery, minimally invasive videothoracoscopy is not yet common practice in military operations [34].

### Abdominal Wounds

Because protective body armour is used on modern battle fields, the incidence of abdominal injuries has decreased. For the surgical management of warfare-related abdominal injuries, it is important to appreciate the difference between surgical resuscitation and definitive treatment for abdominal trauma. Surgical resuscitation implies only that the surgical procedure is necessary to save life by stopping bleeding and preventing further contamination (damage control [35]). Because of high rates of negative laparotomies in the past (15–20%, e.g. Vietnam), effective triage is crucial. Therefore, laparoscopy has been used in attempts to minimise unnecessary laparotomies. It was shown that

- there are areas within the abdominal cavity that cannot be accurately visualised with laparoscopy,
- the evaluation of penetration of the peritoneal cavity from anterior-penetrating injury appears to be accurate and
- a number of injuries were not identified [36].

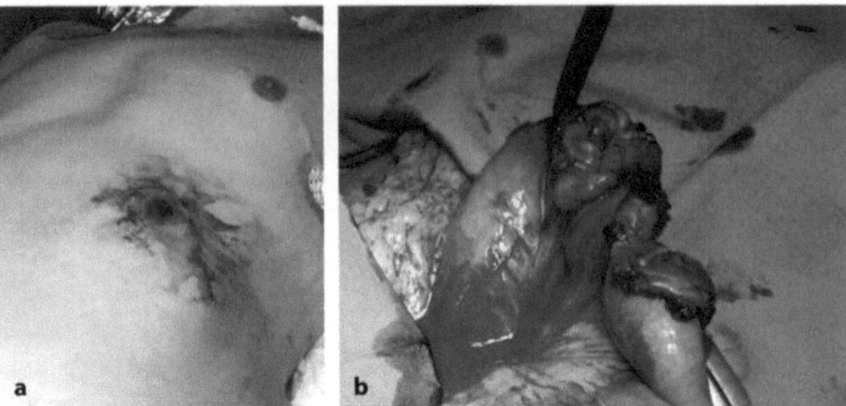

**Fig. 5a,b.** Penetrating abdominal gunshot wound (low-energy transfer injury, Zürich 1999). Entry wound (**a**) and the situs intraoperative (**b**). Therapy: excision of the entry wound at the abdominal wall, primary bowel anastomosis and protective jejunostomy

However, the military surgeon will not have the opportunity of using minimally invasive techniques in an austere military environment [37, 38].

In the case of a haemodynamically unstable patient, signs of peritonitis, significant gastrointestinal haemorrhage with sonographic evidence of free fluidness or radiographic evidence of free gas under the diaphragm or evisceration, a laparotomy should be performed.

The visceral surgery most commonly involves intestinal repair or resection with proximal diversion or exteriorisation when the colon is involved (Fig. 5). For gunshot wounds penetrating the colon, removal of retained missiles should be attempted because these increase the risk of abscess. A brief course of appropriate antibiotic treatment should be initiated as soon as possible after wounding and should be continued for 24 h. Prolonged courses of antibiotic provide no added benefits [39]. Routine primary repair of intestinal injuries should not be preferred because of high rates of major complications due to anastomotic leakage or peritonitis. In some published cases with primary repair, the percentage of complications was high (92%). In patients with the diverting colostomy, it was only 34%. The high complication rate in the cases with primary repair was directly related to the presence of the anastomotic leaks and subsequent peritonitis [40].

### Limb Wounds – Fractures

The determining factor of war injuries with gunshot fractures is the extent of the soft-tissue injury. Therefore, the surgical treatment should be concentrated on the excision of the wound, removing soft tissues and bone – stabilisation of the fracture is secondary. It is important to remember that these wounds are contaminated and that the degree of contamination increases with the severity of the wound. For distal limb wounds, a pneumatic tourniquet is invaluable in the initial operation. The application of the tourniquet before removal of field dressings minimises blood loss and produces a bloodless field which facilitates wound excision.

If the classification of the injury indicates that it is a low-energy-transfer wound, an excision or debridement of the entry wound on the extremity is usually carried out. Fractures that are associated with low-energy-transfer gunshot injuries are usually minimally displaced, with very little destruction of the osseous blood supply. These can be treated as closed fractures with splinting or casting. If there is an indication for external fixation, the fracture should be managed as a grade-I open fracture.

On the other hand, high-energy-transfer wounds must be treated extremely extensively. A wide incision is needed that will allow wide debridement. These wounds are treated as type-III open wounds and must never close during the primary surgical intervention. The fascia is incised and left open because of the risk of development of compartment syndromes. The muscle is likewise debrided, owing to the injury caused by transient-cavitation phenomena. The consequences of missing dead muscle when excising a large wound are unforeseeable. The bone is irrigated copiously, and small, avascular fragments have to be removed. Exposed cortical bone can be left in situ if not stripped of its periosteum by the injury.

If immobilisation by external fixation is not possible, casts, splints or skeletal traction can be the methods to use in the first instance. No screws or plates should be implanted in the wound because of the high risk of dangerous bone infection. Circumferential plasters are best not applied; if they are, they must be split completely down to the skin. In a low-technology environment, it was demonstrated that patients treated by external fixation remained in hospital longer than those treated with traction, and the positional outcome was identical in both groups. As regards tibial fractures, external fixation was of extra benefit only in those of the lower third when compared with simple plaster slabs, unless more complex procedures such as flaps or vascular repair were to be performed. In complex humeral fractures, external fixation resulted in long stays in hospital and a large number of interventions when compared with simple treatment in a sling. Therefore, in an environment where facilities are limited and surgeons have only general experience, very careful initial wound excision is the most important factor determining the outcome. The general application of complex holding techniques is inappropriate in many cases [41].

If projectiles have traversed or remain in a joint, debridement is indicated by an arthrotomy. The joint has to be washed out with saline. After the removal of any foreign matter and loose bone or cartilage fragments, drainage is needed. Then the synovium should be closed. The joint capsule and ligaments should be sutured secondarily as part of the delayed primary closure. Complications usually occur as a result of insufficient debridement, a missed compartment syndrome or an inadequate physical examination which failed to discover primary damage to a joint, nerve, artery or tendon.

### Traumatic Amputation

Traumatic amputation, particularly of the foot or lower leg by a land mine, is a common injury in military conflicts [42]. The surgeon must be aware that injured tissue and earth may be pushed up inside the fascial compartments. Particularly with severe limb injury or traumatic amputation caused by anti-personnel mines, the wound excision element of the primary amputation is complicated and different to civilian amputations. Therefore surgical amputation is at a higher level and may resemble a thorough excision of the original wound or a formal amputation with planned skin and muscle flaps. It is not achieved by amputating tissue that is thought to be viable as far distally as possible. However, where skin is viable, as little as possible is removed. Viable muscle is still identifiable by its colour, contractility and texture. Anti-personnel mines produce a recognisable pattern of injury to the leg, which frequently spares the gastrocnemius muscle. If surgical amputation is indicated, medial gastrocnemius myoplastic below-knee amputation is suitable for these injuries. The technique permits the covering and preservation of a tibial stump that is acceptable for fitting a prosthesis [16, 42]. The amputation wound is left open or can be covered with vacuum sealing as a temporary closure technique (see Fig. 4). Delayed suture is performed after 4 to 6 days when soft tissue can be trimmed. Failure to achieve this is due to the remaining skin being too short in relation to the bone section.

In spite of the advances in treatment and the improved results achieved by modern techniques of wound stabilisation, wound soft-tissue cover and bone and soft-tissue reconstructions, the temptation to try to salvage useless limbs must be resisted. Amputation, judiciously adjudged and correctly timed, remains one of the most successful forms of treatment for these severe injuries, saving the casualty from a physical and spiritual via dolorosa. Enthusiasm for surgical endeavour must be well tempered with mature judgement and realistic clinical acumen [43].

### Vessel Injury

Many deaths in modern conflicts are due to vascular injury, particularly of the iliac and femoral vessels, because the groin is left unprotected by modern body armour [10]. Degiannis et al. showed that in their patients with iliac artery injuries, the majority of patients were admitted with a gross physiological derangement that did not respond to pre-operative resuscitation, so they were taken directly to theatre, with a resulting peri-operative mortality of at least 39%. A prompt operation was mandatory to improve the chances of survival of patients with this injury. All patients with femoral artery injuries responded to preoperative resuscitation and there was an amputation rate of (only) 4% and no mortality [44].

The options for the repair of an iliac or femoral vessel injury include lateral repair, patch angioplasty, end-to-end anastomosis, interposition graft bypass graft, or ligation. Bypass grafting of battlefield injuries using synthetic material has been reported, although autologous vein is most commonly used. Endovascular repairs of femoral vessel injuries have also been described, but the necessary equipment is not available in most battlefield hospitals. Temporary intraluminal shunting (e.g. by a drainage tube) should be used to restore circulation when revascularisation will be delayed due to associated injuries or fracture fixation. Femoral vein injuries should be primarily repaired if possible. Preparation and exposure are identical for venous and arterial injuries. Intraluminal shunting is not indicated in venous injury. Ligation should be performed when primary repair is not feasible. Tourniquets can be used as a last resort when haemostasis is not otherwise achieved. Gosselin et al.

demonstrated that in their patients with acute arterial injury in connection with combat wounds from the Afghan conflict, the overall amputation rate was 65%, but only 22% for patients revascularised within 12 hours of injury and 93% for those undergoing surgery after 12 h. Therefore, the authors recommend attempting revascularisation procedures only in patients seen within 12 h of sustaining a military-type injury to an artery in an extremity [45, 46].

## Summary

The following ten points should be a help for the management of war wounds:
1. Every war wound is dangerous because of the risk that a deep-seated vital structure is injured.
2. All war wounds are contaminated.
3. Missiles do not always travel in straight lines.
4. All dead and contaminated tissue and loose foreign matter must be removed.
5. The objective of wound surgery is to minimise infective complications.
6. In the case of fractures treat the wound, not the X-ray.
7. The wound must be left open.
8. An alternative to closure of the wound is the vacuum sealing treatment (often not possible in a low-technology environment).
9. Not all foreign bodies are visible on X-ray film. Plastic used in small mines, mud and clothing etc. may have entered the wound.
10. Ensure tetanus prophylaxis.

## References


1. Batinica J, Batinica S (1995) War wounds in the Sibenik area during the 1991–1992 war against Croatia. Mil Med 160: 124–128
2. Coupland RM, Samnegaard HO (1999) Effect of type and transfer of conventional weapons on civilian injuries: retrospective analysis of prospective data from Red Cross hospitals. BMJ 319: 410–412
3. Coupland RM (1993) Hand grenade injuries among civilians. Jama 270: 624–626
4. Bowyer GW, Cooper GJ, Rice P (1995) Management of small fragment wounds in war: current research. Ann R Coll Surg Engl 77: 131–134
5. Leedham CS, Blood CG, Newland C (1993) A descriptive analysis of wounds among U.S. Marines treated at second-echelon facilities in the Kuwaiti theater of operations. Mil Med 158: 508–512
6. Biehl JW, Valdez J, Hemady RK, Steidl SM, Bourke DL (1999) Penetrating eye injury in war. Mil Med 164: 780–784
7. Coupland R (1996) Abdominal wounds in war. Br J Surg 83: 1505–1511
8. Coupland RM (1990) War wound excision. Br J Surg 77: 833
9. Coupland RM (1994) Epidemiological approach to surgical management of the casualties of war. BMJ 308: 1693–1697
10. Pearl JP, McNally MP, Perdue PW (2003) Femoral vessel injuries in modern warfare since Vietnam. Mil Med 168: 733–735
11. Ruchholtz S, Waydhas C, Ose C, Lewan U, Nast-Kolb D (2002) Prehospital intubation in severe thoracic trauma without respiratory insufficiency: a matched-pair analysis based on the Trauma Registry of the German Trauma Society. J Trauma 52: 879–886

12. Ruchholtz S (2000) [The trauma registry of the german society of trauma surgery as a basis for interclinical quality management. A multicenter study of the German Society of Trauma Surgery]. Unfallchirurg 103: 30–37

13. Rixen D, Raum M, Bouillon B, Lefering R, Neugebauer E (2001) Base deficit development and its prognostic significance in posttrauma critical illness: an analysis by the trauma registry of the Deutsche Gesellschaft fur Unfallchirurgie. Shock 15: 83–89

14. Larsson E (1993) Diary from the war in Somalia. "One gets so tired of all the gunshot wounds". Vardfacket 17: 36–38

15. Coupland R (1999) Clinical and legal significance of fragmentation of bullets in relation to size of wounds: retrospective analysis. BMJ 319: 403–406

16. Coupland RM (1989) Technical aspects of war wound excision. Br J Surg 76: 663–667

17. Coupland RM (1992) The Red Cross classification of war wounds: the E.X.C.F.V.M. scoring system. World J Surg 16: 910–917

18. Bowyer GW, Stewart MP, Ryan JM (1993) Gulf war wounds: application of the Red Cross wound classification. Injury 24: 597–600

19. Bowyer GW (1996) Management of small fragment wounds: experience from the Afghan border. J Trauma 40: S170–172

20. Bowyer GW, Cooper GJ, Rice P (1996) Small fragment wounds: biophysics and pathophysiology. J Trauma 40: S159–164

21. Dahlgren B, Berlin R, Brandberg A, Rybeck B, Seeman T (1981) Bacteriological findings in the first 12 hours following experimental missile trauma. Acta Chir Scand 147: 513–518

22. Simchen E, Sacks T (1975) Infection in war wounds: experience during the 1973 October War in Israel. Ann Surg 182: 754–761

23. Peters KM, Zilkens KW, Bartsch C (1992) Treatment of osteomyelitis and reconstructive measures in patients with war injuries. Aktuelle Traumatol 22: 72–75

24. Simchen E, Raz R, Stein H, Danon Y (1991) Risk factors for infection in fracture war wounds (1973 and 1982 wars, Israel). Mil Med 156: 520–527

25. Mellor SG, Cooper GJ, Bowyer GW (1996) Efficacy of delayed administration of benzylpenicillin in the control of infection in penetrating soft tissue injuries in war. J Trauma 40: S128–134

26. Czymk KR, Lenz S, Duesel W (1999) Prevention of infection in war wounds. Chirurg 70: 1156–1162

27. Hell K (1991) Characteristics of the ideal antibiotic for prevention of wound sepsis among military forces in the field. Rev Infect Dis 13 [Suppl 2]: S164–169

28. Jacob E, Setterstrom JA (1989) Infection in war wounds: experience in recent military conflicts and future considerations. Mil Med 154: 311–315

29. Coupland RM (1991) The role of reconstructive surgery in the management of war wounds. Ann R Coll Surg Engl 73: 21–25

30. Stanec Z, Skrbic S, Dzepina I et al. (1993) High-energy war wounds: flap reconstruction. Ann Plast Surg 31: 97–102

31. Stanec Z, Skrbic S, Dzepina I et al. (1994) The management of war wounds to the extremities. Scand J Plast Reconstr Surg Hand Surg 28: 39–44

32. Dzepina I, Stanec Z, Skrbic S et al. (1997) One-stage reconstruction of war wounds with free osteocutaneous flaps. Br J Plast Surg 50: 81–87

33. Ordog GJ, Balasubramanium S, Wasserberger J (1983) Outpatient management of 357 gunshot wounds to the chest. J Trauma 23: 832–835

34. Brusov PG, Kuritsyn AN, Urazovsky NY, Tariverdiev ML (1998) Operative videothoracoscopy in the surgical treatment of penetrating firearms wounds of the chest. Mil Med 163: 603–607

35. Eiseman B, Moore EE, Meldrum DR, Raeburn C (2000) Feasibility of damage control surgery in the management of military combat casualties. Arch Surg 135: 1323–1327

36. Rossi P, Mullins D, Thal E (1993) Role of laparoscopy in the evaluation of abdominal trauma. Am J Surg 166: 707–710; discussion 710–711

37. Fabian TC, Croce MA, Stewart RM, Pritchard FE, Minard G, Kudsk KA (1993) A prospective analysis of diagnostic laparoscopy in trauma. Ann Surg 217: 557–564; discussion 564–565

38. Thal ER, Rossi PJ (1996) The role of laparoscopy in the evaluation of abdominal trauma. Semin Laparosc Surg 3: 178–184

39. Fabian TC (1993) Prevention of infections following penetrating abdominal trauma. Am J Surg 165: 14S–19S

40. Saric D, Tudor M, Grandic L, Juricic J, Resic A, Tripkovic A (2001) [Penetrating combat injuries of the colorectal region]. Chirurg 72: 425–432

41. Rowley DI (1996) The management of war wounds involving bone. J Bone Joint Surg Br 78: 706–709
42. Coupland RM (1989) Amputation for antipersonnel mine injuries of the leg: preservation of the tibial stump using a medial gastrocnemius myoplasty. Ann R Coll Surg Engl 71: 405–408
43. Reis ND, Zinman C, Besser MI, Shifrin LZ, Rosen H (1991) A philosophy of limb salvage in war: use of the fixateur externe. Mil Med 156: 505–520
44. Degiannis E, Levy RD, Hatzitheofilou C, Florizoone MG, Saadia R (1996) Gunshot arterial injuries to the groin: comparison of iliac and femoral injuries. Injury 27: 315–318
45. Gosselin RA, Siegberg CJ, Coupland R, Agerskov K (1993) Outcome of arterial repairs in 23 consecutive patients at the ICRC-Peshawar hospital for war wounded. J Trauma 34: 373–376
46. Radonic V, Baric D, Tudor M, Bill B, Kovacevic H, Glavina-Durdov M (1995) [Vascular injuries in war]. Chirurg 66: 883–886

# Animal and Human Bite Wounds

K. Shokrollahi, P.E. Banwell, O.C.S. Cassell

## Introduction

Bite wounds are serious injuries irrespective of the initial degree of trauma caused. One of the contributory factors to poor outcome after minor bites, for example, is commonly a delay in presentation. This is often because injuries may initially seem relatively minor or insignificant. However, the risk of severe infection is high and may result in significant tissue loss or amputation of digits unless treated expediently. Below we highlight important aspects in the management of bites in relation to the most common types of injury, concentrating on presentation, assessment and indications for hospital admission or surgical intervention.

## Classification

Any useful description of a bite injury will include:
- the source of the bite e.g. human or animal;
- the site of bite, most commonly the hand, face and head;
- the type or mechanism of injury, which is particularly relevant in injuries to the hand;
- the time of injury.

Each of the features outlined above has important implications with regards to management. As such, some have warranted consideration and discussion in isolation, in articles on cat bites or human bites to the hand, for example. However, a general understanding of basic principles should provide the basis for management of most of these injuries.

## Presenting Features

Domestic animals, usually cats or dogs, are the most common cause of animal bites. However, on a global scale, the possible perpetrators of such injuries are almost endless (Fig. 1). Appropriate advice regarding microbiology, and sometimes toxicology in situations of possible envenomation, should be sought if necessary.

The anatomical site of injury will have implications with regard to function and cosmesis, and appropriate referral for specialist surgical input.

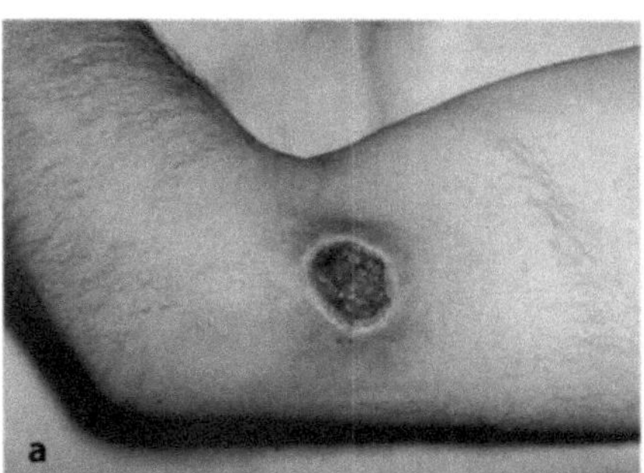 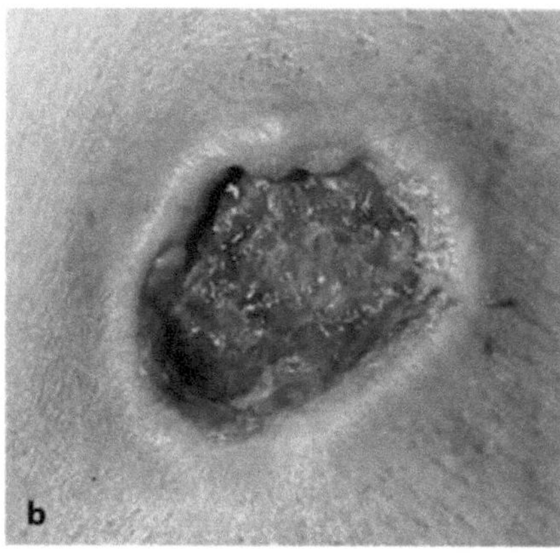

**Fig. 1a,b.** Bite to the arm from a zebra suffered by a doctor on Safari. Such wounds will benefit from surgical debridement and washout after initial microbiological swabs are taken. If possible, antimicrobial treatment should be withheld until swabs and debrided tissue are sent for analysis. If prior antibiotic therapy has been commenced, detailed information regarding the type and duration of therapy should be forwarded to the microbiologist who may be able to maximise the chance of successful culture by the addition of antibiotic inhibitors such as beta-lactamase

A number of common patterns of bite injury exists, each of which has specific implications. Major bite injuries can result in significant tissue damage or loss, and can be immediately life-threatening either if the victim is a small child, a particularly dangerous animal is involved, or a vital structure is damaged. Amputation of digits or facial structures such as ears or nose are also common. Human bites tend to occur most commonly amongst young adults or very young children.

Bites to the hand occur in a number of forms. Any open injury around the metacarpophalangeal joints of the hand should have a high index of suspicion of being punch injuries and thus treated as such. We have not qualified this statement with "unless proven otherwise", because this proof is rarely attainable if patients do not proffer details. Infection in the joint can destroy articular cartilage within hours. Overlying extensor tendons are often inoculated and retract proximally during relaxation of the fist grip, preventing adequate reduction of the microbial load by simple lavage of the original wound.

Similar dispersion of bacteria occurs in even minor bite injuries which involve a deep inoculation, such as can occur during a cat or dog bite. The long syringe-like penetration breaching the tendon sheath can result in proximal spread of infection affecting the whole hand (Fig. 2). It is important to differentiate these tendon sheath infections from superficial cellulitis or abscess, as treatment of the former requires surgical intervention for thorough lavage of the tendon sheath.

As well as simple inoculation of micro-organisms, penetrating injuries from teeth can result in significant injury to underlying structures, such as blood vessels, nerves or tendons. Again, retraction of tendons can mean that surgical exploration is the only means of ensuring structural integrity.

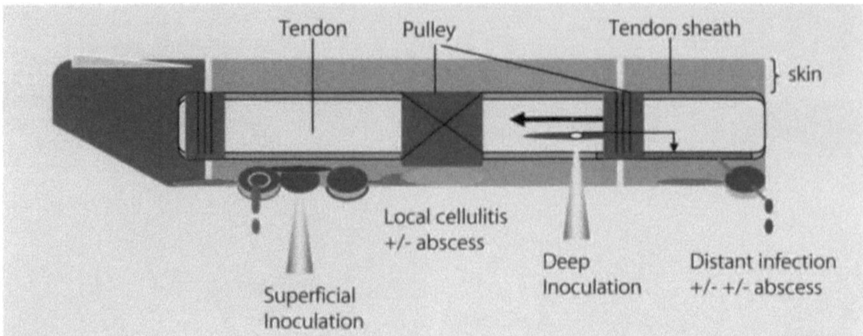



**Fig. 2.** Schematic diagram of inoculation style bite injury to volar aspect of a digit. Deeper injuries that breach the tendon sheath can cause early infection to spread proximally or distally within this space. More superficial injuries can cause a spreading cellulitis or local abscess, which will involve the tendon sheath only if treatment is delayed or inappropriate

Fractures associated with bite wounds are prone to complication from osteomyelitis, and such injuries must be taken seriously. Osteomyelitis can also be a serious complication of bites to the head, which must also be treated with due vigilance.

## Considerations in the History

A number of features in the history are important with regards to management of these injuries. Table 1 below highlights specific points of note, and the implications of these.

## Examination and Investigation

The objectives of assessment include:
- making decisions about hospital admission,
- the aggressiveness of planned management strategy,
- producing a good quality and accurate record of the incident and patient episode.

Principles of examination include assessment of all areas affected for depth of injury, degree of tissue loss, remaining tissue viability and evidence of infection. In addition, special areas will need more detailed inspection. In Fig. 1, we have already discussed the implications of tendon sheath infections of the hand. Figure 3 is a

**Table 1.** History and implications in bite injuries

| | History | Implications |
|---|---|---|
| **History of presenting complaint** | Time of injury | Delayed presentation without signs of infection may potentially be treated conservatively. Early presentation may need more aggressive treatment to prevent infection |
| | Place of injury | Endemic infections e.g. rabies, MRSA |
| | Mechanism of injury | Implications for spread of infection in hand injuries |
| | Source of bite | Selection of antibiotics, patterns of injury, cross infection with hepatitis B or HIV virus |
| | Hand injury – position of hand at time of injury (i.e. flexion or extension) | Wound inspection and cleansing, decisions regarding exploration or admission, and ascertaining possible location of tendon injuries |
| | Possibility of foreign body (tooth) | May require imaging, will require extraction |
| **Past medical history** | Diabetes mellitus | Effects on wound healing and infection. Assessment of peripheral nerve injury may be more difficult in the presence of neuropathy |
| | Hepatitis/HIV status | Cross-infection risk in human bites (all parties) |
| | Arthritis or presence of orthopaedic implants | Presence of joint replacements or other metalwork underlying bite wounds may necessitate removal, prolonged antibiotic treatment or prophylaxis. Rheumatoid joints may be more prone to sepsis, compounded by concurrent immunosuppressants |
| | Cardiac history | Valvular heart disease and the presence of prosthetic valves may be an indication for prolonged intravenous antibiotics, and vigilance for endocarditis |
| | General health/other medical conditions | Anaesthetic considerations |
| **Drug history** | Immunosuppressant drugs and steroids | Impaired wound healing and increased likelihood of infection |
| | Antibiotics | Detailed history of which antibiotics have been taken including duration of treatment and response to treatment will be valuable (1) in guiding further therapy and (2) for microbiologists when culturing tissue samples or wound swabs |

**Table 1.** *Continued*

| | History | Implications |
|---|---|---|
| **Drug history** | Analgesics | Analgesic requirements are a good indicator of pain, which may suggest injuries are more severe than initial appearances. This may be particularly the case with flexor tendon sheath infections |
| | Renal impairment | Many antibiotics are nephrotoxic |
| **Social History** | Occupation | General management decisions |
| | Handedness | Consideration for aggressiveness of treatment when balancing risks with benefits of reconstruction type |
| | Smoking | Implications for success of reconstructive options |
| **Allergies** | Antibiotics | Spurious or doubtful allergies to penicillins may be a difficult problem. In the absence of a history of anaphylaxis in a penicillin allergy, a cephalosporin may be an alternative in appropriate cases, as cross-reactivity is approximately only 15% |
| | Dressings | Allergies to dressings can simulate ongoing infection, often with significant erythema or discharge from a wound. Monitoring of inflammatory markers may help in diagnosis, and frequent wound swabs will often be sterile |
| **General considerations** | Tetanus immunisation | All patients should have appropriate cover for tetanus. In the absence of any previous immunisation, cover with immune globulin will be required with a formal course of immunisation after 3 months |

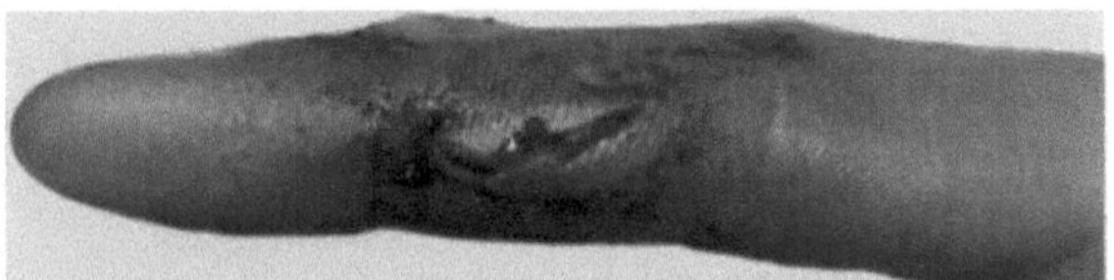

**Fig. 3.** Photograph of a dog bite to the index finger. Principles of management include debridement and washout with delayed primary closure or healing by secondary intention. Thorough clinical examination is required to assess for signs of flexor sheath infection if presentation has been delayed. Such signs are fusiform swelling, flexed posture painful passive extension of the finger and tenderness along the flexor sheath proximally

photograph of a dog bite to the index finger, which can be compared to the schematic one in Fig. 1. This injury has the potential to involve the radial digital nerve, the radial digital artery and the flexor tendon, and appropriate knowledge of the underlying anatomy and relevant techniques of physical and neurological examination is important in the assessment of any such injury.

Similarly, Fig. 4 shows a child who has suffered dog bites to the face. In such cases consideration should be given to the underlying anatomical structures including the facial nerve and parotid duct. Other facial structures, particularly the nose or ears, require specialist input. Bacterial chondritis of cartilaginous structures in the ear or nose can be severe and lead to significant deformity. Such injuries must be assessed carefully, as aggressive treatment with close observation may be required.

Plain radiographs can assist in locating foreign bodies, or in diagnosis of septic arthritis or osteomyelitis. However, radiographic changes, such as a marked periosteal reaction or osteopoenia, occur late in cases of bone infection. The presence of sequestra of dead bone within a surrounding involucrum is a late sign of on-going or previous osteomyelitis that will require debridement to clear the source of harboured bacteria. In early stages, treatment must be guided by clinical suspicion or more detailed investigation such as a bone scan or CT/MRI alone or in combination. If appropriate, samples of bone should be sent for microbiological culture at time of debridement. Ultrasonography may also be useful in assessment of soft-tissue injury, such as tendon injuries or differentiating generalised soft-tissue swelling from an underlying abscess.

Routine phlebotomy is useful for monitoring trends of inflammatory markers, but these should not be interpreted in isolation after surgical intervention, as there is an inevitable rise in these markers for a variable period post-operatively.

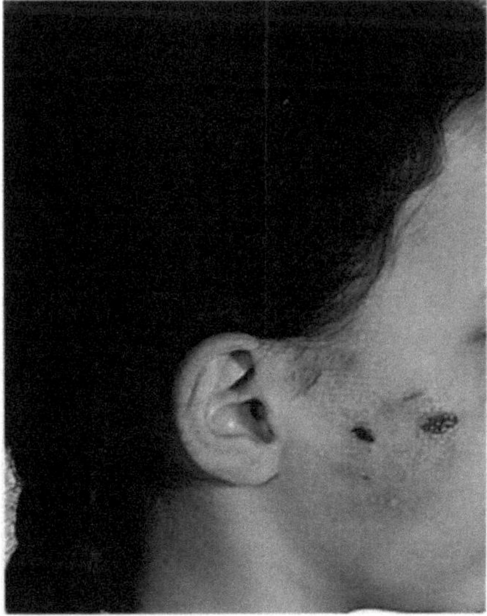

**Fig. 4.** Thorough washout and debridement with primary closure of uncomplicated facial lacerations is acceptable, but early and regular follow-up is required, and antibiotic prophylaxis recommended. Exclusion of injury to underlying structures such as the facial nerve or parotid duct is necessary

A diagram of injuries sustained including functional assessment and depth is the best practice. This is particularly important with the not uncommon scenario of multiple lacerations. In certain circumstances, legal action will ensue against the person (or pet owner) responsible for the bite injury, and good-quality records will be invaluable in such cases.

## Microbiology

Griego and colleagues report the incidence of infection after human bites to be between 10 and 50%, cat bites from between 30 and 50% and dog bites up to 20% [4]. The majority of human and animal bite wounds culture a mixture of aerobic and anaerobic organisms, mainly *Staphylococcus aureus*, Peptostreptococci and *Bacteroides* species.

The majority of organisms causing infection will originate from the oral cavity of the animal or human responsible for the bite. Many of these organisms are anaerobes, the most common being bacteroides. However, there are a number of less common, although classical, organisms associated with bites that will require inclusion for antimicrobial cover. These include *Pasteurella* and *Eikenella* species.

| Potential Pathogenic Anaerobes from the Oral Cavity |
|---|
| *Bacteroides* spp. |
| *Prevotella* spp. |
| *Porphyromonas* spp. |
| *Peptostreptococcus* spp. |
| *Pasteurella multocida* |
| *Eikenella corrodens* |
| *Bartonella henselae* |
| *Capnocytophaga canimorsus* |

This spectrum of organisms is usually covered well with combination therapy using cephalosporins (such as cefotaxime or cefuroxime) and metronidazole or monotherapy with amoxycillin-clavulanic acid. However, a large number of alternatives exist, and local antibiotic guidelines may be in place. Resistant organisms, such as *Eikenella*, will require more aggressive therapy. Intravenous treatment is recommended for complicated infections such as involving the ear, deep infections of the hand or wounds requiring surgical debridement or washout.

If possible, treatment should be delayed to allow wound swabs and tissue samples to be sent for culture.

## Management

Major bites or bites that affect vital structures can be immediately life-threatening. Therefore, the basic principles of acute trauma management should be followed as appropriate.

After major injury has been dealt with or excluded, prevention of infection and achieving optimal cosmetic and functional outcome are the prime objectives. Anti-tetanus immunoglobulin may be required to confer passive immunity to those inadequately or unreliably covered against tetanus. It should be remembered that an ensuing course of tetanus immunisation will require a delay of a number of months to be effective.

Amputated or avulsed digits will need to be transported correctly if replantation is an option. This involves carriage in a container of iced water whilst wrapped in a damp gauze within a plastic bag. Direct contact with ice or immersion in fluid is to be avoided at all cost. Even if replantation is not viable, tissue such as skin or tendon may be useful for reconstruction. In children, especially, composite tissue grafts of amputated tissue such as fingertips are often successfully replanted.

When injuries require referral to other specialists, it is important to undertake as much of the basic treatment of the wound as is possible. Treatment can be significantly delayed at a tertiary referral centre due to transfer time and workload. It is therefore essential that wounds are cleaned and dressed appropriately prior to transfer, as this will have a significant impact on the likelihood of infection.

## Operative Considerations

The objectives of surgical management include:
- debridement of devitalised, infected or non-viable tissue,
- drainage of any pus,
- collection of microbiological specimens,
- removal of foreign bodies (teeth),
- copious lavage,
- primary wound closure (in non-infected wounds, e.g. on face),
- delayed wound closure (infected wounds),
- reconstructive surgery (skin grafts, local flaps or more complex reconstruction).

Surgical debridement may require more than one visit to the operating theatre, and attempts at primary closure of infected wounds will be unsuccessful (Fig. 5). Although many wounds will heal by secondary intention without formal closure, closure is usually possible when the wound is clean and will produce a better cosmetic, and sometimes functional, result.

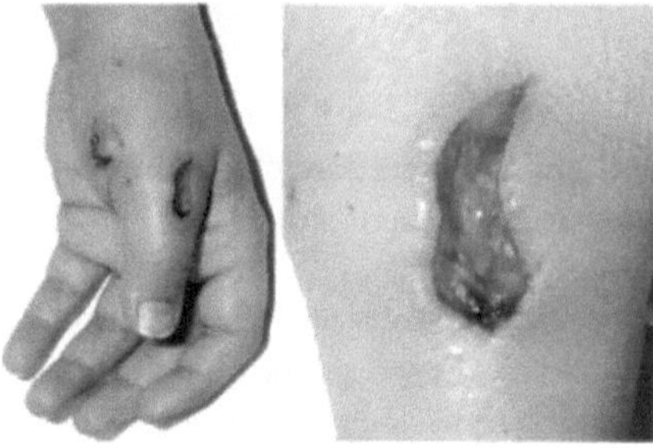

**Fig. 5.** Cat bites to the hand. These have been debrided surgically, as evidenced by the surgical appearance of the wounds. Further debridement is required, as necrotic tissue remains. When the wound is adequately debrided and washed, delayed primary closure can then be undertaken

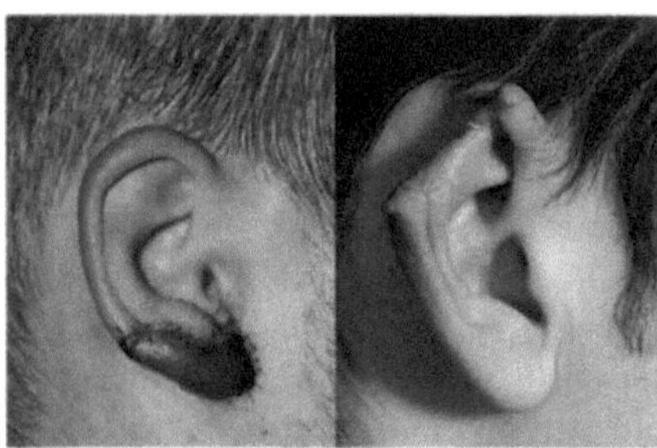

**Fig. 6.** Injuries to the lower pole of the ear (*left*) have a better prognosis in terms of cosmesis due to the wider and simpler range of reconstructive options – here using a local tissue flap. The cosmetic outcome from upper pole injuries is worse, and reconstructive options more limited. Reconstruction should be delayed until such time as wounds are fully healed and all signs of infection are cleared

Reconstructive options will depend on the nature of the injury. Areas of tissue loss on the lower limbs not amenable to primary closure can often be skin-grafted. This is less acceptable on the face due to poor cosmetic outcome. Figure 6 illustrates the outcome after injuries to opposite poles of the ear. The lower pole defect has been covered with a local tissue flap, whereas the upper pole defect has been closed over with adjacent skin as a completion of partial amputation. Reconstruction in this area or for substantial tissue loss from the nose is challenging.

## Summary

Key points in the assessment and management of bite wounds include:
- full assessment of soft tissue and possible underlying bone/joint injury,
- full assessment of the presence or risk of infection,
- adequate surgical debridement and lavage as appropriate,
- appropriate anti-microbial therapy or prophylaxis,
- effective wound closure, wound reconstruction or provision of suitable environment for effective wound healing.

**Acknowledgements.** Department of Medical Illustration, Radcliffe Infirmary, Oxford

## References

1. Dire DJ (1992) Cat bite wounds: risk factors for infection. Ann Emerg Med 21: 1008
2. Bowler PG, Duerden BI, Armstrong DG (2001) Wound microbiology and associated approaches to wound management. Clin Microbiol Rev 14: 244–269
3. Kelly IP, Cunney RJ, Smyth EG et al. (1996) The management of human bite injuries of the hand. Injury 27: 481–484
4. Griego RD, Rosen T, Orengo IF, Wolf JE (1995) Dog, cat and human bites: a review. J Am Acad Dermatol 33: 1019–1029
5. Brook I (1987) Microbiology of human and animal bite wounds in children. Paediatr Infect Dis J 6: 29–32
6. Fleischer GRN (1999) The management of bite wounds. Engl J Med 340: 138–140
7. Periti P, Tonelli F, Mini E (1998) Selecting antibacterial agents for the control of surgical infection. J Chemother 10: 83–90

# Enterocutaneous Fistulae

A.C.J. Windsor

## Definition

Enterocutaneous fistulae are, by definition, abnormal communications between the gastrointestinal tract and the skin, and are associated with regional sepsis, which may be minimal as long-standing established fistulae mature.

## Aetiology

Enterocutaneous fistulae usually occur in the setting of antecedent surgery, although inflammatory bowel disease, diverticulitis, radiotherapy, trauma, ischaemic bowel or malignancy commonly contribute [1–5, 31]. Patients undergoing surgery in the setting of Crohn's disease or radiation enteritis are at the highest risk of developing enterocutaneous fistulae, and the anterior abdominal wall is the most frequent external site of fistulation [6, 7]. Distal intestinal obstruction, persistent local sepsis or inflammation, ischaemia or local neoplasia all play important roles in the persistence of fistulae [8–12]. The incidence of enterocutaneous fistulae remains unclear, although it is not an uncommon problem, and tertiary referral centres have reported large series of patients [13, 14]. Approximately 15% of all Crohn's patients will develop enterocutaneous fistulae, with only 15% of these occurring spontaneously [4].

## Classification

Enterocutaneous fistulae are classified with regard to the gastrointestinal anatomical site of origin, volume of effluent output (with a high-output fistula being regarded as a loss of at least 500 ml of enteric content over 24 h), and complexity (with complex fistulae involving multiple bowel loops or an abscess) [5, 15]. In addition, fistulae may be single or multiple. Their classification helps determine treatment and prognosis, and patients with simple low-output fistulae experience lower mortality and higher closure rates [4]. However, physiological classification into low- and high-output fistulae can be the source of confusion. Whilst an output of 500 ml or more may well lead to significant metabolic disturbance, it should not necessarily mandate parenteral support or nil per os. Many patients with simple ileostomies will experience such outputs and manage without medical intervention, and patients with outputs up to 1500 ml per day can be managed enterally on a strict short-bowel regimen in certain circumstances.

## Investigations

Radiological water-soluble contrast studies in real time are effective at delineating fistulae, allowing fistula classification and planning of future surgical intervention [16]. Antegrade and retrograde studies are often required in order to fully visualise the fistula and to exclude additional intestinal disease and distal obstruction, and to establish the anatomy of unaffected bowel [17]. Useful contrast studies include follow-through studies, contrast enemas, stomography (antegrade and retrograde) and fistulograms (where contrast is introduced via a fine catheter held in place with a small balloon), although all should be delayed until the patient is medically stable. Intra-abdominal abscesses are best assessed using computed tomography (CT) scanning or ultrasonography, which are important in the assessment of the sick patient to direct drainage of foci of sepsis [18–21]. Magnetic resonance imaging (MRI) is gaining more widespread use in the imaging of fistulating disease as it has a high sensitivity for demonstrating sepsis [17, 22, 23]. Its use to visualise the abdominal cavity is, however, limited by visceral and diaphragmatic movement, and its role is more useful within the pelvis.

## Clinical Picture

Favourable outcome relies on early control of sepsis, adequate nutritional support and skin protection [24–26]. A proportion of fistulae will close spontaneously if these issues are addressed adequately, although reported healing rates vary widely from 15% to greater than 80%, most likely reflecting differing patient populations with differing fistula aetiologies [27–32, 43]. Malnutrition and sepsis must be addressed if a fistula is to close without surgical intervention, and active inflammatory bowel disease, regional neoplasia or inadequate blood supply such as in radiation enteritis, are all factors making fistula healing and closure unlikely. Anatomical variables also play a role in spontaneous closure, with distal obstruction or lumen discontinuity precluding healing. Wound maturation resulting in mucocutaneous continuity is another factor preventing closure.

## Treatment

### Non-Operative Treatment

*Fluid and Electrolyte Balance*

Fluid and electrolyte depletion are life-threatening, and can be of rapid onset and difficult to control in high-output fistulae. Big fluid volumes, comprising several litres per day, may require replacement, and careful records of inputs and losses must be maintained. Sick patients with high-output fistulae are often not easily weighed, and measures of urinary sodium loss can be a useful measure of hydration (less than 30 mmol/l is indicative of dehydration).

Losses can be minimised using a treatment regime comprising proton pump inhibitors to reduce gastrointestinal secretions, high doses of loperamide and codeine to slow transit times, separating the intake of liquids and solids by at least an hour (to reduce the osmolarity of the lumen contents) and using oral glucose electrolyte replacement solution [33]. Electrolyte replacement solution comprises 2.5% glucose and 90 mmol/l sodium, and promotes fluid absorption in the proximal small bowel (Fig. 1) [34]. Any oral intake of fluid with a lower sodium concentration results in jejunal loss of sodium, followed by water, resulting in a loss of body fluid (this would be reabsorbed distally in bowel not short-circuited by a fistula) [35]. One litre of electrolyte solution is usually given over 24 h, and the intake of other oral fluids restricted to 500–1000 ml depending on outputs. Loperamide should be given approximately 30 min prior to eating. Octeotride may be useful in reducing losses, but should be continued only if a significant response is observed within 48 h of commencing treatment [25].

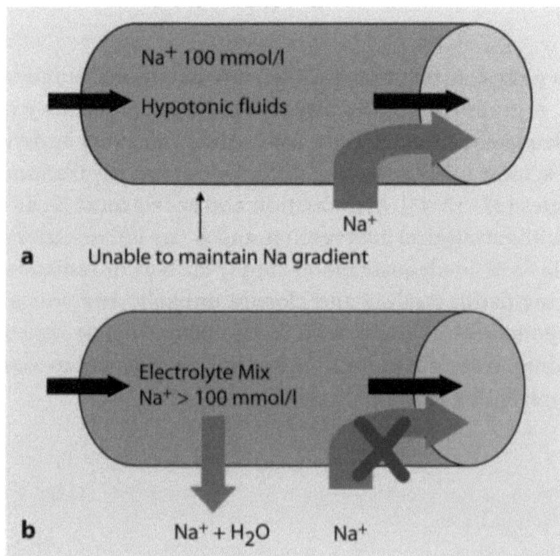


**Fig. 1a,b.** The use of electrolyte solution to prevent loss of sodium ions from the gut. **a** Rehydrating with water. **b** Rehydrating with electrolyte solution

Electrolyte losses require regular monitoring, and magnesium depletion is a common problem in patients with high-output fistulae [36]. In addition to cardiac dysrhythmias, hypomagnesaemia causes disabling symptoms of muscle cramping (tetany) and requires correction before calcium (and sometimes potassium) levels can be corrected [37]. Other electrolytes commonly lost in fistulating disease include sodium and potassium. Excessive loss of bicarbonate from the upper gastrointestinal tract may result in a metabolic acidosis, although this is usually corrected by restoring fluid balance. Sick patients with severe acidosis sometimes require IV bicarbonate replacement however.

Apart from fluids and electrolytes, trace elements and vitamins, such as vitamin $B_{12}$, vitamin D, iron and zinc, are likely to become depleted if significant lengths of intestine are bypassed by fistulae, and these should be measured and replaced accordingly.

### Nutrition

Nutritional support is of great importance in patients with enterocutaneous fistulae. It facilitates more rapid healing and maintains immune function, thereby helping to prevent sepsis, especially in the setting of prolonged non-operative management [32, 38]. Fistula output decreases, and spontaneous closure and mortality rates are improved with nutritional support [27, 39–43]. Many patients require parenteral nutrition, particularly in the early phase of treatment, as they have high calorific requirements that cannot be met by enteric feeding [45]. Careful avoidance of feeding-line sepsis is a key factor [44]. Many will subsequently be able to meet nutritional requirements by enteral feeding, although supplementary parenteral nutrition is sometimes needed long-term [46]. Enteral feeding plays an important role in immune-system preservation and the prevention of bacterial translocation, and should be adopted as soon as it is practical [47, 48]. Enteric feeding has a trophic effect upon the bowel, preventing mucosal atrophy [49]. It also promotes gastrointestinal neurotransmitter release, stimulating mucosal lymphoid tissue (MALT) to produce immunoglobulins, giving immunity against viruses, bacteria and endotoxins [50–52]. Conversely, mucosal malnutrition promotes easier translocation of bacteria, contributing to sepsis [49]. Protein loss through malnutrition contributes to overall loss of immune function efficacy [53, 54].

### Sepsis

Patient outcome has been shown to improve with nutritional support, but it is the control of sepsis which determines survival and is the key to the observed falling mortality rates [43]. Early and aggressive surgery is needed to treat collections or facilitate satisfactory fistula drainage, and is important to prevent overwhelming systemic sepsis [55]. This can sometimes be achieved by the use of interventional radiology [56]. The respiratory tract, urinary tract and feeding lines are other important sites of sepsis, and it is paramount to identify and treat these sources quickly, using appropriate radiological investigation, culturing all sites of potential infection, and discontinuing parenteral feeding until feeding line cultures are proven to be negative. Antibiotics are not routinely required for enterocutaneous fistulae, unless a patient develops systemic sepsis or has a proven site of infection amenable to antibiotic therapy. Patients with a severe systemic inflammatory response may require prolonged intensive-care-unit support in order to manage organ failure, particularly in the form of cardiovascular and/or respiratory support.

### Wound Care

Small-bowel effluent contains digestive enzymes and is corrosive, resulting in auto-digestion and destruction of the skin surrounding the fistula, and causing severe discomfort [57].

The principle of wound management of enterocutaneous fistulae comprises protection of the surrounding skin for comfort and to facilitate healing, and the collection of effluent to allow accurate fluid-balance measurement [58]. Skin protection can be achieved using a variety of skin barriers, adhesives and wound-drainage bags [59–61]. This allows containment and drainage of effluent, and provides a means of facilitating patient mobility, rest and comfort. Wound-drainage bags are able to be connected to drainage tubing in dependent positions, leading to collection bottles. Skin protection is best afforded using adhesive barriers such as Stomahesive, Granuflex or Comfeel sheets, and creases can be filled with Stomahesive paste, providing a watertight seal. A large bag can then be tailored to cover all bowel openings, or, alternatively, additional appliances can be used to cover areas remote from the wound such as mucus fistulae. Areas of healthy skin or granulation tissue contained within a wound-management bag can be protected using a variety of materials including Orobase or Granuflex paste. Healthy skin is best cleaned using warm water and dried using a cool hairdryer, before a new appliance is reapplied, and suction is often needed while attending to the fistula wound [61, 62]. These measures can be labour-intensive, requiring the involvement of specialist nurses, with some patients with high-output complex fistulae requiring up to 2 h of wound care performed by two nurses on a long-term daily basis, although the frequency and duration can be expected to decrease as the fistula wound matures.

### Operative Treatment

The role of early surgery is confined to drainage of radiologically undrainable collections and urgent proximal diversion in situations where it is impossible to protect the skin (Fig. 2). Definitive surgical management or reconstruction is performed only after restitution of normal physiology, usually after up to 6 months. This strategy reduces mortality, as critically unwell patients tolerate major procedures poorly, and even allows spontaneous closure of the fistula in many cases [63]. The cutaneous aspect of a fistula may heal disproportionately quickly, resulting in premature closure and a flare up of sepsis due to inadequate drainage, and minor surgery to prevent this is sometimes important. If the skin heals with a significant residual fistula tract in situ, a collection or fistula recurrence is likely. A significant proportion of spontaneous closures can reoccur for this reason [64].

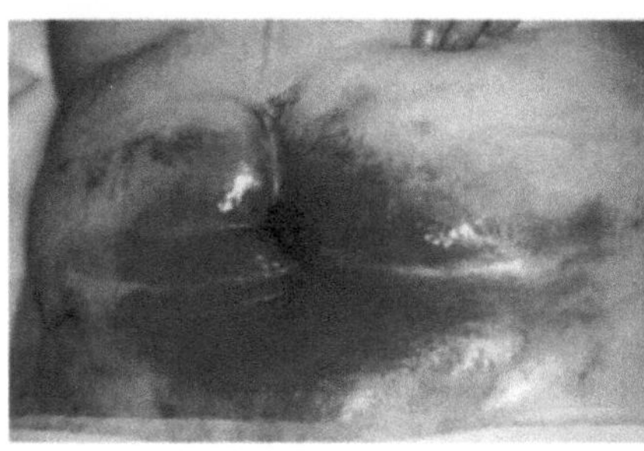

**Fig. 2.** Uncontrolled fistula effluent leading to significant cutaneous injury. Proximal diversion may be the only method of control

Definitive surgery comprises laparotomy, en-bloc resection of the involved bowel and overlying skin and anastomosis, often with temporary defunctioning [13, 65]. It is important to allow time for the fistulae to mature, and for inflammation within the remainder of the peritoneal cavity to resolve, as well as ensuring that the patient is free of residual sepsis and that nutrition has been optimised. A sign that enough time has elapsed is the return of a "soft" abdomen, with induration being limited to the perifistula region only. Re-anastomosis should be performed only between healthy ends of bowel, to minimise the chance of re-fistulation. The rate of re-fistulation can be high, and repeated operations over a number of months or years may be required to achieve fistula healing. Abdominal wall closure can be difficult after fistula excision, particularly if a laparostomy wound was associated with it. If fascial apposition can be achieved, closure is best facilitated using "near-far" interrupted sutures and, if not, an absorbable mesh may be required. Rarely, the abdominal wall has to be left open after excision and re-anastomosis. Non-absorbable mesh should not be considered, due to the high rates of wound infections occurring in these patients post-operatively. Incision and drainage of abdominal wall sepsis is not uncommonly required subsequently, and incisional hernias often result, which may require later repair.

## Survival and Follow-up

Enterocutaneous fistulae have traditionally had a high morbidity and mortality, related to sepsis, malnutrition and fluid, electrolyte or metabolic disturbances [25]. Mortality rates as high as 65% have previously been reported [1]. Overall mortality rates have, however, improved significantly over the past three decades, falling from greater than 30% to approximately 10% [13, 14, 43, 66–68]. Strict adherence to early recognition and control of sepsis, management of fluid and electrolyte imbalances, attentive wound care and the delay of definitive surgery for up to 6 months has resulted in the improvement, as well as advances in intensive-care therapy and nutritional support.

Patients who survive and have healing of the fistulae are unlikely to have further problems, unless the underlying disease process dictates otherwise, such as those with malignancy or aggressive Crohn's disease.

## References

1. Edmunds LH, Williams GM, Welch CE (1960) External fistulas arising from the gastrointestinal tract. Ann Surg 153: 445–771

2. West JP, Ring EM, Miller RE, Burks WP (1961) A study of the causes and treatment of external post operative intestinal fistulas. Surg Gynaecol Obstet 113: 490–496

3. Halversen RC, Hogle HH, Richards RC (1969) Gastric and small bowel fistulas. Am J Surg 118: 968–972

4. Rinsema W, Gouma DJ, von Meyenfeldt MF, van der Linden CJ, Soeters PB (1990) Primary conservative management of external small-bowel fistulas. Changing composition of fistula series? Acta Chir Scand 156: 457–462

5. Berry SM, Fischer JE (1996) Classification and pathophysiology of enterocutaneous fistulas. Surg Clin North Am 76: 1009–1018

6. Harling H, Balslev I (1988) Long-term prognosis of patients with severe radiation enteritis. Am J Surg 155: 517–519

7. Kelly JK, Preshaw RM (1989) Origin of fistulas in Crohn's disease. J Clin Gastroenterol 11: 193–196

8. Deitel M (1976) Nutritional management of external gastrointestinal fistulas. Can J Surg 19: 505–509

9. Thomas RJ (1981) The response of patients with fistulas of the gastrointestinal tract to parenteral nutrition. Surg Gynecol Obstet 153: 77–80

10. Hawker PC, Givel JC, Keighley MR, Alexander-Williams J, Allan RN (1983) Management of enterocutaneous fistulae in Crohn's disease. Gut 24: 284–287

11. Hugh TB, Coleman MJ, Cohen A (1986) Persistent postoperative enterocutaneous fistula: pathophysiology and treatment. Aust N Z J Surg 56: 901–906

12. Chamberlain RS, Kaufman HL, Danforth DN (1998) Enterocutaneous fistula in cancer patients: etiology, management, outcome, and impact on further treatment. Am Surg 64: 1204–1211

13. McIntyre PB, Ritchie JK, Hawley PR, Bartram CI, Lennard-Jones JE (1984) Management of enterocutaneous fistulas: a review of 132 cases. Br J Surg 71: 293–296

14. Lévy E, Frileux P, Cugnenc PH, Honiger J, Ollivier JM, Parc R (1989) High-output external fistulae of the small bowel: management with continuous enteral nutrition. Br J Surg 76: 676–679

15. Fischer JE (1983) The pathophysiology of enterocutaneous fistulas. World J Surg 7: 446–450

16. Alexander ES, Weinberg S, Clark RA, Belkin RD (1982) Fistulas and sinus tracts: radiographic evaluation, management, and outcome. Gastrointest Radiol 7: 135–140

17. Pickhardt PJ, Bhalla S, Balfe DM (2002) Acquired gastrointestinal fistulas: classification, etiologies, and imaging evaluation. Radiology 224: 9–23

18. Elyaderani MK, Skolnick ML, Weinstein BJ (1979) Ultrasonic detection and aspiration confirmation of intra-abdominal collection of fluid. Surg Gynecol Obstet 149: 529–533

19. Koehler PR, Knochel JQ (1980) Computed tomography in the evaluation of abdominal abscesses. Am J Surg 140: 675–678

20. Robison JG, Pollock TW (1980) Computed tomography in the diagnosis and localization of intraabdominal abscesses. Am J Surg 140: 783–786

21. Gandon Y, Mueller PR, Ferrucci JT (1989) Abscess and intra-abdominal fluid collections. Diagnosis and percutaneous drainage. J Radiol 70 : 235–247

22. Semelka RC, John G, Kelekis NL, Burdeny DA, Worawattanakul S, Ascher SM (1998) Bowel-related abscesses: MR demonstration preliminary results. Magn Res Imaging 16: 855–861

23. Rieber A, Aschoff A, Nussle K, Wruk D, Tomczak R, Reinshagen M, Adler G, Brambs HJ (2000) MRI in the diagnosis of small bowel disease: use of positive and negative oral contrast media in combination with enteroclysis. Eur Radiol 10: 1377–1382

24. Williams NM, Scott NA, Irving MH (1997) Successful management of external duodenal fistula in a specialised unit. Am J Surg 173: 240–241

25. Makhdoom ZA, Komar MJ, Still CD (2000) Nutrition and enterocutaneous fistulas. J Clin Gastroenterol 31: 195–204

26. West MAM (2000) Conservative and operative management of gastrointestinal fistulae in the critically ill patient. Curr Opin Crit Care 6: 143–147
27. Kaminsky VM, Deitel M (1975) Nutritional support in the management of external fistulas of the alimentary tract. Br J Surg 62: 100–103
28. Aguirre A, Fischer JE, Welch CE (1974) The role of surgery and hyperalimentation in therapy of gastrointestinal-cutaneous fistulae. Ann Surg 180: 393–401
29. Monod-Broca P (1977) Treatment of intestinal fistulas. Br J Surg 64: 685–689
30. Blackett RL, Hill GL (1978) Postoperative external small bowel fistulas: a study of a consecutive series of patients treated with intravenous hyperalimentation. Br J Surg 65: 775–778
31. Reber HA, Roberts C, Way LW, Dunphy JE (1978) Management of external gastrointestinal fistulas. Ann Surg 188: 460–467
32. Soeters PB, Ebeid AM, Fischer JE (1979) Review of 404 patients with gastrointestinal fistulas. Impact of parenteral nutrition. Ann Surg 190: 189–202
33. Nightingale JM (1999) Management of patients with a short bowel. Nutrition 15: 633–637
34. Nightingale JM, Lennard-Jones JE, Walker ER, Farthing MJ (1992) Oral salt supplements to compensate for jejunostomy losses: comparison of sodium chloride capsules, glucose electrolyte solution, and glucose polymer electrolyte solution. Gut 33: 759–761
35. Spiller RC, Jones BJ, Silk DB (1987) Jejunal water and electrolyte absorption from two proprietary enteral feeds in man: importance of sodium content. Gut 28: 681–687
36. Whang R (1984) Magnesium deficiency. Causes and clinical implications. Drugs 28 [Suppl 1]: 143–150
37. al-Ghamdi SM, Cameron EC, Sutton RA (1994) Magnesium deficiency: pathophysiologic and clinical overview. Am J Kidney Dis 24: 737–752
38. Dudrick SJ, Maharaj AR, McKelvey AA (1999) Artificial nutritional support in patients with gastrointestinal fistulas. World J Surg 23: 570–576
39. Chapman R, Foran R, Dunphy JE (1964) Management of intestinal fistulas. Am J Surg 108: 157–164
40. Wolfe BM, Keltner RM, Willman VL (1972) Intestinal fistula output in regular, elemental, and intravenous alimentation. Am J Surg 124: 803–806
41. Thomas RJ, Rosalion A (1978) The use of parenteral nutrition in the management of external gastrointestinal tract fistulae. Aust N Z J Surg 48: 535–539
42. Anonymous (1979) Nutritional management of entercutaneous fistulas. Lancet 2: 507–508
43. Sitges-Serra A, Jaurrieta E, Setges-Creus A (1982) Management of postoperative enterocutaneous fistulas: the roles of parenteral nutrition and surgery. Br J Surg 69: 147–150
44. Young GP, Alexeyeff M, Russell DM, Thomas RJ (1988) Catheter sepsis during parenteral nutrition: the safety of long-term OpSite dressings. JPEN J Parenter Enteral Nutr 12: 365–370
45. MacFadyen BV Jr, Dudrick SJ, Ruberg RL (1973) Management of gastrointestinal fistulas with parenteral hyperalimentation. Surgery 74: 100–105
46. Lévy E, Frileux P, Sandrucci S, Ollivier JM, Masini JP, Cosnes J, Hannoun L, Parc R (1988) Continuous enteral nutrition during the early adaptive stage of the short bowel syndrome. Br J Surg 75: 549–553
47. Gianotti L, Alexander JW, Nelson JL, Fukushima R, Pyles T, Chalk CL (1994) Role of early enteral feeding and acute starvation on postburn bacterial translocation and host defense: prospective, randomized trials. Crit Care Med 22: 265–272
48. Van Leeuwen PA, Boermeester MA, Houdijk AP, Ferwerda CC, Cuesta MA, Meyer S, Wesdorp RI (1994) Clinical significance of translocation. Gut 35 [Suppl]: S28–34
49. Lubke HJ (2000) Protection of the mucosal barrier by nutritional strategies. What are the therapeutic options? Anaesthesist 49: 455–459
50. Stechmiller JK, Treloar D, Allen N (1997) Gut dysfunction in critically ill patients: a review of the literature. Am J Crit Care 6: 204–209
51. Stallmach A, Zeitz M (1998) The intestine as an immunological organ. Wien Klin Wochenschr 110: 72–78
52. Bengmark S (1999) Gut microenvironment and immune function. Curr Opin Clin Nutr Metab Care 2: 83–85
53. Daly JM, Reynolds J, Sigal RK, Shou J, Liberman MD (1990) Effect of dietary protein and amino acids on immune function. Crit Care Med 18 [Suppl]: S86–93
54. McMahon MM, Bistrian BR (1990) The physiology of nutritional assessment and therapy in protein-calorie malnutrition. Dis Mon 36: 373–417
55. Rolandelli RH, Roslyn JJ (1996) Surgical management and treatment of sepsis associated with gastrointestinal fistulas. Surg Clin North Am 67: 1111–1122
56. MacErlean DP, Owens AP, Hourihane JB (1981) Ultrasound-guided percutaneous abdominal abscess drainage. Br J Radiol 54: 394–397

57. Meadows C (1997) Stoma and fistula care. In: Bruce L, Finlay TMD (eds) Nursing in gastroenterology. Churchill Livingstone, London
58. Irving M, Beadle C (1982) External intestinal fistulas: nursing care and surgical procedures. Clin Gastroenterol 11: 327–336
59. Gross E, Irving M (1977) Protection of the skin around intestinal fistulas. Br J Surg 64: 258–263
60. Dearlove JL (1996) Skin care management of gastrointestinal fistulas. Surg Clin N Am 76: 1095–1109
61. Burch J (2003) The nursing care of a patient with enterocutaneous faecal fistulae. Br J Nursing 12: 736–740
62. Black P (2000) Holistic stoma care. Ballière Tindall, London
63. Irving M (1977) Local and surgical management of enterocutaneous fistulas. Br J Surg 64: 690–694
64. Driscoll RH Jr, Rosenberg IH (1978) Total parenteral nutrition in inflammatory bowel disease. Med Clin N Am 62: 185–201
65. Coutsoftides T, Fazio VW (1979) Small intestine cutaneous fistulas. Surg Gynecol Obstet 149: 333–336
66. Roback SA, Nicoloff DM (1972) High output enterocutaneous fistulas of the small bowel. An analysis of fifty-five cases. Am J Surg 123: 317–322
67. Tarazi R, Coutsoftides T, Steiger E, Fazio VW (1983) Gastric and duodenal cutaneous fistulas. World J Surg 7: 463–473
68. Altomare DF, Serio G, Pannarale OC, Lupo L, Palasciano N, Memeo V, Rubino M (1990) Prediction of mortality by logistic regression analysis in patients with postoperative enterocutaneous fistulae. Br J Surg 77: 450–453

# Pilonidal Sinus Disease

J. TORKINGTON

## Introduction

Pilonidal sinus of the natal cleft is a condition dealt with by general practitioners, accident and emergency departments, general surgeons, colorectal surgeons, plastic surgeons, district nurses and wound-care specialists. It is an unglamorous condition that, despite its prevalence, seldom achieves priority within a busy clinical practice. However, its complex debilitating nature and negative economic effects for the predominantly young working population affected should not be underestimated.

The term pilonidal sinus derives from the Latin words *nidus* meaning nest, *pilus* meaning hair and *sinus* relating to connections to the skin. Its description is confirmed by an increased incidence in hirsute young males although it can occur in relatively hairless women and even in the elderly. The aetiology of the condition is thought to be due to a folliculitis, progressing to a chronic suppurative abscess that draws in hair follicles due to the grinding or shearing nature of the buttocks [1]. A congenital theory is no longer accepted but it is possible that an ingrowing hair or a hair follicle that directly penetrates the skin may be responsible [2].

Macroscopically pilonidal sinus disease can present in a number of ways. It may appear as asymptomatic pits in the midline of the natal cleft, as a chronically discharging lesion or, more commonly, as an acute episode of sepsis with abscess formation often lateral to a visible midline pit. Microscopically, the picture is of chronic sepsis without epithelialisation of the cavity.

This chapter deals briefly with the common modes of treatment but concentrates on the management of the difficult problem of recurrent disease or a nonhealing wound following primary treatment.

## Urgent Treatment

The indication for urgent treatment of a pilonidal sinus is abscess formation. This can cause significant pain and occasionally may cause systemic effects. History and examination should be performed and, as with any condition causing abscess formation, diabetes mellitus should be excluded. Careful examination will usually confirm the diagnosis, but perianal abscess/fistula and hidradenitis suppurativa can occasionally present in a similar manner. Often patients will have had a course of antibiotics prescribed by their family doctor, but evidence regarding the effectiveness of this is lacking. The aim of treatment for an acute pilonidal abscess is to relieve the pain by releasing the pus usually without definitive treatment for the underlying sinus. Attempting to widely excise an inflamed and cellulitic area in order to treat the sinus is likely to result in a larger wound than would be necessary once the acute episode has settled. Drainage of the abscess may be performed by de-roofing the skin over the area of maximum fluctuance often under a general anaesthetic or by making a small stab incision under local anaesthesia. The latter has the advantage of preventing hospital admission [3].

## Elective Treatment

The aims of an ideal treatment for pilonidal sinus disease should be to achieve simple, successful and cost-effective healing with little or no morbidity or recurrence. Secondary aims should be to perform the procedure as a day case, preferably under local anaesthesia. The complex nature of pilonidal sinus disease is illustrated by the fact that no one method of treatment has achieved all these goals and gained widespread acceptance. Treatments range from the simple, for example regular depilation of the area, through to the complex, such as the rotation flap. In between these two extremes there are a range of surgical procedures which are radical yet conceptually easy, such as wide local excision and healing by secondary intention, or conceptually difficult but less disfiguring, such as the so-called Bascom or Karydakis operations (see below). The decision in choosing which operation is suitable for which patient depends mainly on time to healing and the incidence of recurrence, but there may be an influence of the cosmetic result of the procedure and whether day case or inpatient stay is required [4] (Table 1).

**Table 1.** Results of treatments for pilonidal sinus. (After [4])

| Procedure | Time to heal [days] | Non-healing or recurrence [%] | Hospital stay [days] | Scarring |
|---|---|---|---|---|
| Currettage of tract | 21–52 | 3–24 | Day case | + |
| Phenol injection | 14–61 | 0–35 | Day case | + |
| Wide excision and healing by secondary intention | 31–90 | 1–43 | 1–3 | ++ |
| Primary closure | 10–50 | 0–37 | 1–3 | + |
| Asymmetric closure, e.g. Bascom/Karydakis | 8–16 | 0–5 | 1–2 | + |
| Rotation flap | 10–28 | 0–20 | 3–5 | +++ |

## Choosing a Procedure

It appears that some patients having a simple incision and drainage of an acute pilonidal abscess do not require further treatment because either they are cured of the sinus or they have become asymptomatic with a non-troublesome midline pit. This may occur in up to 60% of cases [5].

Such an asymptomatic patient, whether simply being followed up or having been referred with completely asymptomatic disease, needs to think carefully about having a definitive procedure. This is because we know the disease diminishes with age and it is very hard to improve the symptoms of an asymptomatic patient with a benign disease.

In this situation it would seem reasonable to discharge the patient with instructions to get back in touch if problems develop.

In a patient with symptomatic disease, usually a chronic discharging sinus and less than six to eight midline pits, I would favour a Bascom's procedure [1]. Alternatively, a Karydaxis procedure would be suitable [2]. If the number of pits was more than this or if the disease was recurrent, then a rotation flap may be more appropriate. It is increasingly the case that these procedures are preferred to the more traditional wide local excision and healing by secondary intention or primary midline closure.

## Bascom's Procedure

Bascom described his eponymous procedure for the treatment of pilonidal disease in 1980 [1]. He reported a 92% healing rate in 50 cases, 24 of whom had presented with acute abscesses. The principle of the procedure is to avoid a midline wound with its attendant poor healing and to remove the necrotic tissue and foreign body (i.e. hair follicles) from the abscess cavity. At the same time the midline pits and the small amount of epithelialised tissue associated with them are excised. This procedure is described in an uncomplicated case, the patient is placed prone and the buttocks are strapped apart (Fig. 1a). The procedure can be performed under either general or local anaesthetic. An incision is made 2–3 cm away from the midline on the same side as the abscess cavity (Fig. 1b). The abscess cavity is then thoroughly curretted of all debris and hair (Fig. 1c). Next the midline pit(s) are excised with tissue the size of a grain of rice (Fig. 1d). If it is not clear as to which side the abscess cavity lies, the pits should be excised first and the defect probed to either side to localise the cavity. The pit excision is closed with a removable suture and the lateral wound is left open with no packing.

A modification of this procedure involves the mobilisation through the same lateral wound of a flap of subcutaneous fat from the contralateral side that is brought to lie beneath the pit excision site and held using a removable suture. There has been

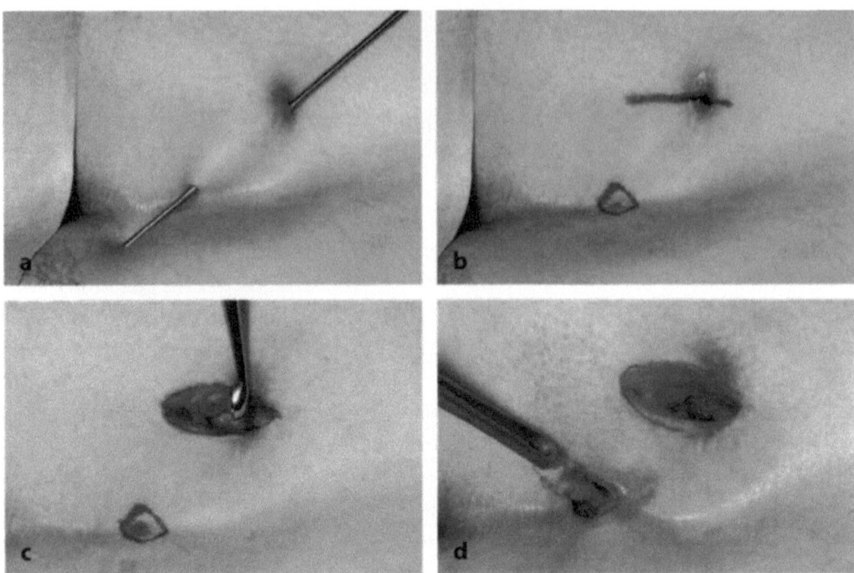

**Fig. 1a–d.** Steps in the Bascom's procedure (see text for details)

no study comparing this additional manoeuvre against the slightly simpler procedure. However, some surgeons have found omission of this step to be a factor in recurrence (Senapati 2003, personal communication).

Sutures are removed at 7 days, and average time to healing is quoted as 28 days. Recurrence rates are among the lowest at 7.3–9.6% [6, 7] (see Table 1).

## Rotation Flap

A rotation flap is an important procedure for the surgeons to have in their repertoire if dealing with a lot of pilonidal sinus disease. It is useful in the case of a non-healing midline wound (see below), in complex recurrent disease and in severe primary disease. It is also useful in a patient for whom cosmesis is not an issue but rapid resolution and a low recurrence rate is important. A number of types of flaps are described including the gluteal flap, the rhomboid flap, the Limberg flap and several others [8]. In reality, the specific type of flap is unlikely to be critical as long as basic principles are adhered to with a wide-based pedicle, no tension and a healthy blood supply. My preference is for the Limberg flap. In this procedure, the area to be excised is marked with the patient prone and again the buttocks strapped apart. This procedure normally necessitates a general anaesthetic. An exact calculation of the dimensions of the area to be excised has been formulated by Grabham and colleagues [9]. They suggest that after measuring the vertical height ($h$) required to excise the affected area, a bisecting line exactly 0.58 its own length will create

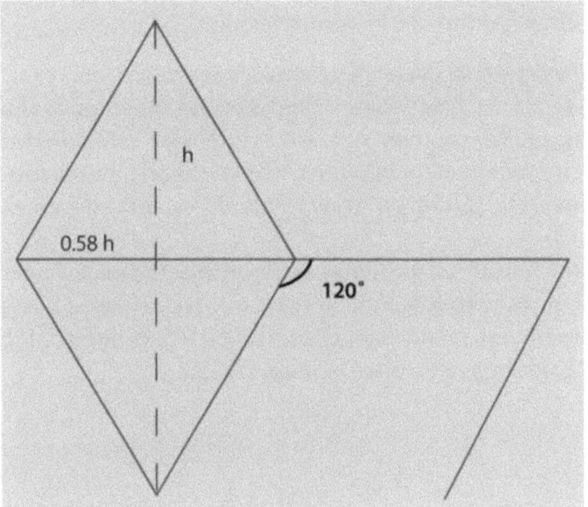

**Fig. 2.** Calculation of the shape of excision in the Limberg flap (see text for details)

two isosceles triangles with angles of 120 degrees. The same length then marks out the flap to be dissected from the buttock (Fig. 2). The fascia overlying the gluteal muscle is dissected with the flap for reasons of mobility and blood supply. The flap is sutured in place using deep absorbable sutures and non-absorbable skin sutures after the placement of a suction drain. It has been most surgeons' policy to keep these patients in hospital for 4 days to observe for wound breakdown and flap viability. Results are impressive, with recurrence rates as low as 0–2% [8, 10] and the patient essentially returning to normal after removal of the sutures at 10 days. These procedures effectively flatten the normal shape of the natal cleft and leave a substantial scar which must be discussed especially in young patients where the current fashion is for low-slung trousers!

## The Non-Healing Wound

The Achilles' heel in the treatment of pilonidal disease is the non-healing wound in the absence of recurrent disease. This occurs when a surgical treatment which leaves an open wound that fails to heal or a wound that was primarily closed breaks down and the wound becomes chronic. These are best avoided in the first place by appropriate initial treatment, but there are two main approaches to this situation should it arise:

- change the wound milieu in order to promote healing;
- surgery (either a rotation flap or Bascom's cleft closure).

### Modifying the Wound Environment to Promote Healing

Unhealed pilonidal wounds have provided a fertile ground for research into the factors that affect wound healing. It has clearly been demonstrated that a pilonidal wound will not heal if infected and the common organisms implicated are skin commensals such as *Staphylococcus aureus*, although it may be the anaerobic contamination which can cause delays in the healing of open pilonidal wounds by a mean of 27 days [11].

The Wound-Healing Unit in Cardiff has produced pathways for the management of these chronic wounds which address this issue of infection, by the use of long-term antibiotics such as erythromycin and metronidazole (Fig. 3). They achieve high success rates in healing, although time to healing remains long.

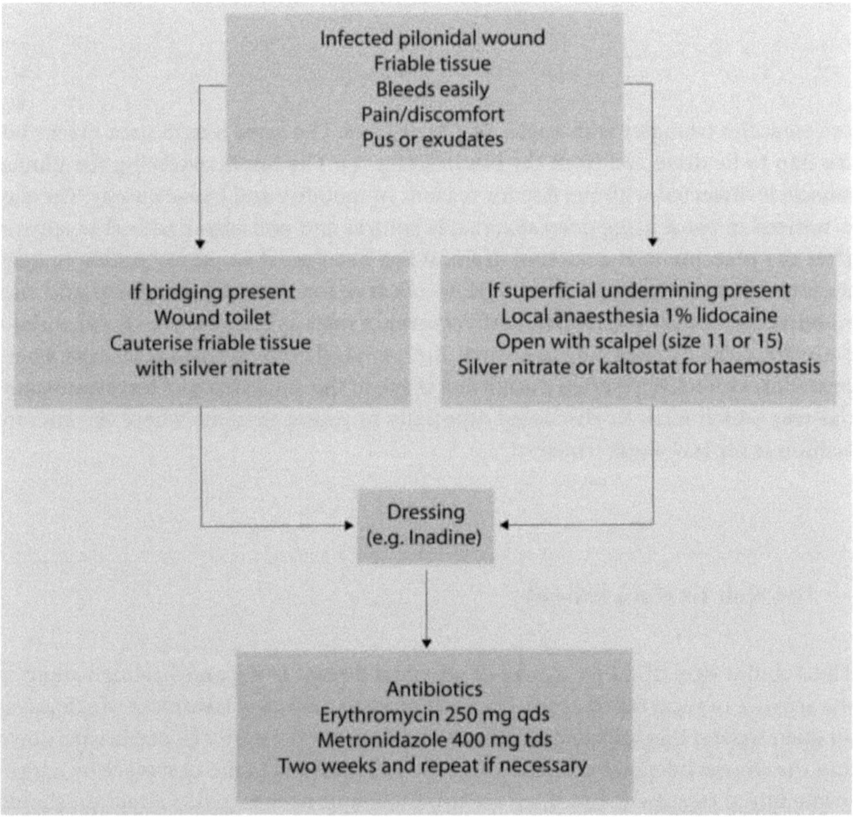

**Fig. 3.** Clinical pathway for management of infected pilonidal sinus wound. (Adapted with permission Wound Healing Research Unit, University of Wales College of Medicine)

## Surgical Solutions

The most obvious surgical solution is to re-excise an unhealed pilonidal sinus wound and to perform a flap in a fashion similar to that described above. The other procedure that has been described specifically for this situation is the Bascom cleft closure procedure [12]. This operation requires the patient to be marked pre-operatively in the upright position with a line showing apposition of the buttocks, since when the patient is positioned prone jack-knife with the buttocks strapped apart this line becomes distorted. With the patient so positioned the procedure is carried out either under local or, perhaps more humanely, under general anaesthetic. In this procedure, the unhealed wound and a peculiar tear drop-shaped flap of skin is excised. Suturing of the underlying fat obliterates the cleft and the skin usually comes together under no tension.

## Conclusions

Patey was somewhat disparaging of the debate that pilonidal sinus disease attracts [13]. He noted that it "is an infected foreign body granuloma" and the treatment should be the same as "is adopted in other similar conditions such as stitch sinus". He suspected that "after the plethora of scholarly thesis on the origin of pilonidal sinus, to reduce it therapeutically to the level of the humble stitch sinus smacks of lèse-majesté." However, he argued convincingly against the use of wide excision of the area and yet this is still commonly practiced over 30 years on.

Pilonidal disease remains a common problem and is seen in many spheres of medical care. The major problems in its treatment are the high recurrence rates of some procedures and the aftermath of a non-healing wound. Preventing this situation involves abandoning wide local excision and healing by secondary intention and by the avoidance of midline wounds. Treatment of a non-healing wound is currently by long-term antibiotics to facilitate healing or using a surgical solution in the form of a rotation flap or the cleft closure technique.

## References

1. Bascom J (1980) Pilonidal disease: origin from follicles of hairs and results of follicle removal as treatment. Surgery 87: 567–572
2. Karydakis G (1992) Easy and successful treatment of pilonidal sinus after explanation of its causative process. Aust N Z J Surg 62: 385–389
3. Senapati A, Cripps N (2000) Pilonidal sinus. In: Johnson CD, Taylor I (eds) Recent advances in surgery 23. Churchill Livingstone, Edinburgh, pp 33–42
4. Allen-Mersh T (1990) Pilonidal sinus: finding the right track for treatment. Br J Surg 77: 123–132
5. Jensen S, Harling H (1989) Prognosis after simple incision and drainage for a first episode acute pilonidal abscess. Br J Surg 75: 9–11

6. Mosquera D, Quayle J (1995) Bascom's operation for pilonidal sinus. J R Soc Med 88: 45P–46P
7. Senapati A, Cripps N, Thompson MR (2000) Bascom's operation in the day-surgical management of symptomatic pilonidal sinus. Br J Surg 87: 1067–1070
8. Tekin A (1999) Pilonidal sinus: experience with the Limberg flap. Colorect Dis 1: 29–33
9. Grabham J, Kelly S et al. (2001) The Limberg flap – a less protracted approach. Colorect Dis 3: 37
10. Bozhurt M, Tezel E (1998) Management of pilonidal sinus with the Limberg flap. Dis Colon Rectum 41: 775–777
11. Marks J, Harding K et al. (1987) Staphylococcal infection of open granulating wounds. Br J Surg 74: 95–97
12. Bascom J (1987) Repeat pilonidal operations. Am J Surg 154: 118–122
13. Patey D (1970) The principles of treatment of saccroxoccygeal pilonidal sinus. Proc Roy Soc Med 63: 939–940

# Acne Inversa

U.E. Ziegler, U.A. Dietz, K. Schmidt

## Introduction

Acne inversa (AI) is a chronically relapsing inflammation of the sebaceous glands and terminal hair follicles [9]. Ecrine and apocrine glands are affected secondarily. AI is characterised by recurrent draining sinuses and abscesses chiefly located in intertriginous areas as axillae, groin and perineum (main localisations), but the annals fold, buttocks, nape of the neck, scalp, genitalia and mammary folds may also be affected (see Fig. 1).

The skin disease was first described by Velpeau in 1839 [21], who reported a peculiar inflammatory process with superficial abscess formation (axillary, mammary, perianal regions). Verneuil considered a disorder of the sweat glands in 1854 [22], Schiefferdecker (1922) and Kierlander (1951) suggested an association with apocrine glands [18, 12]. A dependency on acne of the skin disease was supposed by Lane and Brunsting in earlier times [4, 13], and Gahlen postulated AI as a very serious acne [7]. Different synonyms of AI exist (see following list), but the Anglo-American name hidradenitis suppurativa is incorrect, because of the known pathogenetic process in AI (apocrine glands are affected secondarily). The correct term acne inversa was created by Plewig and Steger 1989 [17].

Synonyms of acne inversa:
- Hidrandenitis suppurativa (Anglo-American)
- Morbus Verneuil
- Hidradenitis axillaries Verneuil
- Pyodermia fistulans significa
- Triad of acne (acne conglobata, hidradentitis suppurativa, perifolliculitis capitis abscedens et suffodiens)
- Tetrad of acne (see above and pilonidal sinus)
- Apocrine acne
- Intertriginous acne
- Chronic-recurrent hidradenitis
- Recurrent abscesses of the sweat glands

## Epidemiology

The disease is very common with an estimated number of unknown cases being probably quite high, because of wrong diagnosis. The correct diagnosis is frequently ignored or missed leading to frustration in both physician and patient. The exact prevalence of the disease is not known, but it has been estimated to range between 1:100 and 1:600 [6, 8, 10]. Point prevalence of 4.1% based on objective findings in a younger adult population and a 1-year prevalence of 1.0% have been reported [10]. There is no evidence for a racial predilection concerning black people [1], although this is supposed by some authors [16].

Both men und women are affected with AI, but the male/female ratio in most published series is 2 to 5:1 [2, 3, 19, 24]. Women are predisposed to axillary lesions, whereas men more frequently show anogenital lesions [11]. The first manifestation of AI may be in puberty (at the age of 12) but also at higher age (up to 88 years) [24].

## Aetiology and Pathogenesis

Acne inversa is a highly chronic disorder, but the pathogenesis of the affection is still not well understood. A histopathomorphologic target of AI was found by Pelwig and Steger [17]. Hyperceratosis of the follicle infundibulum leads to the production of comedos followed by superinfection with segmental rupture of follicle epithelium. This results in an inflammation of the connective tissue and in the development of cutaneous-subcutaneous nodes. Finally, fistulas with epithelium and abscesses are presented with consecutive fibrosis.

Acne vulgaris is a disease of the sebaceous gland follicle, whereas acne inversa affects the terminal hair follicles and the sebaceous gland in intertriginous areas. There are a lot of apocrine glands in the intertriginous areas, but they are only secondarily infected in AI. Patients with AI have no more apocrine sweat glands in comparison to the control group, but this may be the case in patients with AI and hyperhidrosis (Fig. 1).

It is not well understood which factors induce follicle occlusion, but one possible trigger is a local friction trauma. To date, there is no significant evidence that chemical irritations with deodorants, mechanical irritation, hair epilation or shaving are aetiological factors inducing AI. Although skin-to-skin contact is quite common in obesity, there is no positive proof for that aetiology. The individual predisposition for follicle occlusion may be more decisive.

Acne inversa may also be a genetically determined disease. Werth et al. tested the reproducibility of autosomal dominant inheritance for acne inversa [23] by examining the same patients as Fitzsimmons in 1985 [6] and found high penetrance. The association with the HLA system is not constant, but HLA-A1 and HLA-B8 are possibly predispositions for AI to affect more severe diseases [15]. However, further investigations will be necessary to confirm this hypothesis.

It is controversially discussed if there is an influence on the immune system in AI. In several studies, some of the patients showed an increase of T-suppressor (CD8) cell activity and a modified CD4/CD8 ratio [15]. If there are increased levels of testosterone and dehydroepiandrosteronsulphate or an increased ratio of oestrogen/gestagen in women, this will be a predisposition for AI. Lithium therapy has also been implicated in the pathogenesis of AI [14].

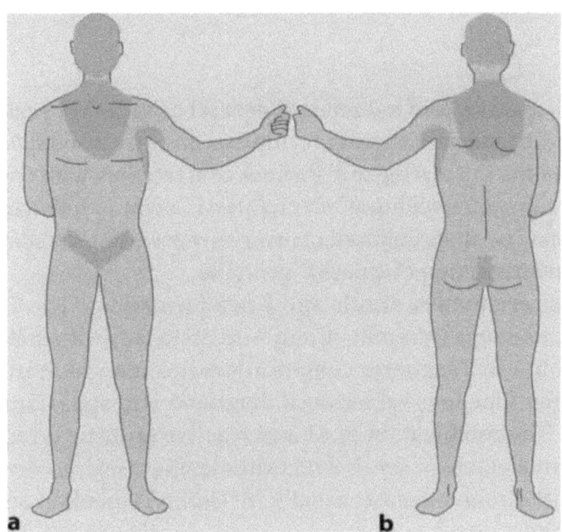

**Fig. 1a,b.** Regions possibly affected with acne inversa

The bacterial burden in AI is very variable and not primarily a pathogenetic problem. In most of the cases, staphylococci, streptococci, Gram-negative and Gram-positive cocci are responsible for the lesions.

The high percentage of active smokers among patients with AI may be evidence for cigarette smoking as a major triggering factor of acne inversa. The pathogenetic mechanisms being responsible for the effects smoking has on the manifestation of AI is still vague, but perhaps the chemotaxis of polymorphic neutrophils plays an important role [2].

In a study by Werth et al., 45% of the patients showed an aggravation in AI with sweat and heat, 35% with stress and 16% with too tight clothes [23].

## Clinic

At an early stage, giant blackheads can be seen and hard, indolent, subcutaneous nodes of the size of a pea can be palpated. These nodes may coalesce into bulging abscesses at a deep level and acute suppuration. In its completely developed form at late stage AI is characterised by dark, broadly infiltrated and indurated areas which are pervaded with nodes, abscesses and fistulas lined with epithelium. If you press on the tissue, pus will evacuate which smells very bad and therefore causes problems in the patient's social interactions. Mostly the patients feel sick, have normally no fever, and feel pain in special affected areas (e.g. when sitting). AI never affects deeper regions or breaks the muscle fascia. In 38–45% of the cases only one preferred localisation is affected, mostly in the groin or in the anogenital region [10]. A spontaneous healing is absolutely rare and progressive disability is the rule.

## Complications

The chronic inflammatory process may lead to a reduced general condition of health in patients suffering from AI, with anaemia, thrombocytopenia and elevated inflammation parameters. It also results in scarring and dermal contractures with constrained movement in special areas. Swelling of elephantiasis nostras following streptococcal complications may be superimposed on acne inversa lesions, leading to monstrous enlargement and distortion of external genitalia.

Uncommon complications are urethra fistula and sinus formations. The development of squamous cell carcinoma (Marjolin ulcera) – occasionally with metastases – is the most serious but rare long-term complication. It comes up mostly in the anogenital area, with the time interval between diagnosis and appearance being an average of 19 years. The combination of AI and reactive arthritis is rare, the development of systemic amyloidose or sepsis with exitus letalis is seldom. Acne inversa can occur together with Crohn's disease; usually, M. Crohn is manifest and AI appears after 3.5 years [5, 20].

### Complications in Acne Inversa

- Reduction of state of health
- Contractures
- Scarring
- Squamous cell carcinoma (Marjolin ulcera)
- Crohn's disease
- Elephantiasis-nostras swelling in anogenital areas
- Fistulas urethral and pararectal
- Reactive arthritis
- Systemic amyloidose
- Sepsis (with exitus letalis)

## Diagnostic and Differential Diagnostic

Acne invera is often a diagnostic challenge. History, total-body examination, fistula assays, blood tests and searching for other signs of the disease will lead to the right diagnosis. Acne inversa must be differentiated from furuncles, carbuncles, vegetating pyoderma, tuberculosis subcutanea et fistulosa, actinomycosis, trichophyts and lymphogranuloma inguinale. In the anogenital region, the differentiation of AI and Crohn's disease needs special attention. Rectoscopy and/or MRI are necessary. If AI is presented over a long period of time, biopsies have to be taken for histomorphology excluding squamous cell carcinoma.

## Treatment

In established acne inversa there is no evidence that treatment other than surgery has any effect on the natural course of the disease. All other therapies are adjuncts to surgery. Only in the early stages can the disease be controlled with medical measures.

---

**Therapy in Acne Inversa**

- Operative
  - Radical excision and healing by secondary intension
  - Split-skin grafts
  - Local cutaneous/subcutaneous flaps
- Conservative (adjunct)
  - Local therapy (antiseptic and antibiotic)
  - Systemic antibiotic
  - Systemic retinoide (Isotretinoin, Acitretin)
  - Hormones (antiandrogens)
  - Dapson (Diaminodiphenylsulfon)

---

Conservative treatment, e.g. with antibiotics, antiseptics, corticosteroids, cyclosporin and retinoides (local or systemic), or radiation, have only temporary and limited benefits as monotherapy. Topical treatment is used pre-operatively with antiseptic substances. Externa with halogen (e.g. polividon-iodine) can deteriorate the local situation. Systemic antibiotics are necessary weeks before and weeks after the surgery (e.g. minocyclin). Although antibiotics are not curative, they can reduce the odour, pain and the secretion of pus. Systemic retinoides (isotretinoin, acitretin) are applied weeks before and after surgery and – with rare exceptions – showed an insufficient stop of the disease. Intralesional and systemic corticosteroids have been used with variable results. Some patients have transient benefits from such treatments. Women in early stage of the disease can benefit from hormonal therapy (antiandrogen – combination of cyproteronacetat with ethinylestradiol) in genital regions. The anti-inflammatory effect of Dapson (Diaminodiphenylsulfon) in acne conglobata and acne fulminans are useful in acne inversa, too, but the studies included only few patients with such a treatment. Anti-tumour-necroses factor alpha was successfully used in one case. Radiotherapy has been used in some series but often fails to eradicate the lesions completely.

In early stages of the disease, surgical interventions are the best methods. Incision, drainage and exteriorisation of individual lesions may be useful, but radical surgical excision can avoid recurrence of AI. In early stage, operations in tumescence anaesthesia or subcutaneous infiltration of local anaesthetics can be performed. Normally, it is necessary to have general anaesthesia to make radical excisions of the fistulas and good haemostasis. All the pre-operatively marked areas have to be removed with wide excision; intra-operatively, all the fistulas have to be detected by filling the canals with methylene blue. The surgical sharp debridement of the areas can be performed with electrosurgery, ultrasound knife or $CO_2$-laser technology for better haemostasis and, additionally, a better overview during the operation.

The wounds can be covered with moist dressings for healing with secondary intention. A new method to control the bacterial burden, exudates and necrosis is the topical negative pressure therapy. It promotes and increases the formation of granulation tissue during a short period of time with polyurethane or polyvinyl-alcohol foam. Coverage of the defects with split-skin or mesh grafts is possible in most cases 1 week after the first surgical intervention. Then, the vacuum containing the foam is used with the grafts. After 3–5 days the vacuum dressing can be removed over the grafts. Topical negative pressure therapy reduces the intervals for coverage from 3–4 weeks to 1 week. Aesthetic and functional results after transplantations of autologous skin are better in certain regions. In the anogenital areas secondary healing processes mostly show good results as grafts, with a longer healing period and more costs for the health-care system. Grafts in the anogenital region are often lost due to local infections of Gram-negative bacteria.

Plastic surgeons prefer a one-stage procedure in certain regions (e.g. axillae, sacrum). Pre-operative antibiotic therapy over 4 weeks to control the pus and inflammation is necessary. Radical wide excision of the infected areas (mostly not deeper than the muscle fascia) and direct coverage of the defect with local rotation/transposition flaps of cutaneous/subcutaneous tissue are standard. The drainages have to be left for a long time, until there is no more secretion in the bottle (sometimes up to 3 weeks). If the drainages are removed too early, consecutive infection will be the result. Suction on the drainages is permanently necessary. Post-operatively, an antibiotic therapy for 4 weeks is recommended. Primary closure of small defects (including drainage) is possible, but this showed high infection rates (personal experience).

Complications are bleeding, infection, delayed wound healing, recurrence, nerve lesions and thrombosis of arm veins. Keloids can produce big plates of scars.

## Prognosis

Wrong diagnosis, inadequate treatment and no radical surgical excision of the involved tissue leads to the consequence that many affected individuals drift away from society. Although spontaneous healing may occur, it is rare. Surgical interventions are sufficient to stop the disease. Surgery in acne inversa leads to a recurrence rate of merely 2.5%. On average, 19 years will pass until a sufficient treatment is started.

# References


1. Banerjee AK (1992) Surgical treatment of hidradenitis suppurativa. Br J Surg 79: 863–866
2. Breitkopf C, Bockhorst J, Lippolda et al. (1995) Pyoderma fistulans sinifica (Acne inversa) und Rauchgewohnheiten. Z Hautkrankheiten 70: 332–334
3. Broadwater JR, Bryant RL, Petrino RA et al. (1982) Advanced hidradenitis suppurativa. Am J Surg 144: 668–670
4. Brunsting HA (1939) Hidradenitis suppurativa: abscess of the apocrine sweat glands. Arch Derm Syphil 39: 108–120
5. Burrows NP, Jones RR (1992) Crohn's disease in association with hidradenitis suppurativa. Br J Dermatol 126: 523
6. Fitzsimmons JS, Guilbert PR, Fitzsimmons EM (1985) Evidence of genetic factors in hidradenitis suppurativa. Br J Dermatol 113: 1–8
7. Gahlen W, Grussendorf EI, Wienert V (1976) Histologischer Beitrag zum Krankheitsbild der sog. Pyodermia fistulans sinifica als Ausdruck einer schweren Akne (= Acne conglobata et sinifica). Z Hautkr 51: 621–626
8. Harrison BJ, Mudge M, Hughes LE (1989) The prevalence of hidradenitis suppurativa in Sotuh Wales. In: Marks R, Plewig G (eds) Acne and related disorders. Martin Dunitz, London, pp 365–366
9. Jansen T, Plewig G (1998) Acne inversa. Int J Dermatol 37: 96–100
10. Jemec GBE, Heidenheim M, Nielsen NH 81996) The prevalence of hidradenitis suppurativa and its potential precusor lesions. J Am Acad Dermatol 35: 191–194
11. Jemec GBE (1988) The symptomatology of hidradenitits suppurativa in women. Br J Dermatol 119: 345–350
12. Kierland RR (1951) Unusual pyodermas (hidradenitis suppurativa, acne conglobata, dissecting cellulitis of the scalp). A review. Minn Med 34: 319–341
13. Lane JE (1933) Hidradenitis axillaries of Verneuil. Arch Derm Syphil 29: 609–614
14. Marinella MA (1997) Lithium therapy associated with hidradenitis suppurativa. Acta Derm Venerol (Stockh) 77: 483
15. O´Loughlin S, Woods R, Kirke PN et al. (1988) Hidradenitis suppurativa. Glucose tolerance, clinical, microbiologic, and immunologic features and HLA frequencies in 27 patients. Arch Dermatol 124: 1043–1046
16. Paletta C, Jurkiewicz MJ (1987) Hidradenitis suppurativa. Clin Plast Surg 14: 383–390
17. Plewig G, Steger M (1989) Acne inverse. In: Marks R, Plewig G (eds) Acne and related disorders. Martin Dunitz, London, pp 345–347
18. Schiefferdecker B (1922) Die Hautdrüsen der Menschen und der Säugetiere, ihre histologische und rassenanatomische Bedeutung sowie die Muscularis sexualis. E. Schweizerbart, Stuttgart
19. Thornton JP, Abcarian H (1978) Surgical treatment of perianal hidradenitis suppurativa. Dis Col Rect 21: 573–577
20. Tsianos EV, Dalekos GN, Tzermias C et al. (1995) Hidradenitis suppurativa in Crohn´s disease. A further support to this association. J Clin Gastroenterol 29: 151–153
21. Velpeau A (1839) In: Bechet Jeune Z (eds) Dictionnaire de Medicine, un Répertoire Général des Sciences Médicales sous la Rapport Théorique et Practique 2, p 91
22. Verneuil A (1854) Études sur les tumeurs de la peau et quelques maladies des glandes sudoripares. Arch Gén Méd 94: 447–468, 693–705
23. Werth von der JM, Williams HC, Raeburn JA (2000) The clinical genetics of hidradenitis suppurativa revisited. Br J Dermatol 142: 947–953
24. Wiltz O, Schoetz DJ, Murray JJ et al. (1990) Perianal hidradenitis suppurativa. The Lahey experience. Dis Col Rect 33: 731–734

# VI  Chronic Wound Problems



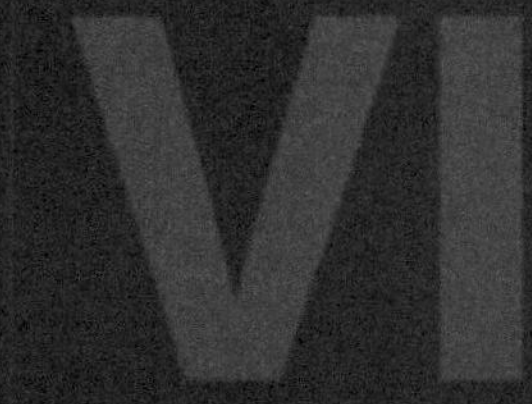

# 32

# Surgery for Arterial Ulcers

S.R. Lauterbach, G. Andros, G. Torres, R.W. Oblath

## Introduction

Although arterial insufficiency may be acute when occurring with an embolus, or chronic-caused by progressive arteriosclerotic obstructive disease, it is the chronic reduction in arterial perfusion that is responsible for most ischemic lesions of the leg. Furthermore, the extent of the occlusive disease spans the clinical spectrum from asymptomatic to functional to critical. Critical limb ischemia is the underlying cause of rest pain, digital gangrene, arterial ulcers and wounds. The relationship of arterial hypoperfusion to distal digital gangrene is well understood; in this chapter we present the role of arterial surgery in chronic wounds including post-traumatic and mixed venous-arterial ulcers.

The clinical significance of this pathophysiological state for recalcitrant wounds is obvious; meticulous wound care alone is too often inadequate to heal the wound. Since chronic wounds tend to progress and become infected, especially in diabetics, the ultimate outcome is too often amputation of the limb.

## Risk Factors

Risk factors for patients developing arteriosclerotic obstructive lesions of the lower extremities are many and include the familiar factors for atherosclerosis: age, cigarette smoking, hyperlipoproteinemia and diabetes mellitus. In addition, hyperhomocysteinemia, elevated plasma fibrinogen, thrombocytosis and increased platelet aggregation contribute to thrombotic occlusion of lower-extremity arteries. Other causes of arterial obliteration include arterial trauma and inflammatory vasculopathies.

Diabetes mellitus deserves special mention because of its high prevalence – more than 17 million persons in the United States. Approximately 15% of diabetics will develop a foot ulcer during their lifetime which may proceed to non-traumatic amputation. Not infrequently, diabetic patients have a history of trauma to the lower extremity. The frequent co-existence of neuropathy may render the patient unaware of the traumatic insult and its associated lesion; moreover, the impaired vision due to diabetic retinopathy may often render the patient blind and unable to see the pedal lesion.

## Clinical Evaluation

The principal evaluation of patients with chronic wounds of the lower extremity is the history and physical examination for the vascular specialist; the former to determine the aetiology of the wound, and the latter to determine the site of the arterial lesion. The majority of wounds can easily be classified as arterial, venous or neuropathic. Mixed patterns also exist. A history of the above-mentioned risk factors and, concerning diabetic patients, neurosensory dysfunction, alerts the practitioner. Since these patients often have significant co-morbidities, attention to the cardiopulmonary, renal and cerebrovascular systems is obligatory.

Claudication (i.e. muscle cramping or pain induced by exercise and promptly relieved by rest) is usually a reliable indicator of chronic lower-extremity arterial insufficiency; unfortunately, in the cohort of patients with chronic wounds, it is seldom manifest. In diabetics, the arterial lesions are commonly infrapopliteal and hence rarely, if ever, cause calf claudication. In non-ambulatory chronically ill people, claudication cannot be used as a marker for arterial occlusive disease.

The essential physical examination begins with a pulse examination of both upper and lower extremities including the carotid arteries and auscultation for bruits. A seasoned clinician can usually note reduced pulses, often graded 0–4, where 0 represents an absent pulse and 4 a full, normal pulse; 1–3 are then grades of reduction [1]. Dependent foot rubor and blanching of the skin on foot elevation are important to document. Neurologic assessment of peripheral sensation and motor function is also important. A dry "autosympathectamised" foot of the diabetic is not uncommon. The wound is categorised for location, size, depth and exposed structures such as tendon and bone. Careful debridement of foot callus and necrotic tissue and sterile probing of the wound is mandatory at the initial assessment because the presence of deep infection cannot be determined by simply looking at the wound. Additionally, plain films of the foot to rule out gas and foreign objects in the soft tissues are helpful. The first priority in wound care is prompt drainage of sepsis and debridement of non-viable tissue at the earliest possible time.

### Wound-Healing Potential

Ulcers and wounds must be assessed for healing potential. The non-invasive vascular laboratory can provide invaluable information by quantifying arterial obstruction and locating the levels of disease in the arterial tree. Reduced segmental limb pressures and Doppler waveforms over the peripheral arteries document peripheral obstruction. Diabetic patients prove to be more challenging as calcification of their medium and small-sized arteries may lead to falsely elevated limb pressures or simply cannot be compressed. Fortunately, the digital arteries are often less calcified than the more proximal plantar and tibial vessels, enabling us to record toe pressures. Toe pressures of at least 30 mmHg appear necessary to heal local toe amputations [2].

Significant venous insufficiency can also be documented in the vascular laboratory. Patients with arterial insufficiency may have significant oedema from prolonged dependent positioning of the feet and legs from chronic rest pain in addition to venous insufficiency. The oedema often complicates treatment because either compression or leg elevation or both are necessary to treat the venous component and leg oedema, but can be hazardous if the arterial component is left unaddressed. Recalcitrant venous ulcers need to be assessed for underlying arterial insufficiency. Finally, ultrasonography of potential bypass venous conduits such as saphenous and arm veins can be accomplished in the vascular lab to assess their size and suitability for surgical bypass, often avoiding unnecessary harvest incisions in the operating room if inadequate [3].

## Therapeutic Decision-Making

The need for vascular intervention to promote wound healing is predicated on weighing the risks and benefits of each of the possible interventions available to patients with critical arterial insufficiency. If it is decided to proceed with a limb-salvaging revascularisation, imaging of the arterial tree is performed. The gold standard of arterial imaging of the lower extremities is contrast angiography, although some surgeons have based therapy on duplex ultrasonography and/or magnetic angiography under certain circumstances, above all in renal insufficiency [4].

The goal of invasive contrast angiography is to precisely define the anatomy of the arterial circulation. When performed properly, risks such as blood vessel injury, embolisation, thrombosis, retroperitoneal haemorrhage and contrast-induced nephropathy are rare. Inflow via the aortoiliac segments is imaged followed by femoral popliteal segments, crural vessels including the tibial and peroneal vessels and foot blood vessels. In the diabetic population, tibial-peroneal disease with sparing of the iliac and pedal systems is a common pattern. Two views of the foot are mandatory to delineate patency of pedal vessels.

## Revascularisation

The goal of arterial revascularisation for critical limb ischemia is restoration of pulsatile flow into the foot. Patients with limb-threatening ischemia often have multi-level occlusive disease (aortoiliac, femoral-popliteal and tibial-peroneal), which offers a variety of therapeutic options for reconstruction. The interventional armamentarium includes percutaneous angioplasty (PTA), placement of stents, surgical thromboendarterectomy, surgical bypass, and combinations of these which are tailored to each individual patient. The vascular surgeon familiar with endovascular procedures, including diagnostic angiography, is the best specialist to care for the patient with arterial insufficiency manifest in chronic wounds.

During the same setting as the diagnostic angiogram, therapeutic endoluminal procedures can be performed if necessary. For example, if patients have reduced femoral pulses and waveforms and if iliac disease is demonstrated, PTA and stenting of the iliac system can be entertained given the large size of the blood vessels and the often short segmental stenoses or occlusions typically present. PTA and stenting of the iliac system is an alternative to direct surgical reconstruction to provide adequate inflow to the femoral levels [5–7].

Shortcomings of PTA and stenting include the creation of intimal flaps, elastic recoil of the vessel, dissection, thrombosis, disease progression within the treated segment, constrictive remoulding of the vessel and the development of intimal hyperplasia which contributes to poorer durability. Although stenting can improve the luminal diameter by sealing intimal flaps and reducing recoil and remoldeling, intimal hyperplasia is often more severe than with PTA alone [8].

Other options for inflow restoration include direct aortoiliac reconstruction in the form of aorto-femoral bypass, which is the most direct and durable reconstruction available. However, it requires open aortic surgery and the inherent risks of general anaesthesia and aortic clamping which can be stressful for patients with compromised cardiac and pulmonary function. Additionally, extra-anatomic bypasses such as axillo-femoral or femero-femoral ones obviate the need for aortic exposure and general anaesthesia which is ideal in compromised patients.

Thrombo-endarterectomy of ilio-femoral segments is most helpful when restoring vessel patency for axillo-femoral/aorto-femoral bypass in addition to providing inflow for more distal bypass procedures. Short segmental stenoses or occlusions of the external iliac, common, superficial and profunda femoral vessels are ideal for local endarterectomy and patching with either synthetic patch material such as Dacron or the hood of the bypass conduit whether synthetic or autologous material.

Without question, the mainstay in infra-inguinal arterial reconstruction for limb salvage is lower-extremity bypass grafting, which provides pulsatile blood flow to arterial targets beyond obstructive lesions maximising tissue perfusion. Lower extremity bypass efforts date back more than 50 years and much has been learned from a technical perspective over the past several decades. Procedures have become standardised, pedal targets are no longer inaccessible and creative use of conduits such as arm veins have become commonplace for the well-trained vascular surgeon [9, 10].

Lower-extremity bypass grafting can be conceptualised in three parts: inflow, conduit and target vessel. After careful review of the angiogram, the inflow and target vessels become evident. Secondly, knowledge of available conduit is crucial when planning the most appropriate procedure. Preoperative vein "mapping" with B-mode ultrasound is most helpful. Often, infra-genicular targets such as tibial or pedal arteries are the desired target, which calls for autologous conduit if available, as the success rate of native veins is better than synthetic grafts [11]. The greater saphenous vein is the first choice in conduit as its patency rate is no doubt the best [12]. Next, lesser saphenous and arm veins such as basilic and cephalic segments are suitable if of adequate size and without sclerosis. We do not hesitate to splice vein segments together (up to three pieces) in an effort to perform an "all autologous" bypass procedure [13].

Autologous veins are sometimes unavailable (previously harvested for coronary or lower-extremity bypass) or are of inadequate size (<2.5 mm), diseased or sclerotic, rendering them unsuitable for use. Either creative efforts using synthetic conduits are required or cadaveric conduits such as cryopreserved saphenous vein are used. Unfortunately, the success rates with these two latter materials are inferior to autologous vein [14, 15].

When forced to use synthetic material to infragenicular postions, the authors' preference has been constructing a venous cuff on the target vessel to which the distal end of the PTFE graft (7 mm Gore stretch; W.L. Gore, Flagstaff, AZ) is then anastomosed. The patency and limb-salvage rates with this procedure have been more favourable than synthetic grafting without the venous cuff [16].

The results of infra-inguinal bypass procedures depend on many factors. It is helpful to distinguish between graft patency and limb salvage because limb salvage is clearly the goal of bypass surgery. When foot necrosis is advanced, for example, maximising arterial flow with a tibial bypass procedure may not save the limb. Patient selection is very important when discussing results. Some patients must undergo leg amputation despite a patent bypass graft; in this example, graft patency does not really provide long-term benefit for the patient.

Another important point to remember when selecting patients for various arterial reconstructive procedures is the patient's life expectancy. Often, patients succumb to their significant co-morbidities long before bypass grafts have had a chance to fail. We have seen the average age of patients presenting with limb-threatening ischemia rise to nearly 80 years over the past decade. Additionally, these aged patients often have more serious co-morbidities. The bottom line is that we are taking care of a much more delicate patient population, which necessitates a firm understanding of the patient's overall clinical condition, significance of the wound, likelihood of healing and available choices for arterial bypass.

Amputation of the leg is often performed in some patients with arterial insufficiency and chronic wounds. Surgical revascularisation has been shown to carry a lower peri-operative mortality rate, shorter hospital length of stay, increased likelihood of regaining ambulatory abilities and a longer survival rate than with primary amputation. Medically compromised patients should not necessarily be denied revascularisation surgery on the basis of presumed greater surgical risk [17].

Probably the most important topic relevant to the care of patients with chronic wounds having undergone arterial surgery in an effort to promote healing is the functional outcome of the patient. A non-ambulatory patient confined to a wheelchair may never ambulate again, despite intervention. However, efforts for wound healing and ultimately limb salvage are important for transferring the patient in and out of a wheelchair, for instance, and for the patients' and their families' emotional well-being, as amputation often is quite difficult for patients to accept. Also, chronic wound care is expensive and demands many work hours from the medical community with nurses, home health aides, etc. When chronic wounds heal and stay healed, resources are spared and patients' quality of life often improves [18].

## References

1. Andros G, Harris R, Dulawa L et al. (1984) The need for arteriography in diabetic patients with gangrene and palpable pulses. Arch Surg 119: 1260–1263
2. Holstein P, Lassen NA (1980) Healing of ulcers on the feet correlated with distal blood pressure measurements in occlusive arterial disease. Acta Orthop Scand 51: 995
3. Salles-Cunha SX, Andros G (1990) Preoperative duplex scanning prior to infrainguinal revascularization. Surg Clinics N Amer 70: 41–59

4. Cambria RP, Kaufman JA, L'Italian GJ et al. (1997) Magnetic resonance angiography in the management of lower extremity arterial occlusive disease: a prospective study. J Vasc Surg 25: 380–389
5. Faries P, Morrissey NJ, Teodorescu V et al. (2002) Recent advances in peripheral angioplasty and stenting. Angiology 53: 617–626
6. Uher P, Nyman U, Lindh M et al. (2002) Long-term results of stenting for chronic iliac artery occlusion. J Endovasc Ther 9: 67–75
7. Nelson PR, Powell RJ, Scheremerhorn ML et al. (2002) Early results of external iliac artery stenting combined with common femoral artery endarterectomy. J Vasc Surg 35: 1107–1113
8. Timaran CH, Stevens SL, Freeman MB et al. (2002) Predictors for adverse outcome after iliac angioplasty and stenting for limb-threatening ischemia. J Vasc Surg 36: 507–513
9. Andros G, Harris RW, Salles-Cunha SX et al. (1988) Bypass grafts to the ankle and foot. J Vasc Surg 7: 785–794
10. Faries PL, Arora S, Pomposelli FB et al. (2000) The use of arm vein in lower-extremity revascularization: result of 520 procedures performed in eight years. J Vasc Surg 31: 50–59
11. Veith FJ, Gupta SK, Ascer E et al. (1986) Six-year prospective multicenter randomized comparison of autologous saphenous vein and expanded polytetrafluoroethylene grafts in infrainguinal arterial reconstructions. J Vasc Surg 3: 104–114
12. Taylor LM, Edwards JM, Porter JM et al. (1990) Present status of reversed vein bypass grafting: Five-year results of a modern series. J Vasc Surg 11: 193–206
13. Faries PL, LoGerfo FW, Arora S et al. (2000) Arm vein conduit is superior to composite prosthetic-autogenous grafts in lower extremity revascularization. J Vasc Surg 31: 1119–1127
14. McCarthy WJ, Pearce WH, Flynn WR et al. (1992) Long-term evaluation of composite sequential bypass for limb threatening ischemia. J Vasc Surg 15: 761–770
15. Farber A, Major K, Wagner WH et al. (2003) Cryopreserved saphenous vein allografts in infrainguinal revascularization: analysis of 240 grafts. J Vasc Surg 38: 15–21
16. Neville RF, Tempesta B, Sidway AN (2001) Tibial bypass for limb salvage using polytetrafluoroethylene and a distal vein patch. J Vasc Surg 33: 266–271
17. Ouriel K, Fiore WM, Geary JE (1988) Limb-threatening ischemia in the medically compromised patient: amputation or revascularization? Surgery 104: 667–672
18. Gibbons GW, Burgess AM, Guadagnoli E et al. (1995) Return to wellbeing and function after infrainguinal revascularization. J Vasc Surg 21: 35–45

# 33

# Interventional Radiology for Revascularisation

R. MOLL

## Introduction

Cardiac and cerebrovascular disease is the most frequent cause of morbidity and mortality in the Western world. Another important form of arterial disease or atherosclerosis is chronic peripheral arterial disease. The prevalence of peripheral arterial disease varies with the age of the patients, with rates of 3.1% at ages 40–59 years, 5.4% at ages 60–69 years and 7.7% at age 70 years and above [18]; 70% of the patients were 65 years and older, and the disease is twice as common in men than in women; with asymptomatic disease the rate is doubled [9].

## Diagnostic

To evaluate peripheral artery disease and to control therapeutic effectiveness of interventional procedures, clinical tests are performed: fontaine stages, walking distance, ankle and thigh brachial index are objective criterions. The special procedures in the diagnosis of atherosclerotic disease are duplex scanning and the colour-flow Doppler (CFD), magnetic resonance angiography (MRA), computertomographic angiography (CTA) and digital subtraction angiography (DSA). Although the CFD is non-invasive and has proven its value in screening aneurysms and carotid stenoses, its value for the lower extremity is limited. MRA and CTA have a lower sensitivity and specificity in grading stenoses than DSA, although they are less invasive; especially MRA is the only possibility in the case of renal failure and hyperthyroidism. Nevertheless, digital subtraction angiography is the gold standard for surgery and above all for percutaneous interventions with the possibilities of catheter-directed thrombolysis, dilatation and stenting.

The different possibilities in the treatment of peripheral arterial disease have the aim to reach a long-term patency of the lesions. Each patient has special characteristics, such as site of lesion, type of lesion (stenosis or occlusion), lesion length, arterial run-off, clinical symptoms and Fontaine stage [5]. Bypass surgery and interventional modalities have shown good results in the therapy of aortoiliac, femoropopliteal and peripheral arterial disease. Surgery has proven higher long-term patency rates, but has a higher rate of morbidity, mortality and hospital stay [13].

## Acute Limb Ischemia

Acute limb ischemia is a sudden decrease in limb perfusion, threatening limb viability. Obstruction is caused by an embolus or a new thrombus, growing on an atherosclerotic disease. In most cases, clinical findings and vascular imaging can differentiate these reasons for ischemia, but vasospasm, low cardiac output, acute deep venous thrombosis and neuropathy can imitate an arterial occlusion. Rapid diagnosis in a severe limb ischemia is correlated with a successful outcome of treatment.

## Thrombolysis

Catheter thrombolysis is an initial treatment, suitable to patients with viable state or marginally threatened ischemia. Absolute contra-indications are an established cerebrovascular event (excluding TIA within the previous 2 months), active bleeding diathesis, recent gastrointestinal bleeding (within the previous 10 days) neurosurgery (intracranial, spinal) and intracranial trauma within the previous 3 months [16]. After performing angiography, the next step is to pass the guide wire through the occluded artery. If the guide wire passes, intra-thrombus thrombolysis can be started; if the passage is not possible, the catheter has to be placed proximal to the occlusion. The most frequently used agents for an intra-arterial drug regime are rt-PA (tissue-Plasminogen-activator: 0.5–5 mg/h), Urokinase (20 000–100 000 mg per hour) and streptokinase. At the same time, intravenous infusion with Heparin (20 000–40 000 IU/day) is necessary to diminish thrombogenity. Dependent on the components and the age of the occlusion, intra-arterial infusion should be performed within 1 hour to 2 or 3 days. Since thrombolysis and revascularisation angiography very often indicate a stenosis, which was the origin of the thrombosis, percutaneous transluminal angioplasty should be performed as an important step to avoid re-thrombosis. In comparison to surgical thrombembolectomy, no difference in limb salvage or mortality could be found [17].

## Percutaneous Aspiration Thrombectomy and Percutaneous Mechanical Thrombectomy

These percutaneous procedures are new helpful options, which can be added to the initial digital subtraction angiography. Percutaneous aspiration thrombectomy (PAT) demands a large-lumen catheter with a thin wall. Aspirating with a 50-ml syringe, thrombotic material can be removed (Fig. 1). Suitable vessels are the femoropopliteal native arteries, bypass grafts and the lower leg arteries. This procedure can be used alone or in combination with a subsequent thrombolysis [12].

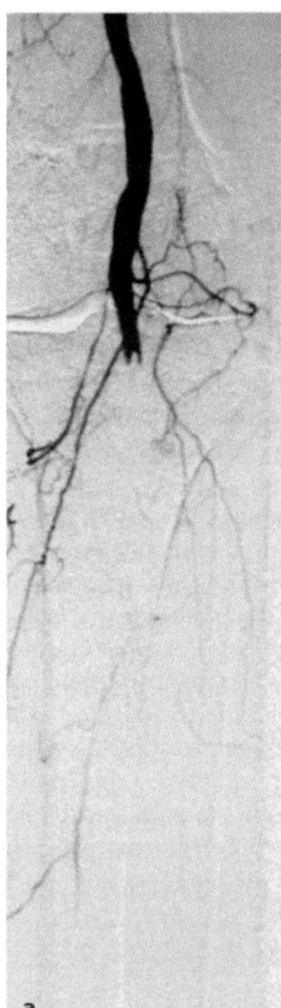
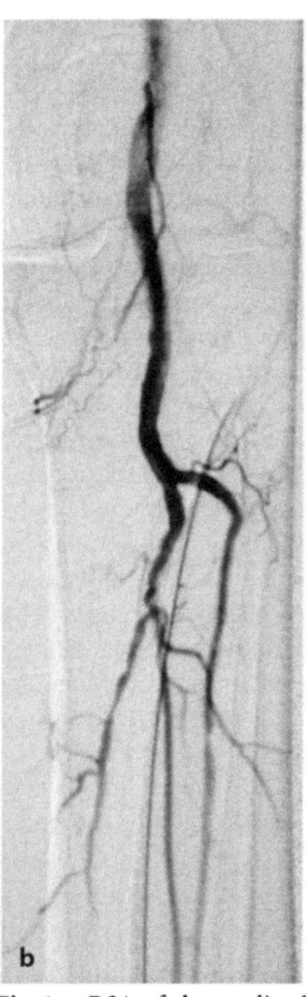

Fig. 1. a DSA of the popliteal and crural artery, occlusion of the trifurcation with an embolus. b DSA after PAT (percutan aspiration thrombectomy), all three calf arteries are free

Percutaneous mechanical thrombectomy (PMT) works with the Venturi principle, and by hydrodynamic recirculation the thrombus will be trapped, dissolved and evacuated in the catheter. Non-recirculation systems like the Amplatz catheter have the disadvantage of a higher risk of embolisation in peripheral vessels and a higher potential for vascular injury [19, 20]. Results of the rotational and hydraulic recirculation systems show the same success rate of 90–95% in the post-interventional period.

For old embolic material, in contrast to the fresh thrombus, success is limited; often thrombolysis or PTA is supplementary. It is an advantage that this fast intervention can be added to the DSA without loss of time. Greater trials to evaluate PAT and PMT in comparison to thrombolysis and surgical thrombembolectomy should be performed to verify the value of these special procedures in interventional radiology.

## Chronic Ischemia

Chronic ischemia is a state with chronic ischemic rest pain (Fontaine III) or patients with ischemic skin, non-healing ulcers and gangrene (Fontaine IV); these patients mostly have passed the stage with intermittent claudicatio (Fontaine IIa und IIb). Chronic limb ischemia includes an ankle systolic pressure of 40 mmHg for patients with rest pain; an ankle systolic pressure less than 60 mmHg is also typical for patients with ulcers and gangrene. The patients in Fontaine stage III and IV would be expected to require a major amputation within the next 6 months to a year, if there is no significant haemodynamic improvement. Critical limb ischemia requires a multidisciplinary approach; before discussing therapeutic strategies a complete angiogram (DSA, MRA or CTA) from the renal arteries to the arcos plantar is necessary. The CFD of the carotids, the coronary situation and also a differential diagnosis for ulcers, gangrene and rest pain should be checked.

In general, a balanced choice of endovascular techniques and surgical procedures should be used, respecting the vessel disease and the comorbidity of the patient. The Transatlantic Inter-Society Consensus (TASC) has edited a definition of types of vascular disease (intermittent claudicatio, acute and chronic limb ischemia), concerning localisation (aortoiliac, femoropopliteal, infrapopliteal) and the division into four groups [5]. Type-A lesions are suited for endovascular treatment, for type-D treatment of choice is surgery, and type B and C are lesions in which no firm recommendation can be made. In type-B lesions endovascular treatment is more commonly used, while surgical procedures will be preferred in type-C lesions. In many cases, patients could be treated by both modalities, but the experience of the institution will play an important role in the choice of procedure. For many patients, a combination of bypass surgery and PTA, especially of the iliac artery, is also a valuable improvement.

## Procedures in Angioplasty

Percutaneous transluminal angioplasty began with Charles Dotter in 1964 [8], who created a new less invasive technique in the therapy of arteriosclerotic disease. He used a coaxial catheter system up to 12 F in diameter with a concept of vessel-sized dilatators. Grüntzig and Hopff [11] described a coaxial balloon catheter that inflated to a fixed diameter for angioplasty in 1974. Since these first steps of interventional therapy, the management of peripheral vascular disease has changed, with advances in technology, particularly in size, track ability, low profile of balloon catheters and hydrophilic guide wires. The technique of percutaneous transluminal angioplasty is standardised and can be performed everywhere, beginning with a balloon catheter; stents can be used as a first choice or in complicated situations like dissection, recoil or occlusion; stent grafts are suitable in the treatment of aneurysms or in the case of an arterial rupture.

## Aortoiliac Region

Aortoiliac disease must be differentiated as aorta and iliac disease. In the majority of patients the aortic disease will be treated by surgery, because it will be associated with widespread disease. For short stenoses of the aorta a balloon dilatation is possible and successful: for good long-time results a stent will be necessary most times. Five-year primary patency was 75%, and most recurrent stenoses (67%) were successfully treated by repeating endovascular procedures [7]. Stenoses and occlusions of the iliac arteries have become a classical localisation for endovascular techniques such as PTA and stent placement (Fig. 2). The technical and clinical success of PTA of iliac stenoses in all series exceeds 90% and approaches 100% for focal iliac stenoses [2]. Profiting from the improved materials like guide wires, balloon catheters and stent developments (Nitinol), limits to recanalisation and reconstruction of occluded arteries have been lowered. The technical success rate of recanalisation of segmental iliac occlusions is 80 to 85% with or without additional fibrinolysis; the complication rate in stenting stenosis or occlusions shows no difference (5–6%) [22]. A 5-year patency rate for stenoses was 61% for PTA and 72% for stents placement [2, 21]; in comparison, a 5-year patency for aorto-bifemoral bypass surgery is 86%. In conclusion, the implantation of stents should be performed if a balloon dilatation has led to a complication (massive dissection) or there remains a rest stenosis of more than 30% (elastic recoil, insufficient haemodynamic result). Other indications for stenting are the treatment of chronic occlusions, ulceration with symptoms,

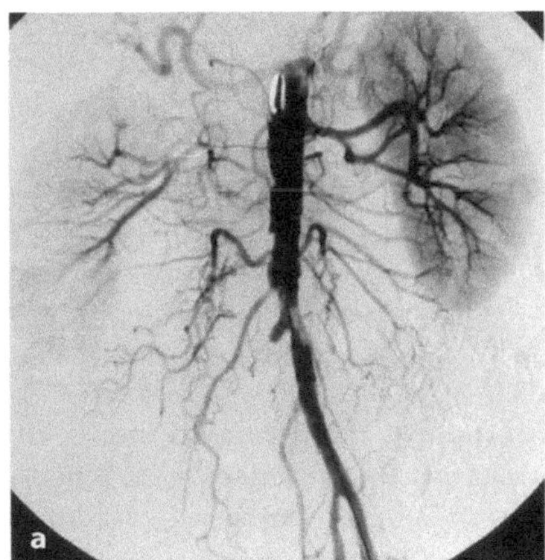

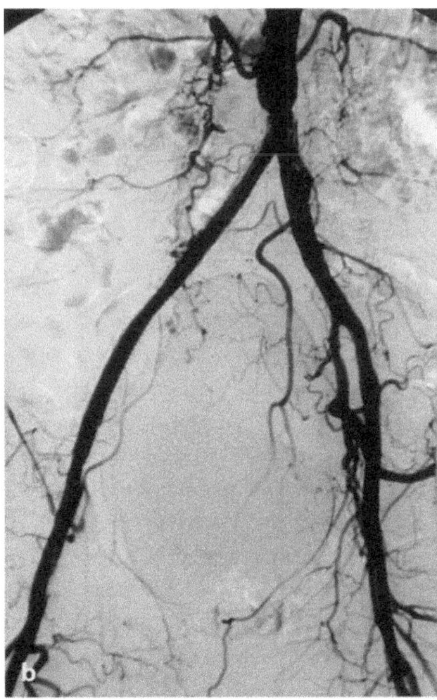

**Fig. 2. a** DSA of the aorta abdominalis from the left side; complete occlusion of the right common and external iliac artery. **b** DSA after recanalisation the occluded iliac artery with two stents, no residual stenosis

restenoses after previously performed PTA and complex lesions. The relative risk of long-term failure after placement of stents was reduced by 39% compared with PTA. Once an iliac artery occlusion has been recanalised successfully, the patency rate for occlusions does not differ from that after PTA of stenoses. The endovascular procedures are generally performed in patients with less severe peripheral arterial disease or unilateral iliac disease. Short iliac lesions (type A, stenosis <3 cm) are suited for endovascular treatment; for long unilateral stenosis, long uni- or bilateral occlusions, surgery should be the treatment of choice (type D), but with modern stent techniques also types C and D have an endovascular therapeutic option in selected patients. Combined surgical and endovascular procedures are used pre- and intra-operatively, especially to ensure the inflow. A special advantage in using these endovascular modalities is the lower morbidity and mortality compared with open surgical revascularisation: mortality 0.8% for PTA, 1% for stents and 3.3% for aortic bifurcation grafts. The complication rate in the endovascular treatment of iliac stenoses is 3.6% for PTA, 6.3% for stents and 8.3% for bifurcation grafts [6].

## Femoropopliteal Region

Percutaneous transluminal angioplasty has its origin in the femoral and popliteal artery, but discussions exist concerning its efficiency and long-time outcome, knowing that PTA in the aorto-iliac segment shows better results than in the femoropopliteal region [23]. Furthermore, patients with peripheral artery disease in the femoropopliteal region, and especially with an infragenicular or multilevel disease, are likely to develop a coronary disease. Preservation of the saphenous vein for coronary bypass grafting could be an important advantage for these patients. The benefit of surgery, endovascular and conservative therapy should be remembered. Results depend on the length of stenosis and occlusion, distal run-off and diffuse disease. The TransAtlantic Inter-Society Consensus has defined a single stenosis up to 3 cm in length as a type-A lesion, suited for PTA, and a complete common femoral artery or superficial artery occlusion or complete popliteal and proximal trifurcation occlusion, as indications for vascular surgery. Technical success for PTA of femoropopliteal lesions (stenoses 90–100% and occlusions 80–85%) is 90%, a 5-year patency about 50%, and a complication rate of 4.3%. Favourable outcome are claudicatio as indication, non-diabetic patients, proximally located short lesions, stenoses, good distal run-off and lack of residual stenoses. If an occlusive lesion is passed and dilated, the same long-term success as for stenosis can be expected [4]. More important is the outcome of femoro-popliteal obstructions; a 5-year patency for PTA of stenosis is 68%, for PTA of occlusions 35%, femoropoliteal bypass with vein 80%, bypass with PTFE above the knee 75% and below the knee 65% [13]. Stents and PTA seem to have the same long-term results for stenoses, and so there is no indication for femoropopliteal stenting as a primary approach in interventional therapy. Nevertheless, stents can play an important role in rescuing failed femoropoliteal PTA like dissection, elastic recoil, eccentric rest stenosis or occlusion after PTA, intimal hyperplasia at graft anastomosis and thrombosis. The initial success is high, but restenosis by intima hyperplasia in the stent segment is quite common in the first 3 to 9 months after stent implantation; also poor outflow and long occlusions appear to increase the frequency of stent thrombosis [24]. Failed PTA did not place the patient at higher risk of limb loss and surgical failure. As in aortoiliac disease, mortality and morbidity of the procedure is an important argument for endovascular treatment; for patients who had undergone surgery, mortality was 2.4%, but only 0% in the PTA group [25]. Short stenoses and occlusions are excellently suited for angioplasty, patients with very long stenoses and occlusions profit from bypass surgery; stents and stent grafts have not shown better results [10, 14].

## Crural and Pedal Disease

Crural arteries often show a three-vessel calf occlusive disease. Patients with diabetes and end-stage renal disease show extensive calcification, which complicates surgical and interventional therapy. The infrapoliteal angioplasty has generally accepted indications like critical acute or chronic limb ischemia and failure of distal bypass grafts; in cases of poor calf run-off after femoropoliteal PTA, tibial angioplasty has shown a better patency in the case of a good distal run-off [3]. The efficacy of infrapopliteal PTA has been substantially improved by technical developments like steerable guide wires and low-profile balloons (Fig. 3). Suitable crural lesions (tibial and peroneal vessels) are short, with a length of 1 cm, and they should have a good run-off. In most cases there are several femoropopliteal and infrapopliteal stenoses; patients who have a dilatation of the proximal stenosis, will get no lasting benefit if a distal stenosis or occlusion is not treated. Recent published technical success rates of infrapopliteal arteries are about 86–100%, complication rate was 2–6%; iatrogenic arterial occlusion responds to local thrombolysis and limb salvage was between 60% and 86% after 2 years. Restoration of the arterial flow from the popliteal region to the crural and pedal arteries is the condition for middle and long-term patency.

## Complications

Interventional procedures in the therapy of peripheral arterial disease include the risks of diagnostic angiography and risks of the therapeutic modalities performed like thrombolysis, angioplasty and stenting. Interventional procedures use larger vascular access, anticoagulation and a lot of additional catheter and guide-wire manipulations. Complications can be classified as major (prolonged hospitalisation, permanent adverse sequel or death) or as minor. Becker [1] published a study with 4662 PTA procedures and observed major complications in 5.6%, in 2.5% surgery was required, limb loss and death were found in 0.2%. Percutaneous interventional therapy can treat 75% of the patients successfully.

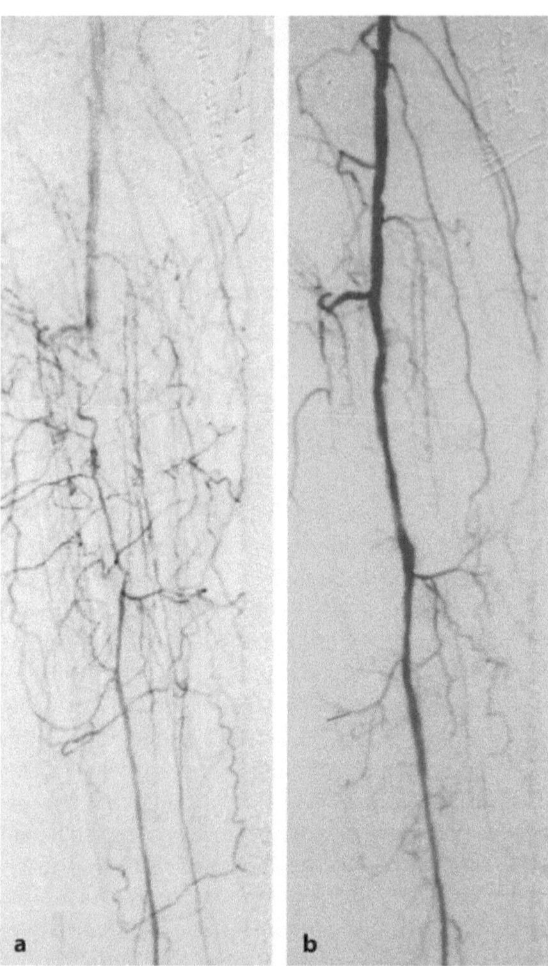

Fig. 3. a Selective angiography of the crural arteries, only fibular artery is filled over collaterals. b DSA after PTA of the fibular artery, normalization of the lumen without rest stenosis

The most common complications are thromboembolic vessel occlusions and puncture site injury like haematoma or false aneurysm. Complications at the PTA site itself, including thrombosis, dissection, perforation and occlusion are less common. Complication rate of the PTA of a stenosis (3.6%) is higher than the PTA of an occlusion (6%); complication rate of PTA of all lesions (stenosis and occlusion) is 4.3%, for stenting of all lesions 5.2%; in femoropoliteal arteries PTA has a complication rate of 4.3%, for stenting of 7.3%. Limb-salvage patients have a 30-day mortality of 10%, whereas patients with claudicatio have 0.5% [15].

Interventional procedures like thrombolysis, percutaneous transluminal angioplasty and stenting play an important role as less invasive treatments between surgery and conservative therapy. Although the Trans-Atlantic Consensus Document (TASC) recommends endovascular treatment as therapy of choice only for short stenosis and occlusions in the aortoiliac and femoropopliteal region, endovascular therapy has proven its potential for acute and chronic ischemia as well as for claudicatio in all regions. Vascular surgery can reach a better patency in severe peripheral artery disease, but interventional procedures have a lower rate of morbidity, mortality and hospital stay, advantages of great importance for elder patients and under economic aspects.

## References


1. Becker GJ, Katzen BT, Dake MD (1989) Noncoronary angioplasty. Radiology 170: 921–940
2. Bosch JL, Hunink MGM (1997) Metaanalysis of the results of percutaneous transluminal angioplasty and stent placement for aortoiliac disease. Radiology 204: 87–96
3. Brown KT, Moore Ed, Getrajdman GI, Saddekni S (1993) Infrapopliteal angioplasty: long-term follow up. JVIR 4: 139–44
4. Capek P, Mc Lean GK, Berkowitz HD (1991) Femoropoliteal angioplasty. Factors influencing long-term success. Circulation 83: 70–80
5. Dormandy JA, Rutherford RB (2000) Management of peripheral arterial disease (PAD). TASC Working Group. TransAtlantic Inter-Society Consensus (TASC). J Vasc Surg 31: 1–296
6. De Vries SO, Hunink MG (1997) Results of aortic bifurcation grafts for aortoiliac occlusive disease: a meta analysis. J Vasc Surg 26: 558–569
7. De Vries JP, van den Heuvel DA, Vos JA, van den berg JC, Moll FI (2004) Freedom from secondary interventions to treat stenotic disease after percutaneous transluminal angioplasty of infrarenal aorta – long-term results. J Vasc Surg 39: 427–431
8. Dotter CT, Judkins MP (1964) Transluminal treatment of arteriosclerotic obstruction. Circulation 30: 654–670
9. Fowkes FG, Housley E, Cawood EH, Macintyre CC, Ruckley CV, Prescott RJ (1991) Edinburgh artery study: prevalence of asymptomatic and symptomatic peripheral arterial disease in the general population. Int J Epidemiol 20: 384–392
10. Gallino A, Mahler F, Probst P, Nachbur B (1984) Percutaneous transluminal angioplasty of the arteries of the lowerlimbs: a 5 year follow-up. Circulation 70: 619–623
11. Grüntzig A, Hopff H (1974) Perkutane Rekanalisation chronischer arterieller Verschlüsse mit einem neuen Dilatationskatheter. Dtsch Med Wochenschr 99: 2502–2510
12. Huettl EA, Soulen MC (1995) Thrombolysis of lower extremity occlusions: a study of the results of the STAR registry. Radiology 197: 141–145
13. Hunink MG, Wong JB, Donaldson MC, Meyerovitz MF, de Vries, Harrington DP (1995) Revascularization for femoro-popliteal arterial disease: a decision and cost-effectiveness analysis. JAMA 274: 165–171
14. Johnston KW (1992) Femoral and popliteal arteries: reanalysis of results of balloon angioplasty. Radiology 183: 767–771
15. Matsi PJ, Manninen HI (1998) Complications of lower limb percutaneous transluminal angioplasty: a prospective analysis of 410 procedures on 295 patients. Cardiovasc Int Radiol 21: 361–366
16. McNamara TO, Bomberger RA (1986) Factors affecting initial and six month patency rates after intra-arterial thrombolysis with high dose urokinase. Am J Surg 152: 709–712
17. Ouriel K, Veith FJ, Sasahara AA (1996) For the TOPAS Investigators. Thrombolysis or peripheral arterial surgery: phase I results. J Vasc Surg 23: 64–73
18. Pentecost MJ, Criqui MH, Dorros G, Goldstone J, Johnston KW, Martin EC, Ring EJ, Spies JB (2003) Guideline for peripheral percutaneous transluminal angioplasty of the abdominal aorta and lower extremity vessels. JVIR 14: 495–515
19. Rilinger N, Gorich J, Scharrer-Palmer R, Vogel J, Tomczak R, Kramer S, Merkle E, Brambs HJ, Sokiranski R (1997) Short term results with use of the Amplatz thrombectomy device in the treatment of lower limb occlusions. JVIR 8: 343–348
20. Sharafuddin MJ, Hicks ME (1997) Current status of percutaneous mechanical thrombectomy. Part 1: General principles. JVIR 8: 911–921
21. Strecker EP, Hagen P, Liermann D, Schneider B, Wolf HR, Wambsganns J et al. (1993) Iliac and femoro-popliteal vascular occlusive disease treated with flexible tantalum stents. Cardiovasc Intervent Radiol 16:158–164

22. Vorwerck D, Günther RW, Schürmann K, Wendt G (1996) Aortic and iliac stenoses: follow-up results of stent placement after insufficient balloon angioplasty in 118 cases. Radiology 198: 45–48

23. Wagner HJ (2002) Zum aktuellen Stellenwert der endovaskulären Therapie im femoropoplitealen Gefäßabschnitt bei chronischer pAVK. Vasa 31: 153–161

24. Wagner HJ, Rager G (1998) Infrapopliteal angioplasty: a forgotten region? Fortschr Geb Rontgenstr Neuen Bildgeb Verfahr 168: 415–420

25. Wilson SE, Wolf GL, Cross AP (1989) Percutaneous transluminal angioplasty versus operation for peripheral arteriosclerosis: report of a prospective randomized trial in a selected group of patients. J Vasc Surg 9: 1–9

# 34

# Venous Ulcer Surgery

F. Gottrup, A. Haabegaard, J.L. Sørensen

## Introduction

Venous ulcerations of the lower extremities represent an increasing socio-economic health-care problem [1]. The main reason is the increased number of elderly people in many countries. The incidence of leg ulcers in the European countries is estimated to range between 0.2 and 0.7% of the whole population and this figure will be three to four times higher after 65 years of age. Females suffer more often from leg ulcer than males, with a ratio of 1.6:1; more than 75% of the patients are over 60 years of age. It has been estimated that the economical burden of treatment in the European Community adds up to about 2% of the total health-care costs [2].

## Pathogenesis and Classification

The cause of venous leg ulcers is traditionally based on the underlying vascular pathology [3]. About 50% of patients with venous leg ulcers show superficial and perforating vein incompetence primarily in the valves [4], while deep venous insuffiency is found in 50–70%. The development of venous insufficiency is not yet fully understood, but different theories have been proposed. Superficial venous insufficiency may be based on increased venous pressure, a weak venous wall, and AV fistulas, while deep venous insufficiency may develop after venous thrombosis with valve destruction or congenital abnormalities. Insufficiency of the perforation veins can be the result of factors influencing both the superficial and deep venous system. These conditions may be related to different conditions of which earlier thrombophlebitis probably is a major cause. The consequence of venous insufficiency is a decreased possibility to reduce pressure in the venous system during exercise. Increased pressure of the foot vein during exercise has shown an increased risk of developing leg ulcers. A connection between total venous reflux based on venous insufficiency and development of venous ulcers has also been shown. Besides the development of an ulcer, the surrounding skin area will develop lipodermatosclerosis, which is a tight fibrotic tissue coloured by haemosiderin pigmentation from extravasation of red blood cells into the interstitial tissue.

The precise pathogenesis resulting in the development of an ulcer is not exactly known. It is generally accepted that venous insufficiency results in changed microcirculation of the lower leg and development of ulcers. The direct link, however, between venous hypertension and ulcer development is still unclear. A number of hypotheses (fibrin-cuff theory, white-cell trapping theory, tissue-pressure theory, trap theory and others) have been suggested, but no general agreement has been achieved. An unfavourable distribution of growth factors and imbalance in proteolytic enzymes has also been mentioned as influencing factor for the development of venous leg ulcers.

Classification of venous leg ulcers has clinically been a problem. The Hawaii Classification [5] is very detailed and is primarily related to diseases in the veins, and it is not usable in normal clinical practice. The most used but very simplistic classification relates to the development of venous insufficiencies in the superficial or deep venous system or in the perforant veins.

In venous ulcer disease the standard conservative treatment is compression bandage and local wound treatment [6–8]. The beneficial effects of compression therapy are well documented [9], and healing in 3 months has been achieved in up to 70% of the patients [7, 10, 11]. However, even when patients are fully compliant and follow the guidelines for optimal conservative treatment, up to 30% of ulcers return within 5 years [12]. The major problems then will be that there will no healing at all using conservative treatment or recurrence after conservative treatment. These patients would be candidates for surgical treatment of their venous leg ulcer.

## Clinic and Considerations

The goal for the surgeons will be a healed wound with stable skin coverage that does not break down over time. This is often difficult to realise in a chronic wound like a venous leg ulcer, where the incompetence of the venous valves still is a major problem. The ideal surgical therapy covering all aspects of the venous ulcer pathology is not yet found, although many procedures have been used. Many of these are purely palliative because they only promote healing but, without other actions, they do not prevent recurrence (see list below) [12]. The only group of patients who can be totally cured by surgery are patients with pure insufficient superficial veins, because the underlying venous dysfunction could be treated. However, in general practice the majority has a mixed superficial and deep insufficiency. In a dedicated wound-healing centre taking care of the most difficult cases, about 80% of the patients had a mixed superficial and deep insufficiency and 66% a poplitea vein sufficiency [13, 14]. For these reasons, also palliative methods have to be used in order to be able to treat a significant part of the patients suffering from venous leg ulcers.

| Surgical Procedures Available for the Treatment of Venous Leg Ulcers [12] |
| --- |

- Palliative
  - General surgery: Revision/debridement, skin grafting, paratibial fasciotomy
  - Vein surgery in legs with DVI: varicose vein surgery, perforator interruption, deep vein reconstruction
  - Arterial surgery for coexisting ischaemia

- Curative
  - Vein surgery in legs with isolated SVI and/or PVI: varicose vein surgery, perforator interruption

  *SVI* Superficial venous incompetence; *PVI* Perforating vein incompetence; *DVI* Deep venous incompetence

To date, there are no clear indications for surgery in venous leg ulcers or the specific procedure to use. An accurate diagnosis of the ulcer, coupled with a definition of the pattern of venous abnormality, is mandatory if surgery is considered [15]. In patients with isolated superficial and/or perforating vein incompetence the ulcers in up to half of the cases are caused by varicose veins [12, 16]. Varicose vein surgery for this reason has to be taken into account, and it must be emphasised that this type of surgery requires surgical skill and should be performed by experienced surgeons [15]. This type of surgery has not generally been highly accepted among vascular surgeons. The results, however, are good, with 90% of ulcers remaining healed after 3–5 years [12]. This and the lacking need for prophylactic compression therapy are benefits of the surgical treatment. The role of varicose vein surgery for patients with deep venous incompetence and coexisting superficial and perforating vein incompetence is still not fully illuminated. If surgery is not followed by prophylactic compression, most ulcers seem to recur.

Recent studies have concluded that non-healing venous leg ulcers can be treated with ulcer excision, meshed split-skin transplantation, and correction of superficial venous insufficiency in the wound area with beneficial results irrespective of underlying pattern of venous insufficiency as determined by colour Duplex scanning [17]. In a group of 385 patients representing 406 chronic leg ulcers treated as described and with venous insufficiency as only aetiology in 64% the overall healing rate was 65% after 1 year [18].

## Diagnostic Methods

The most important issue is to determine the origin of the ulcer in order to institute the correct treatment immediately.

The diagnosis of venous ulceration in primary health care is based on a clinical history including duration of the ulcer, its healing and the type of treatment. Is there a history of deep vein thrombosis? Is claudicatio present? Is oedema present, and what is its aetiology? Is malignancy a possibility?

A patient examination should include palpation of the foot pulses. Most often the symptoms and signs are: varicose veins, oedema, pain and localisation and presentation of the wound and the surrounding skin (lipodermatosclerosis, eczema and atrophy blanche).

The medical history and clinical examination will usually indicate a venous origin of the ulcer. However, further investigations are needed to determine the possibility for surgical intervention.

If the foot pulses are not easily palpated, an ankle-arm index should be performed. In diabetic patients with increased size of media in the vessels the result of this measure often is falsely high in the ankle area, for which reason a toe-pressure measurement should be performed in order to determine the arteriosclerotic component. A colour duplex scan should be performed to determine deep, superficial or combined reflux. This also provides information on deep venous thrombosis, which could be obstructive.

It has been shown that ascending phlebography, continuous-wave Doppler and ambulatory strain gauge plethysmography are of little value in the work-up of patients with deep venous insufficiency, and an triplex ultrasound including anatomical and morphological evaluation is an optimal way to visualise the deep veins, venous valvular competence and the perforating veins [19].

## Surgical Procedures

Surgery in conjunction with venous ulcers is divided into two parts:
- Surgery on the ulcer.
- Surgery on the course of the ulcer, the insufficient veins: surgical treatment of chronic venous insufficiency.

### Ulcer Surgery

Surgical revision/debridement is a one-stage sharp removal of the ulcer and more or less of the changed tissue in its surroundings. Revision is an operation and should therefore be performed with sterile procedures. By surgical revision the ulcer is prepared for immediate healing or closure. Only tissue with sufficient healing potential must be left. An experienced surgeon, for this reason, has to take responsibility for a sufficient revision.

Necrotic tissue must be removed until bleeding to make sure that no inferior tissue is left behind. This is a relatively non-selective procedure since vital tissue may be destroyed (bleeding). The technique should be as atraumatic as possible to reduce the harm of revision, but the procedure will, on the other hand, be in vain if it is not radical. Sharp sweeping cuts are preferred to "chewing" the tissue with a hesitating pair of scissors. The tissue must be gently lifted to be removed and not be ripped off.

The ulcer bed and changed tissue in its surroundings are most often of an inferior quality because they have been fibrotic over time. This lipodermatosclerosis should be eliminated since its blood supply is inferior and reduces the chance for an uncomplicated taking of a split-skin transplant. Concurring diseases and other relevant factors can, however, be an indication for minimising the intervention.

Ideally, all inferior tissue should be removed; however, this can result in a major and blood-consuming operation, and in the case of circular excision there may be postoperative problems with peripheral lymphoedema. The indication for and the extent of an operation therefore has to be assessed carefully before surgery.

Usually the excision is carried out to the deep fascia, but sometimes even deeper excision including exposed tendons and bone is necessary. Tangential excision can usually be performed and may be sufficient. It is carried out with a dermatome slicing the ulcer and the surrounding. The method creates large bleeding surfaces, which should immediately be covered by a split-thickness skin graft.

If calcifications are situated in the soft tissue, if the level of excision is expected to be irregular, or if deep structures are to be excised, direct excision to the fascia or lower should be performed. This method is surgically more demanding but gives less bleeding. Skin grafting usually can be performed directly. Otherwise, a delayed procedure can be performed, preferably using topical negative-pressure therapy (TNP) to reduce the time interval.

Often, an acceptable compromise is to excise the ulcer and the surrounding to obtain an acceptable ulcer bed. The ulcer should be able to accept skin grafting immediately.

If the patient is reluctant to accept more extensive surgery or is in a condition calling for minimising surgery, a tangential excision of the ulcer and its immediate borders can be performed. In this case, only a thin split-skin transplant should be applied, or the transplantation should be postponed until granulation tissue has grown to cover the ulcer. This can be accelerated by applying topical negative pressure (TNP). In all other cases a split-thickness skin graft of intermediate thickness can be applied.

Systemic antibiotics should treat infection in the surrounding living tissue. A positive culture without clinical signs of infection is not an indication for antibiotics unless β-haemolytic streptococcus is found. These bacteria can spread into the tissue, developing erysipelas and lymphatic destruction and should be treated by the use of penicilline.

Usually, the use of local antibiotics is not recommendable. This treatment cannot eliminate infection in the surrounding tissue and bears the risk of developing allergy in the host and resistance in the microorganisms. Local infection is most effectively treated by surgical revision.

Indication for surgery depends on the size of the wound. Normally, keratinocytes can cover a vital defect up to about 3 cm without any problem. If the defect is larger, the quality of the epithelium will in general be of lower quality compared to a healed split-skin transplant regarding strength, amount of scar tissue and cosmetic result. Presuming uneventful healing, a split-skin transplant will cover the ulcer surface faster compared to secondary epithelisation. A deep ulcer also calls for surgical intervention, if deep structures are to be protected or should be removed because of necrosis or infection.

The surgical procedure is performed in the theatre using sterile procedures. A revision is a one-stage procedure with radical elimination of necrosis, e.g. prior to split-skin transplantation.

The aim of revision/debridement is to eliminate all inferior tissue, which will not heal. Lipodermatosclerotic tissue should be removed together with the necrosis in order to supply the ulcer bed with well-perfused tissue fit for healing or receiving a skin transplant. In many cases, the excision must be performed to the deep fascia or deeper to reach tissue of a sufficient quality. Devitalised deep structures must be removed as well.

The process of granulation can be accelerated considerably using topical negative pressure treatment (VAC).

If revision/debridement in the theatre is not possible, it can take place at the bedside or in the outpatient clinic. Clean instruments and procedures are sufficient. Careful handling of the tissue prevents damage to vital tissue and reduces pain. Often several debridements are necessary before the ulcer is totally free of necrosis.

### Alternative Debridement Techniques

Mostly, sharp revision/debridement is quickly performed, and at the bedside it may be even faster and cheaper. However, it is not always possible to be radical (pain, bleeding), and in deep ulcers with fistulas it is often non-sufficient. A lancet or a pair of scissors and a forceps is all that is needed.

Non-surgical revision/debridement can be an option. Several methods are available (see list below) [20]. Further details of these methods would go beyond the scope of this book.

---

**Debridement Techniques**

- Surgical/sharp debridement
- Enzymatic agents
- Chemical agents
- Osmotic debridement
- Autolytic debridement
- Biosurgical debridement
- Wet-to-dry dressings
- Whirlpool and hydrotherapy (mechanical debridement)
- High-pressure irrigations (mechanical debridement)
- Other types

---

### Skin Grafting

A small ulcer with a diameter of less than about 3 cm should be left for secondary healing. In all the other venous ulcers skin grafting should be considered.

In venous ulcer surgery a split-thickness skin graft is the option. If the local perfusion in the wound is satisfactory after revision, an intermediate thickness-skin graft (0.3–0.4 mm) can be used. In the case of dubious blood supply a thin graft (<0.3 mm) is preferred [21].

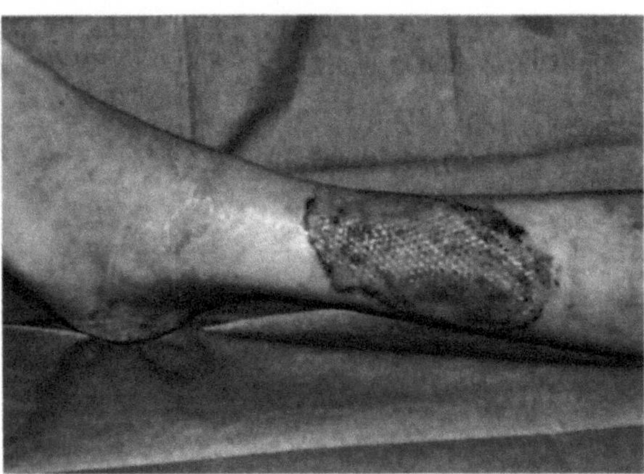

**Fig. 1.** Skin graft/transplant on a revised venous leg ulcer, two weeks old

Split-thickness skin grafts are harvested by dermatomes. They can be constructed to a fixed thickness or, more often, can be individually adjusted. They can be hand-driven or mechanically driven by compressed air or electricity.

Since there will always be a risk of bleeding and infection, grafts immediately applied are meshed. The perforations permit secretion to escape from between the graft and ulcer bed. Any secretion beneath the graft will hamper healing. The meshing procedure increases the area of the graft if it is stretched (usually up to 1.5 times its original size), but this is of no importance in ulcer surgery, where there is no lack of skin for grafting. The graft is fixed to its bed by sutures or staples and kept immobile and compressed against the ulcer bed by a covering bandage. This bandage consists of an inner greasy layer to prevent desiccation of the graft and adherence of the bandage and an outer compressing and absorbing layer to protect and secure the graft. Routinely, the authors remove the bandage after 5 days to check the take of the graft, but even earlier (down to 2 days) removal is possible [18]. The patient is allowed to mobilise freely the day after the operation with a compression bandage. The graft should be healed in 10–14 days (Fig. 1), but minor defects are not uncommon. Usually they can be left for spontaneous healing.

There exist numbers of dressings and routines for donor sites. The authors use a foam bandage or film to protect the donor site and allow a humid environment for healing. The bandage can be removed after 7–10 days depending on the thickness of the graft and the age of the patient.

## Surgical Treatment of Chronic Venous Insufficiency

### Indications for Venous Surgery

Although there is no Cochran-scale level-A evidence to support the superiority of surgery versus conservative treatment, it was shown that 80–90% of patients with ulcers resulting from incompetent perforators benefit from subfacial endoscopic perforator surgery (SEPS). This is performed in patients with or without deep venous insufficiency [22].

The indications for vein surgery in patients with advanced chronic venous insufficiency (CVI, CEAP classification C4 to C6) is reflux in the greater saphenous vein, the smaller saphenous vein and/or reflux in perforators. The diagnosis should be verified by duplex scanning.

Relative contra-indications are thrombosis of the deep veins, arterial occlusive disease with pressures so low that it will compromise healing, severe oedema from reasons other than CVI and medically high-risk patients.

The aim of surgery is to remove superficial veins with reflux. These include varicose veins, greater and smaller saphenous vein and perforators. Ongoing studies will show the need for either perforator surgery together with removal of superficial veins with reflux or removal only of superficial veins with reflux.

### Surgical Procedure

**Pre-Operative.** A duplex scanning to guide the operative procedure is performed. Hereby, the veins and perforators with reflux are marked. In the case of reflux in the smaller saphenous vein, the sapheno-popliteal junction is marked. The varicose veins are likewise marked, which should be done by the surgeon. Patients in general anaesthetics will have local anaesthetics as well to reduce the post-operative pain.

**Peri-Operative.** The procedures should be focused on removing veins with reflux and thereby reduce the ambulatory venous pressure.

If there is reflux in the sapheno-femoral junction and in the greater saphenous vein, a resection of stella venosa should be performed so that all the contributories will be divided, the vena femoralis visualised over approximately 5 cm. Small branches from the deep femoral vein should likewise be divided. The greater saphenous vein should be ligated close to the deep femoral vein. Hereafter, a PIN-stripping to the knee should be performed. This procedure will invaginate the vein and reduce the risk of damage to the saphenous nerve.

With reflux in the smaller saphenous vein, a 4-cm incision in the popliteal region is made. The sapheno-popliteal junction is visualised and the smaller saphenous vein is ligated close to the popliteal vein. After that, PIN-stripping of the smaller saphenous vein is performed.

The varicose veins are removed through stab incisions. A small incision is made over the varicose vein, which is hooked and withdrawn. A few minutes compression will stop the bleeding. These incisions are only plastered.

In the case of reflux in the perforators SEPS (subfascial endoscopic perforator surgery) is performed. This is known as a safe procedure with promising results [23].

We are using a single-port technique with insufflations of carbon dioxide (Stortz). In the past, we used Esmarchs bandage but this was abandoned because of temporary damage to a sensory nerve. A 1-cm transverse incision 15 cm below the knee and 3 cm posterior to the tibial bone is made. The scope is inserted through a small incision in the fascia and visual dissection is performed. All perforators in the widely explored subfacial space are electrocoagulated and divided. The deep posterior compartment is opened by incision of the fascia and perforators are dealt with as mentioned above. Retromalleolar perforators are divided by a small incision. The carbon dioxide is squeezed out after removal of all instruments.

An alternative to SEPS is OPS (open perforator surgery). In this type of surgery the pre-operatively marked perforators are visualised by a skin incision superficial for the perforator, which is divided at the level of the fascia.

**Post-Operative.** Patients are sent home on the same afternoon or the following day, provided with class-I stockings for 3 weeks. Sutures are removed at post-operative day 10 by the family doctor. These patients should be followed annually for 5 years.

## Conclusion

Standard use of surgical treatment in the case of chronic ulcers is increasing. Non-healing wounds based on chronic venous insufficiency should be treated by ulcer surgery, skin grafting and venous surgery. This should consist of correction of the superficial venous insufficiency including insufficient perforators. In the case of ischaemia, arterial reconstruction should be made. A multidisciplinary and multi-speciality set up is needed in most cases.

## References


1. Ruckley CV (1997) Socioeconomic impact of chronic venous insufficiency and leg ulcers. Angiology 48: 67–69
2. Laing W (1992) Chronic venous diseases of the leg. Office of health Economics, London
3. Scriven JM, Hartshore T, Bell PRF, Naylor AR, London NJM (1997) Single-visit venous ulcer assessment clinic: the first year. Br J Surg 84: 334–336
4. Ågren MS, Eaglstein WH, Ferguson MJ, Harding KG, Moore K, Saarialho-Kere UK, Schultz GS (2000) Causes and effects of the chronic inflammation in venous leg ulcers. Acta Derm Venereol 210 [Suppl]: 3–17
5. Porter JM, Monetta GL (1995) International Consensus Committee on chronic venous diseases. Reporting standards in venous disease: An update. J Vasc Surg 21: 635–645
6. Kitahama A, Elliot LF, Kerstein MD, Menendez CV (1982) Leg ulcers. Conservative management or surgical treatment? JAMA 247: 197–199
7. Blair SD, Wright DDI, Blackhouse CM, Riddle E, McCollum CN (1988) Sustained compression and healing of chronic venous ulcers. BMJ 297: 1159–1161
8. Falanga V (1993) Venous ulceration. J Dermatol Surg Oncol 19: 764–771
9. Fletcher A, Cullum D, Sheldon TA (1997) A systematic review of compression treatment for venous leg ulcers. BMJ 315: 576–580
10. Stacay MC, Jopp-Mckay AG, Rashid P, Hoskin SE, Thomso PJ (1997) The influence of dressings on venous ulcer healing – a randomised trial. Eur Vasc Endovasc Surg 13: 174–179
11. Hofman D, Poore S, Cherry GW (1998) The use of short-stretch bandaging to control oedema. J Wound Care 7: 10–12
12. Nelzén O (1995) Surgical options and indications for surgery in the treatment of patients with venous leg ulcers. In: Treatment of venous leg ulcers. The Norwegian Medicines Control Authority and Medical Products Agency, Oslo Uppsala, pp 149–162
13. Gottrup F, Holstein P, Jørgensen B, Lohmann M, Karlsmark T (2001) A new concept of a multidisciplinary wound healing center and a national expert function of wound healing. Arch Surg 136: 765–772
14. Kjaer ML, Jorgensen B, Karlsmark T, Holstein P, Simonsen L, Gottrup F (2003) Does the pattern of venous insufficiency influence healing of venous leg ulcers after skin transplantation? Eur J Vasc Endovasc Surg 25: 562–567

15. Callam M, Ruckley CV (1992) Chronic venous insufficiency and leg ulcers. In: Bell PRF, Jamieson CW, Ruckley CV (eds) Surgical management of vascular diseases. WB Saunders, London, pp 1267–1303
16. Lees TA, Lambert D (1993) Patterns of venous reflux in limbs with skin changes associated with chronic venous insufficiency. Br J Surg 80: 725–728
17. Kjaer ML, Jorgensen B, Karlsmark T, Holstein P, Simonsen L, Gottrup F (2003) Does the pattern of venous insufficiency influence healing of venous leg ulcers after skin transplantation? Eur J Vasc Endovasc Surg 25: 562–567
18. Bitsch M, Saunte DM, Lohmann M, Holstein P, Jorgensen B, Gottrup F (2003) A standardised method of surgical treatment of chronic leg ulcers. (Submitted)
19. Mantoni M, Larsen L, Lund JO, Henriksen L, Karlsmark T, Strandberg C, Ogstrup J, Ribel-Madsen S, Gottrup F, Danielsen L (2002) Evaluation of chronic venous disease in the lower limbs: comparison of five diagnostic methods. Br J Radiol 75: 578–583
20. Gottrup F (2002) Wound Debridement. In: The Oxford European Wound Healing Course Handbook. Positif Press, Oxford, pp 116–120
21. Jankauskas S, Cohen IK, Grabb WC (1991) Skin Grafts. In: Smith JW, Aston SJ (eds) Grabb and Smith's Plastic Surgery. Little, Brown and Company, Boston, pp 20–44
22. Kalra M, Gloviczki P (2003) Surgical treatment of venous ulcers: role of subfascial endoscopic perforator vein ligation. Surg Clin N Am 83: 671–705
23. Nelzén O (2000) Prospective study of safety, patient satisfaction and leg ulcer healing following saphenous and subfascial endoscopic perforator surgery. Br J Surg 87: 86–91

# Diabetic Foot Surgery

D.G. ARMSTRONG

## Introduction

The diabetic foot remains the most common reason for hospitalisation amongst persons with diabetes in the developed and the developing world [1]. With an incidence of up to 68 per 1000 persons with diabetes per year, diabetic foot wounds are exceedingly common and this trend appears to be on the rise [2]. The aetiology of the classic non-infected, non-ischemic neuropathic diabetic foot wound is essentially a pressure-activity imbalance. When discussing the pressure side of this equation, one may modulate this variable externally, through offloading modalities or braces, or internally, through surgical intervention.

The past generation has seen a dramatic increase in interest in reconstructive surgery on the diabetic foot [3–21]. While much of this work began as a rather confusing mixture of indications and types of procedures, recent years have witnessed something of a slow movement toward a more unified parlance. Recently, our group, working out of some frustration with difficulties in intra- and inter-facility communication as regards diabetic foot surgery, proposed a simple classification system which we hope will help to coalesce discourse on this subject [22]. To that end, the purpose of this brief chapter is to discuss proposed risk-based classes of diabetic foot surgery performed on the non-ischemic foot.

A of diabetic foot-surgery classification system should be based on three basic variables:

- The presence or absence of neuropathy. As neuropathy is the permissive event to the development of the vast majority of diabetic foot pathology, the absence of neuropathy should theoretically dramatically reduce risk for ulceration.
- The presence or absence of an open wound. An open wound should theoretically increase the risk for ulceration or amputation. While there are no studies in the literature which specifically confirm or refute this theory, it certainly stands up to trial in the court of common sense. We may also be able to lend credence to this secondarily from some other related works. In a study performed several years ago on simple digital arthroplasty procedures, we reported that persons with a history of a recently healed wound were at higher risk for ulceration than were persons with no history of wound at that site [4]. Additionally, another recent study of first metatarsalphalangeal joint-arthroplasty procedures performed on patients with open hallux wounds, while suggesting a very high rate of success compared with non-surgical therapy, also reported a high rate of post-operative infection (40%) in both treatment and control arms [23].
- The presence or absence of limb-threatening infection.

## What About Ischemia?

Clearly, the presence of profound ischemia is a significant factor associated with failure to heal and subsequent high-level amputation. No non-emergency procedure should be performed without first identifying the patient's overall vascular status. Vascular disease in every case should supersede any prophylactic procedure and should be addressed through pro-active surgical and medical management.

## Classes of Diabetic Foot Surgery

Figure 1 gives an outline of the risk-based classes of diabetic foot surgery.

### Class I: Elective

Elective diabetic foot surgery is performed on the patient with the prime intention of relieving pain or significant impairment of function. It is performed on the patient with intact sensation. This patient, assuming good metabolic control and close medical management, should be at no significantly greater risk for a severe postoperative complication than a similarly aged patient without diabetes. An example of this class of surgery might be a digital arthroplasty for a painful hammer-toe deformity or a bunionectomy for painful hallux valgus.

### Class II: Prophylactic

Prophylactic diabetic foot surgery is that procedure performed on a patient with loss of protective sensation but without an open wound. As this patient does not have the "gift of pain", he or she may have an identical deformity to the patient undergoing class-I (elective) surgery and may undergo the identical procedure. However, the indication for this procedure is the prevention of the occurrence or recurrence of a diabetic foot wound, rather than the alleviation of pain. An example of a prophylactic procedure might be a pan-metatarsal head resection, a Charcot foot reconstruction, an achilles tendon lengthening, or a hammer-toe correction [12, 24–26]. In rare cases, a partial foot amputation might be considered prophylactic. An example of this might be a particularly contracted digit or highly deformed forefoot that has been recalcitrant to previous conservative and/or surgical intervention.

### Class III: Curative

Curative surgery may be identical in nature to prophylactic surgery with one significant difference: the presence of an open wound. The goal of the curative procedure (as opposed to the prophylactic) is to speed healing of the diabetic foot wound. Obviously, a secondary goal would be to prevent recurrence as well. One randomised

| Diabetic Foot Surgery Class | Description | | Potential risk for high-level amputation |
|---|---|---|---|
| Class IV: Emergent | Procedure performed to limit progression of acute infection | | High |
| Class III: Curative | Procedure performed to assist in healing open wound | | Moderate |
| Class II: Prophylactic | Procedure performed to reduce risk of ulceration or reulceration in person with loss of protective sensation but without open wound | | Low |
| Class I: Elective | Procedure performed to alleviate pain or limitation of motion in a person without loss of protective sensation | | Very low |

**Fig, 1.** Risk-based classes of diabetic foot surgery

trial, conducted by Piagessi and co-workers [27], in an amalgam of a 21-patient co-hort with various types of diabetic foot wounds, suggested that the time to wound healing was more rapid than non-surgical therapy. A subsequent case-control study of metatarsophalangeal joint arthroplasties already mentioned above [23] reported significantly faster healing in the surgical group (SG) than patients in the standard therapy (ST) group (ST 67.1±17.1 days vs. SG 24.2±9.9 days), who had fewer recurrent ulcers (ST 35.0 vs. SG 4.8). Both groups had similar rates of infection (ST 38.1 vs. SG 40.0%, $p$=0.9) and short-term amputation (ST 10.0% vs. SG 4.8 vs. $p$=0.5). Numerous other manuscripts have suggested similar results in various case series [11]. Lin et al. [26], in a hybrid case-control study of achilles tendon lengthening, reported rapid healing of previously recalcitrant plantar wounds coupled with a significantly lower rate of recurrence (19% vs. 0%). This procedure is outlined in Fig. 2a–d. Mueller and colleagues, in a recent randomised trial of achilles lengthenings, reported a similar trend toward lower ulcer recurrence (52% reduced risk for reulceration at 2 years) [28].

## Class IV: Emergency

Emergency procedures are performed to limit the spread of acute, limb-threatening infection. Without a doubt, this class of surgery may be performed in the presence of significant ischemia. The potential for vascular intervention should be considered either concomitant with this procedure or in the immediate post-operative hospitalisation period.

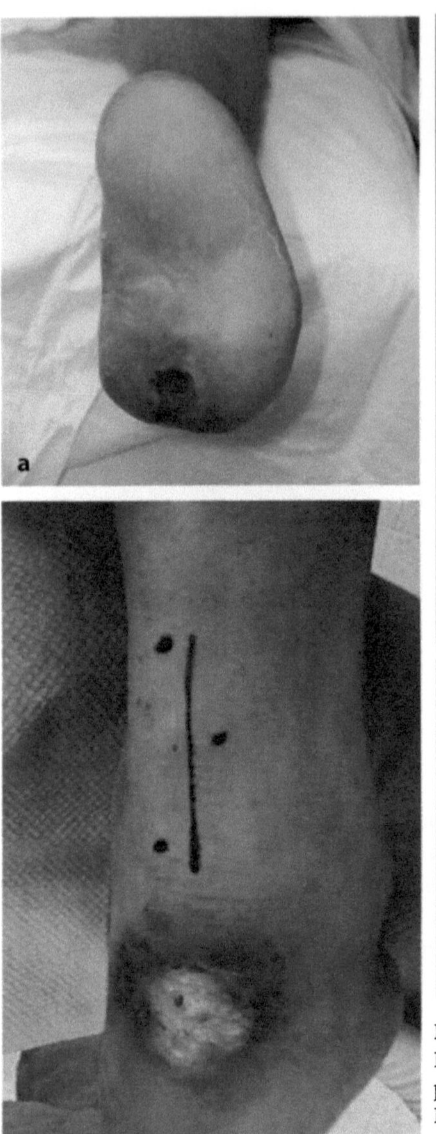

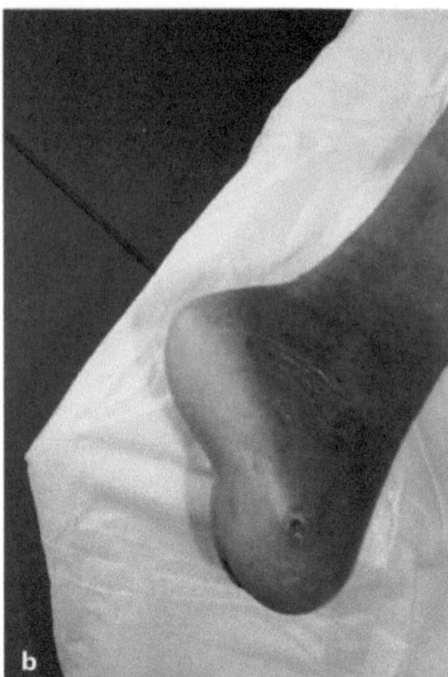

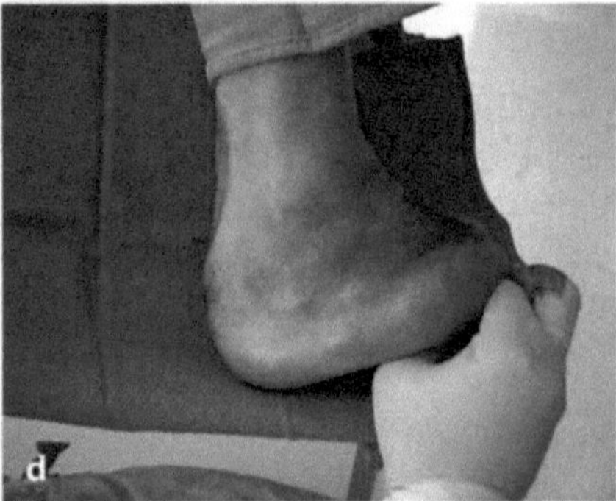

**Fig. 2a–d.** Achilles tendon lengthening. **a,b** Plantar diabetic foot wound with equinus prior to achilles tendon lengthening. **c** Planned sites for two medial and one lateral „stab" incision on the posterior aspect of the leg. **d** Forcible dorsiflexion of foot

## Conclusion

In conclusion, the incidence of diabetic foot wounds is high and continues to increase. Commensurately, our appreciation for the importance of this problem as a significant public-health problem also has increased. With this appreciation, the role of appropriately directed surgery has taken on a high level of importance. With information disseminated throughout the medical community through tomes such as this, it is our hope that we may soon see a decrease in the needlessly high number of wounds and resultant amputations throughout the world.

## References

1. Boulton AJ, Vileikyte L (2000) The diabetic foot: the scope of the problem. J Fam Pract. 49 [Suppl]: S3–8
2. Lavery LA, Armstrong DG, Wunderlich RP, Boulton AJM, Tredwell JL (2003) Diabetic foot syndrome: evaluating the prevalence and incidence of foot pathology in Mexican Americans and non-Hispanic Whites from a diabetes disease management cohort. Diabetes Care 26: 1435–1438
3. Wagner FW (1981) The dysvascular foot: a system for diagnosis and treatment. Foot Ankle 2: 64–122
4. Armstrong DG, Lavery LA, Stern S, Harkless LB (1996) Is prophylactic diabetic foot surgery dangerous? J Foot Ankle Surg 35: 585–589
5. Armstrong DG, Stacpoole-Shea S, Nguyen HC, Harkless LB (1999) Lengthening of the achilles tendon in diabetic patients who are at high risk for ulceration of the foot. J Bone Joint Surg (Am) 81A: 535–538
6. Gudas CJ (1987) Prophylactic surgery in the diabetic foot. Clin Podiatr Med Surg 4: 445–458
7. Catanzariti AR, Blitch EL, Karlock LG (1995) Elective foot and ankle surgery in the diabetic patient. J Foot Ankle Surg 35: 23–41
8. Simon SR, Tejwani SG, Wilson DL, Santner TJ, Denniston NL (2000) Arthrodesis as an early alternative to nonoperative management of Charcot arthropathy of the diabetic foot. J Bone Joint Surg Am 82-A: 939–950
9. Rosenblum BI, Giurini JM, Chrzan JS, Habershaw GM (1994) Preventing loss of the great toe with the hallux interphalangeal arthroplasty. J Foot Ankle Surg 33: 557–566
10. Frykberg R, Giurini J, Habershaw G, Rosenblum B, Chrzan J (1993) Prophylactic surgery in the diabetic foot. In: Kominsky SJ (ed) Medical and surgical management of the diabetic foot. Mosby, St. Louis
11. Wieman TJ, Mercke YK, Cerrito PB, Taber SW (1998) Resection of the metatarsal head for diabetic foot ulcers. Am J Surg 176: 436–441
12. Giurini JM, Basile P, Chrzan JS, Habershaw GM, Rosenblum BI (1993) Panmetatarsal head resection. A viable alternative to the transmetatarsal amputation. J Am Podiatr Med Assoc 83: 101–107
13. Barry DC, Sabacinski KA, Habershaw GM, Giurini JM, Chrzan JS (1993) Tendo Achillis procedures for chronic ulcerations in diabetic patients with transmetatarsal amputations. J Am Podiatr Med Assoc 83: 96–100
14. Giurini JM, Chrzan JS, Gibbons GW, Habershaw GM (1991) Sesamoidectomy for the treatment of chronic neuropathic ulcerations. J Amer Podiatr Med Assn 81: 167–173
15. Fleischli JE, Anderson RB, Davis WH (1999) Dorsiflexion metatarsal osteotomy for treatment of recalcitrant diabetic neuropathic ulcers. Foot Ankle Int 20: 80–85
16. Blume PA, Paragas LK, Sumpio BE, Attinger CE (2002) Single-stage surgical treatment of non-infected diabetic foot ulcers. Plast Reconstr Surg 109: 601–609
17. Frykberg RG, Armstrong DG, Giurini JM et al. (2000) Diabetic foot disorders: a clinical practice guideline. J Foot Ankle Surg 39: S2–S60
18. Laing P (2002) Prophylactic orthopaedic surgery – is there a role? In: Boulton AJM, Connor H, Cavanagh PR (eds) The foot in diabetes, 3rd edn. John Wiley & Sons, Chichester

19. Armstrong DG, Todd WF, Lavery LA, Harkless LB (1997) The natural history of acute Charcot's arthropathy in a diabetic foot specialty clinic. Diabetic Medicine 14: 357–363

20. Ha Van G, Siney H, Danan JP, Sachon C, Grimaldi A (1996) Treatment of osteomyelitis in the diabetic foot: contribution of conservative surgery. Diabetes Care 19: 1257–1260

21. Scher KS, Steele FJ (1988) The septic foot in patients with diabetes. Surgery 104: 661–666

22. Armstrong DG, Frykberg RG (2003) Classification of diabetic foot surgery: toward a rational definition. Diabet Med 20: 329–331

23. Armstrong DG, Lavery LA, Vazquez JR et al. (2003) Clinical efficacy of the first metatarsophalangeal joint arthroplasty as a curative procedure for hallux interphalangeal joint wounds in persons with diabetes. Diabetes Care 26: 3284–3287

24. Cohen M, Roman A, Malcom WG (1991) Pan-metatarsal head resection and transmetatarsal amputation versus solitary partial ray resection in the neuropathic foot. J Foot Surg 30: 29–33

25. Rosenblum BI, Pomposelli FB Jr, Giurini JM et al. (1994) Maximizing foot salvage by a combined approach to foot ischemia and neuropathic ulceration in patients with diabetes. A 5-year experience. Diabetes Care 17: 983–987

26. Lin SS, Lee TH, Wapner KL (1996) Plantar forefoot ulceration with equinus deformity of the ankle in diabetic patients: the effect of tendo-achilles lengthening and total contact casting. Orthopaedics 19: 465–475

27. Piaggesi A, Schipani E, Campi F et al. (1998) Conservative surgical approach versus non-surgical management for diabetic neuropathic foot ulcers: a randomized trial. Diabet Med 15: 412–417

28. Mueller MJ, Sinacore DR, Hastings MK, Strube MJ, Johnson JE (2003) Effect of achilles tendon lengthening on neuropathic plantar ulcers. A randomized clinical trial. J Bone Joint Surg 85A: 1436–1445

# Polyneuropathic Ulcers Surgery

P. Holstein

## Introduction

The Western literature on neuropathic foot ulcers concerns predominantly diabetic patients, who constitute the vast majority with neuropathic foot wounds. Surgery for diabetic neuropathic ulcers has been described in a previous chapter and subsequently the present paper focuses on neuropathic ulcers not related with diabetes.

## Surgical Techniques

Neuropathic ulcers on the feet are caused by local intolerable external pressure or stress, usually in feet with deformities. These ulcers do not heal unless the pressure is relieved, either by external off-loading measures or by surgical correction. A number of surgical techniques are described [1–14]:

- sesamoidectomy,
- condylectomy,
- Keller arthroplasty,
- metatarsal osteotomy,
- pan-metatarsal head resection,
- ulcerectomy with primary or secondary suture,
- exostectomy.

Moreover, there are techniques for functional reduction of the peak plantar forefoot pressure, i.e. Achilles tendon lengthening [15–20].

Recent papers suggest that surgical treatment maintains faster healing [1] and prevents ulcer recurrence [19], as compared to treatment with off-loading.

The treatment of neuropathic foot ulceration in non-diabetic patients is actually the same as in diabetic patients. We adopted surgical interventions for difficult-to-heal neuropathic foot lesions in 1998. About 90% are in people with diabetes mellitus. The rest of the patients suffer peripheral neuropathy from other causes. The results in these patients are documented and discussed in this chapter.

## Material

Pressure ulcer under the forefoot or under the great toe is a common manifestation of peripheral neuropathy [21]. During the past 5 years we have treated 55 feet with bony correction: either an osteotomy in the metatarsal neck or a resection of the prominent metatarso-phalangeal joint. Moreover, in a series of 75 feet with similar lesions, ATL have been tested, and finally 24 feet have had an exostectomy or partial tarsalectomy for protrusion of bone in the plantar mid-foot, in most cases caused by Charcot deformity. Out of these series there were 6, 5 and 3 feet, respectively, with non-diabetic peripheral neuropathy. Details (14 feet in 13 patients) are shown in Table 1.

All ulcers, median duration 19 (3–48) months had been recalcitrant to treatment with off-loading with a walker (Aircast) fitted with individually moulded insoles. Diabetes mellitus had been excluded with fasting blood-sugar determinations and oral glucose-load test. Using Wagner's classification for diabetic ulcers, ten had grade-1 lesion (full-thickness skin ulcer without penetration to deep structures) and four had grade-2 ulcers (penetration to deep structures). Two ulcers were localised to the plantar side of the great toe, nine ulcers were plantar to the metatarsal heads and three ulcers were mid-plantar.

All operations were made in hospital during local infiltration or ankle blockade with 1% Carbocaine plain solution. Prophylaxis with dicloxacillin three times 1 g p.o., possibly with supplement of ciprofloxacin two times 1/2 g p.o., was given for individual periods.

## Resection of MP Joint

Resection of the MP joint was made preferably via a dorsal, dorso-medial or dorso-lateral incision (five cases). Only in one case was a plantar incision used. The joint was exposed, opened and, using a power saw, the metatarsal head and the cartilage of the phalanx was resected. During wound closure, great care was taken to eliminate dead space by interponing soft tissue, closed suction drainage and compression bandage. Only callus was removed from the plantar lesion. The post-operative regimen was non-weight-bearing until the surgical incision was dry and without signs of infection. Then the patient was discharged with Aircast, two crutches and indoor regimen at home. This off-loading was prescribed until the surgical wound as well as the chronic ulcer had healed. The same off-loading inlay as used during the pre-operative treatment was used post-operatively. After healing, extra-depth or custom-made shoes were required.

**Table 1.** Patients' feet with non-diabetic peripheral neuropathy

| Gender | Age | Aetiology of neuro-pathy | Previous Charcot | Previous foot ulcer | Duration of ulcer [months] | Ulcer locali-zation | Wagner classifi-cation | Type of operation | Healing time [weeks] Surgical wound | Healing time [weeks] Ulcer | Compli-cation | Follow-up [months] | Ulcer at follow-up |
|---|---|---|---|---|---|---|---|---|---|---|---|---|---|
| Male | 75 | AA | + | + | 48 | MH 3+4 | 2 | Osteotomy | 2 | 21 | | 26 | Healed |
| Female | 78 | ? | | + | 24 | MH1 | 2 | MP resection | 8 | 8 | | 10 | Healed |
| Male | 51 | AA | + | + | 10 | MH 3+4 | 1 | MP resection | 3 | 7 | | 24 | Healed |
| Male | 43 | ? | | + | 4 | MH 3 | 1 | MP resection | 8 | 8 | | 24 | Healed |
| Male | 80 | AA | + | + | 3 | MH1 | 2 | MP resection | 2 | 5 | Charcot | 27 | Healed |
| Male | 72 | AA | | | 10 | MH1 | 2 | MP resection | 4 | 8 | Transfer ulcer | 22 | Healed |
| Male | 43 | ? | | | 48 | Great toe | 1 | ATL | 2 | 4 | Recurrent ulcer | 16 | Healed |
| Male | 67 | ? | | | 24 | MH3 | 1 | ATL | 2 | 4 | | 18 | Healed |
| Male | 50 | AA | | + | 14 | MH1 | 1 | ATL | 2 | 8 | Recurrent ulcer | 14 | Not healed |
| Male | 61 | AA | | + | 36 | MH1 | 1 | ATL | 2 | 4 | | 12 | Healed |
| Male | 42 | Spinal injury | | | 60 | MH5 | 1 | ATL | 2 | 6 | | 6 | Healed |
| Female | 64 | AA | + | + | 24 | Navi-cular | 1 | Exostec-tomy | 4 | 4 | | 20 | Healed |
| Female (bilateral) | 14 | Myelomen-ingocele | | | 9<br>10 | Base<br>5. metatarsal | 11 | Exostectomy<br>Exostectomy | 2 (right)<br>2 (left) | 32 | | 15<br>16 | Healed<br>Healed |

*AA* alcohol addiction, *MH* metatarsal head.

## Osteotomy

The neck of the metatarsal bone was exposed via incision similar to that used for joint resections (see above). Using a power saw, a wedge-shaped piece of bone was excised leaving a defect in the metatarsal neck, with a dorsal open angle of about 30°. The post-operative regimen was the same as described for joint resection. Only the inlay in the walker was changed to a flat soft insole with the intention of re-aligning the metatarsal heads.

## Achilles Tendon Lengthening (ATL)

With the patient in the prone position, a percutaneous triple hemisection was made. The technique has been described elsewhere [15, 17, 20, 22]. Post-operatively off-loading with two crutches and an Aircast was employed for 6 weeks.

## Exostectomy

An ulcer at an osseous prominence in the mid-plantar region can be treated with exostectomy or partial tarsalectomy [2] (see Fig. 1). The exostosis was exposed sideways through an incision along the circumference of the prominence and at a good distance from the chronic ulcer. With a power saw or with hammer and chisel the bony protrusion was extensively removed. Antibiotics (see above) were given as well as topic gentamycin (Gentacoll) in the cavity. Closed suction, tight suturing of the skin incision, compression bandage and weight-off regimen for 2–3 weeks was employed in order to prevent infection and delayed healing.

## Results

All ulcers healed in median 5.5 weeks (range 2–21 weeks). Four patients had complications: one had a Charcot event following resection of the MP joint of the first ray, treated with a repeated period (3 months) in the Aircast. One had a plantar transfer ulcer at the second metatarsal head following resection of the first metatarsal head. This transfer ulcer healed after resection of the second metatarsal head. Two patients treated with ATL had recurrent ulcers. One healed after removal of the metatarsal head and one is healing slowly during off-loading. During follow-up, four patients have had other foot ulcers not related to the target ulcer, typically an ulcer on the contralateral foot.

The results at follow-up after median 17 (6–26) months was 13 out of 14 ulcers had healed (93%). Two patients are, moreover, being treated almost constantly due to other, varying foot-ulcer problems.

## Discussion

The results in this small series do not justify conclusions regarding preferable techniques. Results were excellent for bony surgery as well as for ATL. This reflects the literature documenting satisfactory healing with the methods described. The relatively fast healing, i.e. in 5.5 weeks, should be compared to the long duration of futile conservative off-loading, i.e. 19 months. These patients are their own control, and document that surgical intervention is effective in recalcitrant cases.

The simple and minor invasive ATL has recently attracted much attention. However, heel transfer ulceration occurred in 11–15% in diabetic patients following ATL [17, 19, 23], in particular when the heel is completely insensate [17]. Heel ulcers are limb-threatening and other techniques for ATL should be studied.

Transfer lesions, recurrent lesions, Charcot foot and infections may complicate more than 50% of the bony foot corrections in diabetic patients. These complications, however, are easily managed, especially in a multidisciplinary diabetic foot unit, and should not detract from the value of the procedures (Fig. 1).

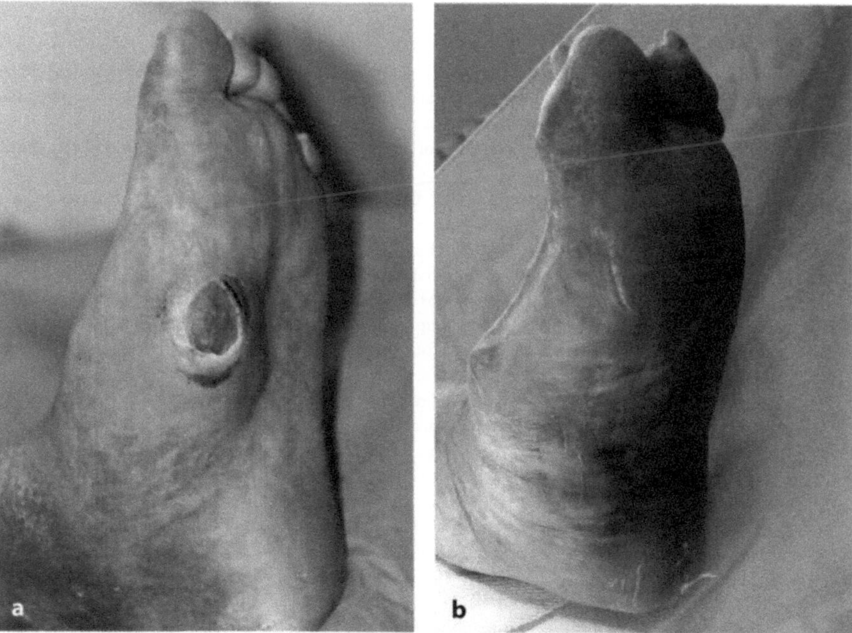

**Fig. 1. a** Charcot foot in 64-year old woman with (neuropathic) ulcer. **b** Healing after exostectomy – photo at 20 months follow-up

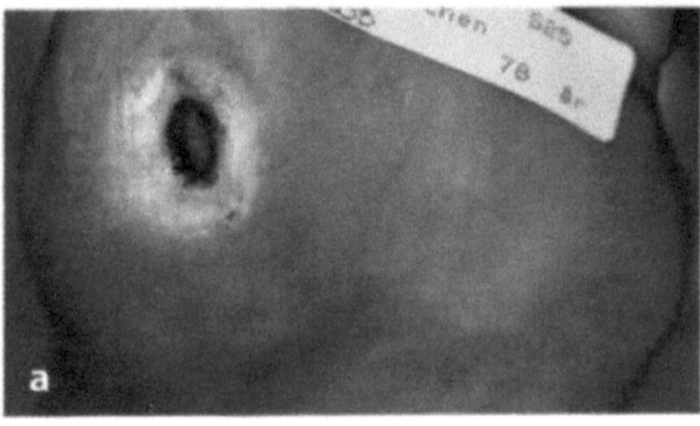
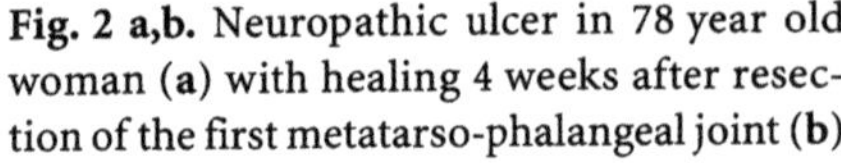
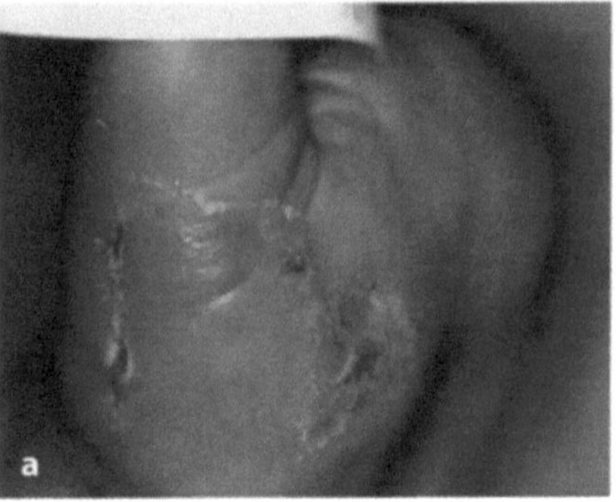

**Fig. 2 a,b.** Neuropathic ulcer in 78 year old woman (**a**) with healing 4 weeks after resection of the first metatarso-phalangeal joint (**b**)

The metatarsal neck osteotomy is now our preferred procedure for grade-1 plantar forefoot lesions. For grade-2 lesions we find resection of the metatarso-phalangeal joint resection (Fig. 2) more attractive, since an osteotomy would maintain a loose fragment of bone in a contaminated area. We have used these methods successfully also in recalcitrant plantar ulcers of the first toe.

In conclusion: surgical treatment of neuropathic foot ulcers recalcitrant to standard off-loading measures maintain healing in diabetic patients as well as in non-diabetic patients. Recent literature suggests faster healing and fewer recurrent ulcerations following surgical intervention compared to conservative off-loading.

## References


1. Armstrong DG, Lavery LA, Vazquez JR, Short B, Kimbriel HR, Nixon BP et al. (2003) Clinical efficacy of the first metatarsophalangeal joint arthroplasty as a curative procedure for hallux interphalangeal joint wounds in patients with diabetes. Diabetes Care 26: 3284–3287
2. Brodsky JW, Rouse AM (1993) Exostectomy for symptomatic bony prominences in diabetic charcot feet. Clin Orthop 296: 21–26
3. Fleischli JE, Anderson RB, Davis WH (1999) Dorsiflexion metatarsal osteotomy for treatment of recalcitrant diabetic neuropathic ulcers. Foot Ankle Int 20: 80–85
4. Giurini JM, Chrzan JS, Gibbons GW, Habershaw GM (1991) Sesamoidectomy for the treatment of chronic neuropathic ulcerations. J Am Podiatr Med Assoc 81: 167–173
5. Giurini JM, Basile P, Chrzan JS, Habershaw GM, Rosenblum BI (1993) Panmetatarsal head resection. A viable alternative to the transmetatarsal amputation. J Am Podiatr Med Assoc 83: 101–107
6. Giurini JM, Rosenblum BI (1995) The role of foot surgery in patients with diabetes. Clin Podiatr Med Surg 12: 119–127
7. Griffiths GD, Wieman TJ (1990) Metatarsal head resection for diabetic foot ulcers. Arch Surg 125: 832–835
8. Holstein P, Lohmann L, Walloe N (2002) Surgical decompression of recalcitrant neuropathic foot ulceration in patients with diabetes. Proceedings DFSG conference, Lake Balaton, Hungary
9. Kumagi SG, Mahoney CR, Fitzgibbons TC, McMullen ST, Connolly TL, Henkel L (1998) Treatment of diabetic (neuropathic) foot ulcers with two-stage debridement and closure. Foot Ankle Int 19: 160–165
10. Patel VG, Wieman TJ (1994) Effect of metatarsal head resection for diabetic foot ulcers on the dynamic plantar pressure distribution. Am J Surg 167: 297–301
11. Petrov O, Pfeifer M, Flood M, Chagares W, Daniele C (1996) Recurrent plantar ulceration following pan metatarsal head resection. J Foot Ankle Surg 35: 573–577
12. Piaggesi A, Schipani E, Campi F, Romanelli M, Baccetti F, Arvia C et al. (1998) Conservative surgical approach versus non-surgical management for diabetic neuropathic foot ulcers: a randomized trial. Diabet Med 15: 412–417

13. Rosenblum BI, Giurini JM, Chrzan JS, Habershaw GM (1994) Preventing loss of the great toe with the hallux interphalangeal joint arthroplasty. J Foot Ankle Surg 33: 557–560

14. Wieman TJ, Mercke YK, Cerrito PB, Taber SW (1998) Resection of the metatarsal head for diabetic foot ulcers. Am J Surg 176: 436–441

15. Armstrong DG, Stacpoole-Shea S, Nguyen H, Harkless LB (1999) Lengthening of the Achilles tendon in diabetic patients who are at high risk for ulceration of the foot. J Bone Joint Surg Am 81: 535–538

16. Barry DC, Sabacinski KA, Habershaw GM, Giurini JM, Chrzan JS (1993) Tendo Achillis procedures for chronic ulcerations in diabetic patients with transmetatarsal amputations. J Am Podiatr Med Assoc 83: 96–100

17. Holstein P, Lohmann M, Bitsch M, Jørgensen B (2004) Achilles tendon lengthening. The Panacea for plantar forefoot ulcerations? Diabetes Metab Res Rev (in press)

18. Lin C-H, Wei F-C, Chen H-C (2000) Filleted toe flap for chronic forefoot ulcer reconstruction. Ann Plast Surg 44: 412–415

19. Mueller MJ, Sinacore DR, Hastings MK, Strube MJ, Johnson JE (2003) Effect of Achilles tendon lengthening on neuropathic plantar ulcers. A randomized clinical trial. J Bone Joint Surg Am 85-A: 1436–1445

20. Nishimoto GS, Attinger CE, Cooper PS (2003) Lengthening the Achilles tendon for the treatment of diabetic plantar forefoot ulceration. Surg Clin North Am 83: 707–726

21. Larsen K, Holstein P, Deckert T (1989) Limb salvage in diabetics with foot ulcers. Prosthet Orthot Int 13: 100–103

22. Lin SS, Lee TH, Wapner KL (1996) Plantar forefoot ulceration with equinus deformity of the ankle in diabetic patients: the effect of tendo-Achilles lengthening and total contact casting. Orthopedics 19: 465–475

23. Barry DC, Sabacinski KA, Habershaw GM, Giurini JM, Chrzan JS (1993) Tendo Achillis procedures for chronic ulcerations in diabetic patients with transmetatarsal amputations. J Am Podiatr Med Assoc 83: 96–100

R. DE ROCHE

## How Pressure Sores Develop

The aetiology of pressure sores is a combination of factors that add to a locally critical ischemia in the soft tissues. Loss of mobility or impaired protective sensation or a combination of both are preconditions for such tissue damage. An interface pressure significantly exceeding the average capillary pressure (2.7 to 6.3 kPa) for more than 2 h will normally result in tissue necrosis [9]. It has been demonstrated that the transcutaneous measurement of oxygen pressure ($pO_2$) in healthy adults decreases rapidly to zero when the subjects are lying motionless on a normal hospital mattress [8]. Many minor factors such as centralisation of blood flow (for instance in shock) or hyperaemia (fever), reduced general condition, especially nutritional deficit, cardiac insufficiency, medications like steroids or catecholamines, prominent pointed bones (ischial or trochanter tuberosities) in rather slim patients and, last but not least, the quality of the mattress or cushion underneath the subject play a role as well.

Pressure sores do have well-defined predilection sites in the human body, strongly dependent on the positioning and the activities of the patient. Specific patterns of pressure sores occur during bed-rest for patients with normal sensation, especially in the elderly patient. Patients with spinal cord injury and lack of protective sensation can develop pressure sores in their wheel chair at quite different sites.

The typical geriatric pressure-sore patient is a weak, malnourished person in a rather bad general condition with significantly reduced amounts of spontaneous movement during sleep.

These patients are unable to move sufficiently in bed to off-load the local pressures that develop over time, which is the normal protective neurologic mechanism to long-lasting interface pressure and ischemic pain in soft tissues. Thus pressure sores occur essentially in the sacral region and the heels, but also over the trochanter in side-lying position.

According to various references, in 9% up to 59% (!) of patients with acute spinal cord-injury pressure sores occur before they are transferred to specialised rehabilitation centres up to 30 days after the accident, usually over the sacrum or the heels [1, 5, 10]. After rehabilitation, in a paraplegic patient in the wheel chair the most common site for pressure sores is under the ischial tuberosity caused while sitting. In the tetraplegic patient pressure sores occur just as frequently under the coccyx as well, as the position of the pelvis is less upright due to an additional weakness of muscular control. Intensive-care patients in coma or patients in extremely catabolic conditions like burn injuries can in addition have ulcers over the posterior spina of the pelvis, the spina scapulae, the elbows and the occipital region of the head.

As a general rule, subcutaneous fat and the muscles underneath are less resistant to ischemia than the skin itself. When a pressure sore is formed, there might be visible damage to the skin in between a fixed reddish stain and an unambiguous necrosis, but the real extent of the tissue damage can only be felt as an extensive hard alteration of the subcutaneous tissue. This dense tissue corresponds to a zone of critical ischemia which is partially reversible if additional pressure is strictly avoided.

## Practical Conclusions for Pressure-Sore Treatment

Pressure sores occurring in the sitting position can be relieved in any horizontal bed-rest position. With early pressure sores resulting from immobility in the bed, the first and most common action plan is turning the patient in a prone position if ever possible, or at least to use a pressure-relieving surface if the patient is unable to stay in bed on his belly, usually because of obesity or respiratory restrictions.

These principles of prevention and treatment of pressure sores above are also valuable for securing the healing process after surgical wide excision of necrotic tissue and flap coverage of pressure sores. Local random-pattern skin flaps as well as big fascio-cutaneous or musculo-cutaneous axial flaps must be protected from any additional compression to their microcirculation during 6 post-operative weeks. This is one of the most important preconditions for the establishment of viability within the flap and undisturbed wound healing. Any critical reduction of microcirculation in the period of wound healing may lead to an increase in fibrosis of the scar tissue. This fibrosis will later restrict shifting because of adherence to the bone beneath or will yield bursa-like tissue alterations, resulting in a lower resistance to pressure and ischemia and thus favouring recurrent pressure sores.

## Who Needs a Pressure-Relieving System?

The need for pressure-relieving systems depends upon the condition of the patient and the site of the pressure sore. Geriatric patients at high risk of pressure sores of sacrum or trochanter are best nursed on a super-soft three-piece foam mattress and turned from the supine position to a left- or right-side 30° oblique back position every 2 h. This type of prevention is very costly because of the nursing personnel being directly involved. Alternatively, a system of alternate automatic turning from one to the other position in a bed like Turnsoft® may be used. Para- and tetraplegic patients with sores in the sitting predilection sites and loss of protective sensitivity can also be put on the super-soft mattress as long as they are in a good general condition and compliant with turning protocols. Nowadays, however, an increasing amount of these patients are – in addition to their spine injury – suffering from diseases of the age, COPD, heart or vascular disease, diabetes and all types of addictions. In a specialised centre like REHAB Basel (Switzerland), a rehabilitation centre for spinal cord injury and brain trauma, we use a risk scale. All patients at high risk of developing pressure sores and all with current ulcers are systematically put on alternating pressure mattresses with an automatic pressure control mechanism (Duo 2®) for prevention and treatment. These new and very effective pressure-relieving systems are easy to handle for the nursing staff and have in the past few years significantly reduced the indication for air-fluidised therapeutic beds like Clinitron®.

## The Turnsoft Principle

Based on research findings of the geriatric department at the University of Basel a list of requirements for an ideal pressure-relief system for patients at risk for pressure sores was defined. The influence of the 30° laterally inclined position was documented and a pressure relief unit developed consisting of a soft foam mattress (Airsoft®) and an automatic bed (Turnsoft) turning the patient continuously from the supine position to a left or right side 30° oblique back position. This unit provides constant pressure relief with peak pressures below 22.5 mmHg simultaneously on all classical pressure-sore areas [8]. The patient immerses in the three-layer soft-foam Airsoft mattress and is not pushed to roll. This allows head elevation without sliding of the patient. Repositioning takes place very gently with a quiet electric drive and does not interrupt the patient's sleep or create disorientation or dizziness and nausea. The system adapts to the patient's body temperature and – very important for wound care – does not dry out moist wound dressings. Auxiliary medical and nursing treatment is as easy as in any normal hospital bed.

Using the Turnsoft principle systematically, the incidence of pressure sores at the geriatric department of the University Hospital Basel was reduced from 23% (1977) to an average of 1 to 3% between 1980 and 1992 – an extremely successful prevention principle, saving enormous amounts of money in geriatric care.

## Air-Fluidised Beds

In contrast to the very simple Turnsoft principle and its enormous benefit in geriatric care, the requirements of pressure-relieving systems for patients with spinal cord injury and impaired protective sensitivity are much more sophisticated. REHAB Basel was founded in 1967; in the first and second decades spinal cord-injured patients were usually young and healthy, most of them could be reintegrated in a professional life after a relatively short period of rehabilitation. Pressure sores after primary rehabilitation were more or less unique episodes that could be cured well

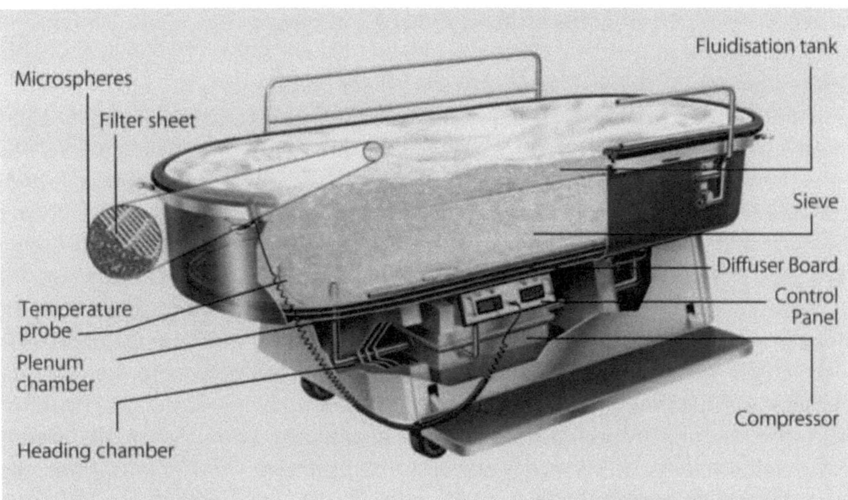


**Fig. 1.** The air-fluidised therapy unit (Clinitron) is an adaptation of the principles of small-particle fluidisation. It provides true flotation on a surface with a density of 1.5 times that of water. No other therapeutic surface provides such low levels of shear friction or pressure

in supine position on a super-soft foam mattress either with or without surgery. This profile of patients has changed dramatically after the third decade of our centre. Life expectancy of our patients has increased due to better general management of their spinal cord injury. They are much older on average, suffering from all the frequent diseases of advanced age like obesity or malnutrition, cardio-respiratory illness, vascular disease, diabetes and other endocrine problems, renal failure and finally long-lasting addictions to alcohol, nicotine and drugs. One in three is admitted to a hospital with a deep pressure sore every year! The incidence of recurrent pressure sores has increased enormously, making surgical treatment and healing a real challenge. Most of these multimorbid patients are unable to endure a period of some weeks in prone position, so that there is an imperative need for perfect pressure relief [2].

The optimal pressure-relieving system has for many years been the air-fluidised therapy in the Clinitron® bed. This system is an adaptation of the principles of small-particle fluidisation. The particles are medical-grade ceramic microspheres which are contained in the fluidisation chamber of the Clinitron unit (Fig. 1). Room air is drawn into the base of the unit, where it is filtered, heated or cooled as required, and channelled through the microsphere beads, setting them in motion and thus creating the fluid effect. This allows a continuous supine position of the patient with optimal pressure relief even after flap surgery because the fluidisation avoids any interface pressure exceeding capillary-closing pressure level. Patients rest comfortably with no constraints on positioning. Pressure is reliably reduced over critical bony prominences and flaps even in the most compromised patients. Because the density of the fluid is approximately 1.5 times that of water, the system provides true flotation and offers a more stable support surface than conventional water beds. The patient is separated from the artificial fluid by a polyester-filter sheet. The sheet is loose-fitting and moves freely with the patient over the fluid. The result is a significant reduction of the destructive forces of shear and friction, the forces often responsible for flap or skin-graft damage. The filter sheet is permeable, allowing an upward stream of air to the patient's skin and a downward flow of fluids. This prevents the softening of tissue caused by prolonged exposure to moisture. As body fluids penetrate the filter sheet, clumping of the microspheres occurs. They form a dry crust that falls to the bottom of the tank, away from the patient. These clumps have to be removed by service technicians. When the fluid system is turned off, the microspheres contour to the body to gently immobilise the patient for dressing changes and other routine care. Cardiopulmonary resuscitation can be performed immediately without a cardiac board. In burns, Clinitron minimises not only the pressure and friction on burn, graft or donor sites, allowing direct placement on them, but also minimises moisture and risk of contamination. Donor-site healing is also enhanced by the warm, dry and clean environment, thereby permitting earlier reharvesting of split-thickness skin grafts.

In REHAB Basel we have used the Clinitron system successfully for many years after flap surgery of the most compromised spinal-cord-injured patients. We have placed patients routinely in the Clinitron for the first 6 weeks after surgery, moving them after that onto a super-soft foam mattress for remobilisation into the wheel chair. In spite of these many advantages, there are also some disadvantages. Patients, whilst receiving such therapy, significantly lose their independence; some of them suffer from the noise of the compressor pumping air into the system, others feel seasick with vertigo, nausea and loss of orientation in space, making mobilisation into the wheel chair considerably more difficult. Many of the patients with cardio-respiratory restrictions are disadvantaged by the reduced resistance of the surface – they have no firm surface to "breathe against" – resulting in poor oxygenation, that means a risk for wound healing. Finally, the continuous airflow through the filter sheet can dry out wounds and grafts. Also, even though patients receive good pressure relief with very good post-operative outcomes, nursing personnel would prefer to have an easier way of bending over the patient and the bed to reduce stress on their backs. No other therapeutic surface can offer the same low levels of shear friction or pressure. On the other hand, the system is quite expensive in leasing and service costs, so that hospitals have started to look for a system with better overall comfort at lower costs [12].

## Alternating-Pressure Mattress Systems

In the past two decades, a great variety of alternating-pressure mattress systems have been developed. Many of them have been tested in our spine injury unit at the REHAB Basel; all of them proved to have the same disadvantages. Conventional alternating-pressure systems exert high peak cushion pressures in their cells during the inflation cycle that can be harmful enough in the post-operative period to leave

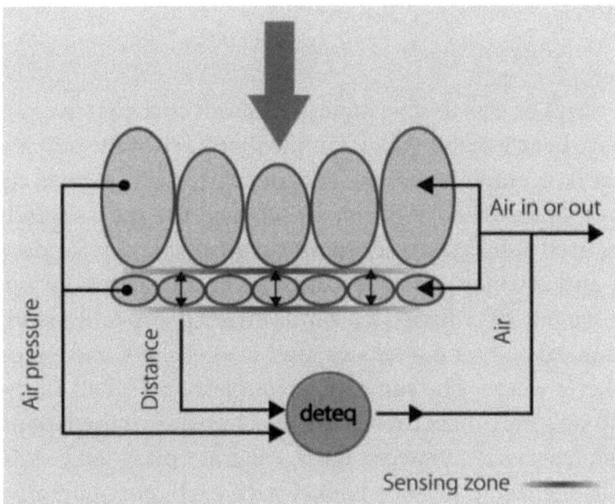


**Fig. 2.** The deteq pressure control technology in Duo 2 mattress constantly monitors the patient's weight and position, providing the lowest possible pressures and optimal pressure relief in all positions

impressions of drains etc. into the skin or flaps, representing a superficial pressure sore. Furthermore, a majority of patients complained about the obtrusive noise of the inflating and deflating mechanism.

The Duo 2® mattress combines the principles of low air loss and alternating pressure with a new technology of pressure control (known as deteq™). This patented intelligent pressure-control module is situated beneath patient and therapeutic mattress and automatically adjusts the pressures in the mattress to accommodate any change of position, weight and size (Fig. 2). This results in cushion peak pressures at least 60% below those found in conventional alternating-pressure mattresses, as low as 15 mmHg internal cushion pressure, giving much softer support than any other mattress available. Additionally, it incorporates a specialised heel zone which ensures that pressure under the heels is always three times softer than the rest of the mattress. The mattress functions are controlled by a small, handy control panel and the mattress is virtually silent in operation. This mattress can be used on almost every standard hospital bed and is able to reduce hospital costs significantly.

Duo 2 provides two clinically proven low-pressure modes: alternating low pressure mode (ALP, relieves pressure by changing the area that supports the patient's weight through the sequential inflation and deflation of air cells, simulating the natural changes in position that occur during sleep) and continuous low-pressure mode (CLP, relieves pressure by distributing the body weight over the supporting surface).

Measurements of transcutaneous $pO_2$ have been shown to be an indicator of risk for pressure sores [3, 6], and the relationship between $pO_2$ values and interface pressures has been previously demonstrated [11]. $PO_2$ measurements on Duo 2 surface over the sacrum were very encouraging in that the 87.5% of the transcutaneous $pO_2$-resting values are the highest ever recorded compared with the literature. They are true for both ALP and CLP modes. Interface pressure maps correlated with transcutaneous $pO_2$ results for each individual [4].

## Clinical Study Results

Risk assessment for pressure sores as well as investigations about cost effectiveness of prevention programmes have been a major subject in the literature of the past few years. On the other hand, there is a complete absence of randomised prospective clinical studies on pressure sores. At the REHAB Basel, we selected the most severely compromised spinal cord-injured subjects undergoing surgical therapy for deep pressure sores between 2001 and 2003 for a clinical study. To find evidence for our post-operative care protocol, we put 20 of them in a randomised prospective study either in the Clinitron air-fluidised bed for 6 weeks or after 2 weeks in Clinitron on the Duo 2 mattress for another 4 weeks. The same surgeon operated on all study-enrolled patients [7]. These 20 surgical procedures included 11 posterior thigh flaps, 5 tensor fasciae latae flaps, 4 gluteal fasciocutaneous flaps, 1 sacral z plasty and 1 VAC therapy for an ischial ulcer. In the group of ten patients with early post-operative transfer on the Duo 2 mattress we had no wound-healing problems at all. In the group where we used Clinitron for the whole post-operative period of 6 weeks, we had three minor wound breakdowns at the donor site of the flaps (12, 13 and 17 days after surgery) that healed spontaneously. One wound breakdown after 31 days at the pressure-sore site itself required further surgery for complete resolution of the wound. Air-fluidised surfaces create such an absence of friction that patients are repositioned extremely fast. We believe that this quickness of movement has repetitively placed stress on the V-Y closure of the donor site of the flaps, where the highest tension occurs, causing the incisional closure to become dislodged and incomplete healing or dehiscence to occur in those areas far from the initial ulcer. We therefore concluded that the easy turning of patients on the air-fluidised surface with almost no resistance was a distinct danger for the undisturbed healing of the incisions.

The equally good outcome of flap healing on the two surfaces will be double-checked in another randomised series comparing a Clinitron (2 weeks) plus Duo 2 (4 weeks) group with a group of patients that are put on Duo 2 mattresses immediately after surgery. Thus the much more comfortable nursing on Duo 2 mattress might become our standard for post-operative care, reducing the costs of our post-operative pressure-relief systems significantly.

## References


1. Aito S et al. (2003) Complications during the acute phase of traumatic spinal cord lesions. Spinal Cord 41: 629–635
2. Colin D, Loyant R, Abraham P, Saumet JL (1996) Changes in sacral transcutaneous oxygen tension in the evaluation of different mattresses in the prevention of pressure ulcers. Adv Wound Care 9: 25–28
3. Colin D, Saumet JL (1996) Influence of external pressure on transcutaneous oxygen tension and laser Doppler flowmetry on sacral skin. Clin Physiol 16: 61 – 72
4. Colin D (1997) Clinical evaluation of an innovative mattress. Poster presentation. 7th European Conference on Advances in Wound Management, Harrogate UK
5. Mawson AR, Biundo JJ Jr, Neville P, Linares HA, Winchester Y, Lopez A (1988) Risk factors for early occurring pressure ulcers following spinal cord injury. Am J Phys Med Rehab 67: 123–127

6. Mawson AR, Siddiqui FH, Conolly BJ, Sharp CJ, Summer WR, Biundo JJ Jr (1993) Sacral transcutaneous oxygen tension levels in the spinal cord injured: risk factors for pressure ulcers? Arch Phys Med Rehabil 74: 745–751

7. de Roche R, Scheel Sailer A, Mäder M (2004) Pressure relief after surgery for pressure sores in high-risk spinal cord injured patients – is there an alternative to the air fluidised bed? (to be published)

8. Seiler WO, Allen S, Stähelin HB (1986) Influence of the 30 degrees laterally inclined position and the "super-soft" 3-piece mattress on skin oxygen tension on areas of maximum pressure – implications for pressure sore prevention. Gerontology 32: 158–166

9. Seiler WO, Stähelin HB (1991) Decubitus ulcers in geriatrics – pathogenesis, prevention and therapy. Ther Umsch 48: 329–340

10. Wanner MB, de Roche R, Lüscher NJ (1995) Chirurgische Therapie des Decubitus. Swiss Med 6-S: 73–79

11. Xakellis GC, Frantz RA, Arteaga M, Meletiou S (1991) A comparison of changes in the transcutaneous oxygen tension and capillary blood flow in the skin with increasing compressive weights. Am J Phys Med Rehabil 70: 172–177

12. Xakellis GC, Frantz RA (1996) The cost-effectiveness of interventions for preventing pressure ulcers. J Am Board Fam Pract 9: 79–85

R. DE ROCHE

## Why Surgical Therapy for Pressure Sores?

Once the general condition of a patient suffering from a pressure sore is stabilised, pressure relief has been optimised and a proper debridement and wound-bed preparation are done, the very first objective for further treatment is a rapid rehabilitation. This is the moment when surgical therapy of pressure sores should be considered. There are two main populations of pressure-sore patients with quite diverging characteristics:

- geriatric patients developing pressure sores of sacrum, trochanter or heels because of a reduced amount of spontaneous movement during sleep and a poor peripheral circulation and oxygenation;
- patients with spinal-cord injury developing pressure sores because of impaired sensation at the sites of elevated interface pressure like ischial tuberosity, coccyx (in tetraplegics with lack of muscular stabilisation of their pelvis), trochanter (quite frequently penetrating and infecting the hip joint and therefore extremely dangerous), less frequently – during bed rest – over sacrum and heels.

For both groups there is strong evidence in favour of surgical treatment. Any spontaneous healing by shrinking of the wound and finally epithelialisation will lead to a fibrous, dense scar tissue with reduced blood supply and poor resistance to further interface pressure and friction exactly at the sites that are at the highest risk for recurrence of the ulcers. Furthermore, time for healing is significantly longer for this spontaneous cicatrisation; it will require a prolonged period of bed rest. This means for the elderly or paraplegic patient loss of independence, reduced incentive for motion, general deterioration, prolonged stay in a nursing home or hospital and an increase of secondary complications like joint contracture, muscular atrophy and thromboembolic complications. The socio-economic impact of prolonged healing is therefore enormous in the geriatric population [11], whereas the risk of recurrence rises dramatically after secondary healing of ulcers in spinal-cord-injured patients.

## Principles of Surgery for Geriatric Pressure Sores

Normally, elderly patients develop pressure sores in an acute period of significantly reduced general condition like, for instance, after a pulmonary infection with high fever or a cerebral stroke, quite frequently at multiple sites. In the first days after admission to a nursing home or hospital they are at high risk of developing additional ulcers at different sites because they are positioned on intact skin only. After treatment of their acute sickness, proper debridement of the necrosis and covering of the pressure sores with a locoregional flap is of highest interest, because every impairment of remobilisation is further weakening their general condition. As soon as there is evidence of an ongoing wound-healing process in the ulcer and the most important parameters in blood check are stabilised [5, 6], flap surgery should be performed in order to reduce the time of bed rest. The surgical aim is to use the simplest surgical technique, whenever possible in regional anaesthesia, that provides a reliable wound healing. As a rule, rhomboid fasciocutaneous flaps [12] and gluteal rotation flaps [1] are the first choice for sacral ulcers; rhomboid fasciocutaneous flaps for the ischial tuberosity [12]; tensor fasciae latae V-Y advancement flaps for the trochanter [15]. Sophisticated technical modifications of axial fasciocutaneous flaps [8, 18], however, rely on intact axial vessels and take an unproportionally elevated risk in a geriatric population; random pattern flaps are certainly more reliable. As these patients should be remobilised to walking later on, it is evident that only fascio-cutaneous flaps must be used. Using musculo-cutaneous gluteal flaps for deep sacral pressure sores with exposed bone, for instance, can end in a severe additional impairment of pelvic stabilisation upon mobilisation, a loss of important muscular force and a Trendelenburg limp that makes independent walking forever impossible.

The simplest technique that secures safe wound healing is a challenge indeed! Even in centres with ample experience, the rate of wound-healing complications in the geriatric pressure-sore population is roughly at 50% [2, 7, 10]. Most of these minor complications resolve by secondary healing without further surgery and in any case allow for mobilisation of the patient into an armed chair in between 3 and 4 weeks post-operatively. Zones of fibrous scarring do not represent a real problem for elevated interface pressure after healing, because these patients still have some protective sensation and are therefore not at significantly elevated risk for recurrence.

## Surgical Tactics for Pressure Sores in Spinal Cord Injury

The treatment principles for pressure sores in the collective of spinal-cord-injured patients diverge significantly from the geriatric group. A para- or tetraplegic patient stays at risk for recurrent pressure sores at the same predilection site for his whole life. In a population of patients over 65 years old with pressure-sore surgery we had no recurrence in the geriatric group at the same site after primary uncomplicated healing, but 18% recurrences in the spine-injured group. With secondary healing after wound complications, the rates were 11% recurrence at the same site in geriatric patients and 34% in the spine-injured population [10]. So even minor complications after flap surgery lead to a massively reduced resistance of the scar tissue against pressure, shear and friction forces; the incidence of recurrence doubled while the tissue left back for further reconstruction was more and more restricted.

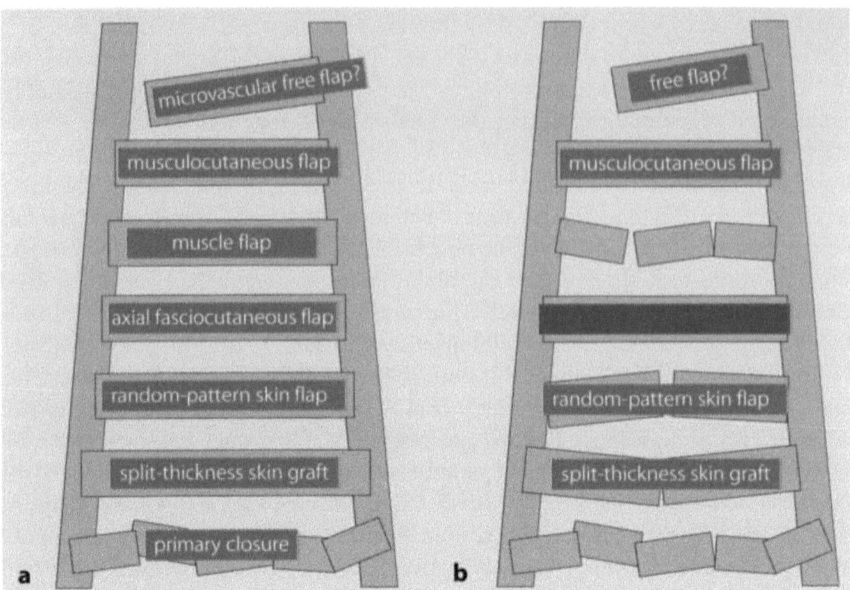



**Fig. 1a,b.** The escalation ladder for surgical repair of pressure sores in spinal cord injury after Lüscher [14] (**a**) has been modified due to a dramatic change in the profile of our spinal cord-injured patient's collective. As wheel chair drivers have a better life expectancy and encounter more recurrences, big fascio-cutaneous flaps from the beginning are the best surgical option (**b**)

This led to a major change of surgical tactics and post-operative management in our institution for rehabilitation of spinal-cord injury, REHAB Basel; our escalation ladder of surgical techniques has been reduced to just a few rungs (Fig. 1). On the other hand, we adhere strictly to a post-operative care protocol with a 6-week period of bed rest in prone position or on pressure-relieving mattresses, and we start with reduced passive motion of the legs not before 4 weeks after surgery. This procedure offers optimal conditions not only for superficial wound healing, but for undisturbed establishment of stable scars both in depth as well as being able to bear pressure and friction when the patient is gradually remobilised into his wheel chair. Only perfect scarring of all tissue layers over the – usually remodelled – bone provides not only resistance to pressure but also shifting and gliding of the tissues; these preconditions guarantee that the flap is a valuable tissue replacement.

The background of these modifications in surgical tactics for pressure-ulcer repair is above all the life expectancy of para- and tetraplegics that has continuously approximated a normal average due to specialised care for these patients. Overall time in the wheel chair has so increased, but the soft tissues – or after prior surgery the scars – exposed to pressure and friction are much more compromised in individuals growing older with, in addition, artherosclerosis, heart failure, obesity or malnutrition, diabetes and other diseases of age. On average, patients with spinal-cord injury are readmitted to a hospital with 0.3 pressure sores per year – those older than 65 years have 1.2 hospital stays for ulcer treatment in a year [10]. Therefore, the need for repetitive surgical repairs taught us to consider multiple recurrences right from the planning of the very first flap, preserving all vascular territories (angiosomes) of neighbouring axial flaps and using a big fascio-cutaneous flap in the beginning even for a small ulcer. Excision of a pressure sore and repair by direct skin closure will always fail because of the dead space underneath that fills with rigid and adherent scar tissue. Skin grafts will lead to recurrent instable scars when under pressure or friction and can, after years, even transform into a scar cancer. Local random pattern flaps lie usually in the angiosome of a bigger flap and are too small to exceed the zone of pressure under ischial tuberosity or coccyx, so that the patient will sit directly on his scars after remobilisation into the wheel chair. Muscle flaps have for many years been considered as the ideal solution to fill dead space and to cover exposed bone, as there is experimental evidence that the well-vascularised muscle tissue is more resistant to infections; but muscle flaps are even much more sensitive to pressure than fascio-cutaneous flaps, so that they lead to the highest recurrence rates of all [20]. Microsurgical free flaps finally, in contrast to some technically spectacular new publications [17, 19], have in our hands never been used for even giant pressure-sore defects of the whole perineum including the anus, as the defect repair with much safer fascio-cutaneous flaps was possible in all our patients. Besides, there is some controversy in the literature about the elective stoma construction for faecal diversion before flap surgery for these big perineal pressure sores. In a collective of spinal-cord-injured and geriatric patients the effect of this preliminary elective operation on healing time was evident, on recurrence rate nevertheless not convincing at all [4]. We have used this procedure only once in a case of simultaneous recurrent ischio-perineal ulcer and septic hip joint. In all other big perineal defects we could cover the pressure sores without stoma and we did not encounter unusual or prolonged wound-healing problems. Even if the elective laparascopic stoma construction is a procedure with low morbidity, the additional damage to the body integrity of a patient with spinal cord injury has to be considered and usually does not rectify this additional surgery.

As a conclusion, out of the failures in more than 500 pressure-sore repairs in our centre, we use in the meantime a very limited choice of flaps, always starting with a generously designed big fascio-cutaneous flap for the first ulcer. All these flaps can be remobilised and advanced without involving neighbouring angiosomes in the case of a recurrence. The standard technique is nowadays the posterior thigh flap [3, 9] for repair of ischial pressure sores (Fig. 2), the tensor fasciae latae flap [15] with V-Y closure for trochanteric ulcers (Fig. 3) and a gluteal fasciocutaneous rotation flap [1] – whenever possible unilateral to preserve the opposite side for an eventual recurrence – for pressure sores over the sacrum or coccyx (Fig. 4). On the other hand, we are very pedantic about resurfacing the bone underneath, removing and smoothing all prominent ischial or trochanteric tuberosities and amputating the coccyx in all tetraplegic patients in the case of a coccygeal ulcer.

There are very few exceptions to our standard procedure for primary ulcers, whereas for recurrent pressure sores rather more improvisation is required. One important exception is the use of a sensory tensor fasciae latae flap for ischial sores in the case of intact sensation of the lateral thigh (N. cutaneus femoris lateralis,

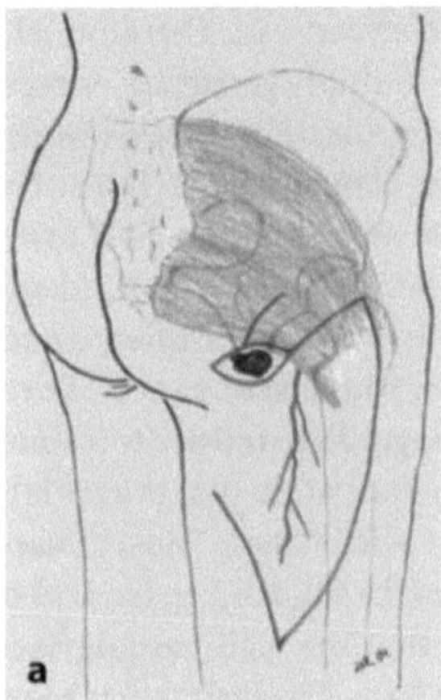 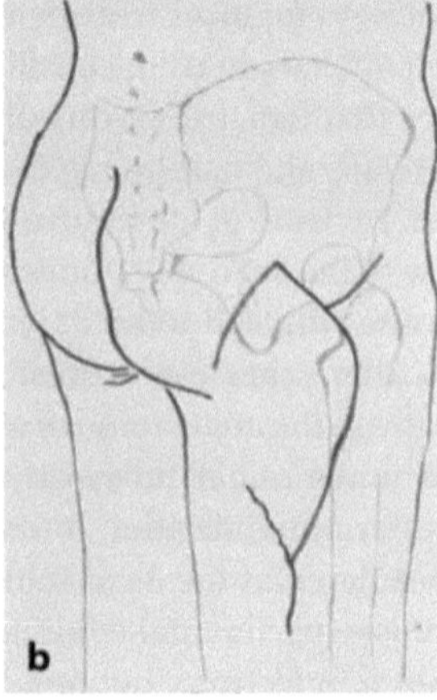

**Fig. 2a,b.** Posterior thigh flap with Z-plasty as best primary option for all pressure sores of the ischial tuberosity in spinal-cord-injured patients. (After Lüscher)

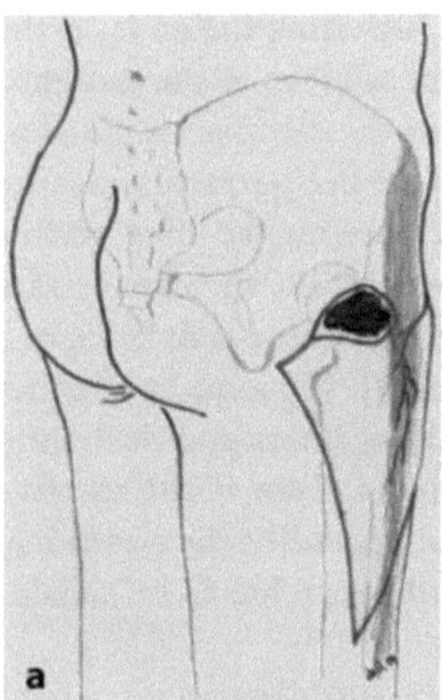 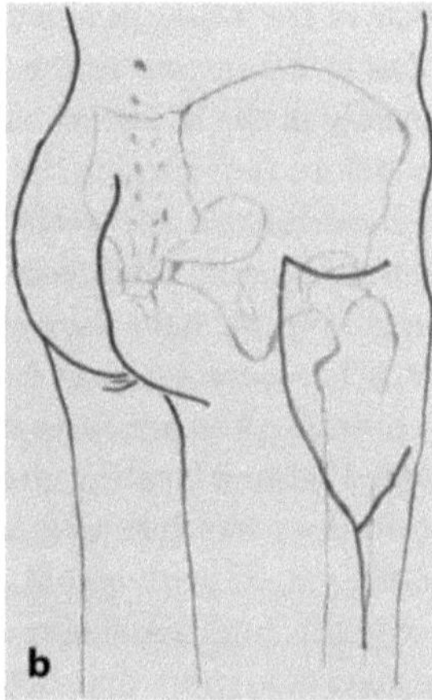

**Fig. 3a,b.** Tensor fasciae latae flap with V–Y closure for pressure sores over the trochanter. (After Lüscher)

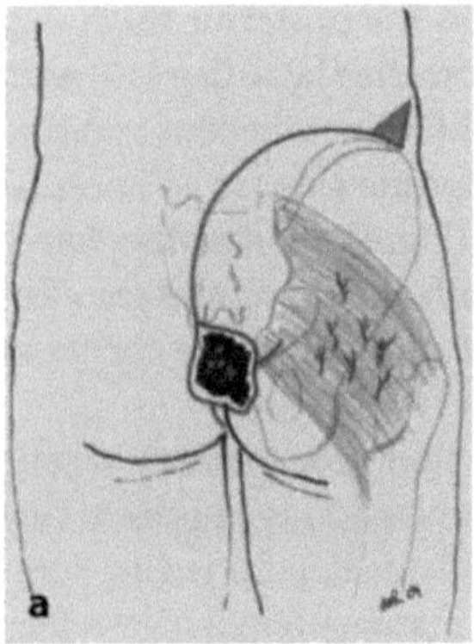 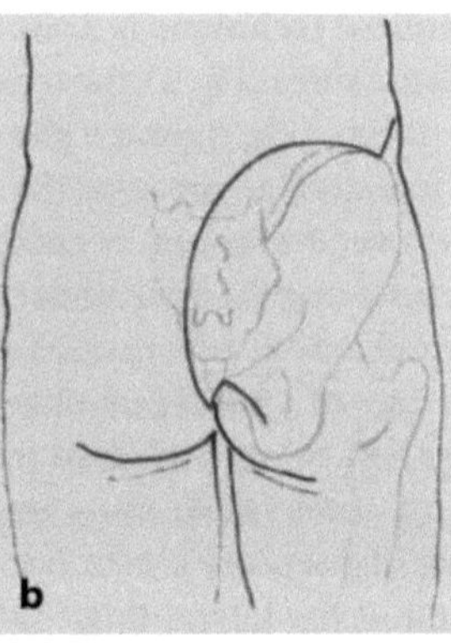

**Fig. 4a,b.** Gluteal fasciocutaneous rotation flap for pressure sores over sacrum and coccyx. (After Lüscher)

L 2/L 3). This technique provides a protective sensibility for the ischial bones and can even allow for a filling control of the rectum when the flap is inserted close enough to the anal skin. This was reported as a terrific new perception, especially for patients with a meningomyelocele [13].

A further exception is the use of a vastus lateralis muscle flap for filling of the cavity after Girdlestone resection of the femoral head in cases of septic hip joints. In a series of 21 septic hips there was a high recurrence rate of trochanteric ulcers and fistula when fascio-cutaneous flaps were used; there was not a single recurrence when we mobilised the vastus lateralis muscle flap into the cavity for improved control of infection in the joint and prevention of ankylosis of the joint [16].

For para- and tetraplegic patients pressure sores represent a continuous threat to their independent daily life, one in three is admitted to a hospital in a year for ulcer treatment, which takes more than 3 months in average, and many of them lose their jobs after repetitive periods in hospitals or nursing homes due to recurrent pressure sores. For this population it would be of highest interest that the standards of care for pressure sores are strictly followed and the tactics of surgical procedure are accepted in all rehabilitation centres. The most important guidelines must be to use for covering the first pressure sore only generously designed fascio-cutaneous flaps that can later on be used repetitively, and to preserve all vascular territories of neighbouring flaps during surgery.

## References


1. Borman H, Maral T (2002) The gluteal fasciocutaneous rotation-advancement flap with V-Y closure in the management of sacral pressure sores. Plast Reconstr Surg 109: 2325–2329
2. Brenner P, Krause-Bergmann A (2002) Das Dekubitalulkus – Entstehung, chirurgische Therapie und Prognose. Zentralbl Chir 127: 527–532
3. Calil JA, Ferreira LM, Neto MS, Castilho HAT, Garcia EB (2001) Clinical application of the V-Y posterior thigh fasciocutaneous flap. Rev Assoc Med Bras 47: 311–319
4. de la Fuente SG, Levin LS, Reynolds JD, Olivares C, Pappas TN, Ludwig KA, Mantyh CR (2003) Elective stoma construction improves outcomes in medically intractable pressure ulcers. Dis Colon Rectum 46: 1525–1530
5. Gengenbacher M, Stähelin HB, Scholer A, Seiler WO (2002) Low biochemical nutritional parameters in acutely ill hospitalized elderly patients with and without stage III to IV pressure ulcers. Aging Clin Exp Res 14: 420–423
6. Guenter P, Malyszek R, Bliss DZ, Steffe T, O'Hara D, LaVan F, Monteiro D (2000) Survey of nutritional status in newly hospitalized patients with stage III or stage IV pressure ulcers. Adv Skin Wound Care 13: 164–168
7. Gusenoff JA, Redett RJ, Nahabedian MY (2002) Outcomes for surgical coverage of pressure sores in nonambulatory, nonparaplegic, elderly patients. Ann Plast Surg 48: 633–640
8. Higgins JP, Orlando GS, Blondeel PN (2002) Ischial pressure sore reconstruction using an inferior gluteal artery perforator (IGAP) flap. Br J Plast Surg 55: 83–85
9. Homma K, Murakami G, Fujioka H, Fujita T, Imai A, Ezoe K (2001) Treatment of ischial pressure sores with a posteromedial thigh fasciocutaneous flap. Plast Reconstr Surg 108: 1990–1996
10. Langauer S (1994) Dekubitus beim geriatrischen Patienten: Stellenwert, Indikationen und Resultate der chirurgischen Therapie. Thesis, University Basel, Switzerland
11. Le Chapelain L, Fyad JP, Beis JM, Thisse MO, Andre JM (2001) Chirurgie précoce de l'escarre pelvienne versus cicatrisation dirigée dans une population de médullo-lésés. Ann Readapt Med Phys 44: 608–612

12. Lüscher NJ, Kuhn W, Zäch GA (1986) Rhomboid flaps in surgery for decubital ulcers: indications and results. Ann Plast Surg 16: 415–421
13. Lüscher NJ, de Roche R, Krupp S, Kuhn W, Zäch GA (1991) The sensory tensor fasciae latae flap: a 9-year follow-up. Ann Plast Surg 26: 306–310
14. Lüscher NJ (1992) Decubitus ulcers of the pelvic region, diagnostics and surgical therapy. Hogrefe, Göttingen
15. Nahai F (1980) The tensor fascia lata flap. Clin Plast Surg 7: 51–56
16. de Roche R., Lüscher NJ, Faulenbach M, Michel D, Mäder M (2001) Surgical tactics for pressure sores with septic hip joint destruction: still "life before limb" or muscle flaps as a reliable alternative? Abstract, 40th IMSOP meeting, Nottwil Switzerland
17. Schoeller T, Shafighi M, Huemer GM, Wechselberger G, Piza-Katzer H (2003) Dekubitalulkusdeckung durch mikrochirurgische Lappenplastiken. Chirurg 74: 671–676
18. de Weerd L, Weum S (2002) The butterfly design: coverage of a large sacral defect with two pedicled lumbar artery perforator flaps. Br J Plast Surg 55: 251–253
19. Yamamoto Y, Nohira K, Shintomi Y, Igawa H, Ohura T (1992) Reconstruction of recurrent pressure sores using free flaps. J Reconstr Microsurg 8: 433–436
20. Yamamoto Y, Tsutsumida A, Murazumi M, Sugihara T (1997) Long-term outcome of pressure sores treated with flap coverage. Plast Reconstr Surg 100: 1212–1217

# VII Burns



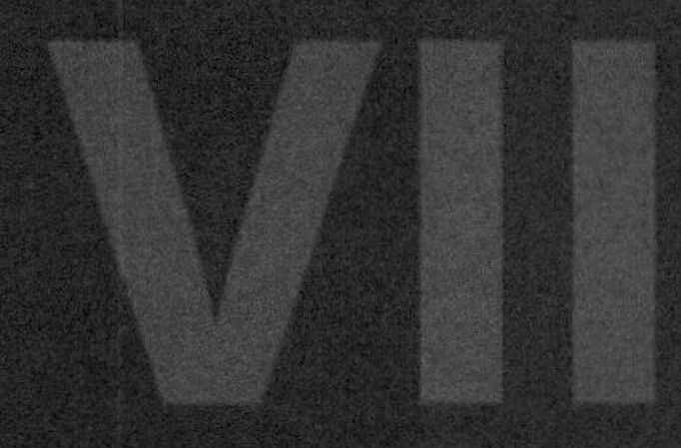

# Thermal Burns Management

L. Téot, S. Otman

## Introduction

Thermal burns are wounds presenting special clinical features, in the initial assessment as well as in the long-term tendency to develop pathologic scars due to an intense inflammatory process. A general consensus emerges considering that a burn wound has to be covered within a period of 2 weeks, a justification for the surgical approach popularised by US surgeons since the 1970s.

New technologies have emerged in the past decade, leading to a new armentarium of therapeutic possibilities, amongst which skin substitutes still form a promising solution. Common dressings proposed for chronic wounds are used in the last stage of minor burns, when skin grafting is not necessary. Prevention of pathologic scars remains a challenge in burn-wound management.

## General Considerations Influencing Thermal Burn-Wound Management

It seems difficult to think about burns without evoking a series of considerations presenting some importance in the wound management. Skin lesions begin to appear after an exposure to heat between 45 °C (1 h) and 70 °C (a few seconds) [1]. Consequences of thermal burns were defined by Jackson [2] in three zones: coagulation, stasis, hyperaemia.

### Types of Burns

Origins of burns can be thermal, electric or chemical. Thermal burns present a specific profile. They are considered not only as wounds but also as a general disease, having consequences on the thermal regulation, glycaemia control, immunological status, myocardial function and pulmonary hypertension. The scars after thermal burns also present a tendency to develop hypertrophy and congestion lasting for a long period of time, more than in electric burns. Chemical burns often present a combination of chemical toxic effects on the skin and thermal consequences.

### Influence of Immediate Care on the Burn Wound

The quality of immediate care has an important influence on the wound [3]. A superficial second-degree burn observed during the initial evaluation can turn into a deep second-degree burn the day after, either due to a poor general management or because the general condition worsens in the resuscitation unit. Problems inherent to immediate burn care will not be developed in this chapter, but it is important to keep in mind the importance of adapted resuscitation measurements during the initial stage. Systemic antimicrobials are also of importance to consider when dealing with general infections coming from the burn wound.

## Burn Wound Assessment

Several key points have to be determined: the extent of the burns over the body surface, the depth of the burns and some important factors like age or pulmonary involvement. These points have to be checked as soon as possible to determine the gravity of the wound in terms of general prognosis, to establish a resuscitation plan as well as for choosing the best local management.

### Extent of Burns

Extent of burns is evaluated following charts derived from the Lund and Browder burn diagram, showing the differences in the respective volumes of the body from birth to adult, or roughly using the rule of nines. Results are expressed in total body surface (TBS) involvement.

### Estimation of Burn Depth

Burn depth is defined by tradition in three degrees, and clinical observation remains the main source of information for the clinician, even if some complementary examinations can be useful to determine the exact extent of deep burns. The surgical indication for excision and grafting depends in the majority of the cases upon the visual evaluation of the wound. This part of burn assessment remains difficult, and cannot be done with precision, even with experience, before the third day after injury. In second-degree burns, the first assessment has been estimated to be accurate in less than 70% of the cases.

### Clinical Evaluation

The first degree corresponds to a shallow wound. The aspect is red, the area is extremely painful, as the sensory endings remain intact. The typical example is sunburn. Only the superficial layer of the epidermis is involved. When total body surface is important, complications like cerebral oedema can be encountered, but the wound remains easy to heal.

Superficial second-degree burns usually present blisters, appearing some hours after the accident. Once the blister has been removed, the wound can be observed. Redness is uniform, and pain is extreme, rarely allowing the physician to touch the lesion. Healing time is short, usually within the first 2 weeks, without aesthetic sequellae. The superficial dermis is exposed, without involving the basal membrane, a guarantee for re-forming quickly the superficial aspect of the skin (Fig. 1).

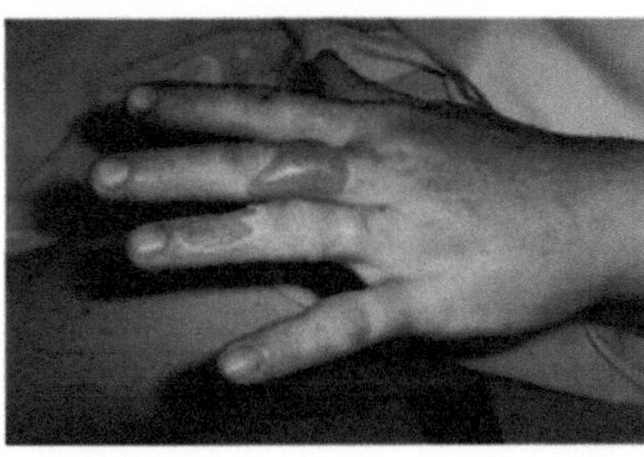

**Fig. 1.** Second-degree burns on the dorsum of the hand. An intact blister can be seen on one digit, the second digit has been cleaned and the base of the wound can really be evaluated

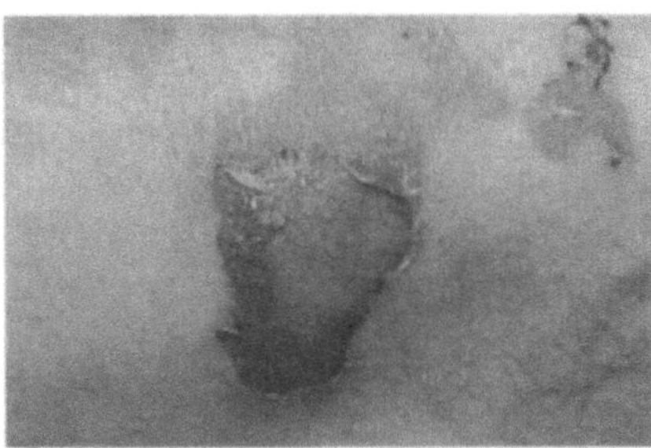

**Fig. 2.** Deep second degree: in this situation, the red colour is not uniform; some discoloured areas can be observed. More than 30% of experts will fail to categorise this wound accurately

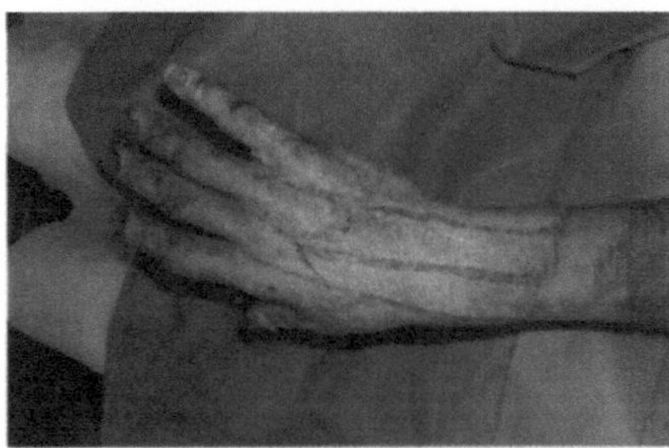

**Fig. 3.** In third-degree burns, risks of compression are important. Incisions of the eschar on the dorsum of the hand are highly recommended in order to prevent ischaemic disorders of the digits. They should be extended distally to the medial and lateral faces in the case of deep burns

Deep second-degree burns also present blisters, but after their removal the aspect is more white or patchwork-like. Sensibility to touch is not as important as in more superficial lesions, due to a partial destruction of sensory endings. Blanching of the skin under digital pressure cannot be obtained. These burns have a tendency to heal spontaneously, except in critical general conditions or if burnt TBS is extensive; the wound will stay unhealed or get worse and transform into a third-degree burn. Usually, healing can be observed within 2 to 3 weeks, but as the deep dermis is exposed, a permanent scar will remain (Fig. 2). These wounds can sometimes require an excision and skin grafting.

Third-degree burns are deep burns involving the subdermal structures. Extent in depth can be important, reaching aponeurosis or even bones. Lesions are sometimes circular on the limbs, a source of ischemia for the distal segments, necessitating emergency surgical procedures of discharge incisions to re-establish a normal distal blood flow (Fig. 3). Lesions present a white colour, tissues are hard. A black eschar will be observed after carbonisation.

## Complementary Examinations

Some complementary examinations have been proposed to determine more precisely the exact depth of the burn:

- Near infrared spectroscopic assessment of haemodynamic changes has been proposed [4]. The principle is to check the tissue-haemoglobin oxygen saturation, total haemoglobin and issue-water content. Significant differences could be observed in the early post-burn period (1 to 3 h after injury).
- Laser Doppler imaging was recently revisited by Pape et al. [5]. In 57 patients presenting an intermediate burn they found that accuracy in classifying lesions as superficial or deep was 97% compared to 60–70% for established clinical methods.
- Non-contact ultrasonography was proposed to determine burn depth. On 15 patients, Iraniha et al. [6] evaluated the differences in ultrasonographic aspects on 78 burn sites compared to 42 normal skin areas, the probe being held 1 inch from the skin. The overall accuracy was estimated to be 96% when predicting that a wound could heal within a period of 3 weeks.
- Pyrophosphate nuclear scan can be considered as a complementary technique. Proposed by Affleck et al. [7], who could determine that in 11 patients with 8 high-voltage electrical injuries, one severe frostbite and two severe infections, Technetium-99 PyP scan showed clear demarcation of viable and non-viable tissue, a key tool to decide amputation. The sensitivity is 94% with a specificity of 100%.
- Diagnosis of burn depth using laser-induced indocyanine green fluorescence was proposed by Still et al. [8] in a preliminary clinical trial, where they could demonstrate the technique.

## Burn-Wound Management

Several options concerning burn-wound management have been proposed all over the world, from open exposure to early surgical excision, from coverage using skin substitutes to the systematic use of anti-infectious topical creams. The consensus is still lacking, except on the fact that burns are difficult to heal and carry a high risk of infection.

### Cooling

Concerning the immediate management, a consensus emerges on the interest of immediate cooling of the burns using tap water at 15 to 18 °C for a period of time varying from 5 to 15 min [9].

## Skin Substitutes

Skin substitutes represent the near future of burns coverage. Some solutions are already available on the market, but all of them show limits [10, 11]:

### Temporary Skin Substitutes

- **Allogenic skin** represents a living tissue, coming from cadavers and pre-mortem situations. Legislation is not universally identical and in some countries this solution is not permitted. Allogenic skin can be used either as a fresh skin or as a cryo-conserved skin; tissue banking allows these products to be frozen and to be stored under suitable conditions. Usually, this skin is submitted to a rejection process, starting during the second week after application. Only the epidermal layer, which presents immunologically active cells, will be submitted to rejection. The dermis will adhere to the underlying wound and create a really good support for any type of epidermal coverage. Usually, autologous keratinocyte cultures are used to cover this alloderm. Potentially, this cadaver allograft can transmit viral diseases.
- Other temporary skin replacement techniques were recently developed: **Transcyte** (Advanced Tissue Sciences) is produced by culturing fibroblasts on a vinyl mesh. Fibroblasts are secondarily extracted, but their local temporary "production" of growth factors remains in the biomaterial. This skin substitute is therefore not cellularised, but contains products of allogenic cells. These cells come from neonates, whose contamination potential is severely controlled. Transcyte was used to cover excised wounds, but also as a temporary material for partial-thickness burns [12–17]. Some studies have proven the efficiency of Transcyte over bacitracine alone [18], or standard therapy in children [19].

### Artificial Dermis

Several collagen-based artificial dermis are available on the market:
- **Alloderm** is based on cadaver skins, from which the epidermal layer is removed, keeping intact the basal membrane. Engraftment of split-thickness meshed grafts is possible. There are reports of improvement in cosmetic results. Alloderm was found useful when covering hand and foot burns [20]. In a control trial, Sheridan et al. did not find any statistical difference following the Vancouver scale test when using Alloderm + skin graft versus skin graft alone [21].
- **Integra** is composed of bovine collagen type I cross-linked with glycosaminoglycans, covered with a silicone film acting as a temporary coverage [22]. A multicentric study report on the use of Integra on recently burned patients confirmed the interest in the product [23]. The technique proposed is a two-step procedure. During the first stage, the burn wound is excised and covered with Integra. The second stage is done after 3 to 4 weeks, consisting of peeling the silicone film, and applying very thin meshed autografts. Aesthetic results are improved, with a less prominent aspect of the mesh and a better pliability of the skin after a period of 1 year.

Other authors described the necessity to protect Integra from infection using a specific protocol including antiseptics applied on the edges of Integra during the revascularisation time of the artificial dermis.

This technique was also proposed in reconstructive surgery to resurface scarred areas [24]. Advantages are the use of thin split-thickness skin grafts, which are prone to heal on the donor-site area within a short period of time, to obtain a dermal support increasing the quality of the scar.

### Cultured Keratinocytes

Keratinocyte cultures were developed in the 1970s [25]. Application on burns was initiated by Gallico et al. [26] and several reports of a high rate of take can be found in the literature. Using Epicel, Odessey [27] reported an overall percent of take close to 60%, but other authors consider the take to be dependent on the severity of burns [28]. Some authors encouraged preparation of the recipient bed using cadaver allografts [29], the epidermal layer being removed. The technique is demanding: harvesting some square centimetres of intact skin, sending them to the laboratory, waiting 3 weeks to have a culture. During this time, excision of the burned area is realised, preparation of the bed site needs the use of allogenic skin, its dermal component not being touched by the rejection process. The team must be familiar with the technique and numerous enough to realise long and difficult pre- and post-grafting dressings, and the rescucitation team has to face the instability of the patient during this period of time. Used in children for extensive burns over 90% of TBS, keratinocyte culture has proven to be a life-saving solution [30].

Cosmetic results have been reported to be at least equivalent to meshed autografts, other reports signalling late severe contractures due to the lack of dermal component.

Attempts to enhance the graft take and maturation have been proposed in different directions and modifications of the support. Presently the support has to be taken down some days after grafting keratinocyte cultures. In order to prevent this take down – a source of possible trauma for the cells – resorbable supports were recently proposed as well as cultivation of keratinocytes on spherical beads.

Despite serious interest in the development of cultured cells to cover large burns, these techniques remain reserved to highly specialised centres.

### Anti-Infectious Topical Creams

Local infection is characterised by growth and development of pathogen germs. Consequences of infection on the burn wound are important, the lesions being more pronounced and the healing delayed, transforming it into a chronic wound. The burn wound presents a permanent risk of infection, even if this risk is more pronounced during the first period. Therefore, local antibacterial products are indicated at the initial stage. After obtaining a granulation tissue, especially in superficial second-degree burns the wound can be managed using dressings which have less action on infection and more effect on moist wound healing.

Prevention of infection is one of the rules when treating a burn wound, and in most cases, a topical cream effective on different germs is proposed. Assessment of infection is another important point. Clinical evaluation is required daily in order to identify signs of infection (colour, odour, aspect, exudation). Bacteriological counts are necessary to demonstrate the presence and virulence of pathogens. $10^5$ germs/g of tissue, a result obtained by tissue biopsy, signals the presence of infection. The specimen must be free from contamination coming from the normal flora, and free of previous application of antiseptics.

Gram-positive (*Staphylococcus aureus, Epidermidis, Streptococcus*) and Gram-negative (*Escherichia coli, Proteus, Pseudomonas aeruginosa*) germs are frequently observed on the burn wound. A consensus emerges on the fact that a burn wound is not infected during the first 3 days. Topical anti-infectious creams should be prescribed immediately after the accident. Monafo et al. [31] recommended that topical antimicrobial therapy should be started initially in order to delay and to minimise wound infection.

The best approach is to clean the wound, to remove debris and necrotic parts, excise as soon as possible and cover the wound using skin grafts. Antimicrobial agents are products being used around this general principle. When a pathogenic germ has been identified as responsible for a massive local infection, the topical antimicrobial to be applied must be specifically active on this germ.

**Silversulfadiazine** is the most commonly used prophylactic topical cream. This white insoluble cream is composed of sodium sulfadiazine and silver nitrate. Painless to apply, it causes a sensation of freshness appreciated by the patient.

This product is effective on *Staphylococcus aureus, Escherichia coli, Klebsiellae, Pseudomonas aeruginosa, Enterobacter, Proteus* and *Candida albicans*, but penetrates poorly into the eschar. Used in a daily application, this topical cream was observed to present some complications (cutaneous rash, methaemoglobinaemia, transient leukopenia).

**Cerium silversulfadiazine**, a modification consisting in addition of 2% cerium nitrate to the original silversulfadiazine, changes the behaviour of the dressing. Reserved for third-degree wounds, this product will create de novo a calcified crust over the burn eschar [32], which protects the area from contamination. Cerium sulfadiazine modifies the local aspect of the wound. Used mainly in Europe, promoted by Wassermann in 1989 [33], this product will actively promote spontaneous healing within a short period, preventing excessive excision, and offers the possibility of sequentially grafting extensive burns, when harvesting the few donor-site areas must be repeated.

However, Hadjiiski et al. [35], could compare in four groups the respective effects of four different topical agents. The best effects were obtained when using flammazine or flammacerium, but the authors could not separate these two last groups in term of results.

**Silver nitrate solution** (0.5%) is effective on *S. aureus*, and *Pseudomonas aeruginosa*; it does not, however, penetrate into the burn eschar. This product causes hyonatremia, colours linen and dressings black. It is more commonly used after surgery to protect a skin graft from infection.

**Mafenide acetate, Sulfamylon**™ is effective on *Pseudomonas aeruginosa*, *Clostridium* and a range of other microorganisms [36]. This product penetrates well the wound eschar, but it was demonstrated to favour the appearance of *Candida albicans*, and to develop a metabolic acidosis if applied on large surfaces. Easy and painless to apply, this cream is used isolated or in combination with others.

**Povidone iodine** has a large spectrum of activity on a series of germs, and is considered also as an antifungal agent (10% solution). Problems due to cytotoxicity, pain and excessive absorption causing thyroid dysfunction limit the use of povidone iodine to temporary use during the dressings, the solution being washed after a few minutes of application.

**Bacitracin/polymixin**, mupirocin, gentamycin sulfate, nitrofuratonin and nystatin have also been proposed as topical agents. They present some indications on specific germs.

**Acticoat:** Silver delivery system is based upon a new technology increasing the surface area between the material and the wound. This nanocrystalline silver is placed on a bilayer of polyethylene, from which ionic silver and silver radicals are released in high concentrations when exposed to water. The system presents a high bactericidal potential, without any described resistance. Some studies recently published demonstrated the interest of such a product in the management of burn wounds [44, 45]. However, this product has to be properly prescribed. In a recent study, Innes et al. (46) compared Allevyn and Acticoat as dressings used for donor-site coverage and the Allevyn was superior to Acticoat in terms of rate of re-epithelialisation and quality of scar. This new product can also be used for prevention of sepsis in burn wounds (Fig. 4).

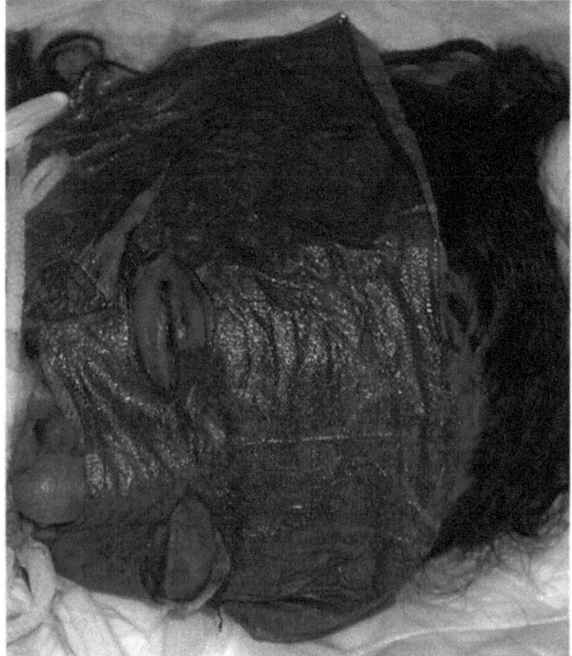

**Fig. 4.** The use of Acticoat claims to permanently provide humidity on the wound but seems promising in the management of local infection

*Alternative Solutions*

**Hydrocolloids** are commonly used on minor burns, as well as hydrogels or hydro-cellular dressings. When there are doubts about a potential infection, it is possible to treat the burn wound as a simple loss of substance. Dressings respecting the moist wound-healing principles can be used to promote granulation tissue formation.

However, hypergranulation can be observed using hydrocolloids after a period of 2 weeks. Usually, the keratinisation process is better obtained using other local treatment, like cortisone-based dressings or films. Experimentally, migration and multiplication of keratinocytes are favoured when using films, compared to other types of dressings. No randomised control trials can be found in the literature; but most of the burn centres commonly use these types of dressings for the last stages of minor burn-wound treatment.

**Moist exposed burn ointment** (MEBO) was described [36] as comparable to silversulfadiazine in terms of results on partial-thickness burns of the face.

**Negative pressure therapy**, proposed by Morykwas and Argenta in 1997, can be used in two different applications on burn wounds:

- In acute burns, vacuum-assisted closure was proposed on deep second-degree burns in an experimental study on pigs. More recently, VAC was applied on third-degree burns that could not be immediately covered, after exposure of vascular pedicles, aponeurosis or nerves. This temporary covering allowed a good healthy germ-free granulation tissue to be obtained within a period of 2 weeks.
- VAC is more commonly used as a means of fixing a skin graft. In this indication, the pressure level must be low (about 55 mmHg). The machine is easy to use, options being the level of pressure and the mode of action, intermittent or continuous. Polyvinyl-perforated pads are cut to the exact size of the area to cover, fixation being done using adhesive films.

### Early Surgical Excision and Skin Grafting

*Excision of the Burn Eschar*

The first report of excision to living tissue followed by split-skin grafting was done by Janzekovic in 1970 [47]. This tangential excision concept still remains the gold standard. Improvement in life saving observed since the 1950s is mainly due to progress in resuscitation, but early excision and grafting represent an important step in reconstructive surgery for burns extending over 30% of the TBS and even less, as this technique is commonly used for deep burns limited in surface.

The technique of eschar debridement is standardised. Tangential excision is usually realised by using a special knife with the possibility to select the depth of tissue to be excised (Watson, Lagrot). The appropriate depth is determined by obtaining a well-bleeding tissue. Excision will be done to the dermis for superficial excision, to the fat for more deep excisions. This technique causes bleeding, and perioperative applications of diluted epinephrine are highly recommended.

Complete excision of the eschar can be done when burns are very extensive in depth (Fig. 5). The excision must in these cases be realised at the aponeurosis of the underlying muscles (fascial excision).

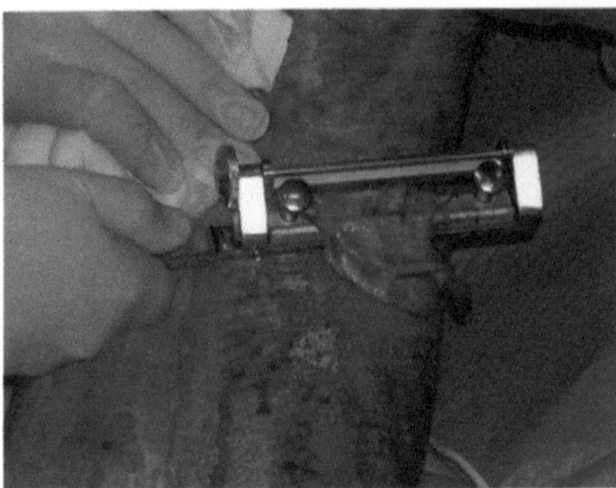

Fig. 5. Tangential excision of the burn eschar is important in the surgical wound-bed preparation before applying skin grafts

### Skin Grafting

Skin grafting can be done using different types of grafts, allografts coming from tissue banking, or autologous skin grafts (partial thickness, expanded or not, full thickness).

Allografts are skin substitutes (see above). **Partial-thickness skin grafts** are harvested usually on a specific donor-site area: the skull represents the area to be used when possible. This technique allows the scar coming from the harvesting to be hidden inside the hair after regrowth. After shaving and injecting some inert liquid (sterile water) between the gala and the subcutaneous area, a thin piece of skin is harvested using a dermatome (2/10 to 4/10 mm). When this zone cannot be used as a donor site, the thighs, the legs, abdomen and the thorax can be alternatives.

The graft can be used with or without skin expansion (×1.5, ×2, ×4) depending on the requirements of the recipient area and the surface of donor site areas available. For small surfaces, especially in children or women, a partial-thickness skin graft coming from the skull is adapted. When dealing with very large surfaces, the "sandwich technique", combining ×6 autografts and ×2 allografts can give satisfactory results in terms of graft take and coverage (Fig. 6).

Complications are peri-operative bleeding, secondary retractions due to the thinness of the skin graft and the low percentage of dermis it contains.

**Full-thickness skin graft** can be harvested in selected areas where complete skin can be harvested, i.e. the anterior folds of the groin area, the elbows or the knees. The amount of skin is limited. This type of skin graft, less subject to secondary retraction, will be promoted when grafting small areas located on mechanically demanding zones, like the feet and the hands.

Colour matching is a very important point to be checked in advance. Brown skins should be analysed with special care, the skin of the thigh presenting a colour poorly compatible with that of the face. One should prefer to use the skin of an available area close to the recipient zone (the shoulder area is sometimes used for the face).

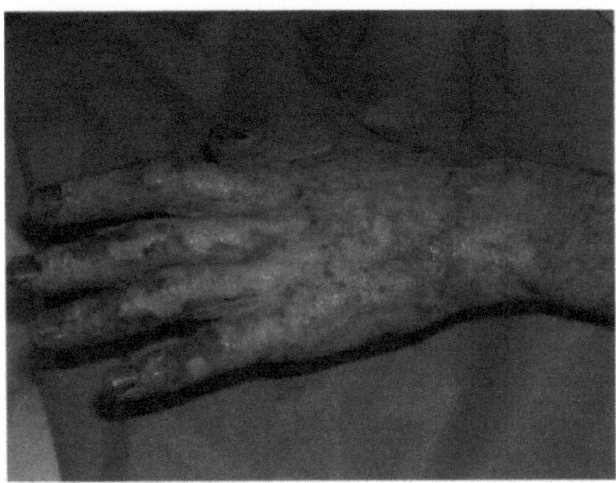

**Fig. 6.** End of keratinisation process on freshly grafted areas on the dorsum of the hand

## Management of Post-Skin-Grafting Infection

Post-operative skin infection is more prominent in burns than in any other surgical activity. Skin-graft infections, clinically assessed on partial loss of freshly healed areas, are not uncommon. In these circumstances, surgeons would promote application of active local antimicrobials. Anti-staphylococci and anti-pseudomonas have already demonstrated some efficiency. Acticoat may become a good indication if confirmed by clinical studies.

## Conclusion

Many efforts are to be developed in management of acute burns , as well as in preventing pathological scars (hypertrophies, keloids) but also in preventing colour disorders and melanocyte reinfiltration of spontaneously healed or grafted skin areas.

## References


1. Moritz AR, Henriques FC (1947)  Studies of thermal injuries II. The relative importance of time and surface temperature in the causation of cutaneous burns. Am J Pathol 23: 695–720
2. Jackson DM (1953) The diagnosis of the depth of burning. Br J Surg 40: 588–596
3. Kim DE, Phillips TM, Jeng JC, Rizzo AG, Roth RT, Stanford JL, Jablonski KA, Jordan MH (2001) Microvascular assessment of burn depth conversion during varying resuscitation conditions. J Burn Care Rehabil 22: 406–416

4. Sowa MG, Leonardi L, Payette JR, Fisch JS, Mantsch HH (2001) Near infrared spectroscopic assessment of hemodynamic changes in the early post-burn period. Burns 27: 241–249

5. Pape SA, Skouras CA, Byrne PO (2001) An audit of the use of Laser Doppler imaging (LDI) in the assessment of burns of intermediate depth. Burns 27: 233–239

6. Irahina S, Cinat ME, VanderKam VM, Boyko A, Lee D, Jones J, Achauere BM (2000) Determination of burn depth with noncontact ultrasonography. J Burn Care Reahabil 2: 333–338

7. Affleck DG, Edelman L, Morris SE, Saffle JR (2001) Assessment of tissue viability in complex extremity injuries: utility of the pyrophosphate nuclear scan. J Trauma 50: 263–269

8. Still JM, Law EJ, Klavuhn KG, Island TC, Holtz JZ (2001) Diagnosis of burn depth using laser-induced indocyanine green fluorescence; a preliminary clinical trial. Burns 27: 364–371

9. Jandera V, Hudson DA, de Wet PM, Innes PM, Rode H (2000) Cooling the burn wound: evaluation of different modalities. Burns 26: 265–270

10. Ozcan C, Ergun O, Celik A, Corduk N, Ozok G (2002) Enzymatic debridement of burn wound with collagenase in children with partial-thickness burns. Burns 28: 791–794

11. Van Zuijlen, Vloemans JF, van Trier AJ, Suijker MH, van Unen E, Groenevelt F, Kreis RW, Middlekoop E (2001) Dermal substitution in acute burns and reconstructive surgery: a subjective and objective long-term follow-up. Plast Reconstr Surg 108: 1938–1946

12. Boyce ST, Kagan RJ, Yabukoff KP, Meyer NA, Rieman MT, Greenhalg DG, Warden GD (2002) Cultured skin substitutes reduce donor skin harvesting for closure of excised, full-thickness burns. Ann Surg 235: 269–279

13. Hansbrough JF, Mozingo DW, Kealey GP (1997) Clinical trials of a biosynthetic temporary skin replacement, Dermagraft-Transitional Covering™ compared with cryopreserved human cadaver skin for temporary coverage of excised burn wounds. J Burn Care Rehabil 18: 43–51

14. Purdue GF, Hunt JL, Still JM (1997) A multicenter clinical trial of a biosynthetic skin replacement, Dermagraft-TC, compared with cryopreserved human cadaver skin for temporary coverage of excised burn wounds. J Burn Care Rehabil 18: 52–57

15. Burd A, Lam PK, Lau H (2002) Allogenic skin: transplant or dressing. Burns 28: 358–366

16. Mackie D (2002) Postal survey on the use of glycerol-preserved allografts in clinical practice. Burns 28 [Suppl] 1: S40–44

17. Noordenhbos J, Doré C, Hansbrough JF (1999) Safety and efficacy of Dermagraft-TC for treatment of partial thickness burns. J Burn Care Rehabil 20: 275–281

18. Demling RH, DeSanti L (1999) Management of partial thickness facial burns (comparison of topical antibiotics and bio-engineered skin substitutes). Burns 25: 256–261

19. Lukish JR, Eichelberger MR, Newman KD et al. (2001) The use of a bioactive skin substitute decreases length of stay for pediatric burn patients. J Pediatr Surg 36: 1118–1121

20. Lattari V, Jones LM, Varcelotti J, Late'nser BA, Sherman HF, Barette RR (1997) The use of a permanent dermal allograft in full-thickness burns of the hand and foot: a report of three cases. J Burn Care Rehabil 18: 147–155

21. Sheridan R, Choucair R, Donelan M, Lydon M, Petras L, Tompkins R (1998) Acellular allodermis in burn surgery: a 1-year results of a pilot trial. J Burn Care Rehabil 19: 528–530

22. Yannas IV (1998) Studies on the biological activity of the dermal regeneration template. Wound Reap Reg 6: 518–524

23. Heimbach D, Luterman A, Burke J et al. (1988) Artificial dermis for major burns. A multicenter randomized clinical trial. Ann Surg 208: 313–320

24. Dantzer E, Braye FM (2001) Reconstructive surgery using an artificial derms (integra): results with 39 grafts. Br J Plast Surg 54: 659–664

25. Rheinwald JG, Green H (1975) serial cultivation of strains of human epidermal keratonicytes: the formation of keratinizing colonies from single cells. Cell 6: 448–451

26. Gallico GG, O'Connor NE, Compton CC, Kehind O, Green H (1984) Permanent coverage of large burn wounds with autologous cultured human epithelium. N Engl J Med 311: 448–451

27. Odessey R (1992) Multicenter experience with cultured epidermal autografts for treatment of burns. J Burn Care Rehabil 13: 174–180

28. Compton CC, Hickerson W, Nadire K, Press W (1993) Acceleration of skin regeneration from cultured epithelial autografts by transplantation to homograft dermis. J Burn Care Rehabil 14: 653–662

29. Hefton JM, Madden MR, Finkelstein JL, Shires GT (1983) Grafting of patients with allografts of cultured cells. Lancet 2: 428–430

30. Sheridan TL, Tompkins RG (1995) Cultured autologous epithelium in patients with burns of ninety percent or more of the body surface. J Trauma 38: 48–53

31. Monafo WW, West MA (1990) Current treatment recommendations for topical burn therapy. Drugs 40: 364–73
32. Koller J, Orsag M (1998) Our experience with the use of cerium sulphadiazine in the treatment of extensive burns. Acta Chir Plast 40: 73–75
33. Wassermann D, Schlotterer M, Lebreton F, Levy J, Guelfi MC (1989) Use of topically applied silver-sulfadiazine plus cerium nitrate in major burns. Burns 15: 257–260
34. Murphy RC, Kucan JO, Robson MC, Heggers JP (1983) The effect of 5% mafenide acetate solution on bacterial contamination of infected rat burns. J Trauma 23: 878–881
35. Hadkiiski OG, Lesseva MI (1999) Comparison of four drugs for local treatment of burn wounds. Eur J Emerg Med 6: 41–47
36. Ang ES, Lee ST, Gan CS, See P, Chan YH, Ng LH, Machin D (2000) The role of alternative therapy in the management of partial thickness burns of the face-experience with the use of moist exposed burn ointment (MEBO) compared with silversulfadiazine. Ann Acad Med Singapore 29: 7–10
37. Vleomans AF, Soesman AM, Sujiker M, Kreis RW, Middlekoop E (2003) A randomized trial comparing a hydrocolloid-derived dressing and glycerol preserved allograft skin in the management of partial thickness burns. Burns 29: 702–710
38. Malpass KG, Snelling CF, Tron V (2003) Comparison of donor-site healing under Xeroform and Jelonet dressings: unexpected findings. Plast Reconstr Surg 112: 430–439
39. Meaume S, Senet P, Dumas R, Carsin H, Pannier M, Bohbot S (2002) Urgotul: a novel non-adherent lipidocolloid dressing. Br J Nurs 11 [Suppl 16]: S42–43, S46–50
40. Téot L, Otman S, Giovannini U (2004) The use of negative pressure therapy in managing wounds. ETRS Annual meeting. Satellite symposium Cardiff Sept 2001. Springer, Berlin Heidelberg New York Tokyo (in press)
41. Webb LX, Schmidt U (2001) Wound management with vacuum therapy. Unfallchirurg 104: 918–926
42. Chang KP, Tsaii CC, Lin TM, Lai CS, Lin SD (2001) An alternative dressing for skin graft immobilization: negative pressure dressing. Burns 27: 839–842
43. Yin HG, Langford R, Tredget EE, Burell RE (1999) Effect of Acticoat antimicrobial barrier dressing on wound healing and graft take. J Burn Care Rehabil 1999 Jan/Frb S231
44. Burell RE, Heggers JP, Davis GJ, Wright JB (1999) Efficacy of silver associated dressings as bacterial barriers in a rodent burn sepsis model. Wounds 11: 64–71
45. Tredget EE, Shankowsky HA, Groenveld A, Burell R (1998) A matched-pair, randomized study evaluating the efficacy and safety of Acticoat silver-coated dressing for the treatment of burn wounds. J Burn Care Rehabil 19: 532–537
46. Innes ME, Umraw N, Fish JS, Gomez M, Cartotto RC (2001) The use of silver coated dressings on donor site wounds: a prospective, controlled matched pair study. Burns 27: 621–627
47. Janzekovic Z (1970) A new concept in the early excision and immediate grafting of burns. J Trauma 10: 1103–1108

J.-C. Castède, V. Casoli, C. Isacu

## Introduction

Electricity is a relatively recent invention (mid 19th century) and its widespread use makes electrical injury a not uncommon problem at work or at home.

Less common than thermal burns, electrical injuries account in the literature from 5 to 10% of all burn casualties. They may lead to death by electrocution. Koumbourlis [1] stated that electrocution is responsible for more than 500 deaths per year in the United States. More than half of them occur in the workplace and constitute the fifth leading cause of occupational injury death [2]. Electrocutions at home are mostly associated with malfunctioning or misuse of consumer products.

On the other hand, electrical injuries are characterised by a high morbidity rate with a significant impact on the functional rehabilitation of the patient. McCauley and Barret [3] noted that the limb amputation rate in high-voltage electrical injuries remains at 45 to 71%.

Typically, the electrically burnt patient is a young active male adult [4–7]. In our experience, over a period of 10 years, electrical injuries represent 6% of all burn unit admissions, 88% were male and the mean age was 27.5 years old with two peaks of frequency between 21 to 30 years old and less than 5 years old.

## Pathophysiology

An electrical injury will occur when a person comes into contact with a source of current. Generally, this source is a home or a workplace installation or appliance, or a power line. There is a possibility of iatrogenic electrical injury during medical examination or treatment in the ICU, the operating room or during electrophysiology procedures. Sometimes, the source of current is a natural one, such as lightning.

Clinicians have arbitrarily divided electrical injuries into low-tension and high-tension injuries. Low-voltage injuries (<1000 V) occur principally at home and result in limited deep cutaneous burns. Electrocution is more frequent in these accidents. High-voltage electrical injuries (>1000 V) are more often work-related, with extensive burns and damages of deeper structures.

## Principles of Electricity

Electricity is a flow of negatively charged electrons through a conductor connecting two points when there is a potential difference or voltage (V) between these points. The flow of electrons creates an electric current (I) measured in amperes (A). Anything that restricts this flow creates a resistance (R) measured in ohms ($\Omega$). Ohm's law relates voltage, current and resistance:

$$V = R \times I.$$

The mechanism for tissue damages was believed to be the conversion of electrical energy into heat, the Joule effect. Heat production is expressed by Joule's law:

$$J = 0.24 \times R \times I^2 \times t,$$

where R is the resistance, I the amount of current and t the duration of contact.

## Determinant Factors of Electrical Injury

Factors determining the type and extent of lesions depend either on the source of current (voltage, type of current) or on the injured patient (tissue resistance, intensity of the current, duration of contact and pathway of the current) [8].

The voltage is specific to the source of the current, 220–240 V for household installations in Europe, 110–120 V in North America.

There are two types of electrical current. The alternating current (AC) is the most common in households, workplaces, industry and outside power lines. The electron flow in the conductor has a cyclic fashion with a frequency of 50 Hz in Europe (60 Hz in North America). The direct current (DC) is produced by batteries and lightning. AC is more dangerous than DC because it causes tetanic muscle contractions that prolong the duration of contact with the source.

The resistance is the main factor which determines the intensity or amount of the current in the body according to Ohm's law. It depends on the type of contact and its duration, the proper resistance of the different tissues of the body and the quality of the skin at the contact points.

Tissue resistance progressively increases from nerves to blood vessels, mucous membranes, muscle, skin, tendons fat and bone.

Skin resistance depends on its thickness and its moisture. The thicker the skin is, the higher its resistance. A dry thick skin may have a resistance of 100 000 Û while the resistance of a wet thin skin drops to less than 1000 Û; this may result in electrocution. Bones have a higher resistance and, according to the Joule effect, produce more heat, which causes necrosis of the deep periosseous tissues.

Globally, the body consists of a resistant envelope, the skin, and a relatively conductive core. According to this, a first theory was that nerves, blood vessels and muscles preferentially conducted the current. Another theory, developed after experimental studies by Hunt et al. [9] and Lee [10], stated that the body conducts the current as a whole, with a composite resistance of all body-tissue components and the cross-sectional diameter of the body part. Since resistance is inversely proportional to the extremity's diameter, heat produced by current passing up through an upper extremity is higher at wrist and elbow.

The pathway of the current through the body determines the type and severity of the injury. A horizontal pathway from hand to hand will affect the brain and the heart and is associated with a high mortality rate. A vertical pathway (from hand to foot) involves virtually all the vital organs. On the contrary, a very short pathway between fingers in one hand may result in deep local lesions without any general disturbance.

## Pathophysiological Effects of Electrical Injury

Our understanding of the pathophysiology of electrical injuries is poor and continues to evolve. Although heat production plays a leading part in the pathogenesis of electrical damages, Lee et al. [11] demonstrated another mechanism named electroporation. Electroporation is an immediate effect of current passing through cellular tissue. This is a cellular phenomenon resulting from the effects of the current on the cell membrane with denaturation of the proteins and creation of pores in the cell membrane which leads to cell death, even in the absence of significant heat production. This phenomenon contributes clinically in large release of arachidonic acid and myoglobin, which indicate intracellular damage.

Electricity can provide a large spectrum of soft-tissue injuries. It should be considered as a multisystem injury.

Electrical injuries may affect the heart, causing cardiac dysrhythmias. Sudden death by asystole and ventricular fibrillation more likely occurs in hand-to-hand pathways and low-voltage injuries. True myocardial infarction or direct necrosis of the myocardium are rare.

The respiratory system may be affected by direct injury of the respiratory control centre or by suffocation, secondary to electrical tetanic contractions of the respiratory muscles. Direct lung injuries or blunt trauma are possible.

The nervous system is affected more commonly. A loss of consciousness and coma are frequent. Spinal cord involvements and peripheral nervous system perturbations cause transient or definitive motor and sensory deficits or paralysis.

Renal injuries may occur as a result of rhabdomyolosis and the massive release of myoglobin, and lead to acute renal failure.

Among other systems cataracts should be mentioned which are a very common but late complication.

## Electrical Burn Injury

Electrical burns result from the heat production according to the Joule effect. They are classified into two types:

- Pure electrothermal burns are produced from a direct contact with an electrical conductor. Skin lesions are located at entry and exit points and are associated with deep hidden burns of internal soft tissues along the pathway of the current.
- Arc injuries are observed when there is no direct contact if the distance is short enough, generally during high-voltage accidents. In addition to the passage of the current, the extremely high temperatures of an arc (2500 to 5000 °C) result in extensive full-thickness burns.

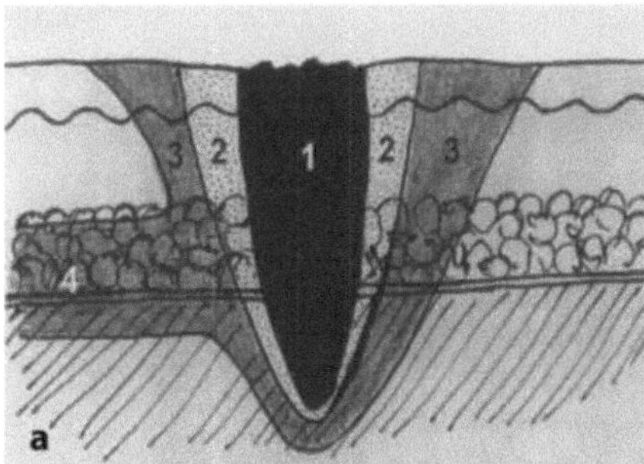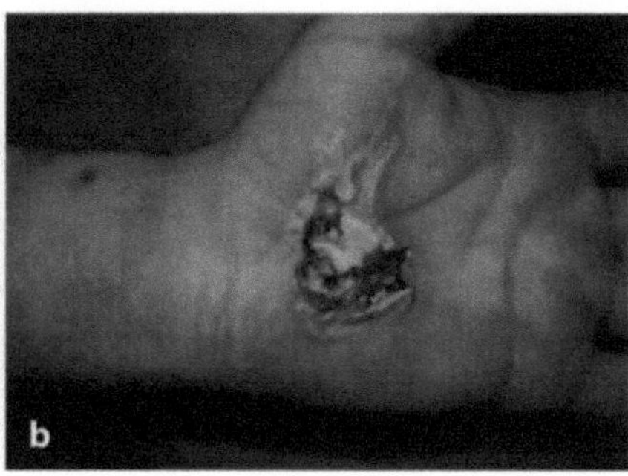

**Fig. 1. a** Schematic representation of the electrical burn injury. *1* Central carbonised area with charred skin craters on the surface of the skin; *2* full-thickness burn area; *3* area of partial necrosis of the skin and soft tissue; *4* deep hidden burn along the pathway of the current. **b** Characteristic aspect of a direct low-voltage contact burn on the palm of the hand

Flash burns with no direct contact or arc involving the patient are not electrical but thermal burns. Sometimes the ignition of clothes and environment may cause associated thermal burns.

Electrical burns are quite different from thermal burns and associate skin lesions and deep soft-tissue damages.

Skin lesions located at entry and exit points represent the elementary electrical burn wound and are characterised by the following [12, 13] (Fig. 1):

- a frequently sharply demarcated and limited burn area,
- a conic shape with deep extension from the surface into the tissues,
- centred by a carbonised area with charred skin craters at the contact sites,
- surrounded by adjacent areas of degressive thickness burns and oedematous skin with microvascular impairment.

However, these skin lesions represent only a part of the burn tissues, like the visible emerged tip of an iceberg.

Deep soft-tissue lesions along the pathway of the current are frequently hidden beneath apparently uninjured skin. They more likely result from high-voltage injuries.

- Secondary burns by arcing in the flexor creases are particularly frequent on the upper limb (wrist, elbow, axilla) (see Fig. 5a). They result from current flowing through the path of least resistance. When the current encounters a relatively resistant joint (small cross-sectional area and highly resistant tissue), helped by the violent tetanic contracture in flexion of the limb, it jumps across the joint. Skoog [14] described this mechanism of re-entry arcing at the anterior face of the wrist when the hand grasps a high-voltage conductor (Fig. 2).
- Muscle damages are very important and the keystone of vital and functional prognosis. Immediate lesions result from heat production, electroporation and periosseous burns. Quinby et al. [15] described the microscopic changes of muscles and emphasised the mixed patchy nature of the electrical injury. Normal muscle cells can be seen immediately adjacent to necrotic cells. These areas of patchy necrosis could be converted into complete tissue loss by the develop-

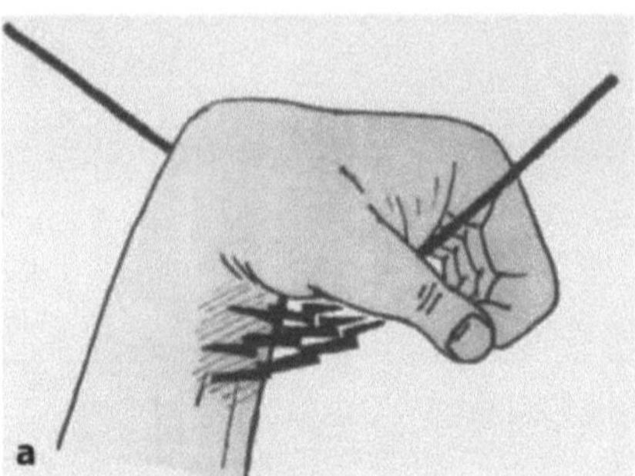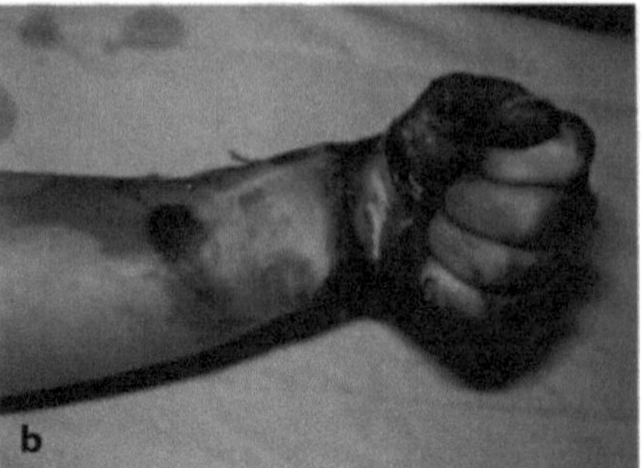

**Fig. 2. a** Mechanism of re-entry arcing at the anterior face of the wrist described by Skoog; **b** clinical aspect

ment of a compartment syndrome due to extensive oedema, progressive small-vessel thrombosis and deterioration of the microvasculature. Bacterial infection and large exposure of muscle by the way of fasciotomies also play an important role.

■ The effects on the vascular bed vary between the size of vessels. Large arteries are not acutely affected but they are susceptible to medial necrosis and secondary rupture. Smaller vessels are acutely affected by coagulation necrosis and most likely participate in muscle necrosis and compartment syndrome.

## Clinical Aspects

### Assessment of Electrical Injuries

Depending on the voltage of current and the conditions of contact, two clinical situations are observed: limited electrical burns and extensive electrical burns.

Limited electrical burns are more commonly due to low-voltage injuries with direct contact. Home accidents are predominant. Burn lesions are essentially located at entry and/or exit points. The most important amount of electrical energy is dissipated into heat at these contact points so that there is a little amount of deep soft-tissue lesions along the pathway of current. Some transient loss of consciousness may be observed. Toddlers, young children and teenagers are particularly involved in these accidents. Skin lesions are sometimes impressive and may involve deep functional structures such as bone and joints, tendons, nerves and main arteries. Even if these contact burns may be located everywhere on the body, hands, mouth and scalp are preferentially affected.

From a surgical point of view, the treatment consists of early and complete excision of damaged tissues and definitive coverage in a one-step procedure.

It is obvious that prolonged wound closure leads to scar contracture, stiff joints, significant functional impairment and sometimes amputation.

Extensive electrical burns are generally due to high-tension injuries. Multiple and extensive skin lesions associated with thermal burns by electrical arc and ignition of clothes and environment are observed.

Associated injuries have been reported, such as head injuries, fractures, dislocations, spinal cord injuries and intra-abdominal traumas [16] when at the time of accident the patient falls from a height (roof, electrical pylon). Similarly, skeletal injury may also occur as a result of a severe muscle contraction due to alternating current.

Massive hidden underlying deep muscle damage dramatically impairs functional and vital prognosis.

Despite the evidence of these skin lesions, a thorough and detailed examination of the patient is necessary, searching for lesions at the flexion creases and evaluating the development of a compartment syndrome by palpation of the limbs.

## Acute Care and Initial Therapy

At the scene of accident, before providing medical care, rescuers must be sure that the source has been cut off or the victim has been extricated safely away from the current source with the use of properly insulated equipment.

Electrocuted patients require immediate cardiopulmonary resuscitation. Continued cardiac monitoring is necessary particularly when the initial ECG findings are abnormal. Patients who sustain electrical injury require admission to a specialised burn unit or to the ICU.

Obviously, the prompt resuscitation of the high-voltage electrical burn patient is of absolute priority. The combination of extensive burns and significant visceral and soft-tissue injuries leads to increased fluid requirements exceeding those predicted by the standard formulas. Ringer-lactate solution is vigorously administered, beginning at about 4 ml/kg/% TBSA burn.

In addition, massive amounts of myoglobin are released from the damaged muscles. Normally, myoglobin is cleared by the kidneys. However, massive amounts may result in the deposition of myoglobin in the renal tubules and lead to acute renal failure. Osmotic diuretic (mannitol) and alkalinisation (sodium bicarbonate) are indicated in order to maintain a urine output near to 2 ml/kg/h. Extra-renal filtration may be necessary.

Standard laboratory tests do not differ from other burn patients. Creatine phosphokinase (CPK) levels are elevated in severe injury. Haemoglobin and myoglobin levels in blood and urine need to be determined.

## Wound Management

The key for managing a patient with electrical injuries lies in the treatment of the wound. Controversy persists whether or not the tissue damage is progressive.

Robson et al. [17] suggested that progressive necrosis does occur and advocated a sequential and conservative approach with cautious debridement and eventual wound coverage. However, in this theory, lesions may be worsened by dessication of the open wounds and infection.

Zelt et al. [18], after experimental studies in a primate model, concluded that progressive tissue necrosis does not occur and suggested that debridement and definitive wound closure could occur much earlier; but this approach is substantially more aggressive and leads to a higher rate of major amputation of the limbs.

Lee and Kolodney [19] suggested that cells not coagulated by heat die by electroporation. This will not be identified at the time of initial decompression and exploration. This inability to assess accurately the real extent of initial tissue damage may be the reason for the progressive tissue necrosis theory.

Various tests have been proposed to examine muscle viability. Technetium-99m pyrophosphate scintigraphy evaluates muscle ischemia [20]. Muscle blood flow can be measured by Xenon-133 scintigraphy [21]. Taking frozen microscopic sections at the time of debridement for histologic examination has been advocated [15]. Magnetic resonance imaging (MRI) also appears as a reliable examination for evaluation of deep necrotic tissue [22]. Unfortunately, because of their expense, time-consuming nature and practical difficulties, these tests have not gained widespread use in the management of patients.

Practically, the first step of the treatment is an early decompression of compartment syndrome of the limbs by fasciotomies. A thorough exploration may be done with debridement of evident necrotic tissue. The initial damage appears less extensive than the damage documented a few days later. Consequently, second-look procedures have become routine to determine the extent of severe electrical in-juries [3].

## Surgical Treatment

The spectrum of anatomic manifestations from electrical trauma is quite varied. Whereas split-thickness skin grafts are almost always sufficient for thermal burn wound closure, flap surgery is frequently required for the closure of electrical burn wounds.

Hand, oral cavity and scalp injuries are more frequent in low-voltage traumas and need early surgical procedures. Extensive high-voltage electrical burns may require specific surgical attention.

### Hand Injuries

More than 50% of electrically burned hands result from low-voltage traumas. Household accidents are predominant, with special mention of wall outlets and electrical cords. In our experience [23], 80% of electrical burn patients sustained hand injuries and 30% of them concerned young children less than 5 years old.

Skin lesions by direct contact may be single or multiple with the characteristic aspect of a well-demarcated deep burn wound, generally located on the palmar face of the hand and fingers or the finger pulp. Commonly, as a result of the grip function of the thumb and the index finger, injuries affect at least these two fingers.

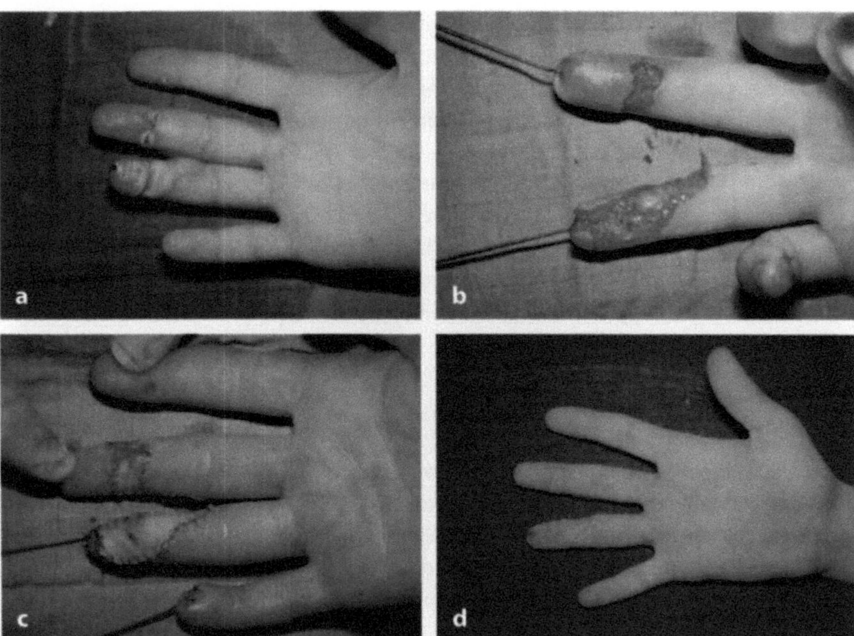

**Fig. 3. a** Deep electrical burn by low-voltage direct contact on the palmar face of the 3rd and 4th fingers. **b** Complete debridement on day 1 extended in the subcutaneous fat tissue. **c** Immediate coverage by a full-thickness skin graft from the groin area. **d** Final result 6 months later

Short or hand-to-hand pathways are predominant, but generally the short duration of contact until the current has been cut off by automatic switches explains that general electrical disturbances are moderate. Some peripheral nervous system dysfunctions may be reported, particularly when the contact site lies on the path of a peripheral nerve. Only very small lesions (Jellinek's marks) do not require surgical treatment.

Due to their functional location and their expected functional impairment, limited electrical burns of the hand require an early surgical treatment in a one-stage procedure on day 1 or 2.

Most of them concern only skin and subcutaneous fat tissue. After complete debridement, the best coverage is obtained with a full-thickness skin graft, harvested from the groin area, for example, and carefully sutured on the edges of the wound. In our experience [23], this technique allows a rapid closure and healing and a good functional recovery of the injured hand (Fig. 3).

When deep functional structures, such as nerves, tendons, bone and joints, are exposed, immediate flap coverage is required even if these structures appear affected by the passage of the current. Only destructive injuries of these functional structures may need a specific surgical treatment during the same procedure. Many local flap procedures, homo- or heterodigital flaps, kite flaps, intermetacarpal and dorsocommissural flaps, are available depending on the extent and the location of the wound.

However, massive destruction may result in amputations that could be carefully assessed in order to minimise their functional impairment.

High-voltage electrical traumas of the hand cause deeper and extensive injuries. The initial clinical appearance largely determines the ultimate outcome of the hand [12, 23–25]. When the hand is charred, ischemic and anaesthetic, held in flexed and contracted posture, amputation is a common result despite early and aggressive management. If the hand can be preserved, the release of the carpal tunnel is almost always necessary to improve blood flow. Flap coverage is more complex and requires regional flap (distally based radial artery forearm flap, posterior interosseous flap, distal ulnar artery flap), distant pedicled flap (groin flap) or free-tissue transfer procedures.

## Mouth and Oral Cavity Injuries

Electrical burns to the mouth are relatively common in young children [26]. They classically result from biting or chewing on electrical cords or sucking electric plugs. Both direct contact and electric arc resulting from saliva bridging may produce the lesions and the lips are deeply marked by wires and plugs. The most frequently affected sites are lips and oral commissures. Partial or total thickness wounds of the lips may be observed. Tongue, gums and alveola, palate and surrounding cheek may also be affected. Extensive and multiple lesions are sometimes very impressive.

The immediate management must ensure an adequate airway prior to the onset of oedema and often requires naso-tracheal intubation.

Classically, the spontaneous wound repair of electrical burns of the mouth consists of a rapid separation of the eschar (10 to 12 days) and a spontaneous healing with wound contraction. Infection is rare. Sometimes, haemorrhage from the labial artery or the tongue artery may occur at the time of eschar separation, but is easily controlled with pressure.

Controversy surrounds the surgical attitude for management of these lesions between early surgical treatment to a more conservative non-surgical approach. The nature of the electrical burn is such that the line of demarcation between non-viable necrotic tissue and the surrounding normal tissue is indistinct and difficult to define. Therefore, surgical excision may be either inadequate or excessive. The local anatomy with its functional requirements is complex. The oral commissure and the modiolus are two problem areas which have a highly specialised function and are extremely difficult to recreate [27].

The goal of the treatment is to maintain or to restore function and to minimise scarring. Scar contracture can lead to microstomia or commissural asymmetry. Aesthetic appearance often has a great priority for the patient.

Several authors [26–28] have reported their experience ranging from the aggressive approach of early debridement and immediate reconstruction to the conservative approach with oral splinting in order to avoid oral commissure contraction and delayed reconstruction, if necessary, after scar maturation about 2 years later.

From a practical point of view, more perioral electrical burns require the latter management. Obviously, it leads to the most satisfactory outcome, and oral splinting is the keystone of these results (Fig. 4).

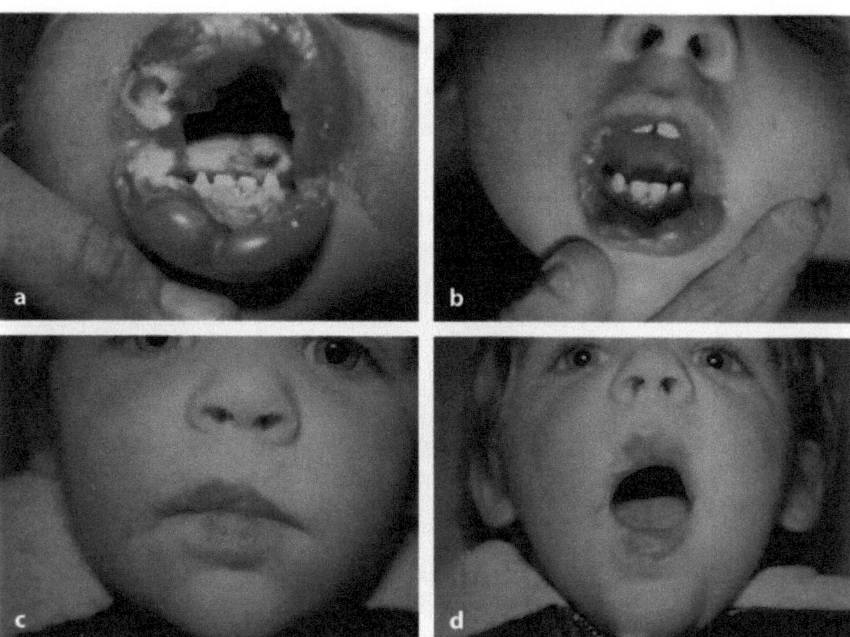

**Fig. 4. a** Extensive electrical burn of the oral cavity in a young child. **b** Spontaneous debridement on day 12. Note the full-thickness defect of the lower lip treated by cuneiform resection and direct suture on day 15. **c,d** Functional and aesthetic result 8 months later after oral splinting during 6 months

However, compliance is the main problem and may affect the final outcome. Hartford et al. [29] first proposed the use of a microstomia prevention appliance. Since then, many devices, standard or custom-made, intra- or extraoral, static or dynamic, have been described. Reisberg et al. [30] suggested that the direction of traction is not as important as its amount. Dugaret et al. [31] reported the use of the Buccinator, a custom-made adjustable intra-oral appliance which may also reduce the negative effects of pressure garments on the maxillary bone development. More recently, McCauley and Barret [3] noted that the use of a custom-fitted intra-oral splint bonded to the maxillary primary molars is a useful method to ensure compliance. Such splints do not inhibit speech or eating but remain in place for the time needed for wound maturation with uniformly satisfactory results.

Reconstructive procedures at the time of complete debridement are indicated to restore an adequate lip seal and avoid saliva leakage (Fig. 4b and c).

When microstomia or commissural asymmetry occurs, delayed commissuroplasty may be performed. Reconstruction of the oral commissure is difficult and needs careful pre-operative planning, re-positioning of the orbicularis oris muscle and sometimes reconstruction of the modiolus [3]. Various types of mucosal flaps have been described. Donelan [32], for example, has used a ventral tongue flap with good results.

## Scalp and Skull Injuries

Electrical injuries to the head result more commonly from high-tension contacts. The damage may range from deep well-demarcated burn of the scalp and partial loss of the outer table of the calvarium to total loss of the cranial bone with underlying brain injury [33]. The surgical attitude hinges on the depth of injury.

If the burn is a full-thickness injury of the scalp through galea and periosteum, the outer table may be exposed and devitalised. Conservative treatment by dressing changes until a sequestrum of the skull could be removed does not offer a good approach because of the risk of infectious complications such as osteomyelitis or epidural abscesses.

A more aggressive surgical procedure consists of the removal of the outer table to expose diploic cavity. The wound is skin-grafted after development of granulation tissue [34]. However, the long-term outcome of these grafted area is sometimes unsatisfactory, with alopecia and recurrent ulcerations for minor traumas. Tissue expansion has become a safe and reliable method for the reconstruction of the scalp.

When the bone injury is full thickness, which may be assessed by drilling holes through the calvarium, early coverage may be obtained with well-vascularised local flaps or free-tissue transfer. Removal of the devitalised skull is not necessary, this bone serving as a bone graft. Secondary evaluation of the fate of the injured bone is necessary. If bony resorption occurs, reconstruction may be done with bone grafts or polymethylacrylate cranioplasty.

## Extensive Electrical Burn Injuries of the Limbs

Extensive injuries of the limbs dramatically exhibit the disastrous effects of high-voltage electrical traumas. In addition to extensive and deep cutaneous burns, there is severe damage to underlying muscles, nerves and blood vessels. Upper limbs are more often affected. Deep visceral injuries may be associated.

Consequently, they usually result in high mortality (5 to 15%), a high rate of proximal amputations and important definitive functional impairment which may compromise social and professional rehabilitation [35, 36].

Muscle damage is the keystone of vital and functional outcome. Rhabdomyolysis and massive release of myoglobin may lead to acute renal failure. The rapid development of a severe compartment syndrome worsens the initial lesions [37, 38]. Immediate fasciotomies must be performed as soon as possible (within 6 h after injury), even before the development of evident clinical signs of compression, associated with a thorough evaluation of the deep damage. All potentially involved muscle compartments are explored, including deep muscle groups adjacent to bone (Fig. 5). Mann et al. [39] documented that this is the best way to reduce the risk of severe amputation.

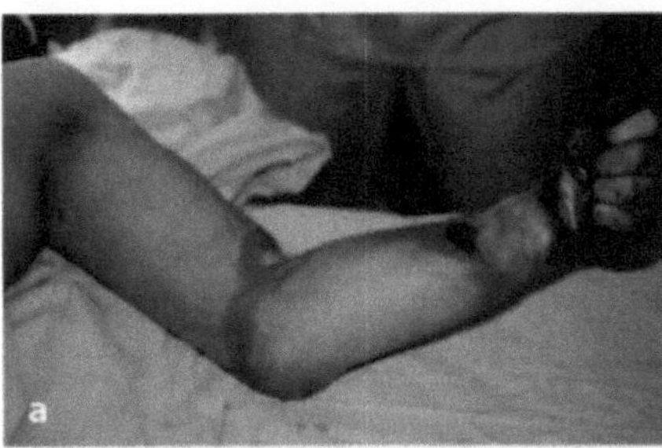
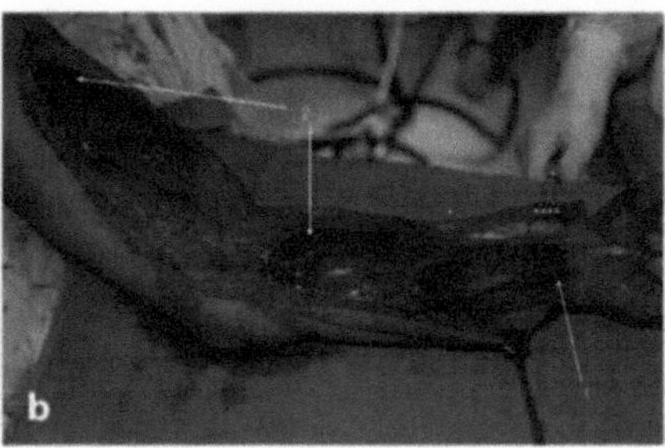
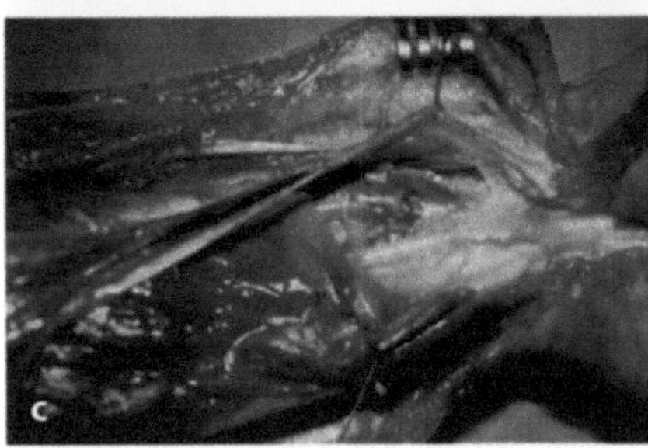

**Fig. 5. a** Extensive high-voltage electrical burn of the upper extremity. Note the deep burns on the flexion creases of elbow and axilla by a secondary electrical arc. **b** Large fasciotomy. *1* Deep burn on the palmar face of the wrist; *2* muscle damage. **c** Closing view of the anterior face of the wrist showing severe damages of deep muscles and devitalisation of the median nerve

The conservative surgical treatment is based on early debridement of obviously necrotic tissue. Second-look procedures have become routine, 48 to 72 h later, for reassessment of tissues with questionable viability. Nerves and tendons should be preserved even if they appear devitalised. Repeated debridements are usually necessary in order to excise all necrotic tissue. Definitive coverage may be achieved with split-thickness skin grafts. Flap coverage of injured deep functional structures may reduce further functional impairment.

Because this approach results sometimes in prolonged wound closure and significant functional limitation, several authors have emphasised the interest of early and complete debridement and immediate closure of the wound with flaps or free-tissue transfer in order to enhance blood supply [40, 41].

A difficult remaining problem is to decide when to perform amputation and its level, which depends on the severity of lesions and the possibilities of prosthetic compensation. Completely devitalised, charred and not salvageable extremities require immediate amputation. In the other cases, amputation should be carried out as soon as it becomes clearly necessary, maintaining length as maximal as possible, both to lessen the local risk of invasive infection and to lessen the vital risk.

High-voltage electrical injuries particularly involve the upper limb, with subsequent injury of the median and ulnar nerves [6, 42]. Achauer et al. [24] outlined the principles for staged reconstruction of the upper extremity. Adequate soft-tissue coverage is the first step in the reconstruction with well-vascularised regional flaps or free-tissue transfer (Fig. 6). Nerve injury can be reconstructed later using sural nerve grafts on a suitable graft bed with good overlying soft-tissue coverage.

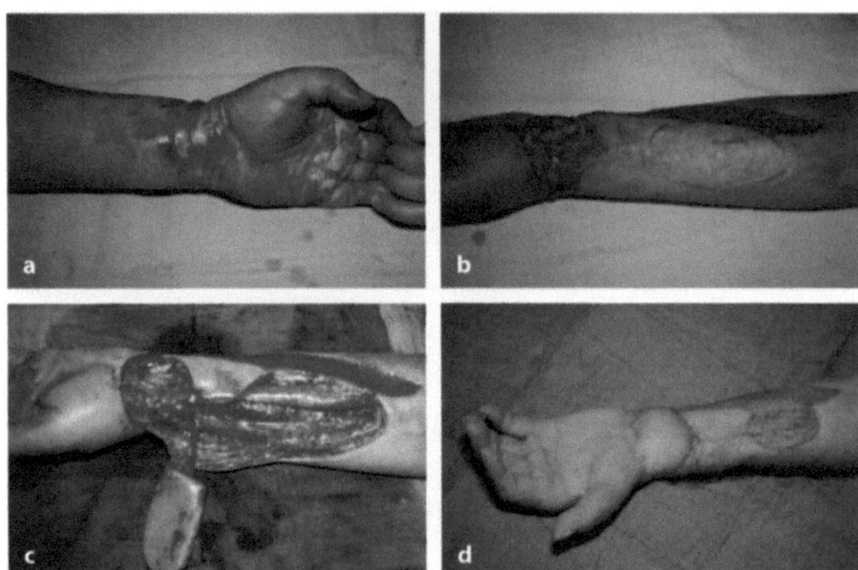

**Fig. 6 a** Initial aspect of a high-voltage electrical burn of the upper extremity. **b** Clinical aspect 15 days later with deep wound of the wrist exposing the median nerve. **c** Distally based radial artery forearm flap. **d** Result 6 months later before nerve grafting of the median nerve

## Conclusion

The low incidence of electrical injuries is offset by the high short-term and long-term morbidity rates. Low-voltage injuries particularly affect hand and mouth of young children and require specific surgical procedures. High-voltage injuries result frequently in extensive tissue damage with high amputation rates and severe functional impairment.

Prevention remains the essential action in order to reduce the initial severity and the sequelae of electrical trauma.

## References


1. Koumbourlis AC (2002) Electrical injuries. Crit Care Med 30: S424–430
2. Taylor AJ, McGwin G Jr, Valent F, Rue III LW (2002) Fatal occupational electrocutions in the United States. Inj Prev 8: 306–312
3. McCauley RL, Barret JP (2000) Electrical injuries. In: Achauer BM, Eriksson E, Guyuron B et al. (eds) Plastic surgery, vol I. Mosby, St Louis
4. Haberal M (1986) Electrical burns: a five-year experience – 1985 Evans lecture. J Trauma 26: 103–109
5. Haberal M (1995) An eleven-year survey of electrical burn injuries. J Burn Care Rehabil 16: 43–48

6. Ugland OM (1967) Electrical burns: a clinical and experimental study with special reference to peripheral nerve injury. Scand J Plast Reconstr Surg 2 [Suppl]: 1–74

7. Wallace BH, Cone JB, Vanderpool RD, Bond PJ, Rossell JB, Caldwell FT Jr (1995) Retrospective evaluation of admission criteria for paediatric electrical injuries. Burns 21: 590–593

8. Folliot D (1982) Les accidents d'origine électrique. Masson, Paris

9. Hunt JL, Mason AD, Masterson TS, Pruitt BA (1976) Pathophysiology of acute electrical injuries. J Trauma 16: 335–340

10. Lee RC (1992) Electrical trauma. Cambridge Press, Cambridge, UK

11. Lee RC, Gzylor DC, Brett D, Israel DA (1988) Role of cell membrane rupture in the pathogenesis of electrical trauma. J Surg Res 44: 709–719

12. Peterson RA (1966) Electrical burns of the hand. J Bone Joint Surg 48A: 407–424

13. Rougé D, Polynice A, Grolleau JL, Nicoulet B, Chavoin JP, Costagliola M (1994) Histologic assessment of low-voltage electrical burns: experimental study with pigskin. J Burn Care Rehabil 15: 328–334

14. Skoog T (1970) Electrical injuries. J Trauma 10: 816–830

15. Quinby WC, Burke JF, Trelstad RL, Caulfield J (1978) The use of microscopy as a guide to primary excision of electrical burns. J Trauma 18: 423–431

16. Rouse RG, Dimick AR (1978) Treatment of electrical injury compared to burn injury. J Trauma 18: 43–47

17. Robson MC, Murphy RC, Heggers JP (1984) A new explanation for the progressive tissue loss in electrical injuries. Plast Reconstr Surg 73: 431–437

18. Zelt RG, Daniel RK, Ballard PA, Brissette Y, Heroux P (1988) High voltage electrical injury: chronic wound evolution. Plast Reconstr Surg 82: 1027–1041

19. Lee RC, Kolodney MS (1987) Electrical injury mechanisms: dynamics of the thermal response. Plast Reconstr Surg 80: 663–671

20. Hunt JL, Lewis S, Parkey R, Baxter C (1979) The use of technetium-99 m stannous pyrophosphate scintigraphy to identify muscle damage in acute electric burns. J Trauma 19: 409–413

21. Clayton JM, Hayes AC, Hammel J, Boyd WC, Hartford CE, Barnes RW (1977) Xenon-133 determination of muscle blood flow in electrical injury. J Trauma 17: 293–298

22. Nettelblad H, Thuomas KA, Sjoberg F (1996) Magnetic resonance imaging: a new diagnostic aid in the care of high-voltage electrical burns. Burns 22: 117–119

23. Castède JC, De Bonfils C (1992) Brûlures électriques des mains. Ann Medit Burns Club 5: 216–219

24. Achauer B, Applebaum R, Van der Kam VM (1994) Electrical burn injury to the upper extremity. Br J Plast Surg 47: 331–340

25. Butler ED, Gant TD (1977) Electrical injuries, with special reference to upper extremities. A review of 182 cases. Am J Surg 134: 95–101

26. Barone CM, Hulnick SJ, Grigsby de Linde L, Sauer JB, Mitra A (1994) Evaluation of treatment modalities in perioral electrical burns. J Burn Care Rehabil 15: 335–340

27. Thomas SS (1996) Electrical burns of the mouth: still searching for an answer. Burns 22: 137–140

28. De la Plaza R, Quetglas A, Rodriguez E (1983) Treatment of electrical burns of the mouth. Burns 10: 49–60

29. Hartford CE, Kealey GP, Lavelle WE, Buckner H (1975) An appliance to prevent and treat microstomia from burns. J Trauma 15: 356–360

30. Reisberg DJ, Fine L, Fattore L, Edmonds DC (1983) Electrical burns of the oral commissure. J Prosthet Dent 49: 71–76

31. Dugaret I, Capron B, Roques C et al. (1998) Premiers résultats sur l'expérimentation de l'appareil buccinator. In: Dhennin C, Griffe O, Baux S (eds) Brûlures. Sauramps médical, Montpellier

32. Donelan MB (1995) Reconstruction of electrical burns of the oral commissure with a ventral tongue flap. Plast Reconstr Surg 95: 1155–1164

33. Benito-Ruiz J, Baena-Montilla P, Navarro-Monzonis A, Bonanad E, Cavadas P (1994) Severe electric burn of the skull. Burns 20: 553–556

34. Spies M, McCauley RL, Mudge BP, Herndon DN (2003) Management of acute calvarial burns in children. J Trauma 54: 765–769

35. Hussmann J, Kucan JO, Russell RC, Bradley T, Zamboni WA (1995) Electrical injuries: morbidity, outcome and treatment rationale. Burns 21: 530–535

36. Xiao J, Cai BR (1994) A clinical study of electrical injuries. Burns 20: 340–346

37. Block TA, Aarsvold JN, Matthews KL II, Mintzer RA, River LP (1995) The 1995 Lindberg award. Nonthermally mediated muscle injury and necrosis in electrical trauma. J Burn Care Rehabil 16: 581–588

38. Téot L, Griffe O, Brabet M, Gavroy JP, Thaury M (1992) Severe electric injuries of the hand and forearm. Ann Hand Surg 11: 207–216
39. Mann R, Gibran N, Engrav L, Heimbach D (1996) Is immediate decompression oh high voltage electrical injuries to the upper extremity always necessary? J Trauma 40: 584–587
40. Luce EA (2000) Electrical burns. Clin Plast Surg 27: 133–143
41. Zhu ZX, Xu XG, Li WP, Wang DX, Zhang LY, Chen LY, Liu T (2003) Experience of 14 years of emergency reconstruction of electrical injuries. Burns 29: 65–72
42. Haberal M, Gurer S, Akman N, Basgoza O (1996) Persistent peripheral nerve pathologies in patients with electrical burns. J Burn Care Rehabil 17: 147–149

# 41 Chemical Burns Management

L. Téot, U. Giovannini

## Introduction

Chemical burns are less frequent in routine practice, but can be very serious owing to the complexity and severity of their actions [1, 2]. They are specific wounds at several points. According to epidemiological data, management during the acute stage is particularly intense and there are difficult-to-manage sequellae in some mucosal areas like eyes or mouth. Some chemical agents can create intense general disorders. The intensity of the lesions depends on the concentration of the product, some alkaline agents remaining active locally for several hours due to remnant action, in spite of suitable management. Large surfaces are rarely touched [3].

Influx of casualties after a civil disaster (industrial explosion) or military (war or terrorism) is possible. The action of these agents could be prolonged and deep. In addition to the skin, respiratory lesions and general intoxication could be observed [4]. The urgent local treatment relies essentially on prolonged washing [5]. Chemical splashes on the eye/skin are a significant problem [6, 7]. Diphoterine is a hypertonic, polyvalent, amphoteric compound developed in France as an eye/skin chemical splash water-based decontamination solution. In vitro and in vivo, it actively decontaminates approximately 600 chemicals, including acids, alkalis, oxidizing and reducing agents, irritants, lacrimators, solvents, alkylating agents and radionuclides. Its chemical bond energy for such agents is greater than that of tissue receptors. Its hypertonicity impedes chemical tissue penetration and may remove some amount of skin/cornea-absorbed toxicants not already bound to tissue receptors. Diphoterine chemical reactions are not exothermic. Diphoterine and its acid/alkali decontamination residues are not irritating to the eyes or skin; it is essentially non-toxic. Diphoterine can prevent eye/skin burns following chemical splashes and results in nearly immediate pain relief [8, 9]. Prevention and adequate emergency care can limit the serious consequences of these accidents.

## Epidemiology and Causes

The exact determination of the causing agent is fundamental. Its basic or acid character, the degree of corrosion (concentration and molar mass, its nature, the length of exposure to the agent) have to be established as soon as possible.

Some chemical agents will have to be determined and discovered behind a fierce trademark or a common appearance, an uncoloured, non-odour cleaning liquid [10].

Products susceptible to provoke burns are numerous. Miller had established a classification based on the mode of action, ranging them into five groups:

- **Corrosive agents:** Acid and alkali act by coagulation of proteins with mitotic inhibition. Alkali causes also a lipid soaping, increasing its possibilities of penetration. Burns are deeper and more serious than with acids. To this group are added hydrocarbon phenoric agents.
- **Tearing agents:** These are classified into two groups, one including a halogen (chloraceton, bromaceton) or a not-saturated component (acrogens, acid chloride).
- **Solvents:** Numerous products or families, whose causticity is variable, belong to this group: hydrogen carbons aliphatic or aromatic (toluene, benzene) halogen hydrogen carbon (derived from methane, ethane, ethylene and propane), alcohols in concentrated solutions, aldehydes and acetones.
- **Detergents and emollients:** These provoke an irritative action, but can favour transcutaneous penetration of other substances.

Burns are more prone to occur on some localisation like the hands and the feet but all areas are open to chemical projections. Shoes usually protect the feet. Immersions in a caustic agent being exceptional, chemical burns are commonly seen as riddling burnt areas.

The aspect, depth and surface of burns depend on the length of contact, the composition and the concentration of the product. The clinical aspect varies with time and is often the cause of errors [11].

Acids present initially as lesions showing a white, apparently superficial, aspect, which progressively darkens until it is represented by dry and retractile eschars (Fig. 1).

Strong alkali liquefies tissues and creates soft eschars, deep and extensive. Pain is varying and is often more intense with acids than alkali. Pain is often delayed and appears later.

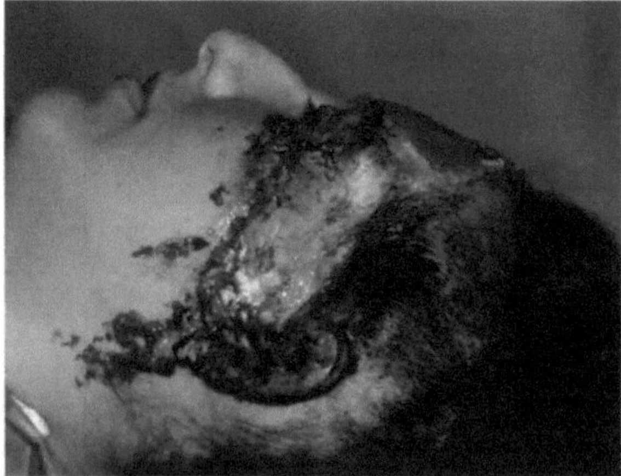

Fig. 1. Acid burn

## Acute Management

### Cooling

Cooling remains the best initial management, the easiest to obtain in commonly not professional surroundings [11]. Cooling has several benefits:

- Pain is reduced during the time of water circulation over the burnt area.
- The patient is stabilised during this period of time, a crucial moment when the patient can be submitted to some degree of stress or panicking.
- Cooling must be realised properly, using fresh tap water (18 °C) for a period of time of 5 to 10 min.
- Even if most of the authors recommend cooling during the initial period, the real effect of cooling on the evolution of the healing process has not yet been determined.

### Neutralisation

Neutralisation can be obtained by local application of a chemical antagonist after determination of the exact composition, nature and concentration of the chemical burning agent. It has been progressively rejected as an efficient management of chemical burns, mainly because of the complications occurring afterwards. Neutralisation causes an important increase in local temperature during the chemical process – a source of thermal burns not compatible with ethical issues [12].

### Splash Decontamination

The use of amphoteric solutions was proposed in the 1990s to prevent this inconvenience from occuring; the principle of the application of amphoteric solutions is the combination of the product to all kinds of chemical agents, whatever their origin, acid or alkali. The product is presented under a gel formulation, the gel being compatible for application on burnt skin but also under mucosa like the anterior chamber of the eye. Several publications can be found in the literature concerning interesting results using amphoteric products in ophthalmology. This product, named Diphoterine, can be applied also in the mouth and the upper digestive track, in children as well as in adults [9]. Diphoterine does not seem to present any toxicity or side effect.

## Specific Situations

### Hydrofluoric Acid

Hydrofluoric acid (HF) is one of the strongest inorganic acids and is used widely in industry. It differs from other acids in the mechanism of injury. The hydrogen ion readily penetrates the skin and causes destruction of deep-tissue layers and even bone. An accurate occupational history and physical examination are important aspects in patient assessment. Hydrofluoric acid can provoke specific lesions. Skin contact usually occurs by application of cleaning and detergent products in incorrect domestic use (without glove protection). Lesions usually observed are local necrotic areas at the fingertips. If contact time is prolonged, general complications such as hypocalcaemia can occur, mainly due to the decrease of calcium blood levels, the fluorine ion combining with the circulating calcium [12]. Cardiac failures have been described on massive exposure to hydrofluoric acid.

Calcium gluconate gel, applied after initial rinsing with water, has a documented effect as first-aid treatment for hydrofluoric acid burns [13]. Hexafluorine is a novel liquid compound developed especially for emergency decontamination of hydrofluoric acid eye and skin exposures. However, scientific documentation of the effect of hexafluorine is insufficient. Hexafluorine showed a consistent trend towards a worse outcome, both in comparison to water plus topical calcium and to water rinsing alone. Based on these observations, it is concluded that water rinsing followed by topical calcium should remain the standard first-aid treatment for skin exposure to hydrofluoric acid [14].

### Alkaline Burns

Alkali drain cleaners are one of the main causes of domestic chemical burns. The mechanism of injury is almost identical in the majority of patients: few seconds after pouring the cleaner into the clogged drain, a backflow of the poured cleaner causes burns of the dominant hand and forearm. Literature reports dating as far back as 1927 have lured clinicians into the belief that alkaline skin burns are best treated by water dilution and that neutralisation attempts should be avoided. Although this belief has never been substantiated, neutralisation of an alkaline burn of the skin with acid was thought to increase tissue damage secondary to the exothermic nature of acid-base reactions. Furthermore, immediate water lavage is rarely done for domestic chemical burns [15]. When washing was started within 1 min of injury, the tissue pH values did not exceed 8.0. Washing had virtually no effect on lowering the raised pH levels when the delay between injury and the start of washing was 10 or 30 min. It is nowadays proposed that neutralisation of an alkaline substance with household vinegar (i.e. 5% acetic acid solution) would result in rapid neutralisation and thus reduce the extent of tissue injury. The observed benefits of treating alkaline burns with 5% acetic acid in animal models are significant and may be proposed for standard human treatment [16].

Demarcation of the wound following alkali burns occurs over a period of several days and the surgical treatment should be delayed till the necosis is stable (Fig. 2) [17]. Timing of surgery for minor alkali burns (less than 5% TBSA) is still controversial. It is difficult to determine the depth of tissue damage soon after injury, but the burn depth can be judged beginning a few days post-injury. The eschar in full-thickness burns feels like leather without any sensation of pain, and thrombosed veins are frequently seen. However, clear demarcation of the deep aspect of the eschar and the underlying healthy tissue takes several days to occur. A waiting period of 7–9 days contributes to the development of the deep demarca-

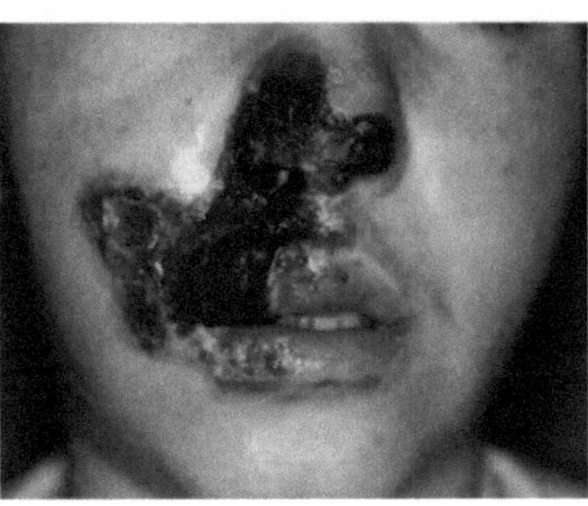

**Fig. 2.** Alkali burn

tion plane which makes excision easier and the underlying bed more suitable for the take of the skin graft [18]. This waiting period did not result in any incidence of eschar infection. Other authors have also noticed that bacterial colonisation of the wound did not occur early following alkali burns [11, 19].

## Cement Burns

Cement burns are rarely reported, particularly considering the heavy skin exposure and high frequency of use [20]. They may, however, lead to severe illness needing intensive therapy.

The skin, eye and respiratory tract are the organ systems most prone to be damaged by ready-mixed cement or cement dust. Damage to the respiratory epithelium may become life-threatening. So-called cement burns do not relate to skin damage caused by thermal effects, but are instead due to irritation or alkaline burns of the upper skin layers. Explosions in cement plants may cause emission of hot cement powder [21].

Apart from the alkalinity of cement (pH 12), relevant factors for developing cement burns are occlusion and abrasion: the skin surface is damaged by the abrasive properties of added particulates, such as sand, and penetration of alkaline cement, mostly used ready-mixed, is thus facilitated. This effect is increased by occlusion due to wet clothes. A few hours after exposure, burning sensations, pain, erythema and vesicles occur as the initial symptoms; 12–48 h later, partial- to full-thickness burns characterise the clinical picture.

Differences are found in therapeutic management between Anglo-American and European authors. Full-thickness burns were treated by surgery and skin grafting without delay in the former countries, resulting in short duration of complaints and hospitalisation, with, however, not always satisfactory cosmetic results. Partial-thickness burns were treated conservatively on an outpatient basis [11, 19].

Cement burns are avoidable by means of adequate protective measures, such as suitable gloves and appropriate protective boots and clothes, as well as immediate first aid. For prevention of these injuries, information and training in risk management is recommended especially for employees and apprentices in the construction industry [1].

## White Phosphorus Burns

Such burns combine the heat of chemical combustion with the corrosiveness of phosphoric acid as phosphorus is oxygenated and hydrated in tissues. Phosphorus has several allotropic forms, namely white, red and black, with the yellowish discolouration often seen in white phosphorus due to impurities. When exposed to air, white phosphorus spontaneously oxidises to phosphorus pentoxide and hydrolyses in water to form potentially corrosive phosphoric acid, capable of producing chemical injury in tissues. Adherence of phosphorus to clothing and skin will often cause thermal injury because white phosphorus ignites spontaneously if the temperature exceeds 34 °C .

Systemic effects including hypoproteinaemia, haematuria, oliguria, generalised petechiae, icterus, acute yellow atrophy of the liver, seizures, impaired glycogenolysis, hypocalcaemia and ischemic-like ECG changes can arise quickly [22].

Burning phosphorus is easily extinguished with water, but re-ignites after drying, producing smoke. A lethal human dose ranges between 50 and 100 mg.

The initial treatment of a white phosphorus burn consists of prompt removal of contaminated clothing followed by immediate irrigation with water. Phosphorus will keep burning if exposed to air. Lavaging of cutaneous wounds with water or saline is indispensable as it can stop combustion.

Several treatment protocols have been proposed for phosphorus burn [1, 2, 22]. The main goal is always prompt removal or neutralisation of active phosphorus from the burn site. Our protocol for the management of phosphorus burn includes the application of 1% copper sulphate solution, which on contact with phosphorus forms copper phosphate ($CuPO_3$), both allowing easy identification of retained white phosphorus particles and impeding further white phosphorus oxidation. Excessive copper sulphate should be removed immediately by water irrigation to prevent the systemic effects of copper intoxication, which include vomiting, diarrhoea, haemolysis, haematuria, oliguria, hepatic necrosis and cardiorespiratory collapse.

The systemic effects of phosphorus burns include calcium-phosphorus shifts, which are believed to be due to absorption of phosphorus compounds from the burn area. These burns can rapidly develop hypocalcaemia and hyperphosphataemia, which have been shown to be the major cause of sometimes fatal cardiac arrhythmias. Abnormalities seen on the electrocardiogram include prolongation of the QT interval, bradycardia and ST-T wave changes. Excision of the burned wounds within 1 hour of injury does not improve survival, suggesting that metabolic changes may occur earlier. The dehydrating effects of phosphorus pentoxide can be ignored since 6.06 mg of phosphorus as phosphorus pentoxide combines with only 2.18 mg of water to form acid, which is negligible. Other complications include deep-lying shrapnel fragments in soft tissues. They are usually contaminated with the phosphorus particles, which will react continuously with tissue fluid. Removal of stained phosphorus particles on the wounds is essential for prevention of further ignition, absorption into the circulation and possible systemic effects.

The smoke generated is the result of combustion or oxidation, and is strongly irritant to mucosal surfaces, where it combines with water to form phosphoric acid. Ensuring airway patency was particularly important in patients rescued from phosphorus explosions occurring in close confinement. Patients should be assessed for life-threatening injuries as soon as a pertinent history is obtained, and fiberoptic bronchoscopy should be performed if there is a history of smoke exposure and symptoms or signs suggesting the possibility of inhalation injury [22]. Phosphorus-induced systemic intoxication and hypocalcaemia can be reversed with intravenous infusion of 10% calcium gluconate solution, but intensive monitoring of electrolytes is still necessary.

Phosphorus burns have aspects that differ from other burns and are often combined with explosion injury. The retention of shrapnel fragments often produces associated injuries of nerves, tendons or open fractures (Fig. 3). The first priority for reconstruction should be restoration of function, followed by cosmetic considerations. Consequently, skin grafts are not always appropriate, as flaps may allow better preservation and restoration of function. For example, groin flaps can be used to cover exposed digital nerves, arteries and thenar muscle groups. Doing this also allows the first web space to be maintained after burns to the hands. Finger tips with compromised circulation after severe burns can be left to auto-amputate. Although this can take several months, the patient is able to begin rehabilitation more quickly provided that the flexor digitorum profundus is uninvolved.

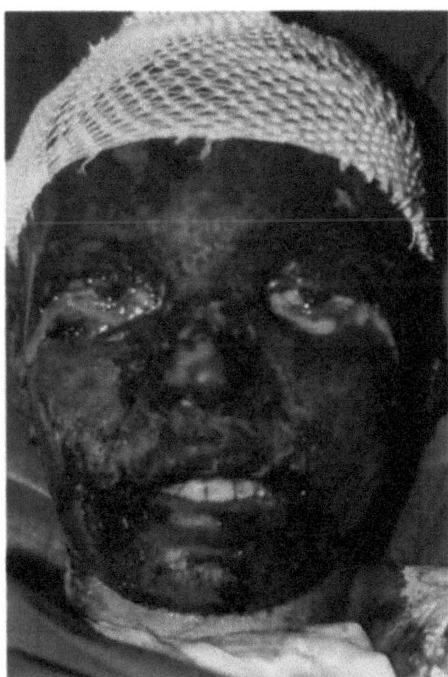

**Fig. 3.** Phosphorus burn

# References


1. Cartotto RC, Peters WJ, Neligan PC, Douglas LG, Beeston J (1996) Chemical burns. Can J Surg. 39: 205–211
2. Ricketts S, Kimble FW (2003) Chemical injuries: the Tasmanian Burns Unit experience. ANZ J Surg 73: 45–48
3. Chien WC, Pai L, Lin CC, Chen HC (2003) Epidemiology of hospitalized burns patients in Taiwan. Burns 29: 582–588
4. Al-Qattan MM, Pitkanen J (2001) Delayed primary excision and grafting of full thickness alkali burns of the hand and forearm. Burns 27: 398–400
5. Henderson P, Mc Conville H, Hohlriegel N, Fraser JF, Kimble RM (2003) Flammable liquid burns in children. Burns 29: 349–352
6. Schrage NF, Kompa S, Haller W, Langfeld S (2002) Use of an amphorique lavage solution for emergency treatment of eye burns. First animal type experimental clinical considerations. Burns 28: 782–786
7. Bendeddouche K, Assaf E, Emadisson H, Forestier F, Salvanet-Bouccara A (2003) Air bags and eye injuries: chemical burns and major traumatic ocular lesions- a case study. J Fr Ophtalmol 26: 819–823
8. Gerard M, Gosset P, Louis V, Menerath JM, Blomet J, Merle H (2000) Is here a delay in bathing the externat eye in the treatment of ammonia eye burns ? Comparison of two ophthalmic solutions: physiological serum and Diphoterine. J Fr Ophthalmo 23: 449–458
9. Hall AH, Blomet J, Mathieu L (2002) Diphoterine for emergent eye/skin chemical splash decontamination : a review. Vet Hum Toxicol 44: 228–231
10. Wibbenmeyer LA, Morgan LJ, Robinson BK, Smith SK, Lewis RW 2nd, Kealey GP (1999) Our chemical burn experience: exposing the dangers of anhydrous ammonia. J Burn Care Rehabil 20: 226–231
11. Eldad A, Weinberg A, Breiterman S, Chapuat M, Palankar D, Ben-Bassat H (1998) Early nonsurgical removal of chemically injured tissue enhances wound headline in partial thickness burns. Burns 24: 166–172
12. Sanz-Gallen P, Nogue S, Munne P, Faraldo A (2001) Hypocalcaemia and hypomagnesaemia due to hydrofluoric acid. Occup Med (Lond) 51: 294–295
13. Beiran I, Miller B, Bentur Y (1997) The efficacy of calcium gluconate in ocular hydrofluoric acid burns. Hum Exp Toxicol 16: 223–228
14. Hojer J, Personne M, Hulten P, Ludwigs U (2002) Topical treatments for hydrofluoric acid burns: a blind controlled experimental study. J Toxicol Clin Toxicol 40: 861–866
15. Andrews K, Mowlavi A, Milner SM (2003) The treatment of alkaline burns of the skin by neutralization. Plast Reconstr Surg 111: 1918–1921
16. Sekundo W, Augustin AJ, Stremped I (2002) Topical allopurinol or corticosteroids and acetylcysteine in the early treatment of experimental corneal alkali burns : a pilot study. Eur J Ophtalmo 12: 366–372
17. Erdmann D, Hussmann J, Kucan JO (1996) Treatment of a severe alkali burn. Burns 22: 141–146
18. Acikel C, Ulkur E, Guler MM (2001) Prolonged intermittent hydrotherapy and early tangential excision in the treatment of an extensive strong alkali burn. Burns 27: 293–296
19. Graham JS, schomaker KT, Glatter RD, Briscoe CM, Braue EH Jr, Squibb KS (2000) Efficacy of laser debridement with autologous split-thickness skin grafting in promoting improved headline of deep cutaneous sulfur mustard burns. Burns 28: 719–730
20. Spoo J, Elsner P (2001) Cement burns: a review 1960–2000. Contact Dermatitis 45: 68–71
21. Morley SE, Humzah D, McGregor JC, Gilbert PM (1996) Cement-related burns. Burns 22: 646–647
22. Chou TD, Lee TW, Chen SL, Tung YM, Dai NT, Chen SG, Lee CH, Chen TM, Wang HJ (2001) The management of white phosphorus burns. Burns 27: 492–497

# The Meek–Wall Micrograft Technique

F.R.H. Tempelman, A.F.P.M. Vloemans, E. Middelkoop, R.W. Kreis

## Introduction

Extended areas of full-thickness burns require, after surgical excision or debridement of non-viable tissue, specific grafting techniques for closure of the wound surface.

During the 1960s, techniques for the expansion of split skin autografts became available. The first of these expansion techniques was the Meek-Wall method [1], in which a regular distribution of postage stamp autografts was produced by expanding cut squares of split-skin autograft on specially prefolded gauze. The technique was cumbersome, but the expansion of 1:9 achieved by this method remains unsurpassed by the mesh-graft techniques introduced later [2]. However, the open, grafted wounds were prone to dehydration and infection, and the average take with expanded autografts was unsatisfactory.

In patients with burns of up to 35% of the total body surface area (TBSA), early excision and primary coverage with autografts, meshed if necessary, is technically straightforward, as sufficient donor sites are generally available. With burns of 35–65%, a lack of donor sites might require an intermediate phase, in which areas that cannot be directly covered with autograft may be temporarily protected by the application of allograft skin, while donor sites heal sufficiently to be harvested again. For patients with injuries greater than 65%, Burke proved that long-term wound coverage with allografts could be achieved by administering immunosuppressant drugs to prevent allograft rejection, providing time for repeated harvesting of the limited donor sites available for autografts [3].

In the last two decades of the 20th century, the use of mesh grafts has been further improved by the introduction of the so-called sandwich technique, in which the (widely) expanded split skin autografts were covered with a layer of (meshed) split skin allograft [4].

## Cryopreserved Allografts

When cryopreserved allografts became available, fears of immunological reactions restricted the use of allografts to their short-term application as a biological dressing. Thus, allografts were initially employed as a temporary cover for partial skin thickness burns, and a marked improvement in cosmetic results was obtained [5]. Allografts were also used on excised wounds on which autografts had failed to take [6]. Wounds treated in this way improved and became free from infection.

However, despite an initial satisfactory take of both autograft and allograft layers, epidermal outgrowth was frequently disrupted during the second or third week by immunological rejection of the allograft component, which occasionally resulted in loss of the entire graft. These experiences suggested that results might be improved if the allografts could be modified to reduce their antigenicity.

## Glycerol-Preserved Allografts

Interest in the use of glycerol as a preservative for allografts was prompted by observations that allografts lyophilised by freeze-drying displayed reduced antigenicity [7]. However, the technique of freeze-drying was complex and expensive, and, in a series of laboratory experiments in collaboration with the Dutch Skin Bank, it was found that lyophilisation could be achieved more simply by 98% glycerol. By replacing tissue water by glycerol, the structural integrity of the allografts remained optimally preserved [8]. Studies on a porcine model confirmed that the inflammatory response evoked by glycerol-preserved allografts was milder than that evoked by viable donor skin. Encouraged by favourable results obtained elsewhere with glycerol-preserved xenografts [9], non-viable glycerol-preserved allografts were introduced in the clinic [10].

More recently, different artificial products have been manufactured to achieve wound coverage in extensive burns. These products are, among others: Biobrane®, a semi-permeable silicone membrane bonded to nylon to which peptides of porcine collagen have been added [11, 12] and Integra®, a bilayer membrane system of a bovine tendon collagen and glycosaminoglycan layer on a silicone layer [13, 14]. Although Integra seems to be the most promising skin substitute presently available, its use is limited by costs and complications during the ingrowth phase of the treatment [15, 16].

## Skin (Meek) Micrografting

An ingenious method for obtaining widely expanded postage-stamp autografts was described by Meek, in which prefolded gauzes were used to achieve a regular distribution of autograft islands cut with a Meek–Wall dermatome [1, 17]. Despite the ninefold expansion obtained by this method, the technique became eclipsed by the introduction of mesh skin grafts [2]. Manufacture of the dermatome and pre-folded gauzes was eventually discontinued, and the method was in danger of fading into obscurity.

However, with the improved early survival of patients with extensive burn injuries, lack of autograft donor sites was increasingly encountered as a limiting factor in achieving wound closure. Mesh grafts required the presence of suitable donor sites, and epithelisation was delayed with expansion ratios of greater than 1:6. In collaboration with the Dutch instrument manufacturer HUMECA (Enschede, The Netherlands), the Meek technique was reintroduced in our clinic. The materials were modified and improved considerably, and the dermatome was adapted to run on compressed air. Furthermore, the components were enlarged to allow expansion of larger pieces of autograft [18].

## Patients and Methods

### Operative Procedure

At operation, wounds to be grafted were excised down to the underlying fascia and haemostasis was secured.

Split-skin autografts were obtained following standard procedures. A cork square, measuring 4.2×4.2 cm, was dampened, and the graft spread, dermis side down, on the cork and – if necessary – was trimmed to size (smaller graft remnants are also suitable). The cork containing the graft was placed in the carrier block of the dermatome and was secured by a grill. The carrier block was then passed through the dermatome, containing 13 parallel blades, spaced 3 mm apart. The blades cut through the graft and into, but not through, the cork. After the first pass, the grill was carefully removed; the cork with the graft was rotated 90° reclamped, and passed through the dermatome once more, thus cutting the graft into 14×14 small squares measuring 3×3 mm (materials: HUMECA) (Fig. 1).

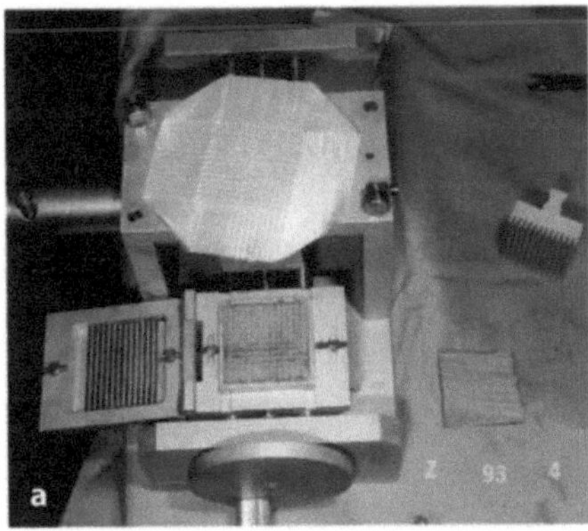
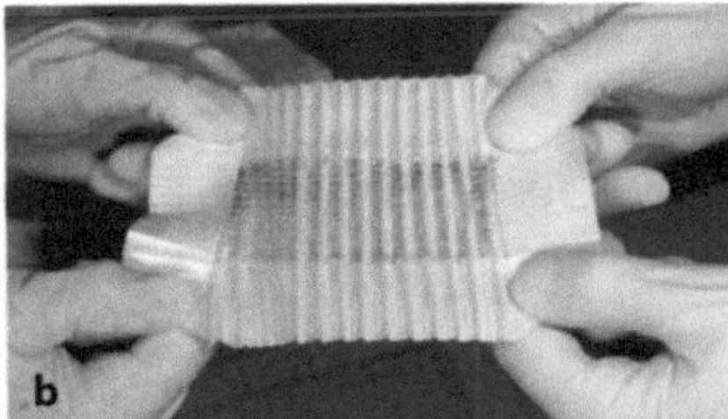
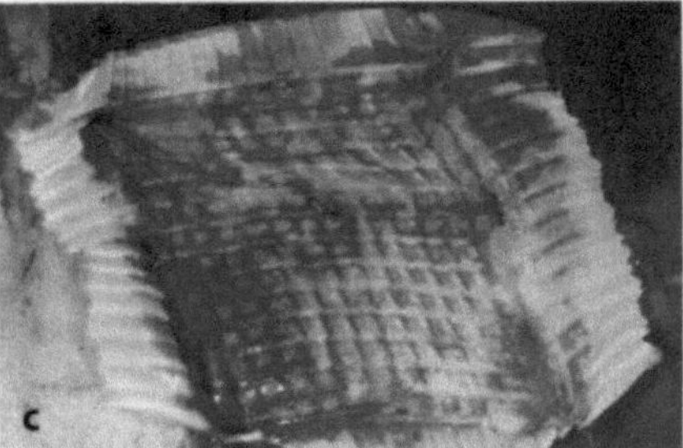

**Fig. 1. a** Surgical equipment to acquire the Meek–Wall grafts. **b** Micrografts on the pre-folded gauze that is being unfolded. **c** Totally unfolded gauzes with micrografts stapled to the excised wound

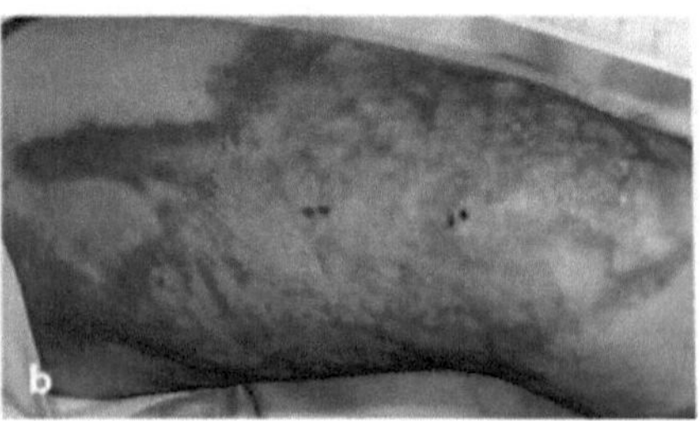

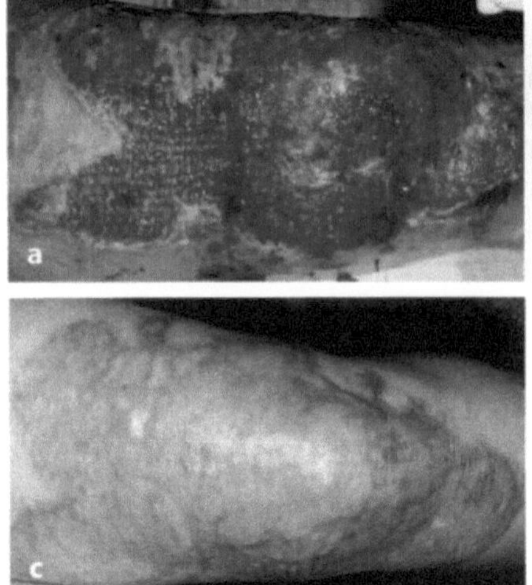

Fig. 2. a Wound with micrografts in situ after removal of the gauze. b Result after 9 months. c Result after 17 months

The grill was carefully lifted off. A specially serrated wedge, supplied with the dermatome, was used to hold the grafts in place on the cork while the grill was loosened.

The cork, with the cut graft in place, was removed. The upper (epidermal) surface of the graft was sprayed with an adhesive dressing spray, and allowed to become tacky. The pre-folded polyester gauze, which is folded on an aluminium foil backing into a series of square pleats corresponding to the cuts in the autograft, was pressed onto the graft for a few seconds, after which the cork square was gently removed, leaving the graft islands adhering to the gauze. The gauze was pulled out by firm traction on all four sides, until the pleats became completely unfolded. Finally, the aluminium backing was peeled off, to leave the expanded gauze with the separated, adherent autograft islands ready for transplantation. After trimming the margins, the gauze was applied, graft side down, to the wound bed, and secured with surgical staples (Fig. 2).

The gauzes were covered with dressings soaked in different local therapeutics, such as silvernitrate in polyethyleneglycol, Betadine in polyethyleneglycol or Furacine depending on the wound cultures taken. The dressings were changed on a daily base.

After six days the grafts had grown sufficiently into the wound bed to allow removal of the gauze. At operation, the staples were removed and, using blunt forceps, the gauze was gently detached, leaving the autograft islands in situ on the wound bed. The grafts were covered with an overlay of glycerol-preserved allografts, meshed 1:1.5, and secured with either Adaptic or Cuticerin. After a further 6 days, when the allografts were firmly adherent to the wound, this dressing was removed. Daily dressings were continued until epithelisation was complete. Details of the general surgical procedure have been described previously [18].

## Patient group

A total of 128 Meek–Wall procedures were analysed retrospectively in 49 patients. In this patient group, 7 of the 49 patients suffered from diabetes mellitus, 8 patients had inhalation trauma. Mean TBSA was 34±20% (range 5–84%), with a percentage of third-degree burns of 25±17% (range 4–83%).

Since it was impossible to systematically obtain end results, e.g. cosmetic results, from retrospective data analysis, we have chosen the take rate of the graft as the primary effect parameter. An experienced surgeon of the burn-care unit performed the estimation of the take rates between the fifth and the seventh post-operative day. Take rate was defined as the percentage of the transplanted area, adherent to the wound bed, which retained a vital appearance [19].

Earlier clinical observations suggested that the percentage of total body surface area burned and the percentage of third-degree burns (TBSA3) could have an effect on wound condition and wound healing in general. The TBSA percentage treated was determined peri-operatively in each procedure.

The semi-quantitative laboratory testing of culture swabs on the presence of bacteria provided a grading ranging from – (none) to +++ (multiple colonies of a species). Only culture swabs taken in a period ranging from 4 days before till 7 days after the surgical procedure were evaluated. Different bacterial species pose different threats to normal wound healing [20, 21]. A wound was considered to be contaminated, when its swab culture identified one or more of the species of *Pseudomonas*, *Staphylococcus* or *Streptococcus* in sufficient (estimated +++) amounts. Slight contamination was defined as a comparable or less extensive (estimated – to ++) wound-bed contamination with other species.

## Statistics

Statistical analysis was performed with SPSS. A multiple linear regression analysis was performed using the graft take rate as the dependent variable. Statistical significance level was determined at $p<0.05$.

## Results

The influence of various independent variables, such as TBSA, level of contamination of the wound, method of debridement, presence or absence of inhalation trauma and expansion of the grafts on the take of the grafts was evaluated retrospectively in a total of 128 Meek–Wall procedures in 49 patients. The primary effect parameter, the average graft take rate, was 76.6±18% and ranged from 20 to 100%.

Multiple linear regression analysis showed a difference of 12.4% in take rate, favouring avulsion over tangential excision. This relation, however, was just outside the defined limits for statistical significance ($p=0.059$). The presence of diabetes as a systemic disorder resulted in a significant reduction in take rate of 14.5% ($p=0.008$).

**Table 1.** Graft expansions with respective take-rate percentages

| Expansion Ratio | Mean take rate [%] | Standard deviation [%] | Frequency in n=128 [%] |
| --- | --- | --- | --- |
| 4/1 | 76 | 14 | 13 |
| 6/1 | 76 | 18 | 73 |
| 9/1 | 78 | 20 | 14 |

Other independent variables, including bacterial contamination, TBSA as well as inhalation trauma, failed to prove a statistically significant relationship with the dependent variable take rate.

Also the influence of the expansion ratio, an important aspect of the Meek–Wall procedure, on the take rate of the grafts was investigated. In this patient population the following ratios were used: 4/1, 6/1 and 9/1, their averaged take rates are summarised in Table 1. The differences in take rate between the different expansions were not statistically significant.

## Discussion

The regression analysis showed that the take rate of grafts applied to a wound bed after avulsion was slightly, but not statistically significantly, better than when used on a wound bed prepared by tangential excision. One could envisage that debridement by avulsion is more extensive than by tangential excision, resulting in a wound bed that is essentially free of necrosis. The presence of diabetes as a systemic disorder resulted in a significant reduction in take rate of 14.5% ($p=0.008$). This is not surprising, since impaired wound healing is a well-known phenomenon in diabetes mellitus [22, 23]. All the other independent variables enrolled in this analysis did not show a statistically significant effect on the take rate of the micrografts.

It is remarkable that factors such as TBSA (TBSA3) and inhalation trauma did not show a significant relation to the take rate. Apparently, the modern intensive care meets the needs for an adequate maintenance of wound-bed perfusion in the more extensively burned patients. Taking into account that no grafts were placed when a clinical wound infection was obvious, we still expected lower take rates whenever the wound was bacterially contaminated in the peri-operative period. Apparently, these subclinical infections posed no real threat to the take of grafts since no significant effect on the take rate could be demonstrated.

The small areas of donor site needed when using Meek–Wall grafts is seen as its biggest advantage. Therefore, the expansion ratios were examined to determine which ratio resulted in the best take rate. Also here no statistically significant differences could be found, suggesting that the choice of a specific expansion ratio does not affect the take of the graft. It should be realised, however, that less skin is applied on the wound by a largely expanded graft, so the healing time will be longer.

The results reported suggest that, in combination with an overlay of glycerol-preserved allografts, the Meek technique provides reliable wound healing with auto-grafts expanded to a ratio of 1:9. The delay in applying the allograft overlay did not appear to affect graft take. Although the need for a second operative procedure is a relative disadvantage, we found in practice that the application of allografts could often be staged to coincide with some other procedure in these extensively injured patients.

Furthermore, our results, as well as those from others, indicate that micro-island grafts, in contrast to mesh grafts, show a remarkable survival under poor wound conditions [24, 25].

In conclusion, the sandwich Meek micro-graft technique has proved to be a prac-tical and reliable method for obtaining widely expanded autograft islands when donor sites are scarce. The technique has reached a wide area of acceptance [26, 27] and has become the method of choice when insufficient donor sites are available to achieve primary wound coverage with mesh grafts. Meek–Wall micro-grafting can be used in patients with large TBSA, patients with an inhalation trauma, in the case of a contaminated wound bed, or particularly when large graft expansion ratios (up to 9/1) are needed. These conditions do not significantly affect the take rate of this procedure.

Intriguing are efforts in the combined use of Integra® and Meek micrografts after ingrowth of the dermal part of Integra and removal of the silicon outer sheet [28].

**Acknowledgements.** The help of O.P.M. Teernstra, I.A. Brussé, State University of Maastricht, the Netherlands, in the retrospective data analysis is greatly appre-ciated.

## References

1. Meek CP (1958) Successful microdermagrafting using the Meek-Wall microdermatome. Amer J Surg 96: 557–558
2. Tanner JC Jr, Vandeput J, Olley JF (1964) The mesh skin graft. Plast Reconstr Surg 34: 287–292
3. Burke JF, Quinby WC, Bondoc CC (1978) Early excision and prompt wound closure supplemented with immunosuppression. Surg Clin N Amer 58: 1141–1150
4. Alexander JW, MacMillan BG, Law E, Kittur DS (1981) Treatment of severe burns with widely meshed skin autografts and meshed allograft overlay. J Trauma 21: 433–438
5. Hermans RP (1983) The use of human allografts in the treatment of scalds in children. Panminerva Medica 25: 155–156
6. Vloemans AFPM, Schreinemachers MCJM, Middelkoop E, Kreis RW (2002) The use of glycerol-preserved allografts in the Beverwijk Burn Centre: a retrospective study. Burns 28: S2–S9
7. Abbott WM, Hembree JS (1970) Absence of antigenicity in freeze-dried skin allografts. Criobiology 6: 416–418
8. Hoekstra MJ, DuPont JS, Kreis RW (1994) History of the Euro Skin Bank: The innovation of preser-vation technologies. Burns 20 [Suppl 1]: S43–47
9. Basile ARD (1982) A comparative study of glycerinised and lyophilised porcine skin in dressings for third-degree burns. J Plast Reconstr Surg 69: 969–974
10. Kreis RW, Vloemans AF, Hoekstra MJ, Mackie DP, Hermans RP (1989) The use of non-viable glycerol-preserved cadaver skin combined with widely expanded autografts in the treatment of extensive third degree burns. J Trauma 29: 51–54

11. Hartford CE, Wang X-W, Peterson VM, Rodgers CM, Ketch LL (1989) Healing characteristics of expanded autografts on wounds covered with homografts and Biobrane temporary wound dressing. J Burn Care Rehab 10: 476–480

12. Yang J-Y, Tsai Y-C, Noordhoff MS (1989) Clinical comparison of commercially available Biobrane preparations. Burns 15: 197–203

13. Yannas IV, Burke JF (1980a) Design of an artificial skin. I. Basis design principles. J Biomed Mater Res 14: 65–81

14. Yannas IV, Burke JF, Gordon PL, Huang C, Rubenstein RH (1980b) Design of an artificial skin. II. Control of chemical composition. J Biomed Mater Res 14: 107–131

15. Heimbach DM, Warden GD, Luterman A et al. (2003) Multicenter Postapproval clinical trial of Integra dermal regeneration template for burn treatment. J Burn Care Rehabil 24: 42–48

16. Peck MD, Kessler M, Meyer AA, Bonham Morris PA (2002) A trial of the effectiveness of artificial dermis in the treatment of patients with burns greater than 45% total body surface area. J Trauma 52: 971–978

17. Meek CP (1963) Extensive severe burn treated with enzymatic debridement and microdermagrafting: case report. Am Surg 29: 61–64

18. Kreis RW, Mackie DP, Vloemans AFPM, Hoekstra MJ (1993) Widely expanded postage stamp skin grafts using a modified Meek technique in combination with an allograft overlay. Burns 19: 142–145

19. Demling RH, La Londe C (1989) Management of the burn wound. In: Demling RH, Lalande C (eds) Burn trauma.Thieme Stuttgart New York, pp 179–192

20. Lawrence JC (1985) The bacteriology of burns. J Hosp Infect 6: 3–17

21. Mozingo DW, Pruitt BA (1994) Infectious complications after burn injury. Curr Opin Surg Infect 2: 69–75

22. Morain W, Colen L (1991) Wound healing in diabetes mellitus. Clin Plast Surg 17: 493–501

23. Loots MAM (2002) Wound healing in diabetic ulcers. University of Amsterdam, Amsterdam, the Netherlands. Thesis, pp 21–27

24. Benmeir P, Eldad A, Weinberg A, Neuman A, Rotum M, Lusthaus S, Wexlar MR (1991) Use of buried skin implants after recurrent failure of conventional grafting in massive burn: the renewal of an old technique. Burns 17: 342–343

25. Raff T, Hartmann B, Wagner H, Germann G (1996) Experience with the modified Meek technique. Acta Chir Plast 38: 142–146

26. Hadjiiski O (2000) The method of micrografting in the treatment of large area full-thickness burns. Ann Burns Fire Disasters XIII: 155–158

27. Lari AR, Gang RK (2000) Expansion techniques for skin grafts (Meek technique) in the treatment of severely burned patients. Burns 27: 61–66

28. Papp A, Härmä M (2003) A collagen based dermal substitute and the modified Meek technique in extensive burns. Report of three cases. Burns 29: 167–171

# Skin Substitutes – an Overview of Cultured Epithelia to Treat Wounds

R.E. HORCH

## Introduction

Skin-wound healing is the prototype of a defence mechanism against environmental lesions and may be regarded as the elementary process of tissue repair. The primary destination of skin-wound healing is the re-epithelialisation of the wound surface [1]. In massive burns the mere extent of wound surfaces and the considerable loss of skin made the invention of skin substitutes necessary since the body's own resources cannot allow for recovery. Therefore, the evolution of biological and synthetic dressings and skin substitutes began with the recognition that extensive wounds require a barrier protection to prevent infection and desiccation, and cell guidance by dermal elements to maximise healing. Properties of both layers of skin are important to incorporate. Use of cultured skin substitutes for wound closure has reduced the amount of donor skin required by more than ten times compared with conventional skin grafts. Effective wound closure with these skin substitutes has reduced the number of surgeries to harvest donor skin and decreased the time of recovery of severely burn-injured patients. From experiences in burn-wound treatment, cultured skin substitutes have also been used to treat chronic wounds and problem wounds which are difficult to heal. This latter field of skin-substitute application is constantly evolving and is still under discussion.

## Basic Overview of the Most Popular Currently Available Skin Substitutes

Currently available biological and synthetic skin substitutes may be categorised regarding the principal action of the materials into three groups:
- temporary (material designed to be placed on a fresh wound (partial thickness) and left until healed);
- semi-permanent (material remaining attached to the excised wound, and eventually replaced by autogeneous skin grafts);
- permanent (incorporation of an epidermal analogue, dermal analogue, or both as a permanent replacement.

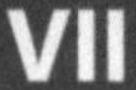

### Currently Available Biologic and Synthetic Skin Substitutes

- Biologicals (naturally occurring tissues)
  - Cutaneous allografts (γ-irradiated, deep frozen, glycerolised)
  - Cutaneous xenografts
  - Amniotic membranes
- Skin substitutes
  - Synthetic bilaminate
  - Collagen-based composites (Biobrane, TransCyte, Integra®)
- Collagen-based dermal analogues
  - Deepithelised allograft (Alloderm)
- Culture-derived tissue (see also list p. 438)
  - Cultured autologous keratinocytes (sheet grafts, cell suspensions)
  - Bilayer human tissue (Apligraf)
  - Polyglycolic or acid mesh
  - Fibroblast-seeded dermal analogues
  - Collagen-glycosaminoglycan matrix
  - Epithelial-seeded dermal analogues

The application of and indications for some of the materials that are used as a skin substitute have been modified over the years with regard to clinical experiences that were different from the original intention. As an example, Biobrane, which is made of an inner dermal analogue composed of a three-dimensional irregular nylon filament weave upon which type-I collagen peptides are bonded, has been shown to be very efficient in superficial burn wounds, but did not perform equally when used in combination with cultured cells (Fig. 1) [2].

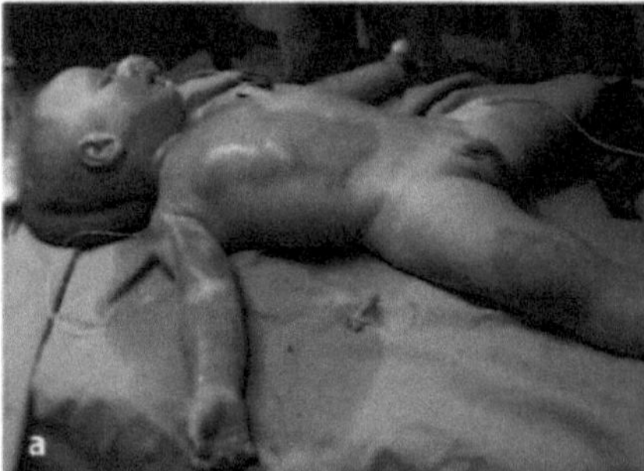
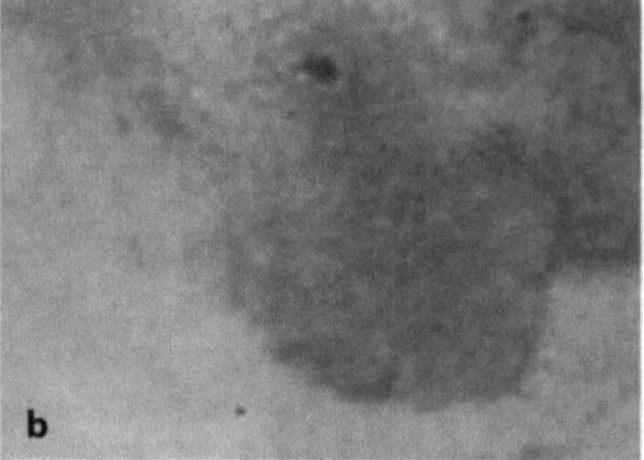

**Fig. 1. a** Second-degree scald in a child as an ideal candidate for temporary skin substitute application. **b** Healing of second-degree scald on the trunk after temporary Biobrane skin substitute application

## Specific Problems of the Burn Wound

Modern treatment concepts in extensive burn surgery are based on the perception that early surgical removal of heat-denatured proteins and devitalised tissue from a wound (staged serial debridement between the second and tenth day after the injury = early necrectomy) turns the burn into an excisional wound which can heal faster [3–6].

Primary excision has reduced mortality, morbidity and later reconstructive measures by a factor of 50% when compared to results obtained by awaiting spontaneous separation of eschar with later grafting. Early excision and reconstitution of a functional skin as early as possible is considered to be crucial for the further course and for the patient's survival [7–9] and leads to a better wound healing with improved functional results [10].

Today, standard autologous split-thickness skin autografts still represent the gold standard to re-surface large wounds. In massive burns the available skin-donor sites for auto-grafting may be very limited. This has been the initial stimulus for the development of skin substitutes. The increasing emphasis on rehabilitation and quality of skin cover has further accelerated this field. A skin substitute which has properties of a dermis is the marker for gauging a permanent substitute.

Allogeneic or alloplastic skin-substitute coverage as a temporary solution is necessary until definitive cover can be achieved [7, 8, 11–18]. Allogenic skin grafts may be completely integrated into the healing wound initially and bridge the critical time gap in the early phase of burn treatment, but in the further course irrevocably undergo immunogenic rejection [7, 8, 12, 16, 19–24]. Theoretically, the application of in vitro cultivated autologous skin substitutes is able to overcome this specific deficit of today's burn treatment and reconstructive surgery.

## Skin-Cell Culture-Based Developments

The possibility to rapidly multiply a large number of epithelial cells under culture conditions with intervals of cell multiplication less than 24 h based on the breakthrough technique by Rheinwald and Green in 1975, that allowed keratinocytes to be successfully cultured and subcultured in clonal cell densities on a feeder layer of lethally irradiated mouse fibroblasts [25], renders the chance to grow epidermis in the quantity of the complete body's surface within 3 to 4 weeks out of a single small skin biopsy. Numerous and outstanding research efforts of various groups led to the formulation of perfectly defined commercially available media, which enable keratinocytes to be cultured without a feeder layer, and serum-free. The combination of the concepts of early-staged burn debridement with temporary skin cover and the technique of keratinocyte multiplication in culture gave rise to the hope that each burn wound, no matter how extensive, may be covered within 3 to 4 weeks [7, 22, 26–33].

The further development of in-vitro cultured skin substitutes since the first clinical applications can been characterised by two principally different ways of culture ideas:

- the construction of multilayered epithelial transplants (so called sheet grafts) [2, 25, 30–32, 34–44];
- the construction of composite dermal–epidermal analogues [18, 26, 27, 29–32, 36, 40, 41, 45–56].

An overview of the best-known techniques to produce and apply cultured skin substitutes and most of the currently available methods and research directions can be found in the list below. Regarding these different approaches, some implications for the further development and research can be deduced which are mainly based on clinical problems with cultured skin.

The list below gives an overview of some of the most popular currently used cultured skin substitutes and experimental developments using cultured keratinocytes.

### Cultured Skin Substitutes and Keratinocytes

**Autologous keratinocytes**
- Autologous epidermal sheet transplants
- In-vitro cultured and constructed dermo-epidermal autologous transplants:
  - Keratinocytes on a collagen gel + fibroblasts
  - Keratinocyte sheets + collagen-glycosaminoglycan membrane + fibroblasts
  - Keratinocyte sheets on a layer of fibrin gel
  - Keratinocyte sheets on cell-free pig dermis
  - Keratinocyte sheets on cell free human dermis
  - Keratinocytes on bovine or equine collagen matrices
  - Keratinocyte sheets on micro-perforated hyaluronic acid membranes
  - Keratinocyte sheets on collagen + Chondroitin-6 sulfate with silicon membrane coverage (living skin equivalent)
- Combination of allogenic dermis (in vivo) with epidermal sheets
- Non-confluent keratinocyte suspensions (as a spray in saline solutions, in a fibrin matrix)
  - Exclusively
  - In combination with fresh or preserved allogenic skin
  - In combination with bovine collagen matrices or hyaluronic acid membranes
  - In combination with collagen-coated nylon on silicone backing
  - Dissociated keratinocytes without culture
  - Outer root sheath cells non-cultured
  - Outer root sheath cells cultured
- Three-dimensional cell cluster cultures (spherocytes)
  - Cultured on microspheres as carrier systems (dextrane, collagen, hyaluronic acid)
  - Cell seeded microspheres + allografts/biomaterials

**Allogeneic keratinocytes**
- Keratinocyte sheets – temporary cover
- Allogeneic keratinocyte suspensions (experimentally)
- Syngenic-allogeneic keratinocytes
- In-vitro-constructed dermo-epidermal composites/analogues
  - Keratinocytes and fibroblasts in collagen matrices

## Conventional Sheet-Graft (CEA) Skin Substitutes

Despite the fascinating feasibility of grafting cultured sheets of human autologous epithelium (sheet grafts), there are ongoing controversies about the optimal indications and the pros and cons of this exciting technique [11, 35, 57]. Among the disadvantages especially the high costs have tempered a more widespread use. In a clinical trial, conventionally meshed autografts were found to be superior to CEA concerning hospital cost, diminishing length of hospital stay and decreasing the number of re-admissions for reconstruction of contractures. In a survey of burn survival costs after treating a patient with 88% TBSA burn with CEA an amount of ca. 450 000 Euro (currently US $ 403 751) has been specified for the successful primary care of this patient [58]. According to the literature, the cost for a successful treatment of 1% of TBSA with CEA accounted for US $ 13 000 in 1995. Reported take rates of CEA and the necessity to repeatedly graft the areas again are extremely variable and differ considerably [49, 59].

Wound infection, that is clinically significant bacterial contamination, is the main cause of graft failure. Particularly in the first few days following grafting, the fragile non-cornified epithelium and dermo-epidermal junction are much more susceptible to the damaging effects of bacterial infection than a meshed graft.

Single-centre experiences with a larger number of CEA-grafted patients report lower take rates (between 15 and 65%) than the other earlier literature data of multicentre trials revealed [11, 26, 27, 30, 45, 49, 60–64]. The true take rate from the cumulative literature data may therefore reach an average value of 50% or less. This is consistent with the original data of the pioneering works, which varied considerably between 0% and more than 80% take in adults and 50% take in children [45, 47].

The sheet grafts consist of three to five cell layers and the surgical handling with secondary devices is delicate [47]. The lack of adherence and the tendency to form blisters even months after the engraftment when exhibited to shearing forces is another unsolved problem. In CEA-grafted areas therefore no mechanical stress may be allowed.

One of the reasons for the uncertain take rates of sheet grafts could be related to the abnormal structure of the anchoring fibrils [26]. Until now, only parts of the body have been successfully covered with sheet grafts in extensive burns. One more critical problem is the lack of dermis when resurfacing third-degree burns and chronic wounds. Several research efforts therefore aim towards the development of dermal equivalents or combinations of keratinocytes and dermal analogues or matrix cells such as fibroblasts [11, 21, 48, 49, 54, 56, 65–67]

Alternatively, the temporary coverage of debrided wounds has been propagated and relies on the engraftment of at least parts of the allograft dermis that remain after the immunogenic rejection process or after surgical removal of the allogenic epidermis. In burn patients, clinical experience has shown that early excision and covering with allograft that temporarily engrafts may keep the wound bed clean and well-vascularised and enhance the likelihood of sheet graft take [7, 8, 23, 35, 65, 68, 69]. Allogenic temporary skin coverage may serve as a biological and infection-preventing in-vivo culture environment after surgical debridement and consequent autografting until the allogenic epidermis is rejected. There is, however, a major problem in availability. Xenografts (tissue from another species) are more accessible than allografts. However, xenografts cannot be re-vascularised from the wound, so the tissue breaks down and sloughs off the wound.

In burns, the allografts allow for a stable temporary wound cover until further harvesting of the already-used donor sites is possible. The autologous split skin is then subsequently mechanically expanded by different means. Therefore, even with limited donor sites, extensive burn areas may sequentially be covered with a definite result [10]. Among other reasons, the limited resources in various health systems have recently favoured the further development of these conventional techniques to circumvent cultured skin substitutes whenever possible leading to the propagation of microskin grafting [7, 8, 23, 35, 65, 68, 69].

## Single Cell Suspensions

Epithelial cell seeding to chronic wounds and wound cavities was a technique described in 1895 by von Mangoldt, who showed astoundingly good clinical results [70]. He harvested epithelial cell or cell clusters by scraping off superficial epithelium from a patient's forearm with a surgical blade "until fibrin was exudated from the wound". The cells were dissolved in natural serum or blood components and applied to wounds. The advantages compared to the method of Reverdin, which was the common method at this time, were seen in a reduced donor-site morbidity and a more regular aspect of the resurfaced wounds. Due to his exact clinical and histological observations he noted that single cells or cell clusters "better stick to the wound bed" than pieces of skin.

Pels-Leusden further modified this technique at the beginning of the 19th century. He mixed the scraped-off epithelial cell-serum/blood suspension and injected it into the wound bed of chronic wounds. The method was not widely adopted because other surgeons feared the induction of epithelial cell cysts [71].

During the 1950s epidermal cell suspensions were transplanted without a binding matrix, such as fibrin sealant, but yielded inconsistent clinical results only [72]. In 1988, Hunyadi and coworkers reported upon the successful application of non-cultured keratinocytes gained by trypsinisation from biopsies and suspended in a fibrin matrix to heal chronic venous leg ulcers, while at the same time trypsinised keratinocyte suspensions without fibrin sealant did not lead to re-epithelialisation in a control group [31]. Fibrin, as a naturally occurring substrate, leads to haemostasis and plays a key role in wound healing. The use of fibrin sealant to fix skin grafts on burn and other wounds has been shown by various authors [31, 36, 73].

In clinical trials our group successfully demonstrated for the first time that extensively burned areas up to 88% TBSA can be covered with a cultured keratinocyte-fibrin-sealant suspension in 6 patients and 14 transplantations using a commercially available two-component fibrin sealant [31, 32, 42, 58, 74, 75] (Fig. 2). The KFGS (keratinocyte-fibrin-glue suspension) was available after 10 days since no epidermal differentiation was needed for the single cell suspensions, while the CEA were available after 3 weeks only. The initial attempts at KFGS grafting without meshed allograft overlays led to re-epithelialisation within 1 week when applied to long-lasting and non-spontaneously healing wounds, but showed mechanical instability similar to CEA-grafted areas.

The technique was therefore modified by preliminary wound-bed preparation with allograft skin and subsequent KFGS transplantation together with meshed split-thickness allograft skin overlays. While the allografts healed initially showing signs of revascularisation like autologous skin grafts, a slight and progressive immunogenic rejection period was noted after 12 to 14 days and was followed by stable wound coverage within 2 more weeks. It seems notable that a stable wound closure was achieved even over stress-prone areas like knees and elbow joint regions without signs of mechanical instability, as was seen after simple epithelial grafting without allografts [31, 32, 42, 58, 74, 75].

Other groups try to provide readily available sources of cultured epithelium using allogenic keratinocytes, which are of special interest for large burns. In extensive burns superficial wounds are thought to be immediately covered, or third-degree wounds may be covered with a biological skin substitute until enough autologous grafts are available. Skin-donor sites are described as healing faster, and thus repeated harvest of thin skin grafts may be facilitated. However, the duration of persistance of such allogenic cells or substitutes in the wound and the timely course of rejection is unclear and controversely discussed [7, 8, 13, 22, 26–30, 32, 33, 35, 48, 57, 60, 61, 76, 77].

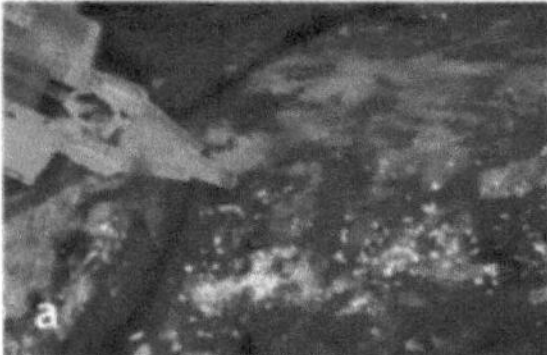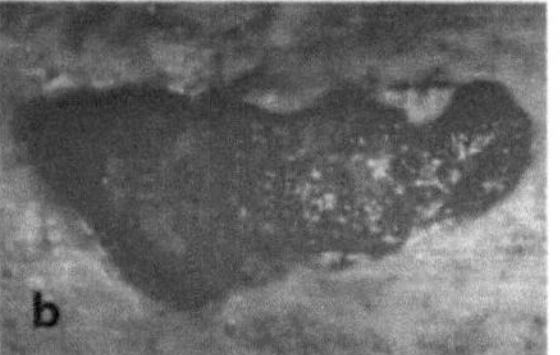

**Fig. 2. a** Grafting of cultured autologous keratinocyte-fibroblast-fibrin-sealant suspension onto muscle fascia after surgical excision of third-degree burn wound. **b** Chronic wound in arterial and venous ulcer disease not responding to conventional therapy. **c** Healing chronic wound after repeated transplantation of cultured autologous keratinocyte-fibrin-sealant suspension

## Cultured Cells and Biological Carriers

Since only the proliferating basal cells are responsible for the initial reconstitution of an epithelium, it seems logical that only these cells may be needed to re-surface wounds. Differentiation of cells in vitro has not been proved to be necessary for re-epithelialisation. Differentiated cells are not likely to actively contribute to the process of re-epithelialisation since they do not divide themselves any longer. From our previous studies and clinical trials, the concept was delineated that it is more natural to shorten the time of skin-substitute production in the laboratory and to bring cultured epidermal cells back to the more natural wound-healing environment as early as possible. The combination of allografting with simultaneously delivered cultured human keratinocytes in fibrin sealant as a carrier and matrix vehicle both clinically and experimentally is also feasible.

One of the unsolved problems is the constant and reliable delivery of cultured cells to the recipient wound bed. Using fibrin sealant as a biological cell carrier, some groups now have introduced spray techniques. This enables the dispersion and distribution of cultured cells to a maximum surface compared to our initial traditional approach without spray systems. The fact that cultured keratinocytes do survive this procedure has recently been shown in vitro by our group [48] experimentally as well as clinically by others. Another way to optimise keratinocyte growth and delivery is the method of Ronfard and co-workers, who cultured keratinocytes on a stabilised fibrin sealant in the gel phase. After sufficient multiplication, the whole fibrin-keratinocyte graft can be mechanically removed from the culture systems and be transplanted to the recipient. By this elegant technique a reliable and simple delivery of keratinocytes is enabled, as was shown experimentally and clinically [35].

The enzymatic detachment from the culture dishes – necessary in the delivery of CEA sheets – is potentially harmful to the cultured cells and has been accused to be the main reason for the lack of adherence of sheets to the wound. Attempts at mounting cultured epithelia on dermal matrices have been a possible way to facilitate handling, to avoid enzymatic treatment before grafting and at the same time to deliver a dermal analogue. Various templates have been used. One of the most common materials has been collagen in combination with glycosaminoglycane (C-GAG), with or without a cover of a gas-permeable silastic membrane, that serves as a barrier to fluid loss [76]. The question whether dermal fibroblasts seeded into such composites are necessary or not has not been definitively answered up to now [20, 76, 78–80].

Due to a possible barrier function of the matrix material towards nutrients necessary for keratinocyte survival on top of such composites, questions of survival of such grafts in wounds have remained open and the clinical long-term success has yet to be shown (Fig. 3).

To avoid such obvious barrier functions of biological or synthetic carriers we transplanted composite grafts with the keratinocyte layer in an upside-down direction towards the wound bed, so that the collagen component serves as a carrier and as a biological dressing on top. Subsequently we used subconfluent monolayers of cultured human keratinocytes instead of multilayered sheet grafts. Collagen as a

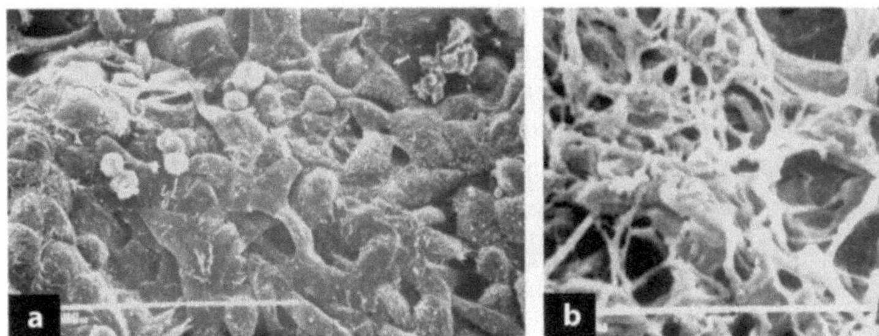

**Fig. 3. a** Confluent culture of human epithelia on collagen type-I carrier. **b** Ultrastructure of collagen type-I carrier resembling dermis structures

normal part of wound healing is an obvious material to be used in dermal substitutes and has been applied in various forms to resurface full-thickness wounds as a cell-carrier material or dermal template. Our experimental data with this upside-down grafting technique in full-thickness nude-mice wounds reveal the feasibility of this new approach [48]. In contrast to known standard composite grafts, there is no time required until revascularisation is established and nourishment is re-established, so that a high number of transplanted cells can survive in the natural wound environment, similar to buried chip skin grafting [23]. Until now it is not known if parts of the biological carrier are integrated into the newly reconstituted skin. This method combines the in-vitro expansion of graftable cells with advantages of the transplantation of actively proliferating cell populations on appropriate biological carriers. Clinically it may become one more valuable tool to treat burns or chronic wounds.

## Outlook

At the moment scientific principles and practical approaches to replace skin temporarily or permanently are advancing at a rapid rate. Although research in this area as well as the clinical application of cultured human skin substitutes is an expensive modality, we definitely need further progress to optimise skin substitute performance by tissue-engineering procedures. Improved cosmesis and the ultimate regaining of lost skin functions including sensitivity, elasticity, normal physiological sweat gland and dermal appendage function, as well as normal pigmentation with invisible scars, are the goals of future endeavours in this field. Research in this field may lead to improvements in skin reconstitution while at the same time today's limits of donor sites and donor-site morbidity in afflicted patients may be overcome.

Through both basic and clinical research there will be major improvements in the understanding and ability to deal effectively with the problems of wound healing and to replace a truly functional skin with dermal appendages; but perhaps the major improvement will come through the ability to replace worn-out, defective or damaged body parts through technologies that resemble regeneration. The concepts of tissue engineering applied to dermal replacement following burn injury or dealing with chronic wounds may well overcome many of today's limits in skin substitution.

## References


1. Slavin J (1996) The role of cytokines in wound healing. J Pathol 178: 5–10
2. Bannasch H et al. (2004) A semisynthetic bilaminar skin substitute used to treat pediatric full-body toxic epidermal necrolysis: wraparound technique in a 17-month-old girl. Arch Dermatol 140: 160–162
3. Ehrlich HP (1995) Control of wound healing from connective tissue aspect. Chirurg 66: 165–173
4. Demling RH, DeSanti L (1999) Management of partial thickness facial burns (comparison of topical antibiotics and bio-engineered skin substitutes). Burns 25: 256–261
5. Achauer BM, Martinez SE (1985) Burn wound pathophysiology and care. Crit Care Clin 1: 47–58
6. Prasanna M, Singh K, Kumar P (1994) Early tangential excision and skin grafting as a routine method of burn wound management: an experience from a developing country. Burns 20: 446–450
7. Horch R et al. (1994) Cologne Burn Centre experiences with glycerol-preserved allogeneic skin: Part I: Clinical experiences and histological findings (overgraft and sandwich technique). Burns 20 [Suppl 1]: S23–26
8. Horch RE et al. (1998) Reconstitution of basement membrane after 'sandwich-technique' skin grafting for severe burns demonstrated by immunohistochemistry. J Burn Care Rehabil 19: 189–202
9. Nanchahal J, Ward CM (1992) New grafts for old? A review of alternatives to autologous skin. Br J Plast Surg 45: 354–363
10. Alexander J et al. (1981) Treatment of severe burns with widely meshed skin autograft and meshed skin allograft overlay. J Trauma 21: 433–438
11. Nanchahal J, Dover R, Otto WR (2002) Allogeneic skin substitutes applied to burns patients. Burns 28: 254–257
12. Rouabhia M et al. (1995) Allogeneic-syngeneic cultured epithelia. A successful therapeutic option for skin regeneration. Transplantation 59: 1229–01235
13. Rouabhia M (1996) In vitro production and transplantation of immunologically active skin equivalents. Lab Invest 75: 503–517
14. Shakespeare P (2001) Burn wound healing and skin substitutes. Burns 27: 517–522
15. van Luyn MJ, Verheul J, van Wachem PB (1995) Regeneration of full-thickness wounds using collagen split grafts. J Biomed Mater Res 29: 1425–1436
16. Zhao YB (1992) Primary observation of prolonged survival of cultured epidermal allografts. Zhonghua Wai Ke Za Zhi 30: 104–106, 125–126
17. Phillips TJ (1993) Biologic skin substitutes. J Dermatol Surg Oncol 19: 794–800
18. Gallico GG 3rd (1990) Biologic skin substitutes. Clin Plast Surg 17: 519–526
19. Suzuki T et al. (1995) Mixed cultures comprising syngeneic and allogeneic mouse keratinocytes as a graftable skin substitute. Transplantation 59: 1236–1241
20. Wu J, Barisoni D, Armato U (1995) An investigation into the mechanisms by which human dermis does not significantly contribute to the rejection of allo-skin grafts. Burns 21: 11–16
21. Alsbjorn B (1984) In search of an ideal skin substitute. Scand J Plast Reconstr Surg 18: 127–133
22. Heimbach D et al. (1988) Artificial dermis for major burns. A multi-center randomized clinical trial. Ann Surg 208: 313–320
23. Horch R, Stark GB, Spilker G (1970) Treatment of perianal burns with submerged skin particles. Zentralbl Chir 119: 722–725
24. Kohnlein HE (1970) Skin transplantation and skin substitutes. Langenbecks Arch Chir 327: 1090–1106

25. Rheinwald JG, Green H (1975) Serial cultivation of strains of human epidermal keratinocytes: the formation of keratinizing colonies from single cells. Cell 6: 331–343
26. Compton CC et al. (1989) Skin regenerated from cultured epithelial autografts on full-thickness burn wounds from 6 days to 5 years after grafting. A light, electron microscopic and immunohistochemical study. Lab Invest 60: 600–612
27. De Luca M et al. (1989) Multicentre experience in the treatment of burns with autologous and allogenic cultured epithelium, fresh or preserved in a frozen state. Burns 15: 303–309
28. Green H, Kehinde O, Thomas J (1979) Growth of cultured human epidermal cells into multiple epithelia suitable for grafting. Proc Natl Acad Sci USA 76: 5665–5668
29. Herndon DN, Rutan RL (1992) Comparison of cultured epidermal autograft and massive excision with serial autografting plus homograft overlay. J Burn Care Rehabil 13: 154–157
30. Hickerson WL et al. (1994) Cultured epidermal autografts and allodermis combination for permanent burn wound coverage. Burns 20 [Suppl 1]: S52–55; discussion S55–56
31. Horch RE et al. (1998) Single-cell suspensions of cultured human keratinocytes in fibrin-glue reconstitute the epidermis. Cell Transplant 7: 309–317
32. Horch RE, Bannasch H, Stark GB (2001) Transplantation of cultured autologous keratinocytes in fibrin sealant biomatrix to resurface chronic wounds. Transplant Proc 33: 642–344
33. Yannas IV et al. (1982) Wound tissue can utilize a polymeric template to synthesize a functional extension of skin. Science 215: 174–176
34. Grossman N, Slovik Y, Bodner L (2004) Effect of donor age on cultivation of human oral mucosal keratinocytes. Arch Gerontol Geriatr 38: 114–122
35. Ronfard V et al. (2000) Long-term regeneration of human epidermis on third degree burns transplanted with autologous cultured epithelium grown on a fibrin matrix. Transplantation 70: 1588–1598
36. Pellegrini G et al. (1999) The control of epidermal stem cells (holoclones) in the treatment of massive full-thickness burns with autologous keratinocytes cultured on fibrin. Transplantation 68: 868–879
37. Meana A et al. (1998) Large surface of cultured human epithelium obtained on a dermal matrix based on live fibroblast-containing fibrin gels. Burns 24: 621–630
38. Wright KA et al. (1998) Alternative delivery of keratinocytes using a polyurethane membrane and the implications for its use in the treatment of full-thickness burn injury. Burns 24: 7–17
39. Ronfard V et al. (1991) Use of human keratinocytes cultured on fibrin glue in the treatment of burn wounds. Burns 17: 181–184
40. Foyatier JL et al. (1990) Clinical application of grafts of cultured epidermis in burn patients. Apropos of 16 patients. Ann Chir Plast Esthet 35: 39–46
41. Bannasch H et al. (2000) Treatment of chronic wounds with cultured autologous keratinocytes as suspension in fibrin glue. Zentralbl Chir 125 [Suppl 1]: 79–81
42. Horch RE et al. (2000) Gene therapy perspectives in modulation of wound healing. Zentralbl Chir 125 [Suppl 1]: 74–78
43. Tanczos E et al. (1999) Keratinocyte transplantation and tissue engineering. New approaches in treatment of chronic wounds. Zentralbl Chir 124 [Suppl 1]: 81–86
44. Gallico GR et al. (1984) Permanent coverage of large burn wounds with autologous cultured human epithelium. N Engl J Med 311: 448–451
45. Compton CC et al. (1998) Cultured human sole-derived keratinocyte grafts re-express site-specific differentiation after transplantation. Differentiation 64: 45–53
46. Gallico GG 3rd, O'Connor NE (1985) Cultured epithelium as a skin substitute. Clin Plast Surg 12: 149–157
47. Gallico GG 3rd et al. (1984) Permanent coverage of large burn wounds with autologous cultured human epithelium. N Engl J Med 311: 448–451
48. Horch RE et al. (2000) Cultured human keratinocytes on type I collagen membranes to reconstitute the epidermis. Tissue Eng 6: 53–67
49. Kopp J et al. (2004) Applied tissue engineering in the closure of severe burns and chronic wounds using cultured human autologous keratinocytes in a natural fibrin matrix. Cells Tissue Banking 5: 212–217
50. Burke JF et al. (1981) Successful use of a physiologically acceptable artificial skin in the treatment of extensive burn injury. Ann Surg 194: 413–428
51. Harriger MD et al. (1997) Reduced engraftment and wound closure of cryopreserved cultured skin substitutes grafted to athymic mice. Cryobiology 35: 132–142
52. Kogan L, Govrin-Yehudain J (2003) Vertical (two-layer) skin grafting: new reserves for autologic skin. Ann Plast Surg 50: 514–516
53. Sheridan RL, Moreno C (2001) Skin substitutes in burns. Burns 27: 92

54. Voigt M et al. (1999) Cultured epidermal keratinocytes on a microspherical transport system are feasible to reconstitute the epidermis in full-thickness wounds. Tissue Eng 5: 563–572
55. Yannas IV et al. (1981) Prompt, long-term functional replacement of skin. Trans Am Soc Artif Intern Organs 27: 19–23
56. Xu W et al. (1996) Permanent grafting of living skin substitutes: surgical parameters to control for successful results. J Burn Care Rehabil 17: 7–13
57. Munster AM (1997) Whither [corrected] skin replacement? Burns 23: v
58. Horch R (2001) Economy of skin grafting in burns. Hospital – J Eur Assoc Hosp Man 3: 6–9
59. Yasushi F et al. (2004) Treatment with autologous cultured dermal substitutes (CDS) for burn scar contracture in children. Wound Repair Regen 12: A11
60. Munster AM, Weiner SH, Spence RJ (1990) Cultured epidermis for the coverage of massive burn wounds. A single center experience. Ann Surg 211: 676–679; discussion 679–680
61. Munster AM (1996) Cultured skin for massive burns. A prospective, controlled trial. Ann Surg 224: 372–375; discussion 375–377
62. Raghunath M, Meuli M (1997) Cultured epithelial autografts: diving from surgery into matrix biology. Pediatr Surg Int 12: 478–483
63. Shakespeare PG (1999) Cost effectiveness of skin substitutes. A commentary on the debate at the 10th ISBI Congress, Jerusalem 1998. International Society for Burn Injuries. Burns 25: 179–181
64. Shakespeare P (2001) Skin substitutes – benefits and costs. Burns 27: vii–viii
65. Munster AM, Smith-Meek M, Shalom A (2001) A cellular allograft dermal matrix: immediate or delayed epidermal coverage? Burns 27: 150–153
66. Eaglstein WH, Iriondo M, Laszlo K (1995) A composite skin substitute (graftskin) for surgical wounds. A clinical experience. Dermatol Surg 21: 839–843
67. Andree C et al. (2001) Plasmid gene delivery to human keratinocytes through a fibrin-mediated transfection system. Tissue Eng 7: 757–766
68. Zhao Y, Wang X, Lu S (1995) Identifying the existence of cultured human epidermal allografts with PCR techniques. Zhonghua Wai Ke Za Zhi 33: 387–389
69. Kopp J et al. (2003) Ancient traditional Chinese medicine in burn treatment: a historical review. Burns 29: 473–478
70. Mangoldt F (1895) Die Überhäutung von Wundflächen und Wundhöhlen durch Epithelausaat, eine neue Methode der Transplantation. Dtsch Med Wschr 21: 798–799
71. Pels-Leusden F (1905) Die Anwendung des Spalthautlappens in der Chirurgie. Dtsch Med Wschr 31: 99–102
72. Billingham R, Reynolds J (1952) Transplantation studies on sheet of pure epidermal epithelium and of epidermal cell suspensions. Br J Plast Surg 23: 25–32
73. Archambault M, Yaar M, Gilchrest BA (1995) Keratinocytes and fibroblasts in a human skin equivalent model enhance melanocyte survival and melanin synthesis after ultraviolet irradiation. J Invest Dermatol 104: 859–867
74. Bell E, Sher S, Hull B (1984) The living skin-equivalent as a structural and immunological model in skin grafting. Scan Electron Microsc Pt4: 1957–1962
75. Stark GB et al. Biological wound tissue glue systems in wound healing. Langenbecks Arch Chir Suppl Kongressbd 115: 683–688
76. Orgill DP, Straus FH 2nd, Lee RC (1999) The use of collagen-GAG membranes in reconstructive surgery. Ann N Y Acad Sci 888: 233–248
77. Munster AM, Smith-Meek M, Sharkey P (1994) The effect of early surgical intervention on mortality and cost-effectiveness in burn care, 1978–91. Burns 20: 61–64
78. Pruitt BA Jr (1997) The evolutionary development of biologic dressings and skin substitutes. J Burn Care Rehabil 18: S2–5
79. Supp DM et al. (2000) Enhanced vascularisation of cultured skin substitutes genetically modified to overexpress vascular endothelial growth factor. J Invest Dermatol 114: 5–13
80. Dubertret L, Coulomb B (1994) Reconstruction of human skin in culture. C R Seances Soc Biol Fil 188: 235–244

# 44

# Skin Equivalents – Integra® in Acute Wounds

C. Wicke, H.D. Becker

## Introduction

Wound healing is a dynamic, interactive process involving soluble mediators, blood cells, extracellular matrix and parenchymal cells. The healing process includes haemostasis and inflammation, re-epithelialisation, granulation-tissue formation, fibroblast proliferation, angiogenesis and wound contraction. All of these processes must occur in proper sequence for optimal results. Ideally, permanent skin equivalents can be integrated into this healing cascade. Skin equivalents should be easily handable, adherent to the wound bed, durable, biocompatible, elastic, uniform in composition when prepared in vitro, non-toxic and non-antigenic [34]. When developing or selecting permanent skin equivalents, their functional and structural properties should match the basic qualities of epidermis and dermis as closely as possible. Components of engineered skin range from cultured parenchymal cells to tissue derivates or synthetic materials. Commercial products and experimental models have been configured from individual and combined materials [1–3, 6]. There have been two major approaches to the provision of a cell-free matrix for permanent replacement of the dermal component of skin [22]. One has been to use allogeneic human dermis rendered cell-free and preserved, such as AlloDerm®. The second has been to fabricate a matrix with the required physical and chemical structure. One example of this approach is the material developed in the 1980s by Yannas and Burke which is now in use as Integra® Dermal Regeneration Template (Integra LifeSciences Corporation, US) [38].

## Characteristics of Integra®

Integra® Dermal Regeneration Template was designed to reduce the time needed to achieve final wound closure in the treatment of major burn wounds, to optimise the sparse autologous skin resources and to improve the durable mechanical quality of the skin equivalent [24]. Integra® is a bilayer membrane system for skin replacement. The dermal replacement layer is made of a porous matrix of fibres of cross-linked bovine tendon collagen and glycosaminoglycan (chondroitin-6-sulfate) which gives it controlled porosity and a defined degradation rate. The temporary epidermal substitute layer is made of a thin silicone layer to control moisture loss from the wound and to protect the wound from bacterial invasion. Integra® Dermal Regeneration Template facilitates the formation of a neodermis. The collagen/glycosaminoglycan dermal portion serves as a template for the infiltration of the

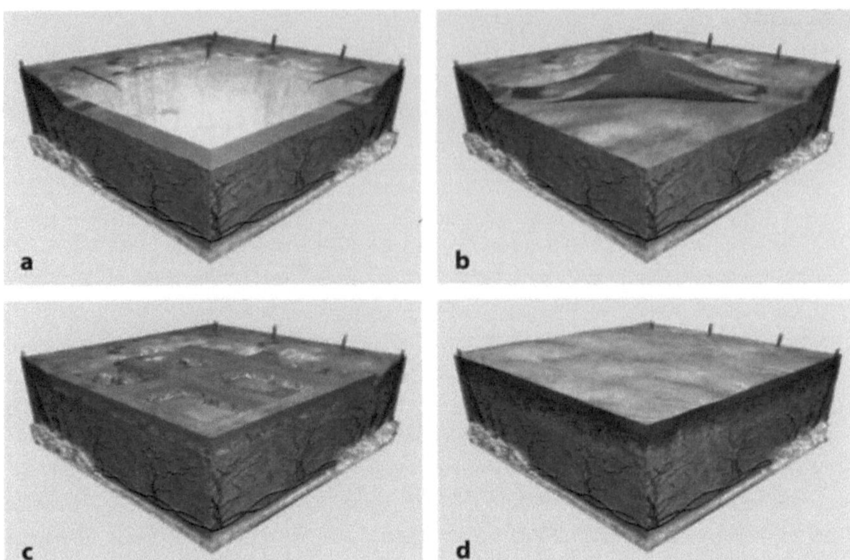

**Fig. 1a–d.** Integra® actively interfaces with the open wound surface inducing the migration of fibroblasts and endothelial cells into the material. The dermal layer of the dermal regeneration template becomes degraded, and an endogenous collagen matrix is deposited, forming a neodermis (**a**). Once engraftment is complete, the patient is returned to the operating room, where the silicone layer is removed (**b**) and a thin, meshed epidermal autograft is placed over the neodermis (**c**). **d** Regenerated skin. (With permission from Integra Lifes Sciences 2004)

recipient's lymphocytes, macrophages, fibroblasts and endothelial cells. As healing progresses, collagen is deposited by the fibroblasts, which replaces the collagen/glycosaminoglycan portion of Integra® as it biodegrades. After adequate vascularisation of the neodermis (approximately 21 days) and the availability of donor autograft, the silicone layer is atraumatically removed and an ultrathin layer of epidermal autograft is placed over the neodermis. Cells from the epidermal autograft grow and form a confluent stratum corneum, thereby closing the wound and reconstituting a functional dermis and epidermis (Fig. 1a–d).

## Handling of Integra®

Integra® Dermal Regeneration Template is aseptically processed. Reconstruction with Integra® is a two-stage procedure. The first step creates a neodermis, the second step creates an epidermis on the newly formed neodermis. Integra® should be applied to fresh, clean, surgically excised wounds on the day of excision. It is critical to meticulously remove all devitalised tissue on and around the area to be grafted. Complete haemostasis must be achieved before application of Integra® Dermal Regeneration

Template. Integra® should be shaped accurately to fit the excised wound margins to minimise scarring. Integra® is secured by staples or sutures placed in an interrupted fashion under slight tension. Within 2 to 3 weeks, a neodermis forms and an ultra-thin autograft can be placed over the neodermis. A well-vascularised wound bed is a prerequisite for this second surgical step. Ultrathin split-thickness skin grafts should be obtained with a calibrated dermatome set to 0.006 inches (0.15 mm) to obtain translucent grafts [18]. Typically, the epidermal autograft is meshed up to a 3:1 ratio and anchored by sutures or staples. Continuous wound care and infection control during the first and the second stage of the reconstruction are crucial for the success of the reconstruction [13]. Potential problems during post-operative care include haematoma and seroma formation, infection, separation of the matrix from the wound bed, premature silicone layer separation, and difficult removal of the silicone layer. At later stages of the reconstruction epidermal autograft failure and progressive epithelial loss (melting) can occur [25].

## Indications for Integra®

Integra® Dermal Regeneration Template is indicated for the post-excisional treatment of partial-thickness and full-thickness injuries and defects. The bilayer dermal regeneration template has been examined in both animal and human studies. Burke et al. reported covering full-thickness skin wounds in guinea pigs without histological evidence of inflammation or rejection [38]. The application of the bilayer membrane delayed the onset and the extent of wound contraction [37]. After publication of the first results on ten patients with third-degree burns grafted with the dermal regeneration template, the material has been widely used in the treatment of major burn wounds, showing satisfactory functional and cosmetic results, lack of scar hypertrophy, and improved survival over conventional autografting [4, 9–12, 15, 19, 35]. Heimbach et al. published the results of a multicentre randomised trial of Integra® use in major burns in 1988 [20]; 106 patients with life-threatening burns who underwent primary excision and grafting within 7 days of injury had comparable sites randomised to receive either the artificial dermis or the investigator's usual skin-grafting material including autograft, allograft, xenograft, or a synthetic dressing. Mean burn size was 46.5 ±15% mean total body surface. Median artificial dermis take was 80% compared with 95% for all comparative sites, but the take was equivalent to that of all non-autograft control materials. At the completion of the study, there was less hypertrophic scarring of the artificial dermis, and more patients preferred the artificial dermis to the control graft. The study, however, used a very heterogenous control group for comparison. Sheridan et al. reported similar results with 121 burn patients grafted over an 11-year period [29]. However, infection rates associated with Integra®-grafted sites were higher than in those sites that had been covered with autograft. The US Food and Drug Administration therefore requested a post-approval study to obtain additional data on infection rates associated with Integra® use. The results of this study were published in 2003 by Heimbach et al., who studied 216 burn-injury patients treated at 13 burn-care facilities in the United States [21]. The study showed a comparatively low infection incidence with an incidence of invasive infection at Integra®-treated sites of 3.1% and that of superficial infection 13.2%. Mean take rate of Integra® was 76.2%; the median take rate was 95%. Stern et al. examined the histological phases of the vascularisation of the template and the establishment of a neodermis when Integra® was used in acute burns [30]. Serial biopsy specimens were obtained from 131 patients during a period of 7 days to 2 years after application. In this study, six sequential phases of repair were discerned. There were occasional unusual histological features, eosinophilic infiltration, and/or macrophage-derived giant cell formation in the wound area; however, such findings did not clinically correlate with a negative response to Integra®. An intact dermis was achieved as well as definitive closure of a complete epidermal layer with a minimum of scarring. The use of Integra® has also been studied in patients undergoing reconstructive surgical procedures for release of contractures [26]. In this study of 20 patients the scar tissue was excised or released, the subcutaneous fat was left undisturbed, and the matrix sheet was directly applied to it, in contrast to the fascial excision of acute burn wounds, in which a more significant contour defect is created. Consecutive punch biopsies showed four phases of dermal regeneration: imbibition with wound fluid and blood cells, fibroblast migration, neovascularisation and remodelling and maturation. Full vascularisation of the neodermis occurred after 4 weeks. Patients reported a 72% increase in range of movement, a 62% improvement in softness, and a 59% improvement in appearance compared with their pre-operative states. Pruritus and dryness were the main patients' complaints, and neither was much improved post-operatively. Integra® has also been used in the treatment of severe purpura fulminans when skin and extremity necrosis occurred [5]. The use of cultured epithelial autografts instead of epidermal autografts has emerged as an alternative strategy [27]. In animals, composite grafts of Integra® and human keratinocytes engineered in a perfusion culture system reconstituted an organised epidermis within 10 days [23]. Boyce et al. treated patients with full-thickness burns of greater than 50% total body surface areas with a combination of Integra® and cultured fibroblasts and keratinocytes obtained from skin biopsies [7, 8]. They showed that the combination of cultured skin substitutes and Integra® can accomplish functi onally stable and cosmetically acceptable wound closure. This approach is expected to reduce the time to definitive closure of wounds and to reduce the morbidity associated with the harvesting of donor sites for split-thickness skin autografts.

## Conclusions

Management of large or difficult-to-heal wounds due to burns, surgery, trauma or comorbidities poses a challenge to health-care professionals. Engineering of permanent skin equivalents provides a prospective source for treatment of acute and chronic wounds combining the replacement of skin defects with the promotion of wound healing. In addition to their wide use in treating burn wounds, bioengineered skin equivalents have been successfully used in the treatment of venous and diabetic foot ulcers [17, 36]. In vitro, bioengineered skin acts as a living tissue, capable of appropriately responding to wounding injury in a staged and specific pattern of cell migration, re-epithelialisation, and cytokine expression [16]. Skin equivalents may employ different mechanisms of action for acute and chronic healing. Further improvement of skin equivalents might include additional cell types, such as melanocytes, carrier systems for growth factors, biopolymer substrates, or gene therapy [14, 31–33]. Uniform standards for quantitative analysis of skin equivalents must be established for evaluation of material composition and outcomes [6, 28]. Advantages of individual materials must be weighed against the cost of the product, the meticulous surgical technique and post-operative care required, and the functional and cosmetic results.

## References

1. Bell E, Ehrlich HP, Buttle DJ, Nakatsuji T (1981) Living tissue formed in vitro and accepted as skin-equivalent tissue of full thickness. Science 211: 1052–1054
2. Bell E, Ehrlich HP, Sher S, Merrill C, Sarber R, Hull B, Nakatsuji T, Church D, Buttle DJ (1981) Development and use of a living skin equivalent. Plast Reconstr Surg 67: 386–392
3. Bell E, Ivarsson B, Merrill C (1979) Production of a tissue-like structure by contraction of collagen lattices by human fibroblasts of different proliferative potential in vitro. Proc Natl Acad Sci USA 76: 1274–1278
4. Berger A, Tanzella U, Machens HG, Liebau J (2000) [Administration of Integra on primary burn wounds and unstable secondary scars]. Chirurg 71: 558–563
5. Besner GE, Klamar JE (1998) Integra Artificial Skin as a useful adjunct in the treatment of purpura fulminans. J Burn Care Rehabil 19: 324–329
6. Boyce ST (2001) Design principles for composition and performance of cultured skin substitutes. Burns 27: 523–533
7. Boyce ST, Kagan RJ, Meyer NA, Yakuboff KP, Warden GD (1999) The 1999 clinical research award. Cultured skin substitutes combined with Integra Artificial Skin to replace native skin autograft and allograft for the closure of excised full-thickness burns. J Burn Care Rehabil 20: 453–461
8. Boyce ST, Kagan RJ, Yakuboff KP, Meyer NA, Rieman MT, Greenhalgh DG, Warden GD (2002) Cultured skin substitutes reduce donor skin harvesting for closure of excised, full-thickness burns. Ann Surg 235: 269–279
9. Burke JF, Yannas IV, Quinby WC, Jr., Bondoc CC, Jung WK (1981) Successful use of a physiologically acceptable artificial skin in the treatment of extensive burn injury. Ann Surg 194: 413–428
10. Cedidi C, Hartmann B, Schepler H, Raff T, Germann G (1999) Grafting of deeply burned problem zones in the lower extremity with a dermal substitute. Eur J Plast Surg 22: 119–124
11. Cedidi C, Hierner R, Wilkens L, Berger A (2002) The deeply burned upper extremity: functional graft distribution concept with selective use of a synthetic dermal substitute (Integra) and split-thickness skin grafts. Eur J Plast Surg 25: 226–230
12. Chou TD, Chen SL, Lee TW, Chen SG, Cheng TY, Lee CH, Chen TM, Wang HJ (2001) Reconstruction of burn scar of the upper extremities with artificial skin. Plast Reconstr Surg 108: 378–384: discussion 385
13. Clayton MC, Bishop JF (1998) Perioperative and postoperative dressing techniques for Integra Artificial Skin: views from two medical centers. J Burn Care Rehabil 19: 358–363
14. Coulomb B, Dubertret L (2002) Skin cell culture and wound healing. Wound Repair Regen 10: 109–112
15. Dantzer E, Braye FM (2001) Reconstructive surgery using an artificial dermis (Integra): results with 39 grafts. Br J Plast Surg 54: 659–664
16. Falanga V, Isaacs C, Paquette D, Downing G, Kouttab N, Butmarc J, Badiavas E, Hardin-Young J (2002) Wounding of bioengineered skin: cellular and molecular aspects after injury. J Invest Dermatol 119: 653–660

17. Falanga V, Margolis D, Alvarez O, Auletta M, Maggiacomo F, Altman M, Jensen J, Sabolinski M, Hardin-Young J (1998) Rapid healing of venous ulcers and lack of clinical rejection with an allogeneic cultured human skin equivalent. Human Skin Equivalent Investigators Group. Arch Dermatol 134: 293–300

18. Fang P, Engrav LH, Gibran NS, Honari S, Kiriluk DB, Cole JK, Fleckman P, Heimbach DM, Bauer GJ, Matsumura H, Warner P (2002) Dermatome setting for autografts to cover INTEGRA. J Burn Care Rehabil 23: 327–332

19. Fitton AR, Drew P, Dickson WA (2001) The use of a bilaminate artificial skin substitute (Integra) in acute resurfacing of burns: an early experience. Br J Plast Surg 54: 208–212

20. Heimbach D, Luterman A, Burke J, Cram A, Herndon D, Hunt J, Jordan M, McManus W, Solem L, Warden G, et al. (1988) Artificial dermis for major burns. A multi-center randomized clinical trial. Ann Surg 208: 313–320

21. Heimbach DM, Warden GD, Luterman A, Jordan MH, Ozobia N, Ryan CM, Voigt DW, Hickerson WL, Saffle JR, DeClement FA, Sheridan RL, Dimick AR (2003) Multicenter postapproval clinical trial of Integra dermal regeneration template for burn treatment. J Burn Care Rehabil 24: 42–48

22. Kearney JN (2001) Clinical evaluation of skin substitutes. Burns 27: 545–551

23. Kremer M, Lang E, Berger A (2001) Organotypical engineering of differentiated composite-skin equivalents of human keratinocytes in a collagen-GAG matrix (INTEGRA Artificial Skin) in a perfusion culture system. Langenbecks Arch Surg 386: 357–363

24. Kremer M, Lang E, Berger AC (2000) Evaluation of dermal-epidermal skin equivalents ('composite-skin') of human keratinocytes in a collagen-glycosaminoglycan matrix(Integra artificial skin). Br J Plast Surg 53: 459–465

25. Matsumura H, Meyer NA, Mann R, Heimbach DM (1998) Melting graft-wound syndrome. J Burn Care Rehabil 19: 292–295

26. Moiemen NS, Staiano JJ, Ojeh NO, Thway Y, Frame JD (2001) Reconstructive surgery with a dermal regeneration template: clinical and histologic study. Plast Reconstr Surg 108: 93–103

27. Pandya AN, Woodward B, Parkhouse N (1998) The use of cultured autologous keratinocytes with integra in the resurfacing of acute burns. Plast Reconstr Surg 102: 825–828; discussion 829–830

28. Shakespeare P (2001) Skin substitutes – benefits and costs. Burns 27: vii–viii

29. Sheridan RL, Hegarty M, Tompkins RG, Burke JF (1994) Artificial skin in massive burns – results to ten years. Eur J Plast Surg 17: 91–93

30. Stern R, McPherson M, Longaker MT (1990) Histologic study of artificial skin used in the treatment of full-thickness thermal injury. J Burn Care Rehabil 11: 7–13

31. Supp DM, Bell SM, Morgan JR, Boyce ST (2000) Genetic modification of cultured skin substitutes by transduction of human keratinocytes and fibroblasts with platelet-derived growth factor-A. Wound Repair Regen 8: 26–35

32. Supp DM, Boyce ST (2002) Overexpression of vascular endothelial growth factor accelerates early vascularisation and improves healing of genetically modified cultured skin substitutes. J Burn Care Rehabil 23: 10–20

33. Swope VB, Supp AP, Boyce ST (2002) Regulation of cutaneous pigmentation by titration of human melanocytes in cultured skin substitutes grafted to athymic mice. Wound Repair Regen 10: 378–386

34. Tavis MJ, Thornton J, Danet R, Bartlett RH (1978) Current status of skin substitutes. Surg Clin North Am 58: 1233–1248

35. Tompkins RG, Burke JF (1990) Progress in burn treatment and the use of artificial skin. World J Surg 14: 819–824

36. Veves A, Falanga V, Armstrong DG, Sabolinski ML (2001) Graftskin, a human skin equivalent, is effective in the management of noninfected neuropathic diabetic foot ulcers: a prospective randomized multicenter clinical trial. Diabetes Care 24: 290–295

37. Yannas IV, Burke JF, Gordon PL, Huang C, Rubenstein RH (1980) Design of an artificial skin. II. Control of chemical composition. J Biomed Mater Res 14: 107–132

38. Yannas IV, Burke JF, Orgill DP, Skrabut EM (1982) Wound tissue can utilize a polymeric template to synthesize a functional extension of skin. Science 215: 174–176

# 45

# Rehabilitation and Post-Burn Care

C. ROQUES

## Introduction

Burns set a problem of reanimation and cutaneous recovering in the acute phase; when this phase is finished, the difficulty of scar maturation arises for about 18 months. Around the second month scar inflammation appears, until at approximately the sixth month its intensity increases. This period is characterised by redness of the scar, hypertrophic tendency, induration of the burnt skin and, sometimes, disorders of the pigmentation; during this period cutaneous retractions appear – contractions which limit joint mobility. From the sixth to the ninth month the inflammation is stabilised and this stage is completed. Finally, these phenomena decrease, to be replaced by after-effects which persist when the inflammation has stopped. These phenomena occur on areas treated by directed cicatrisation, all the more if the cicatrisation was long, on the periphery of the grafts, the mesh grafts in net and sometimes on the donor sites.

Histologically, this maturation is marked by a hypervascularisation, anarchistic accumulation of collagen fibres, reduction in the apoptosis and the presence of myofibroblasts. The evaluation is difficult; it is carried out on the Vancouver scale and with the in vitro pressure test.

## Problems Arising from Burns

Various problems appear in the course of time. Oedema is present at the acute phase; it contributes to delay in scarring, stiffness, adherence and complicated rehabilitation. Pain decreases gradually; it must always be treated by analgesics during the three OMS stages; at the time of dressing, baths, use of interfaces under the bandages, techniques of distraction and mixed $NO_2/O_2$ often help the patient's comfort. Itching is very frequent, and leads to scratching wounds, which delays the pressure therapy and often disturbs sleep. This can be decreased by antihistaminic drugs, but it is sometimes necessary to use benzodiazepines. Pressure therapy, thread-like showers and hydration of the skin reduce this manifestation. Inflammation appears precociously at the time of scar maturation; it causes redness of the skin – more or less intense according to individual factors – thickness and induration of the burnt skin, which becomes hardbound. Hypertrophy can evolve to a cheloïd scar, a development which is facilitated by racial origin, topography and non-compliance with the treatment. To control these phenomena, we use pressure therapy and silicone gels; massage, thread-like showers and physiotherapy are auxiliary treatments. When hypertrophy is developing, a corticoid injection in the scar often brings an improvement.

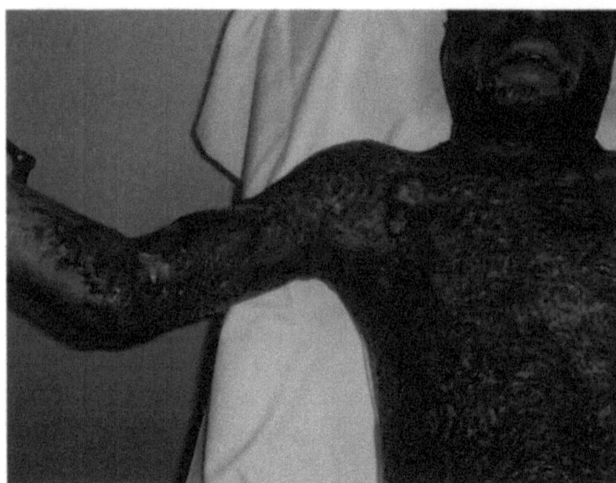

**Fig. 1.** Hypertrophic scar, contractures and wound on axilla and anterior face of elbow

These scars are responsible for aesthetic problems on the exposed parts, as cutaneous restrictions in the areas near a joint or around orifices and contractions limit mobility; in the adult patients these contractions sometimes produce capsular restrictions which are difficult to reverse (Fig. 1). Adherences in the deep planes can decrease the mobility of the skin. Here, massage, positioning and splints complete the pressure therapy.

Burns are sometimes responsible for algodystrophies or paraosteoarthropathies which increase the functional disorders. Secondary amputations are an additional incapacitating factor. Pigmentation can be affected, skin areas appearing hyper- or hypo-colorated. These changes in colour do not respond well to various therapies; only avoiding sunlight prevents their aggravation. Rehabilitation makes it possible to limit the aesthetic and functional after-effects, and thus to limit secondary surgical repair.

## Therapeutic Methods

Various methods of treatment exist and must be combined, depending on the state of the scar.

### Pressure Therapy

Pressure therapy is the basic treatment for burn scars; it decreases oedema and congestion, allows a better organisation of collagen fibres and a reduction in the number of myofibroblasts. An average pressure therapy is 24 mmHg with variations, according to the authors, from 5 to 50 mmHg. It is applied early as soon as the cicatrisation allows it. At the beginning, flexible compression is carried out by

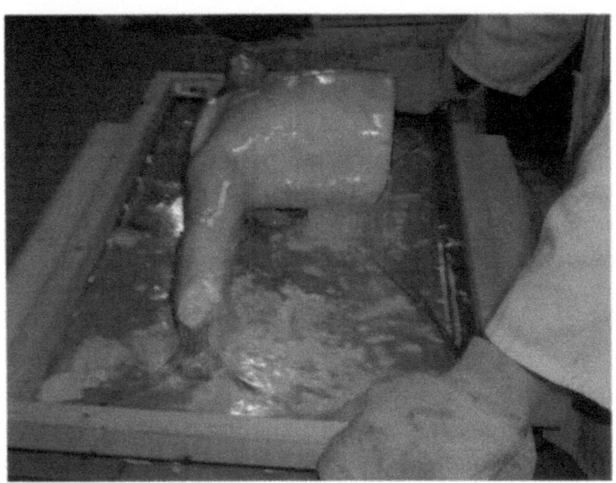

**Fig. 2.** Thoraco-brachial orthesis modelling

adhesive tapes (hypafix®, méfix®, etc.), cohesive elastic tapes (cohéban®, etc.), biflex tapes, tubular rubber bands (tournier bottu®, rocopress®, tubigrip®, etc.), pressure garments made in rehabilitation institutes or standard pressure garments. In the second phase, it is applied by final pressure garments (cicatrex®, medical Z®, céréplast®, jobst®, lymed ® etc); the fit of garment is determined using a measuring tape according to the manufacturers' specific indications. Pressure therapy is applied for 23 h a day.

Pressure therapy can also be rigid; it is then carried out starting from precise moulds, equipment being made in orlene® on a plaster positive. Here the pressure is applied perpendicularly to the skin and its effect can be controlled by the transparency of material. Its principal use is as a mask or facial conformator, but also in splints for the hand, splints applied to joint areas or folds for additional positioning and hyperhydration; this hypersudation may be uncomfortable for the patient.

Additions can be applied to improve pressure therapy: we use foam (varico®) or bandages (allevyn®); mineral oil copolymers (medigel®) or silicone gel (cicacare® etc.) have the effect of occlusion and thus of hyperhydration on the scar. To obtain good tolerance, it is recommended to increase the time of application gradually.

### Postures

Physiotherapists or the occupational therapists carry them out manually in a slow and progressive way to put the skin under maximum tension; the wearing of splints of the correct joint size completes them.

### Orthesis

Orthesis keeps the parts of limbs in good position to avoid deformation and improve mobility of the joints; they are made of thermoplastic materials or plaster by the occupational therapists (Fig. 2).

### Massage

Massage will be adapted to the state of the scar; at the beginning we apply hydrating or thermal creams, then according to the age of the scar and its state of inflammation, the intensity is increased by stretching, crushing operations, circular crushing, rolled pleat and Morice technique. To control the oedema, some teams apply lymphatic drainage very early. Massage will always be adapted to the state of the skin, but if it is too aggressive, it can increase the local inflammation.

### Physiotherapy

Physiotherapy is the treatment of the scar by physical agents. Medicalised compressed air is used in a child, in the early stages, to prepare with thread-like showers and to carry out a skin pleat and thus mobilise the skin compared to the underlying plan; the pressure is 8 to 10 kg/cm$^2$. Secondarily, when the skin is stronger, thread-like showers are used at higher pressure, 20 kg/cm$^2$ approximately, and make it possible to decrease itching, soften the scar, and drain the oedema; the risk from the showers is superficial wounds. These showers are carried out with water in the rehabilitation establishments or thermal water in the specific dermatological stations. Ultrasound makes it possible to control hypertrophy and induration in auxiliary treatment. Finally, vacuotherapy apparatuses help the therapist to carry out the rolled pleat operation , to mobilise the cutaneous plane on the underlying planes; this is applied after 45 days.

## Indications

### In the Acute-Care Centre

Rehabilitation is difficult to implement because of the requirements for reanimation; however, the fight against oedema can be begun early, if possible, with inclined positioning; retraction is prevented by mobilisation several times daily, manual postures associated to a good positioning of the parts of limbs. As soon as possible, autonomy must be ensured by early standing upright and walking practice, according to the topography of the burns with pressure garments on the lower limbs. The requirements of rehabilitation must thus be adapted to the reanimators' and the surgeons' requirements.

### After the Acute-Care Centre

Sometimes, two contradictory objectives must be combined to obtain cicatrisation and begin pressure therapy and rehabilitation. The control of hypertrophy begins with the early wearing of a flexible or rigid compressive garment together with the silicone gel, possibly the orlene® orthesis (pressure therapy and positioning), compressed air and, after the third month, thread-like showers. A combination of massage on the contraction, manual and orthesis positioning together with ultrasound and LPG, is used to treat the restrictions. To control adherences we use cutaneous mobilisation, positioning and active muscle training. Finally, the quality of life of the "survivors" needs psychological support, taking into account social problems, autonomisation and the demands of training.

When the inflammation is finished, the after-effects can be decreased by plastic surgery; this treatment by plastic surgery often requires secondary treatment by pressure therapy, physiotherapy and sometimes orthesis.

## Specific Problems of the Child

The treatment of children requires the participation of the family to obtain good compliance, teams specialised in child physiotherapy and an educational, social and pedagogical assistance; the psychomotrician and the speech therapist also play an important role. The treatment applied has effects on the growth, particularly on the facial skeleton; this element should not be forgotten and often a secondary orthodontic treatment is necessary. Finally, on the hands it can cause problems with change of laterality; there the positioning must be adapted and liberalised, accompanied by occupational therapy and psychomotor rehabilitation. The slower growth of the contractions compared to the healthy skin can increase deformations and require secondary repairing surgery.

## Conclusion

Post-burn care requires strict observance of the rehabilitation treatment to limit the after-effects of burns and secondary surgery acts; the co-operation of the patient or the child's family is fundamental to allow a good compliance of the treatment. A regular follow-up is essential to adapt the treatment to the evolution of the scars, especially when the child is young.

## References

1. Costa AM, Peyrol S, Porto LC, Comparin JP, Foyatier JL, Desmoulière A (1999) Mechanical forces induce in scar remodelling. Study in non-pressure treated hypertrophic scars. Am J Pathol 155: 1671–1679
2. Costagliola M, Rougé D, Gavroy JP, Ster F (1994) Quantitative and qualitative aspect of the vitro pressure test. 9. Congrès de l'International Society for Burn Injury, Paris, 27 Jun 1994
3. Descamp H, Baze Delecroix C, Jauffret E (2001) Rééducation de l'enfant brûlé. In: Kinésithérapie – Médecine physique – réadaptation, 26–275-D-10, Elsevier, Paris, p 10
4. Desmoulière A, Comparin P La cicatrice hypertrophique. JPC 7: 50–51
5. Poveda A, Campech M, Gavroy JP, Ster F (1998) Le massage «en brûlure»: formes topographiques et chronologiques. 18. Congrès de la Société Française d'Etude et de Traitement de la Brûlure, SFETB Saint Gervais 1998

6. Roques C (2002) Massage applied to scars. Wound Repair Regen 10: 126–128

7. Roques C (2002) Pressure therapy to treat burn scars. Wound Repair Regen 10: 122–125

8. Teot L, Griffe O, Brabet M, Gartner R, Léandris M (1995) Troubles de croissance, séquelles de brûlures chez l'enfant. In: Actualités SFETB. Editions Masson

9. Scott Ward R (1991) Pressure therapy for the control of hypertrophic scar formation after burn. Car Rehabil 12: 257–262

10. Staley MJ, Richard RL, Marlys J (1997) Use pressure to treat hypertrophic burn scars. Adv Wound Care 10: 44–46

11. Stewart R, Bhagwanjee AM, Mbakaza Y, Binase T (2000) Pressure garment adherence in adults patients with burn injuries: an analysis of patient and clinician perception. Am J Occup Ther 54: 598–606

# 46

# Compression Therapy

N. FRASSON

## Introduction

Compression is commonly used for the treatment of pathological scars (hypertrophy, inflammation). In the 17th century Ambroise Paré was the first who wrote on compression and described remedies for the deformity of scars (Johnson 1678): "If the scare is be too big, or high, it shall be plained by making convenient ligation and straddle binding to the part a plate of lead rubbed over with quick-silver..." [22].

The pioneering work on compression goes back to the years 1960–1970 and was published by the team of Shriner's Burns Institute, Galveston, under the control of Doctor Larson [21]. This work demonstrated that compression could have a positive effect on prevention and treatment of hypertrophic scars, so the first splints in thermoplastic material and the first pressure garments were made.

## Action Mechanism

The action mechanism of compression is still badly known. Hypoxy plays an important role in increasing the degradation of fibroblasts and myofibroblast which results in a reorganization of the extra-cellular matrix [4, 7, 15, 18, 27].

The most recent works in vitro suggest that the presence of PGE2 could be important for the normal process of repair, and low levels of PGE2 are possible key factors in the development of hypertrophy [30].

Production, release and activation of MMP-9 in hypertrophic scars could be responsible for hypertrophic regression induced by mechanical compression [29]. Finally, elastic compression was able to strongly increase apoptosis in the hypertrophic scar dermis [30].

## Method of Compression

Compression can be applied either by a pressure garment, temporary or definitive, or by a rigid thermoplastic splint. The correct pressure to exert in regard to the scar areas is not yet clear. Pressure measurement with pressure sensors gives different results from the in vivo use because of the great variations in pressure due to the anatomical site (bone, soft tissue etc.) [11, 14, 23, 33].

Pressure at ca. 15 to 20 mm of mercury appears sufficient to obtain an effective response on the scars [12].

The pressure applied obeys the law of Laplace; it is proportional to the tension of tissue and inversely proportional to circumference (P = T/C) [34]. The larger the diameter, the lower is the pressure. The concave areas are less compressed.

## Compression Tissue

Tissue compression can be provisional or definitive. It makes it possible to compress at an early stage and in patients who are not yet healed, while waiting for delivery of final clothing. Early compression (in the first 14 days) can decrease the pathological risk of scarring after a burn [13].

### Provisional Compression

#### Elastic Band

Provisional compression is carried out with elastic bands such as Koeban® and Thuasne®. Elastic binding makes it possible to begin compression on non-epidermised lesions. In addition to its compressive effect, it also allows a veno-lymphatic drain which supports the speed of cicatrisation [1].

Binding is performed according to different techniques. It always starts at the base from the toes, is rolled up the foot by, maintaining a constant pressure, and is taken around the ankle up to the knee in whorls, covering 2/3 or half of the preceding whorls.

Each whorl is parallel to the others, being tighter at the lower edge, and with more space on the upper.

#### Adhesive Band

Adhesive bands (Gazofix®) permit starting early compression and at the same time veno-lymphatic drainage on the hands [28]. They must be changed every day by an experienced kinesitherapist. This kind of compression can be accompanied by a dressing.

#### Tubular Bandage

Tubular band (Raucopress®, Tournier-Bottu®) is available as a roll of differing diameter and can be cut into the necessary length according to the scar to be compressed. This kind of band is sold by the metre. Its pressure effect decreases quickly and the tissue must be washed daily to preserve this effect.

*Standard Clothing*

Standard clothing (Thuasne®, Jobst®) permits starting with compression as soon as epidermisation has begun and while waiting for the final compression. By using initially less pressure than the final compression, the patient can be prepared for the final clothing.

## Custom-Fitted Garment

A custom-fitted garment starts as an epidermisation of the wounds, without any local trophic trouble (oedema) and when the patient's weight is stabilized. Taking the measurement is standardized according to the kind of clothing with some differences in manufacturing. (Jobskin®, Thuasne®, Medical Z®, Ottimedi®, Cereplast®) [2, 39]. The measurement is taken by measuring tape or slide calibre, and requires a certain experience. The first fitting must be made in the presence of the physician to ensure good adaptability of clothing (good tension tissue, good tolerance after a few hours, bleaching of the skin after removal) [32]. This clothing must be worn for 23/24 h during the period of scar healing (18 to 24 months).

## Rigid Compression

This is made on a mould and has to be perfectly adapted to the area to be compressed. This allows compression of difficult areas such as face, neck and thorax [9, 19].

### Thermoplastic Low Temperature

This is presented as a thermoplastic sheet (Polyflex®, Aquaplast®), heated in a drying oven at 70 or 80 °C and moulded on the pathological scar area (Fig. 1). It is used most of the time additionally under a compressive clothing to increase the pressure in a particular area [19, 33].

### Thermoplastic High Temperature

The moulding is made of orlene (heated up to 160 °C) on a plaster positive moulded on the patient (Fig. 2). Orlene is transparent and thus any bleaching of the compressed area can be seen. The positive allows increased compression in a particular area, especially in hypertrophy of the face [2, 9].

The conformator must be worn for 12/24 h since the maceration under this mask makes wearing it for 23/24 h impossible.

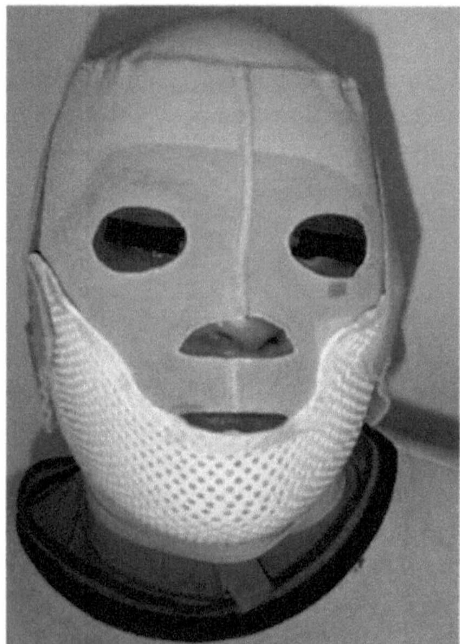

**Fig. 1.** Thermoplastic low temperature

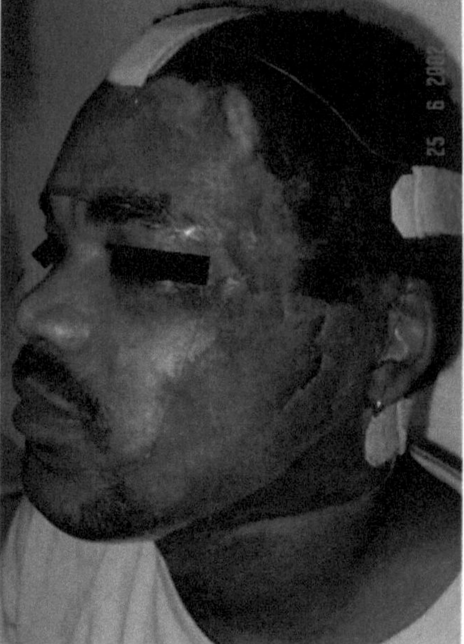

**Fig. 2.** Thermoplastic high temperature

## Interfaces

Interfaces are products used to increase the pressure on a hypertrophic area or to improve compression in areas difficult to compress. The materials used are foams of different density (Allevyn®, TP Foam®), neoprene, silicone (Cicacare®) or comparable material (Medigel®). Some foams are expanded (Cavicare®), compressing zones with a cavity. The sheets of silicone must be worn for at least 12 h each day – if possible even for 24/24 h, with washing twice a day [3].

## Indications

The principal indications are pathological scars, particularly hypertrophic postburn scars. Compression is used to improve the speed of cicatrisation, and especially because of its effect on the veno-lymphatic drain. It should also be used on scars of the face to decrease the risk of aesthetic damage. Compression must be continued until the scar is healed, which means for a period of 18–24 months.

## Secondary Effect

There is a risk of maceration under rigid compression which can involve wounds (desepidermisation by rubbing). Daily monitoring is indispensable. The wearing of compressive clothing is decisive in the patient's mobility and thus an important factor for a successful treatment [10, 17].

In rare cases, allergies to one of the components of the clothing are possible, and these endanger the continuation of treatment. Apnoea was described during face pressure in dental anomalies in children, but this remains exceptional [16, 20]. In patients with burns, in addition to the effect on cicatricial hypertrophy, compression decreases the pruritus.

## Conclusion

Compression remains the treatment of choice for pathological cicatrisations. It must be started as soon as possible even before complete epidermisation, using provisional and then final clothing. It must be correctly explained to the patient to improve his compliance during the long treatment. Interface addition is often useful to increase compression in a difficult area. Even today, the mechanisms of action are not completely understood. The regulation and the monitoring of compression, especially of rigid compression, must be rigorous and should be made by trained teams.

## References


1. Bardot J (1994) [Cutaneous cicatrix, natural course, anomalies and prevention]. Rev Prat 44: 1763–1768
2. Blaha J, Pondelicek I (1997) Prevention and therapy of post burn scar. Acta Chir Plast 39: 17–21
3. Borgognoni L et al. (2000) Hypertrophic scars and keloid: immunoprophenotypic features and silicone sheets to prevent recurrences. Ann Burn Fire Desasters 8: 164–169
4. Carr-Collins JA (1992) Pressure techniques for prevention of hypertrophic scar. Clin Plast Surg 19: 733–743
5. Brown CA (2001) A comparison of the outcomes of two clinical audits of burn pressure garment satisfaction and compliance in Saudi Arabia. Burns 27: 342–348
6. Chang P, Laubenthal KN, Lewis RW 2nd, Rosenquist MD, Lindley-Smith P, Kealey GP (1995) Prospective, randomized study of the efficacy of pressure garment therapy in patients with burns. J Burn Care Rehabil 16: 473–475
7. Cheng W, Saing H, Zhou H, Han Y, Peh W, Tam PK (2001) Ultrasound assessment of scald scars in Asian children receiving garment therapy. J Pediatr Surg 36: 466–469
8. Johnson J, Greenspan B, Gorga D, Nagler W, Goodwin C (1994) Compliance with pressure garment use in burn rehabilitation. J Burn Care Rehabil 15: 180–188
9. Dantzer E, Dias Garson MT, Queruel P (1995) [Device of the burnt face. Role of compression and splints. Ann Chir Plast Esthet] 40: 293–301

10. Gallagher JM, Kaplan S, Maguire GH, Leman CJ, Johnson P, Elbaum L (1992) Compliance and durability in pressure garments. J Burn Care Rehabil 13: 239–243

11. Gavroy et al. (1998) Un outil informatique d'assistance à la pressothérapie dans le traitement de la brûlure. Actualités SFETB brûlure Sauramps Médical, 246–250

12. Giele HP, Liddiard K, Currie K, Wood FM (1997) Direct measurement of cutaneous pressures generated by pressure garments. Burns 23: 137–141

13. Giele HP, Currie K, Wood FM, Hansen H (1995) Early use of pressure masks to avoid facial contracture during the pregrafting phase. J Burn Care Rehabil 16: 641–645

14. Giele H, Liddiard K, Booth K, Wood F (1998) Anatomical variations in pressures generated by pressure garments. Plast Reconstr Surg 101: 399–406; discussion 407

15. Hambleton J, Shakespeare PG, Pratt BJ (1992) The progress of hypertrophic scars monitored by ultrasound measurements of thickness. Burns 18: 301–307

16. Hubbard M, Masters IB, Williams GR, Chang AB (2000) Severe obstructive sleep apnoea secondary to pressure garments used in the treatment of hypertrophic burn scars. Eur Respir J 16: 1205–1207

17. Johnson J, Greenspan B, Gorga D, Nagler W, Goodwin C (1994) Compliance with pressure garment use in burn rehabilitation. J Burn Care Rehabil 15: 180–188

18. Johnson CL (1984) Physical therapists as scar modifiers. Phys Ther 64: 1381–1387

19. Jordan RB, Daher J, Wasil K (2000) Splints and scar management for acute and reconstructive burn care. Clin Plast Surg 27: 71–85

20. King SD, Blomberg PA, Pegg SP (1994) Preventing morphological disturbances in burn-scarred children wearing compressive face garments. Burns 20: 256–259

21. Larson z et al. (1970) Development and corrections of burn scar contracture. In: Matter P (ed) Transactions of the Third International Congress on Research in Burns. Hans Huber, Bern, p 403

22. Linares HA, Larson DL, Willis-Galstaun BA (1993) Historical notes on the use of pressure in the treatment of hypertrophic scars or keloid. Burns 19: 17–21

23. Mann R, Yeong EK, Moore M, Colescott D, Engrav LH (1997) Do custom fitted pressure garments provide adequate pressure. J Burn Care Rehabil 18: 247–249

24. Mann R, Yeong EK, Moore ML, Engrav LH (1997) A new tool to measure pressure under burn garment. J Burn Care Rehabil 18: 160–163; discussion 159

25. Palmieri TL, Kayden D, Greenhalgh DG (2000) The effect of medical insurance coverage on the obtainment of pressure garments. J Burn Care Rehabil 21: 414–416

26. Silfen R, Amir A, Hauben DJ, Calderon S (2001) Effect of facial pressure garments for burn injury in adult patients after orthodontic treatment. Burns 27: 409–412

27. Reid WH, Evans JH, Naismith RS, Tully AE, Sherwin S (1987) Hypertrophic scarring and pressure therapy. Burns Incl Therm Inj 13 [Suppl]: S29–32

28. Reiffel RS (1995) Prevention of hypertrophic scars by long term paper tape. Plast Reconstr Surg 96: 1715–1718

29. Reno F, Grazianetti P, Stella M, Magliacani G, Pezzuto C, Cannas M (2002) Release and activation of matrix metalloproteinase-9 during in vitro mechanical compression in hypertrophic scars. Arch Dermatol 138: 475–478

30. Reno F (2003) In vitro mechanical compression induces apoptosis and relate cytosines release in hypertrophic scars. Wound Repair Regen 11: 331–336

31. Reno F, Grazianetti P, Cannas M (2001) Effects of mechanical compression on hypertrophic scars: prostaglandin E2 release. Burns 27: 215–218

32. Rochet z (1998) Rééducation de l'adulte brûlé. In: Kinésithérapie Médecine Physique Réadaptation. Elsevier, Paris, p 27

33. Sawada Y (1993) Pressure developed under pressure garment. Br J Plast Surg 46: 538–541

34. Staley MJ, Richard RL (1997) Use of pressure to treat hypertrophic burn scars. Adv Wound Care 10: 44–46

35. Stewart R, Bhagwanjee AM, Mbakaza Y, Binase T (2000) Pressure garment adherence in adult patients with burn injuries: an analysis of patient and clinician perceptions. Am J Occup Ther 54: 598–606

36. Thompson R, Summers S, Rampey-Dobbs R, Wheeler T (1992) Color pressure garments versus traditional beige pressure garments: perceptions from the public. J Burn Care Rehabil 13: 590–596

37. Whitestone JJ, Richard RL, Slemker TC, Ause-Ellias KL, Miller SF (1995) Fabrication of total-contact burn masks by use of human body topography and computer-aided design manufacturing. J Burn Care Rehabil 16: 543–547

38. Wienert V (1999) Compression and treatment after burns. Wien Med Wochenschr 149: 581–582

39. Williams F, Knapp D, Wallen M (1997) Comparison of the characteristics and features of pressure garments used in the management of burns scars. Burns. 24: 329–335

# 47

# Frostbite: Current Concepts in Pathophysiology and Management

T.R. Palser, A.R. Barnard, P. Banwell

## Introduction and Historical Perspective

Frostbites are localised tissue injuries resulting from exposure to temperatures below the freezing point of skin. Their severity is proportional to the amount of heat lost from the tissues and is therefore related to both duration of exposure and the temperature gradient at the skin surface. Its consequences are serious, frequently resulting in permanent loss of function or amputation of the affected areas.

Historically, frostbite was almost exclusively a military problem, affecting armies throughout the ages. From the Roman Army manning Hadrian's Wall, through Napoleon's infamous retreat from Moscow in 1812, to the horrific winters on the Eastern Front in the Second World War, soldiers have suffered from cold injury. Even in the mechanised, modern environment of the Allied heavy bomber force in World War II, more injuries were inflicted by frostbite than by all other causes combined [1]. However, frostbite is now an increasing problem in the general civilian population.

## Epidemiology

Over the past two decades, increasing numbers of homeless people and the rising popularity of outdoor pursuits have increased the frequency of frostbite in the civilian population [2]. Several studies have identified the major risk factors for frostbite in civilians [3–6]. These are alcohol consumption (~46%), psychiatric illness (~17%), vehicular trauma (~19%), vehicular failure (~15%) and drug misuse (~4%).

Tissue damage is related to the length of time the tissue remains frozen. These risk factors generally exert their effect by increasing the duration of cold exposure or delaying presentation. Indeed, a retrospective review by Urschel [4] implicated impaired cerebral function as the major predisposing factor to frostbite in a civilian population. In her study, 53% of patients were under the influence of alcohol and 17% were psychiatrically ill. The role of psychiatric illness has been further explored: in one study of 20 cases all had overt or covert psychiatric disease [7]. This finding prompted the authors to perform a retrospective review, which placed the incidence of psychiatric illness in frostbite at between 61 and 65%. They therefore advocate psychiatric screening of all hospital admissions for frostbite [7].

Other factors that have been identified include homelessness, fatigue, lack of protective clothing or wet clothing, altitude above 17 000 feet, prior cold injury and outdoor activity lasting longer than 1 h [5, 6, 8–10]. Systemic conditions that decrease blood flow to the peripheries, such as peripheral vascular disease and tobacco smoking, have also been shown to increase the risk of tissue injury [5, 8]. Likewise, diabetes mellitus has been associated with frostbite, due both to its role in peripheral vascular disease [3], and to peripheral neuropathy reducing awareness of pain [4, 5].

The relationship between ambient temperature and the risk of frostbite has been shown by experimental studies and epidemiological observation. Danielsson found a linear relationship between frostbite risk and decreasing air temperature, with the risk being minor when air temperature was above –10 °C [12]. Below –25 °C, the risk was especially high, a conclusion confirmed by a retrospective study of frostbite injuries in Antarctica [10]. Both studies found wind velocity to be far less important [10, 12].

Males are far more susceptible to frostbite, probably due to social and occupational factors. The male-female ratio is 10:1 or more [5, 8]. Presumably for similar reasons, the peak incidence is between ages of 30 and 49 years (3, 6, 13–15]. As might be expected, hands and feet are most commonly affected, accounting for around 95% of all recorded injuries [5]. The other main sites are the head and neck and the perineum [3, 5, 6, 13–18].

The concept of physiological adaptation to cold is interesting but controversial. It is known that the vasoconstrictive response to cold decreases in fishermen who consistently work in freezing waters [19]. It has also been suggested that Eskimo people "feel the cold" less than others, although many authors believe that this is due to simple experience of arctic conditions [20, 21].

Likewise, although several studies have reported that individuals of African racial origin are more susceptible to freezing injuries than Caucasians, to state that this is for physiological rather than behavioural reasons can only be conjecture. Certainly, Eskimos freeze at the same rate as others in the same contact situation [22], and in Hashmi's study in the Karakoram Mountains, a large proportion of the patients were experienced local porters and guides [5]. With the exception of the "Fisherman's hand" phenomenon, there seems little convincing evidence that physiological adaptation to cold exists.

## Pathophysiology

The first description of the pathophysiology of frostbite was made by Baron Dominique Larrey, surgeon to Napoleon during the retreat from Moscow in 1812. He wrote: "The natural heat is absorbed and a discharge of caloric takes place, the pores close and the capillary vessels fall into a state of contraction; the fluids are condensed and flow more slowly [23]." During that horrendous campaign, Larrey had ample opportunity to study the condition and was the first to recognize similarities with burn injuries. He also noted the deleterious effects of the freeze-thaw-freeze cycle, in which men marching for continuous periods froze their feet, thawed them in the evening, and then refroze them the following day.

## Physiological Response to Cold

The initial response to cold is vasoconstriction, with cycles of transient vasodilatation at roughly 10-min intervals: the so-called "hunting reaction" [24]. This response warms the extremity and hence prevents frost damage. However, in releasing blood to the peripheries, core temperature falls, so at extremely cold temperatures the hunting response is blunted, leading to a critical temperature drop in the tissues. Freezing injury then follows.

Since Larrey's time, the pathogenesis of frostbite has been well investigated, but it still remains controversial. Several mechanisms have been recognised: direct cellular damage occurring at the time of freezing, indirect ischaemic necrosis secondary to vascular stasis [25–28] and reperfusion injury.

### Direct Cellular Damage

Direct cellular damage is due to the formation of extracellular ice crystals, which change the osmotic gradient across the cell membranes, directly damage the cell membrane and impede blood flow. The change in osmotic gradient is by far the most important as the resulting intracellular dehydration causes rising intracellular enzyme, electrolyte and protein concentrations, and hence cell death [29]. As the temperature falls further, intracellular ice crystals form and expand, contributing to cell death [30]. Most ice crystals form outside the vascular space, thus reducing circulating blood volume and increasing tissue ischaemia.

However, although ice crystallization definitely causes tissue damage, it does not account for the progressive tissue loss seen after cold injury. This was elegantly demonstrated by Weatherley-White, who transplanted frostbitten rabbit-skin grafts to normal recipients and vice versa [25]. The frostbitten grafts (which had undergone direct injury through ice crystallization) survived when applied to normal sites, whereas the uninjured tissue transplanted to frostbitten ears died. Therefore, indirect injury mechanisms are of crucial importance in the pathogenesis of frostbite. This is analogous to the process of "burn-depth progression" in thermal burn injuries.

### Post-Thaw Ischaemic Damage

Two causes of post-thaw ischaemia have been described: local arterial vasoconstriction [31, 32], and microcirculatory damage causing inflammation and progressive thrombosis [25, 33, 34].

### *Vasoconstriction*

Several studies have shown that inhibition of the sympathetic nervous supply to frostbitten areas can improve prognosis, using either sympathetic antagonists or surgical sympathectomy (see section Management below). This implies a significant vasospastic contribution to tissue loss in frostbite, a theory strengthened by studies showing increased tissue-blood flow following reserpine administration [35, 36].

Furthermore, vasoparalysis and sympathetic nerve degeneration was demonstrated in an experimental rabbit ear model by Arvesen et al. [37]. However, the exact nature and role of this vasospastic response is unclear, as sympathectomy performed within the first few hours of injury actually accelerates tissue destruction and worsens oedema [25, 38], while if performed 24–48 hours later, it appears to decrease tissue loss and hasten oedema resolution and ulcer healing [38]. Likewise, whether the vasoconstriction is due primarily to the sympathetic nervous system or to vasoconstricting cytokines such as thromboxane $A_2$ (see below), is unknown.

### Microcirculatory damage and the inflammatory response

Evidence for the role of the inflammatory response in frostbite comes from several sources. The successful clinical use of anti-inflammatory agents, such as acetylsalicylic acid and ibuprofen [39–41], is supported by experimental studies, which show that inhibition of the inflammatory response is beneficial in animal frostbite models [42, 43]. Inflammatory mediators such as thromboxane have also been demonstrated in frostbite-blister fluid [44].

There are two arms to this inflammatory reaction: the humoral response, mediated by inflammatory mediators, and the cellular response, mediated primarily by neutrophils.

**Humoral Response.** The initial investigations into the role of inflammatory mediators stem from studies into the pathophysiology of thermal burn injuries. The progressive ischaemic necrosis that occurs in frostbite shows definite similarities to that seen in burns [39, 44], and there is considerable evidence of the role of inflammatory mediators (e.g. prostaglandins, thromboxanes and bradykinin) in burn pathophysiology. These similarities prompted Robson and Heggers to investigate frostbite blister fluid. They found markedly elevated levels of prostaglandin $F_{2\alpha}$ and thromboxane $B_2$ (a stable metabolite of thromboxane $A_2$) [44]. Both molecules are known to mediate dermal ischaemia in burns and pedicle flaps [45–48]; levels of prostaglandin E (a vasodilator and platelet anti-aggregant) were also decreased. Supporting this, a study in rabbits found increased levels of prostaglandin $I_2$ [49],which is anti-thrombogenic. Importantly, however, this increase (188%) was significantly lower than the increase in thromboxane $B_2$ (249%). Further evidence supporting the role of eicosanoids comes from the demonstration that inhibitors of eicosanoids significantly improve dermal perfusion, tissue survival and prognosis in both burn and frostbite injuries [40].

**Cellular Response.** In addition to the humoral response described above, there is evidence that the extravasation of neutrophils at the injury site worsens tissue damage. This is likely to occur both at the time of acute injury and later following reperfusion [50]. It is well established that neutrophils (PMN) are an integral part of the acute inflammatory response [51], and mediate tissue damage through the production of oxygen-free radicals and destructive enzymes [52, 53]. It is known that the numbers of PMN increase in frostbitten tissue [54], and their importance was first demonstrated by Manson et al., who showed that superoxide dismutase (a free radical scavenger enzyme) given at thawing reduced tissue damage in the rabbit ear model [55]. This was reinforced by Mileski et al., who used a monoclonal antibody to block neutrophil aggregation and neutrophil-endothelial cell adherence. This resulted in significantly reduced oedema and tissue loss compared to control animals [42].

Further, albeit indirect, evidence comes from other conditions in which ischaemic tissue damage is followed by reperfusion. For example, neutrophils are thought to be increasingly important in burns [56–58], and they are also believed to have a significant role in the reperfusion injury seen after myocardial infarction [59–61].

The inflammatory response appears to be triggered by damage to endothelial cells. Marzella et al. used the classic rabbit ear model and electron microscopy to investigate the vascular endothelium in frostbite [54]. They found that within an hour of freezing, the entire microvasculature of the affected area showed endothelial damage. This triggered two processes crucial in the pathophysiology of frostbite: inflammation as described above with leukocyte adhesion and oedema formation, and the clotting cascade with thrombosis and platelet aggregation. Histological changes characteristic of inflammation followed [54].

These studies therefore support the hypothesis that the progressive tissue loss seen in frostbite is due, at least in part, to an imbalance between the pro-thrombotic, pro-inflammatory cytokines (such as thromboxane $A_2$ and $PGF_{2\#a\#}$) and the anti-aggregant, anti-inflammatory cytokines (such as $PGI_2$) [49]. This imbalance is triggered by endothelial damage and leads to an inflammatory reaction (with leukocyte adhesion and oedema formation) and intravascular thrombosis (along with platelet aggregation). Combined, these two mechanisms lead to intravascular arrest and progressive dermal ischaemia. Modification of this balance (for example by thromboxane inhibitors) could reduce this tissue loss.

## Clinical Presentation and Classification of Frostbite Injuries

Historically, classification of frostbite was based on clinical observations and was similar to that of burn injuries [50, 62–64]. However, this system could not predict the extent of tissue ischaemia, and so was not useful for predicting prognosis [65, 66]. There are two main reasons for this. Firstly, as described above, frostbite is a progressive injury that continues to evolve after re-warming. Secondly, it damages deeper structures such as soft tissue and bone, as well as the skin [67, 68]. Therefore, any classification scheme based purely on initial surface appearance will be inherently inaccurate, because it does not take into account these two factors.

Workers in France have therefore recently suggested a new classification scheme based on both clinical appearance and the results from early two-phase bone scans [65], which investigate the level of viability. They claim three advantages over previous schemes: firstly, earlier prediction of final outcome is possible. Secondly, the approximate level for amputation is known at day 2 as opposed to after several weeks, and thirdly they believe that the new scale can be used to manage the patient even in a non-specialist setting. However, it is not in widespread use due to widespread concerns regarding the imaging modality [67–71]. Further studies are awaited to confirm the validity of this system.

Chillblains represent a mild form of cold injury that should be considered separately from true frostbite [72]. They consist of itchy, red lesions, usually on the dorsum of the foot and are self-limiting. Rest and moisturising lotions may accelerate recovery. True frostbite damages the affected tissues in even its mildest forms.

## Radiological Evaluation

As described above, clinical examination is very poor at predicting the necessity and degree of surgical debridement. In addition, there is often a discrepancy between skin lesions and the damage to underlying structures. As a result, there is usually a "holding" period of between 1 and 6 months before amputation is advised [73–75], resulting in great psychological stress for the patient, a long, expensive hospital stay, a significantly increased risk of infection and often substantially delayed and impaired rehabilitation [50, 71, 76]. Several imaging techniques have therefore been used in attempts to provide early, accurate assessment of tissue viability and more speedily delineate the level of injury, thus improving early management. These techniques include plain radiographs, angiography, magnetic resonance imaging and radioisotope scanning.

Plain radiographs are of little use in the acute setting, as bony changes are not evident for several weeks and are of no use in determining the ultimate level of demarcation [30, 50, 77]. Xenon (Xe) 133 injections have been used to try and define the extent of soft-tissue injury, but cannot assess bone perfusion, are complicated by the presence of subcutaneous adipose tissue and require highly specialised personnel for the interpretation of the results. Also, the technique is not suitable for use in fingers, as the injection of the xenon fluid may compress the blood vessels, causing a tourniquet effect and worsening tissue ischaemia [50, 76, 78]. Fluorescein is easy to use, but is unreliable in this setting [79]. Angiography, used early post-injury, does not sufficiently clarify levels of viability, and does not appear to be useful in early management [80]. It may be used to define the limits of vascular injury [81] but does not allow the imaging of vessels at arteriolar or capillary levels [50]. Likewise, although digital plethysmography and Doppler ultrasonography accurately assess local blood flow, neither technique is able to assess the microcirculation; Doppler studies are also highly operator-dependent [71].

Technetium (Tc)-99 scintigraphy has become the standard imaging technique for the assessment of the extent of tissue damage [67–70]. Two techniques of technetium scanning have been described: two-stage and triple-phase scanning. Two-phase bone scanning has been advocated for the purpose of predicting amputation risk. Cauchy et al. reported that a scan performed 3 days post injury has a sensitivity for bone necrosis of 98%, which allows early reassurance for the patient. This sensitivity is further improved by a second scan on day 7, which also helps to determine the eventual level of amputation (positive predictive value 84%) [82].

However, other authors advocate triple phase scanning (arterial phase, venous phase and bone-pool images), which allows evaluation of the microcirculation of both bone and soft tissue. Using this technique, Mehta and Wilson [76] found 3 patterns of frostbite injury:

- Essentially normal blood and bone pool images.
- No blood pool but normal bone uptake images.
- No blood pool and no bone uptake

In the first case, both the soft tissue and bone are viable. In the second case, bone is viable but the soft tissues are not; this may later lead to bone necrosis and full amputation. In the latter case, both bone and soft tissues are necrotic and amputation is inevitable.

The area of lack of bone uptake was found to delineate the extent of bone infarction very accurately (confirmed histologically following amputation [68]). This accuracy in the early evaluation of tissue viability enables different management strategies to be followed, something that was not possible with earlier techniques. This shall be further discussed in the "Surgical Management" section below.

Finally, MRI and magnetic resonance angiography (MRA) have also been employed in frostbite. Barker et al. compared the MR techniques to Tc-99 scanning in two patients, and found them to be superior by allowing direct visualisation of occluded vessels and surrounding tissues [83]. Interestingly, they found the level of demarcation of ischaemic tissue to be more distinct using this modality. However, there are some problems with the technique. The fact that the fingers and toes contain little or no striated muscle may limit the technique to more proximal injuries [84], and there is also a cost implication. As the study by Barker et al. is the only study so far reported, further work is required before definite conclusions can be drawn.

## Management

The management of cold injury is extremely controversial, with only a few principles being universally accepted. Treatment can be broadly divided into three phases: pre-thaw field care, management in the emergency department, and post-thaw care that continues for several weeks or months (see below).

### Early Management

- Pre-thaw field care stage
  - Resuscitate
  - ATLS survey
  - Keep extremity frozen during transport
  - Pad and splint to protect the limb, but avoid rubbing.

- Emergency department care
  - Refer to specialist Burns Unit (if possible).
  - Resuscitate and stabilise according to ATLS guidelines
  - Rapid re-warming in a waterbath with antibacterial agent (aim for 40–42 °C)
  - Continue until vasoconstriction resolves (approx. 30 min)
  - Commence post-thaw care

### Pre-thaw Field Care

The initial management of frostbite is focused on protecting the injured tissues and on avoiding thawing until definitive, rapid re-warming can be performed in hospital. Repeated thawing and freezing or inadequate re-warming will worsen the injury [30, 50, 85], so during transport, the extremity must be kept frozen. Rubbing the affected tissue with hands or snow, once the mainstay of treatment, does not actually augment local blood flow and may cause mechanical trauma [41, 86]. It should be padded and splinted for protection, but no other treatment for the injured limb should be initiated. Since frostbite may be associated with hypothermia and other forms of trauma, a rapid ATLS survey should be carried out and any necessary resuscitation (e.g. with warm intravenous fluid) carried out.

### Emergency Department Management

Ideally, all patients should be admitted to a specialised treatment centre, usually a burns unit. The initial management is the stabilisation of the patient according to the standard ATLS guidelines. In particular, close attention should be made to the patient's fluid balance. The hypothermic patient may exhibit a cold diuresis due to suppression of antidiuretic hormone secretion at low temperatures [87]. In addition, cases of rhabdomyolysis and subsequent renal failure have been reported in frostbite patients [88].

When the patient is stabilised, definitive and rapid re-warming should take place [39, 50, 62]. It is only since the second world war that the importance of re-warming a frostbitten extremity rapidly has been appreciated [64]. Before then, it had been believed that rapid re-warming would increase the metabolic demands of the tissue to an extent that would increase, rather than limit, the level of tissue necrosis [26].

Studies by Fuhrman and Crimson [89, 90], and later by Finneran and Schumacker [91] have shown this not to be the case. Both experimental evidence and clinical experience have indicated that the definitive temperature for re-warming is 40–42 °C [39, 50, 62, 92]. Re-warming should be done by placing the extremity in a waterbath, containing a mild anti-bacterial agent (povidone-iodine or hexachlorophene) at this temperature. Close attention should be paid to ensure that this temperature range adhered to as re-warming at lower temperatures is less beneficial to tissue survival, while re-warming at higher temperatures may worsen the injury by producing a burn injury [64]. Re-warming should continue for around 30 min to ensure complete thawing. A red/purple appearance and pliable texture of the involved body part signal the end of vasoconstriction and are signs that re-warming should cease [86, 93].

### Post-Thaw Care

Post-thaw care can be broadly divided into two categories: medical and surgical. We will discuss each in turn although it should be emphasised that a combined approach is usually necessary.

**Medical Management of Frostbite.** Re-warming reverses the direct effects of ice-crystal formation within the tissue but does not prevent the progressive dermal ischaemia seen in the post-thaw phase, and may actually contribute to it. The first definitive management algorithm based upon frostbite pathophysiology was the "Chicago protocol" published two decades ago by McCauley et al., that forms the basis of many specialist unit protocols [40]. However, several points warrant discussion (see below).

> **New Suggested Algorithm for the Medical Management of Frostbite**
>
> 1. Debride white blisters but leave haemorrhagic blisters intact
> 2. Institute topical aloe-vera treatment every 6 hours
> 3. Elevate the affected part
> 4. Administer anti-tetanus prophylaxis
> 5. Analgesia: opiate, intravenously or intramuscularly as indicated
> 6. Administer ibuprofen 400 mg orally every 12 h
> 7. Perform daily hydrotherapy for 30–45 min at 40 °C
> 8. Prohibit smoking
> 9. Refer for psychiatric screening
> 10. Strongly consider
>     - LMW dextran
>     - Thrombolysis
>     - Topical negative pressure
>     - Hyperbaric oxygen therapy
>     - Antibiotic prophylaxis

White blisters represent superficial damage and require immediate debriding to prevent further exposure to the high levels of prostaglandin F2A and thromboxane A2 in the inflammatory exudates. However, haemorrhagic blisters represent damage to the superficial dermal plexus and the management of these is controversial. Some authors recommend that they should also be excised, for the reasons that it allows rehabilitation to begin earlier (thus limiting functional sequelae), and that it decreases the risk of local superinfection, which can lead to septic shock [82, 94]. However, the act of excision itself carries a risk of infection and also introduces the risk of dessication. As a result, most [13, 30, 95] although not all [82, 86] authors recommend that they are left intact. Unfortunately, there is little clinical data supporting either method. This dilemma is similar to that encountered in burn management.

The Chicago protocol includes aspirin as a systemic antithromboxane agent [39, 85]. However, the appropriate dose has not been established [22], and aspirin also inhibits the synthesis of some prostaglandins that are beneficial to wound healing [39]. Ibuprofen has therefore superseded aspirin as the drug of choice [2, 9, 50, 86].

Elevation and the subsequent minimisation of oedema is beneficial for two reasons: Firstly, oedema formation has been implicated in the pathogenesis of progressive dermal ischaemia [96–98]; secondly, oedema has been found to inhibit the skin's own streptococcicidal properties.

Most centres use penicillin prophylactically to reduce the risk of superimposed streptococcal infection [9, 13, 39, 50], but some authors reserve antibiotics for specific infectious complications [2]. One retrospective review of 125 patients found that prophylactic antibiotics did not decrease the incidence of wound infection [3].

The regime of daily hydrotherapy has two functions: aiding debridement of devitalized tissues [39, 86] and, most importantly, maintaining active and passive ranges of movement. It has been shown to be essential for the preservation of function [99].

Many adjunctive therapies not included in the Chicago protocol have also been used to improve tissue survival. These are discussed below.

**Psychiatric Screening.** Psychiatric illness is a very strong risk factor for cold injury [3, 4, 7] with up to 65% of patients having some form of psychiatric illness. Thus psychiatric screening seems wise [7].

**Low-Molecular Weight Dextran.** Studies in other thromboembolic diseases have shown that haemodilution improves blood flow by decreasing the haematocrit and hence the viscosity of the blood. It also decreases the coagulability of the blood and hence reduces intravascular thrombosis [99–101]. It was therefore suggested that low-molecular weight (LMW) dextran may be effective in reducing the dermal ischaemia and hence the degree of tissue necrosis. Although still to be confirmed by clinical trials, some excellent animal studies have demonstrated significantly reduced tissue loss following LMW dextran administration [25, 102]. It is therefore an extremely promising new therapy and should be considered.

**Thrombolysis.** The importance of intravascular thrombosis and the resulting dermal ischaemia in the pathogenesis of frostbite [25, 34] (see above) has led to suggestions that thrombolytic agents may be an effective treatment for cold injury. Investigations in animal models showed striking improvements in the degree of tissue survival, even when begun 12–24 h after injury [103]. So far, the only clinical data is from a small pilot study in 1992 in which ten patients received supportive treatment only (as described above), while four others received infusions of tissue plasminogen activator. All ten patients in the control group had amputations at or near the level of vascular cut-off. In contrast the thrombolysed group showed significant reperfusion distal to the vascular cut-off level, and three of the four patients avoided surgery altogether [104]. These studies are inconclusive, but certainly present thrombolysis is a very promising new treatment option, which (like haemodilution) may actually alter the condition's prognosis.

**Topical Negative Pressure.** Topical Negative Pressure (TNP) is a novel, non-pharmacological method of enhancing wound healing that has been shown to improve the prognosis of many different types of injury. These include traumatic injuries [105, 106] (also those involving open tibial fractures [107] and large skin/muscle loss [105, 108]), pressure ulcers [109, 110], abdominal wound dehiscence [111–113], post-sternotomy infections [114] and, most relevantly, thermal burn injuries [107]. The role of tissue ischaemia in burns and frostbite has been discussed above; it is interesting therefore that in an experimental deep dermal burn model, TNP was shown to significantly increase dermal blood flow [115]. Furthermore, TNP diminished the inflammatory response [116] and prevented the progression of partial thickness wounds [117]. It was also shown to significantly improve the survival of skin flaps [118], which could have an impact on surgery for limb salvage. Its use in frostbite care is yet to be reported, but it is a novel therapy with a sound experimental basis, that is of proven benefit in the treatment of many other wounds. Its use should be strongly considered.

**Anticoagulation.** Since thrombosis is observed in the superficial dermal plexus in the first few days after thawing, it was suggested that anti-coagulation would be a possible treatment for frostbite. Unfortunately, despite investigation [119] there is no evidence that heparin or any other anti-coagulant alters the natural history of frostbite [22].

**Sympathectomy.** As discussed above, there is a significant vasospastic component in the pathogenesis of frostbite. While the exact role of regional sympathectomy remains controversial, there is good evidence that pain resolution, sensation return, gangrene demarcation and ulcer healing is more rapid following surgical sympathectomy [8, 38, 120, 121]. Several studies (e.g. Golding et al.) evaluated the operation by performing unilateral sympathectomy in patients with bilateral injuries. The sympathectomised side was less painful, had less oedema and an improved rate of healing compared with the control side [38]. The timing of the procedure is especially controversial. Experimentally, sympathectomy within the first few hours in creases oedema formation and worsens tissue loss [25, 38]. If delayed until 24–48 h, the operation appears to be beneficial [38]. Some authors advocate even later intervention [121]. A randomised control trial is needed to determine the indications and timing of sympathectomy. It should be emphasised, however, that none of these studies found that sympathectomy decreased tissue loss, so although it appears highly effective for symptomatic relief, it appears to be ineffective in improving the prognosis.

**Hyperbaric oxygen.** Hyperbaric oxygen (HBO) therapy was first reported by Ledingham in 1963 [122]. Although based on outdated concepts of frostbite pathophysiology, it does increase local oxygen tension and so may abrogate the tissue

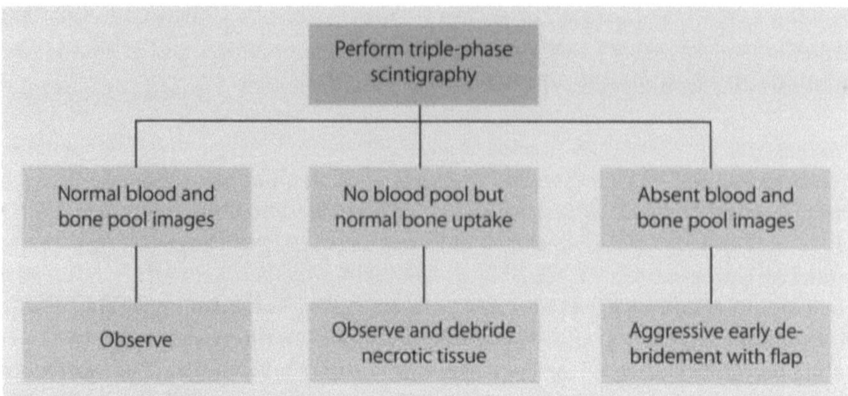


**Fig. 1.** Algorithm for the surgical management of frostbite. (Adapted from Greenwald et al. [71])

ischaemia. Numerous case reports suggest an apparent benefit [122–126], although control data are few. Animal experiments have been contradictory [127–130]. However, in one recent report, laser Doppler flowmetry and vital capillary microscopy were used to measure local blood flow, which indicated that HBO therapy seemed to improve the local microcirculation [126]. Since only one patient was involved, results should be interpreted cautiously. Again, no definite conclusions can be drawn about HBO therapy due to the lack of data, but it certainly seems worthy of further investigation.

### Surgical Management of Frostbite

Traditionally, frostbite has been managed conservatively, with surgery delayed until mummification and tissue demarcation has occurred. This takes many months and is the source of the adage "frostbite in January, amputate in July". Early surgical intervention involved only escharotomy (or fasciotomy in the rare cases of secondary compartment syndrome). Traditionally, the disadvantages of delay seemed outweighed by the risk of losing potentially viable tissue.

However, with the advent of triple-phase scintigraphy, which can provide early, accurate assessment of tissue viability [71, 76], many authors advocate an aggressive surgical approach to patients with severe injuries [69, 70, 76, 131–133]. In patients for whom aggressive surgical management is advocated, the aim is to restore blood supply to devascularised bone, thereby avoiding amputation and restoring function. Salimi et al. showed new bone formation around necrotic areas and the ingrowth of osteocytes, demonstrating that the structural integrity of bone may be preserved if surrounded by viable tissue [131].

Surgery involves debridement of avascular soft tissues and immediate closure of the defect with well-vascularised soft-tissue flaps. The new blood supply to the underlying tissues should prevent frank necrosis, preserving limb length and optimising eventual recovery. Several case reports exist where amputation was avoided or minimised [69, 70, 131, 132]. Flaps have also been shown to aid salvage of tissues rendered avascular by high-dose local radiation injury [134] and electrical injury [135]. Based on these results, Greenwald et al. devised an algorithm for the surgical management of frostbite (Fig. 1) [71], which we strongly advocate.

## Late Sequelae

Frostbite has a poor long-term prognosis with around 20% of patients having some form of chronic disability [136]. Most commonly this is residual pain and cold intolerance, mainly due to vasomotor dysfunction resulting from ischaemic neuropathy. Other late sequelae are localised osteoporosis, joint contracture, skin atrophy and hyperhidrosis [50, 137, 138]. In children, epiphyseal closure is a particularly serious complication as it commonly leads to growth limitation or angular deformity, and therefore to functional impairment [139, 140].

## Conclusion

The incidence of frostbite injury in the civilian population is increasing. Knowledge of frostbite management is therefore crucial for physicians in both rural and urban areas. Research over the past 20 years has led to a greater understanding of the pathophysiology of frostbite, particularly of the importance of inflammatory mediators in intra-vascular thrombosis and dermal ischaemia. As a result, new management strategies designed to combat this process have evolved. New imaging methods allow early delineation of the extent of necrosis, and aggressive surgical management is now a realistic strategy. For the first time in the history of frostbite treatment, surgery can now be aimed at the salvage, rather than just the amputation, of necrotic tissue. Other novel pharmacological and non-pharmacological techniques have also made an impact. Although the limited numbers of patients involved in trials mean that controversy still exists in many areas, frostbite management is now aimed at altering the wound environment and therefore at improving prognosis, rather than merely limiting damage.

## References

1. Dembert ML, Dean LM, Noddin EM (1981) Cold weather morbidity among US Navy and Marine Corps personnel. Mil Med 146: 771–775
2. Edlich RF, Chang DE, Birk KA et al. (1989) Cold injuries. Compr Ther 15: 13–21
3. Valnicek SM, Chasmar LR, Clapson JB (1993) Frostbite in the prairies: a 12 year review. Plast Reconstr Surg 92: 633–641

4. Urschel JD (1990) Frostbite: predisposing factors and predictors of poor outcome. J Trauma 30: 340–342

5. Hashmi MA, Rashid M, Haleem A et al. (1998) Frostbite: epidemiology at high altitude in the Karakoram mountains. Ann R Coll Surg Engl 80: 91–95

6. Boswick JA, Thompson JD, Jonas RA (1979) The epidemiology of cold injury. Surg Gynecol Obstet 149: 326–332

7. Pinzur MS, Weaver FM (1997) Is urban frostbite a psychiatric disorder? Orthopedics 30: 43–45

8. Kysola K (1974) Clinical experiences in the management of cold injures: a study of 100 cases. J Trauma 14: 32–36

9. Bracker MD (1992) Environmental and thermal injury. Clin Sports Med 11: 419–436

10. Cattermole TJ (1999) The epidemiology of cold injury in Antarctica. Aviat Space Environ Med 70: 135–140

11. Candler WH, Ivey H (1997) Cold weather injuries among US soldiers in Alaska: a 5 year review. Mil Med 162: 788–791

12. Daanielsson U (1996) Windchill and the risk of tissue freezing. J Appl Physiol 91: 2666–2673

13. Pulla RJ, Pickard LJ, Carnett TS (1994) Frostbite: an overview with case presentations. J Foot Ankle Surg 33: 53–63

14. Antti-Poika I, Pohjolainen T, Alaranta H (1990) Severe frostbite of the upper extremities: a psychosocial problem mostly associated with alcohol abuse. Scan J Soc Med 18: 59–61

15. Hermann G, Schecter DC, Owens JC (1963) The problem of frostbite in civilian medical practice. Clin North Am 43: 519–536

16. Lehmuskallio E, Lindholm H, Koskenvuo K et al. (1995) Frostbite of the face and ears: epidemiological study of risk factors in Finnish conscripts. BMJ 311: 1661–1663

17. Rosen L, Eltvik L, Arvesen A et al. (1991) Local cold injuries sustained during military service in the Norwegian Army. Arctic Med Res 50: 159–165

18. Ervast E (1969) Frostbite of the extremities and their sequelae. Acta Chir Scand 299: 1–69

19. Nelms JD, Soper DJ (1962) Cold vasodilatation and cold acclimatization in the hands of British fish filleters. J Appl Physiol 12: 444–448

20. Vaughn PB (1980) Local cold injury: menace to military operations. Mil Med 145: 305–309

21. Taylor MS, Kulungowski MA, Hamelink JK (1989) Frostbite injuries during winter manoeuvres: a long-term disability. Mil Med 154: 411–413

22. McCauley RL, Smith DJ, Robson MC et al. (1995) Frostbite and other cold-induced injuries. In: Auerbach PS. ed. Wilderness Medicine 3rd edn. Mosby, St Louis, pp 129–145

23. Larrey DJ (1814) Memoirs of military surgery and campaigns of the French armies. Cushing, Baltimore, pp 156–164

24. Lewis T (1930) Observations upon the reaction of vessels of human skin to cold. Heart 15: 177–208

25. Weatherly-White RC, Sjostrom B, Paton BC (1964) Experimental studies in cold injury II: the pathogenesis of frostbite. J Surg Res 4: 17–22

26. Weatherly-White RC, Sjostrom B, Paton BC (1965) Experimental studies in cold injury III: observations on the treatment of frostbite. Plast Reconstr Surg 36: 10–18

27. Quintanilla R, Krusen FH, Essex HE (1947) Studies on frostbite with special reference to treatment and the effect on minute blood vessels. Am J Physiol 149: 149–161

28. Granberg PO (1991) Freezing cold injury. Arctic Med Res 50 [Suppl 6]: 76–79

29. Meryman HT (1956) Mechanics of freezing in living cells and tissues. Science 124: 515–521

30. Heggers JP, Robson MC, Manavalen K et al. (1987) Experimental and clinical observations on frostbite. Ann Emerg Med 16: 1056–1062

31. Rakower SR, Shahgoli S, Wong SL (1978) Doppler ultrasound and digital plethysmography to determine the need for sympathetic blockage after frostbite. J Trauma 18: 713

32. Snider RL, Porter JM (1975) Treatment of experimental frostbite with intra-arterial sympathetic blocking drugs. Surgery 77: 557

33. Reite OB (1965) Functional qualities of small blood vessels in tissue injured by freezing and thawing. Acta Physiol Scand 63: 111

34. Bourne MH, Piepkorn MW, Clayton F et al. (1986) Analysis of microvascular changes in frostbite injury. J Surg Res 40: 26

35. Espinosa GA (1981) Management of frostbite injuries. J Nat Med Assoc 73: 1125–1131

36. Porter JM, Wesche DH, Rosch J et al. (1976) Intra-arterial sympathetic blockade in the treatment of clinical frostbite. Am J Surg 132: 625–630

37. Arvesen A, Meahlen J, Rosen L et al. (1999) Early and late functional and histopathological perturbations in the rabbit ear artery following local cold injury. Vasa 28: 85–94

38. Golding MR, DeJong P, Sawyer PN et al. (1963) Protection from early and late sequelae of frostbite by regional sympathectomy: Mechanism of "cold sensitivity" following frostbite. Surgery 53: 303–308
39. McCauley RL, Hing DN, Robson MC et al. (1983) Frostbite injuries: a rational approach based on the pathophysiology. J Trauma 23: 143–147
40. McCauley RL, Hing DN, Robson MC et al. (1983) Frostbite injuries: a rational approach based on the pathophysiology. J Trauma 23: 143–147
41. Vogel JE, Dellon AL (1989) Frostbite injuries of the hand. Clin Plast Surg 16: 565–576
42. Mileski WJ, Raymond JF, Winn RK et al. (1993) Inhibition of leukocyte adherence and aggregation for treatment of severe cold injury in rabbits. J Appl Physiol 74: 1432–1436
43. Raine TJ, London MD, Goluch L (1980) Antiprostaglandins and antithromboxanes for treatment of frostbite. Surg Forum 31: 557–559
44. Robson MC., Heggers JP (1981) Evaluation of hand frostbite blister fluid as a clue to pathogenesis. J Hand Surg (Am) 6: 43–47
45. Heggers JP, Ko F, Robson MC et al. (1980) Evaluation of burn blister fluid. Plast Reconstr Surg 65: 798–804
46. Heggers JP, Loy GL, Robson MC et al. (1980) Histological demonstration of prostaglandins and thromboxanes in burned tissue. J Surg Res 28: 110–117
47. Robson MC, Del Beccaro EJ, Heggers JP (1979) The effects of prostaglandins on the dermal microcirculation after burning and the inhibition of the effect by specific pharmacological agents. Plast Reconstr Surg 63: 781
48. Del Beccaro EJ, Robson MC, Heggers JP (1980) The use of specific thromboxane inhibitors to preserve the dermal microcirculation after burning. Surgery 87: 137
49. Ozyazgan I, Tercan M, Melli M et al. (1998) Eicosanoids and inflammatory cells in frostbitten tissue: prostacyclin, thnromboxane, poloymorphonuclear leukocytes, and mast cells. Plast Reconstr Surg 101: 1881–1886
50. Su CW, Lohman R, Gottlieb LJ (2000) Frostbite of the upper extremity. 16: 235–247
51. Baumann H, Gauldie J (1994) The acute phase response. Immunol Today 15: 74–80
52. Weiss SJ (1989) Tissue destruction by neutrophils. N Engl J Med 320: 365–376
53. Badwey JA, Karnovsky ML (1980) Active oxygen species and the functions of phagocytic leukocytes. Annu Rev Biochem 49: 695–726
54. Marzella L, Jesudass RR, Manson PN et al. (1989) Morphologic characterization of acute injury to vascular endothelium of skin after frostbite. Plast Reconstr Surg 83: 67–76
55. Manson PN, Jesudass R, Marzella L et al. (1991) Evidence for an early free radical-mediated reperfusion injury in frostbite. Free Radic Biol Med 10: 7–11
56. Tyler MP (1998) A study of acute leukocyte extravasation in human burns [ChM Thesis]. Aberdeen University, United Kingdom
57. Eriksson E, Straube R, Robson MC (1979) White blood cell consumption in the microcirculation after a major burn. J Trauma 19: 94–97
58. Xia ZF, Hollyoak M, Barrow RE et al. (1995) Superoxide dismutase and liepeptin prevent delayed reperfusion injury in the rate small intestine during burn shock. J Burn Care Rehabil 16: 111–117
59. Hansen PR (1998) Inflammatory alterations in the myocardial microcirculation. J Mol Cell Cardiol 30: 2555–2559
60. Engler RE (1989) Free radical and granulocyte-mediated injury during myocardial ischaemia and reperfusion. Am J Cardiol 63: 19E–23E
61. Hansen PR (1995) Role of neutrophils in myocardial ischaemia and reperfusion. Circulation 91: 1872–1885
62. Murphy JV, Banwell PE, Roberts AH et al. (2000) Frostbite; pathogenesis and treatment. J Trauma 48: 171–178
63. Orr KD, Fainer DC (1952) Cold injuries in Korea during Winter of 1950–1951. Medicine 31: 177–220
64. Mills WJ, Whaley R, Fish W (1960) Frostbite: experience with rapid re-warming and ultrasonic therapy. Alaska Med 2: 114–122
65. Cauchy E, Chetaille E, Marchand V et al. (2001) Retrospective study of 70 cases of severe frostbite lesions: a proposed new classification scheme. Wild Environ Med 12: 248–255
66. Mills WJ (1993) Summary of treatment of the cold injured patient; frostbite. Alaska Med 35: 61–66
67. Lisbona R, Rosenthall L (1976) Assessment of bone viability by scintiscanning in frostbite injuries. J Trauma 16: 989–992
68. Mehta RC, Wilson MA (1989) Frostbite injury: prediction of tissue viability with triple-phase bone scanning. Radiology 170: 511–514

69. Ikawa G, dos Santos PA, Yamaguchi KT et al. (1986) Frostbite and bone scanning: the use of 99m-labelled phosphates in demarcating the line of viability in frostbite victims. Orthopedics 9: 1257–1261

70. Salimi Z (1985) Frostbite: assessment of tissue viability by scintigraphy. Postgrad Med 77: 133–134

71. Greenwald D, Cooper B, Gottlieb L (1998) An algorithm for early aggressive treatment of frostbite with limb salvage directed by triple-phase scanning. Plast Reconstr Surg 102: 1069–1074

72. Duffill MB (1993) Milker's chillblains. N Z Med J 24: 101–103

73. Christenson C, Stewart C (1984) Frostbite. Am Fam Physician 30: 111–122

74. Page RE, Robertson GA (1983) Management of the frostbitten hand. Hand 15: 185–191

75. Knize DM, Weatherly-White RC, Paton BC et al. (1969) Prognostic factors in the management of frostbite. J Trauma 9: 749–759

76. Mehta RC, Wilson MA (1989) Frostbite injury: prediction of tissue viability with triple phase bone scanning. Radiology 120: 511–514

77. McCauley RL, Heggers JP, Robson MC (1990) Frostbite: Methods to eliminate tissue loss. Postgrad Med 88: 67–68

78. Sumner DS, Boswick JA, Criblez TL et al. (1971) Prediction of tissue loss in human frostbite with xenon-133. Surgery 69: 899–903

79. Ristkari SK, Vorne M, Mokka RE (1988) Early assessment of amputation level in frostbite by $^{99m}$Tc-pertechnate scan. Acta Chir Scand 154: 403–405

80. Purdue GF, Hunt JL (1986) Cold injury: a collective review. J Burn Care Rehabil 7: 331–342

81. Gralino BJ, Porter JM, Rosch J (1976) Angiography in the diagnosis and therapy of frostbite. Radiology 110: 301–305

82. Cauchy E, Marsigny B, Allamel G et al. (2000) The value of technetium 99 scintigraphy in the prognosis of amputation in severe frostbite injuries of the extremeties: a retrospective study of 92 severe frostbite injuries. J Hand Surg 25A: 969–978

83. Barker JR, Haws MJ, Brown RE et al. (1997) Magnetic resonance imaging of severe frostbite. Ann Plast Surg 38: 275–279

84. Fleischmann W, Becker U, Bischoff M et al. (1995) Vacuum sealing: indication, technique and results. Eur J Orthop Surg Traumatol 5: 37–40

85. Washburn B. Frostbite (1962) N Engl J Med 266: 974–989

86. Britt LD, Dascombe WH, Rodriguez A (1991) New horizons in the management of hypothermia and frostbite injury. Surg Clin North Am 71: 345–370

87. Broman M, Kallskog O, Nygren K et al. (1998) The role of antidiuretic hormone in cold-induced diuresis in the anaesthetized rat. Acta Physiol Scand 162: 475–480

88. Schechter DS, Sarot RA. Historical accounts of injuries due to cold. Surgery 1968;63:527–530

89. Fuhrman F, Crimson JN (1947) Studies on gangrene following cold injury, VII: rapid re-warming after injury. J Clin Invest 6: 476–479

90. Fuhrman F, Crimson JN (1947) Studies on gangrene following cold injury, II: the general course of events in rabbits' feet and ears after cold injury. J Clin Invest 26: 236–242

91. Finneran JC, Shumacker HG (1950) Studies in experimental frostbite, V; further evaluation of early treatment. Surg Gynecol Obstet 90: 4–10

92. Entin MA, Baxter H (1952) The influence of rapid re-warming on frostbite in experimental animals. Plast Reconstr Surg 9: 511–515

93. Fritz RL, Perrine DH (1989) Cold exposure injuries: prevention and treatment. Clin Sports Med 8: 111–128

94. Marsigny B (1998) Mountain frostbite. The Newsletter of the International Society for Mountain Medicine 8: 8–10

95. Reamy BV (1998) Frostbite: review and current concepts. J Am Board Fam Pract 11: 34–40

96. Zawacki BE (1974) The natural history of reversible burn injury. Surg Gynecol Obstet 139: 867–872

97. Boykin JV, Eriksson E, Pittman RN (1980) In vivo microcirculation of a scald burn and the progression of postburn dermal ischaemia. Plast Reconstr Surg 66: 191–198

98. Remensnyder JP (1972) Topography of tissue oxygen tension changes in acute burn oedema. Arch Surg 105: 477–482

99. Borgo J, Chevreaud C, Laxenaire MC et al. (1983) Hemodilution et prevention de la maladie thromboembolique post-operatoire. Agressologie 24: 621–627

100. Chevreaud C, Thouvenot P, Durdin D et al. (19686) Hemodilution normovolemique intentionelle dans la traitement medical de l'arterite des members inferieurs. Annales Francaises d'Anesthesie-reanimation 5: 223–228

101. Oriani G, Sacchi C, Borghi B (1995) From low hematocrit physiology to isovolemic hemodilution. Int J Artif Organs 18: 143–149

102. Martinez-Villen G, Garcia Bescos G, Rodriguez Sosa V et al. (2002) Effects of haemodilution and rewarming with regard to digital amputation in frostbite injury: an experimental study in the rabbit. J Hand Surg (Br) 27B: 224–228

103. Salimi Z, Wolverson MK, Herbold DR et al. (1987) Treatment of frostbite with streptokinase: an experimental study in rabbits. Am J Roentgenol 149: 773–776

104. Skolnick AA (1992) Early data suggest clot-dissolving drugs may help save frostbitten limbs from amputation. JAMA 267: 2008–2010

105. Argenta LC, Morykwas MJ (1997) Vacuum-assisted closure: a new method for wound control and treatment: clinical experience. Ann Plast Surg 38: 563–576

106. Mullner T, Mrkonjic L, Kwasny O et al. (1997) The use of negative pressure to promote the healing of tissue defects: a clinical trial using the vacuum sealing technique. Br J Plast Surg 50: 194–199

107. Banwell PE, Teot L (2003) Topical negative pressure (TNP): the evolution of a novel wound therapy. J Wound Care 12: 22–28

108. Banwell PE (2002) The Role of TNP in Burns. 2nd European Vacuum Therapy Symposium. Salisbury, UK, June 2002

109. Azad S, Nishikawa H (2002) Topical negative pressure may help chronic wound healing. BMJ 324: 1100

110. Baynham SA, Kohlman P, Katner HP (1999) Treating stage IV pressure ulcers with negative pressure therapy: a case report. Ostomy Wound Manag 454: 25–28

111. Garner GB, Ware DN, Cocanour CS et al. (2001) Vacuum-assisted closure provides early fascial re-approximation in trauma patients with open abdomens. Am J Surg 182: 630–638

112. Erdmann D, Drye C, Heller L et al. (2001) Abdominal wall defect and enterocutaneous fistula treatment with the Vacuum-Assisted Closure (VAC) system. Plast Reconstr Surg 1087: 2066–2068

113. Bonnamy C, Hamel F, Leporrier J et al. (2000) Use of the vacuum-assisted closure system for the treatment of perineal gangrene involving the abdominal wall. Ann Chir 125: 982–984

114. Giovannini UM, Demaria RG, Otman S et al. (2002) Treatment of post-sternotomy wounds with negative pressure. Plast Reconstr Surg 1095: 1747

115. Banwell PE, Morykwas MJ, Jennings DA et al. (2000) Dermal microvascular blood flow in experimental partial thickness wounds: the effet of sub-atmospheric pressure. J Burn Care Rehabil 21: s161

116. Banwell PE, Morykwas MJ, Jennings DA et al. (1999) Application of topical sub-atmospheric pressure modulates inflammatory cell extravasation in experimental partial thickness injury. Wound Rep Regen 74: A287

117. Morykwas MJ, David LR, Schneider AM et al. (1999) Use of subatmospheric pressure to prevent progression of partial thickness burns in a swine model. J Burn Care Rehabil 201: 15–21

118. Morykwas MJ, Argenta LC, Shelton-Brown EI et al. (1997) Vacuum-assisted closure: a new method of wound control and treatment: animal studies and basic foundation. Ann Plast Surg 38: 553–562

119. Schumaker HB (1947) Studies in experimental frostbite: the effect of heparin in preventing gangrene. Surgery 22: 900–905

120. DeJong P, Golding MR, Sawyer PN et al. (1962) The role of regional sympathectomy in the early management of cold injury. Surg Gynecol Obstet 115: 45–48

121. Schumaker HB (1951) Sympathectomy in the treatment of frostbite. Surg Gynecol Obstet 93: 727–734

122. Ledingham I (1963) Some clinical and experimental applications of high pressure oxygen. Proc Roy Soc Med 56: 999–1002

123. Perrin ER, Bossinnette R (1965) Frostbite: a new adjunct in treatment. JAMA 194: 99

124. Ward MP, Garnham JR, Simpson BR et al. (1968) Frostbite: general observations and report of cases treated by hyperbaric oxygen. Proc Roy Soc Med 61: 787–789

125. von Heimburg D, Noah EM, Sieckmann UP et al. (2001) Hyperbaric oxygen treatment in deep frostbite of both hands in a boy. Burns 27: 404–408

126. Finderle Z, Cankar K (2002) Delayed treatment of frostbite injury with hyperbaric oxygen therapy: a case report. Aviat Space Environ Med 73: 392–394

127. Gage AA, Ishikawa H, Winter PM (1970) Experimental frostbite: the effects of hyperbaric oxygen on tissue survival Cryobiology 7: 1–8

128. Hardenburgh E (1972) Hyperbaric oxygen treatment of experimental frostbite in the mouse. J Surg Res 12: 34–40

129. Obukoye JA, Ferguson CC (1968) The use of hyperbaric oxygen in the treatment of experimental frostbite. Can J Surg 11: 78–84

130. Gage AA, Ishikawa H, Winter PM (1969) Experimental frostbite and hyperbaric oxygenation. Surgery 66: 1044–1050

131. Salimi Z, Wolverson MK, Herbold DR et al. (1986) Frostbite: experimental assessment of tissue damage using Tc-99 m pyrophosphate. Radiology 161: 227–231

132. Leonard LG, Daane SP, Sellers DS et al. (2001) Salvage of avascular bone from frostbite with free tissue transfer. Ann Plast Surg 46: 431–433

133. Classen DA (2000) Free flap coverage of bilateral frostbite of the feet. Plast Reconstr Surg 106: 1316–1320

134. Krizek TJ, Ariyan S (1973) Severe acute radiation injuries of the hands. Report of two cases. Plast Reconstr Surg 51: 14–22

135. Hartford CE (1989) Preservation of devitalized calvarium following high-voltage electrical injury: case reports. J Trauma 29: 391–394

136. Orr KD, Fainer DC (1952) Cold Injuries in Korea during winter of 10501951. Medicine 31: 177–220

137. Suri ML, Vijayan GP, Puri HC et al. (1978) Neurological manifestations of frostbite. Indian J Med Res 67: 292–299

138. Tischler JM (1972)The soft-tissue and bone changes in frostbite injuries. Radiology 102: 511–513

139. Bigelow DR, Ritchie GW (1963) The effects of frostbite in childhood. J Bone Joint Surg Br 45(B): 122–131

140. Reed MH (1988) Growth disturbances in the hands following thermal injuries in children 2. Frostbite. J Can Assoc Radiol 39: 95–99

# VIII Treatment of Scaring

# Fundamental Aspects of Extracellular Matrix

R.H. DEMLING

## Introduction

It has been well established that an extracellular matrix in the dermis containing active dermal elements, is critical for the orchestration of a normal healing process, and the absence of dermal elements will lead to excess scar [1–4]. The role of the extracellular matrix, responsible for orchestration of healing, can be divided into its structural component and its biologically active component.

## Structural Function

The scaffolding or structure of the matrix is made up of the collagen lattice, mainly collagen type I and ground substance [5–8]. Collagen is the major building block of connective tissue, accounting for 30% of total body protein [5–7]. The mature collagen fibre found in dermis is composed of collagen units which form a very strong filament. The fibres are formed outside the fibroblast, oriented by matrix signals and through proteoglycan contact. Of the many types of collagen, type I is the most abundant in normal skin. Type III is less pliable and more common in scar [5–7]. Besides dermal structure, type I provides a contact orientation for dividing and migrating epithelial cells. This cell-guidance system allows for a more organised, less abundant scar. Elastin, another structural protein, provides elasticity.

The matrix or ground substance is composed of glycosylated proteins found both on cell surfaces and in the extracellular tissue space [5–9]. Other key factors include hyaluronic acid and heparin sulphate produced by the fibroblast. The glycosaminoglycans (GAGs) are polysaccharides composed of repeating disaccharide units. The GAGs are attached to a core protein producing a proteoglycan. Chondroitin sulphate and heparin sulphate are two such matrix elements. Glycosaminoglycans (GAGs) are essential for normal dermal structure and function. Functions of the ground substance include a scaffold for protein deposition, a conduit for nutrients, a de-activator of proteases and a guidance system for cell migration.

## Biologically Active Matrix Function

A number of biologically active compounds are present in matrix which direct the healing process. The main active components are fibronectin, hyaluronic acid and growth factors [10–14].

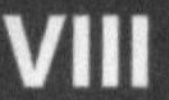



Fibronectin is an adhesion protein, produced mainly by fibroblasts and macrophages. It is a large glycoprotein found in all tissues and plasma [11, 12]. One of its key functions is as an attachment protein for skin cells via collagen type I. In addition, this protein is the key adherence molecule attaching epithelial and endothelial cells at cell junctions. Fibronectin also stimulates epithelial cell migration, spreading and orientation, as well as acting as a chemoattractant for fibroblasts.

Hyaluronic acid (HA) is a major carbohydrate component composed of a simple repeated disaccharide in a co-polymer structure [16, 17]. Hyaluronic acid, in its native macromolecular form, does provide a structural property. However, it also affects cell behaviour by directing proper cell alignment. HA is also found as fragments which have direct actions on all dermal cells, affecting all phases of wound healing through receptor-binding events [16, 17].

## Dermal Matrix Components

- Collagen (protein)
    - Scaffold for cell migration and matrix deposition
    - Cell guidance
- Elastin (protein)
    - Tissue elasticity
- Glycosaminglycan (glycosylated protein)
    - Cell adherence properties
    - Conduit for healing factors
    - Deactivator of proteases
    - Scaffold or foundation for dermal elements
- Fibronectin (protein)
    - Cell to cell adherence
    - Contact orientation for cells
    - Increases epithelial cell division, migration
    - Chemoattractant for fibroblasts, macrophages
- Hyaluronic acid (complex carbohydrate)
    - Maintaining matrix moisture
    - Decreases inflammation
    - Stimulates healing
    - Proper cell alignment
- Growth factors (proteins)
    - Stimulate all phases of wound healing

The healing process within the matrix is also directed by a group of macrophage-produced polypeptides (protein fragments). These polypeptide growth factors have many actions including the stimulation of cell proliferation and cell migration [18–21]. These messages cause the cells to react to product structures. For example, these messages cause epithelial cells to produce epidermis and cause fibroblasts to make collagen.

A large variety of polypeptide growth factors have been identified and named [20]. Although each has a predominant function on a specific cell, it now appears that essentially all growth factors have a multitude of actions. Monocytes and macrophages are thought to be the main producers of growth factors; however, all skin cells, including fibroblasts and keratinocytes, play an important role in secreting growth factors.

Once formed, the growth factors can be rapidly deactivated by wound proteases; i.e. those released from white cells, mainly neutrophils. The wound is activated to produce excess proteases, probably in an attempt to break down surface dead tissue. Surface exudates developing on an open wound are a rich source of such proteases, especially the class of metalloproteases.

## Collagen-Matrix Products

Because of the importance of the extracellular matrix in healing, a number of collagen-matrix products have been developed which are designed to restore some of the dermal-like properties when placed on a clean, usually full-thickness, wound bed [22, 23]. The addition of these dermal-like properties should allow for a more normal healing process, thereby potentially decreasing scar, while also maintaining a moisture layer on the wound bed. Most of the matrix wound dressings provide a simple collagen scaffold to help organise new tissue formation [21, 22]. New cells can migrate on the collagen fibres into the healing wound. The addition of a glycosaminoglycan component provides absorptive properties as well as providing a conduit for nutrients to the new wound tissue [24]. The collagen used in most products is denatured so that the active biological properties are missing. Only the structural properties remain. The collagen is usually incorporated into the wound bed over a matter of days.

A unique wound matrix product has been developed from porcine small intestinal submucosa (OASIS® Wound Matrix – Healthpoint) [26–29]. This tough wound matrix contains biologically active collagen type I in a natural lattice form. In addition, the matrix contains biologically active glycoproteins, fibronectin and growth factors including fibroblast growth factors. Application onto a full-thickness wound bed provides a more natural matrix-like layer which incorporates into the wound in several days and should lead to less scar with more rapid re-epithelialisation from the edges or, in the case of a partial-thickness wound, from the wound bed itself. Preliminary data from clinical trials have demonstrated a more rapid wound-healing rate in full-thickness venous and diabetic ulcers compared to standard of care [30].

Providing an extracellular matrix-like layer to a full-thickness wound bed should improve healing and help control scarring, especially if the components maintain the biological activity of normal dermal elements.

## References


1. Raghow R (1994) The role of extracellular matrix in post inflammatory wound healing and fibrosis. FASEB J 8: 823–831
2. Badylak SF (2002) The extracellular matrix as a scaffold for tissue reconstruction. Cell Develop Biol 13: 377–383
3. Verani J, Nickoloff B, Riser B, Mitra R, Dixit V (1988) Regulation of keratinocyte motility and proliferation by extracellular matrix components and cytokines. FASEB 2: 1821
4. Makatsuki T (2003) Reciprocal interactions between cells and extracellular matrix during remodeling of tissue constructs. Biophys Chem 100: 593–605
5. Park S (2003) Biological charaterization of EDC-crosslinked collagen hyaluronic acid matrix in dermal tissue reconstruction. Biomaterials 24: 1631–1641
6. Pilcher B (1998) Collagenase 1 and collagen in epidermal repair. Arch Dermatol Res 290: 37–46
7. Woodley D (1985) Cutaneous wound healing: a model for cell-matrix interactions. J Am Acad Dermatol 12: 420–433
8. Soloman D (2002) An in vitro examination of an extracellular matrix scaffold for use in wound healing. Int J Exp Pathol 83: 209–216
9. Suzuki K et al. (2003) Cell matrix and cell-cell interactions during epithelial wound healing. Prog Retin Eye Res 22: 113–133
10. Donaldson D, Mahan J (1983) Fibrinogen and fibronectin as substrates for epidermal cell migration during wound closure. J Cell Sci 62: 117–127
11. Mudera V (2002) Evidence for sequential utilization of fibronectin, vitronectin and collagen during fibroblast mediated collagen contraction. Wound Repair Regen 10: 397–408
12. Sottile J (2002) Fibronectin polymerization regulates the composition and stability of extracellular matrix fibrils and cell-matrix adhesion. Mol Biol Cell 10: 3546–3469
13. Sclmidinger G (2003) Effect of tenascin and fibronectin on the migration of human corneal fibroblasts. J Cataract Refract Surg 29: 354–360
14. Posposilov J, Reibelov V (1986) Fibronectin – its significance in wound re-epithelialization. Acta Chir Plast 28: 96–102
15. Pieper JS, Hafmans T, van Wachem PB, van Luyn MJ, Brouwer LA, Veerkamp JH, van Kuppevelt TH (2002) Loading of collagen-heparan sulfate matrices with bFGF promotes angiogenesis and tissue generation in rats. J Biomed Mater Res 62: 185–194
16. Chen W (1999) Functions of hyaluron in wound repair. Wound Rep Regen 7: 79–89
17. Noble P (2002) Hyaluron and its catabolic products in tissue injury and repair. Matrix Biology 21: 25–29
18. Frazur K (1996) Stimulation of fibroblast cell growth, matrix production and granulation tissue formation by connective tissue growth factor. J Invest Dermatol 107: 404–411
19. Ignotz R (1986) Transforming growth factor beta stimulates the expression of fibronectin and collagen and their incorporation into the extracellular matrix. J Biol Chem 261: 4337–4345
20. Robson M (1998) The future of recombinant growth factors in wound healing. Am J Surg 176: 80–82
21. Marks M (1991) Effect of fibroblasts and basic fibroblast growth factor on facilitation of dermal wound healing by type I collagen matrices. J Biomed Mater Res 25: 683–696
22. Jones I, Currie L, Martin R (2002) A guide to biologic skin substitutes. Br J Plast Surg 55: 185–193
23. Boykin J, Molnar J (1992) Burn scar and skin equivalents in wound healing. In: Cohen K, Deigelmann I (eds) Wound Healing. WB Saunders, Philadelphia
24. Yamas I, Burke J, Orgill D (1982) Wound tissue can utilize a polymeric template to synthesize a functional extension of skin. Science 215: 174–178
25. Heimbach D, Luterman A, Burke J et al. (1988) Artificial dermis for major burns. A multicenter randomized clinical trial. Ann Surg 208: 313–320
26. Hodde JP, Badylak SF, Brightman AO et al. (1996) Glycosaminoglycan content of small intestinal submucosa: a bioscaffold for tissue replacement. Tissue Engineering 2: 209–217
27. McPherson TB, Badylak SF (1998) Characterization of fibronectin derived from porcine small intestinal submucosa. Tissue Engineering 4: 75–83
28. Hodde JP, Hiles MC (2001) Bioactive FGF-2 in sterilized extracellular matrix. Wounds 13: 195–201
29. Chen W (1999) Functions of hyaluron in wound repair. Wound Rep Regen 7: 79–89
30. Demling R, Niezgoda J, Haraway G, Mostow E (2004) Small intestinal submucosa wound matrix and full-thickness venous ulcers; preliminary results. Wounds 16: 18–22

# Prevention of Excessive Scar Formation – a Surgical Perspective

R.H. Demling

## Introduction

Scar is defined as the normal process of repairing a wound with new collagen deposition instead of restoring the normal architecture of the lost tissue [1–3]. Hypertrophic or proliferative scarring is excessive scar formation over and above the required scarring for normal healing.

## Characteristics and Causes of Excess Scaring

The characteristics of proliferative or hypertrophic scar are shown in the list below. Proliferative scar in a cutaneous wound is characteristically red, raised, rigid and painful. Itching is also common on stretching. Increased collagen content is evident. In addition, there is more random orientation and less cross-linking of the collagen present. Type-III collagen is also more prominent compared to type-I collagen in the well-healed wound [1–5].

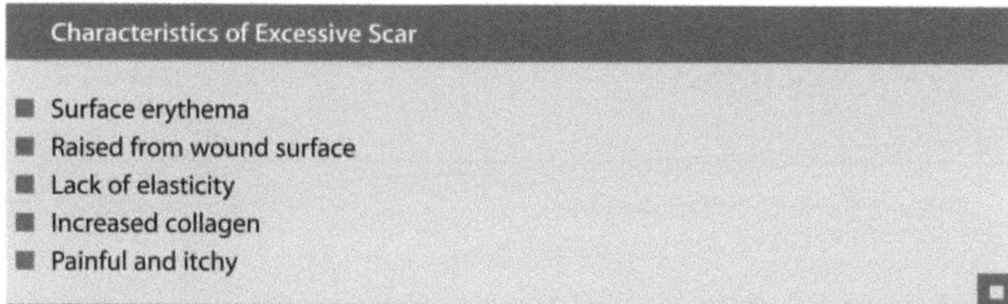



Hypertrophic or proliferative scar is seen in approximately 50% of wounds after surgery and more than 50% in healed deep burns. The increased scar is particularly prominent around joints, where tension is more common.

There are a number of recognised causes of excess scarring (see list next page). This list in turn leads to a number of potential preventative measures [1–9].

The causes most readily manipulated are tension on the wound edges during healing, excess inflammation, wound remaining open for a prolonged period and lack of any dermal elements to help orchestrate normal healing.

## Causes of Proliferative Scar in a Cutaneous Wound

- Tension on the wound
- Excess inflammation in wound bed
    - Inflammatory stimulus
    - Infection
    - Foreign body
- Wound open for more than 3 weeks
- Lack of dermal elements
- Genetic predisposition

## Tension at the Wound Edges

Tension at the wound edges has long been recognised as a factor causing increased scar production [1–4]. The mechanism is multifactorial. First of all, tension leads to a decrease in microvascular blood and nutrient flow to the wound, prolonging the healing process and resulting in increased fibroplasias. Local immune defences will be impaired by the decreased blood flow, leading to the risk of infection and further inflammation. There also appears to be a stimulation of excess collagen deposition in response to continued wound tension.

Avoiding tension is an obvious preventative measure. In cases where some tension is inevitable, techniques such as deep-tissue suture or zipper support or procedures such as Z plasty appear to decrease the amount of scar.

## Wound Surface Inflammation

Excess wound inflammation caused by a number of factors will delay the normal healing process and accentuate scar formation [5–7]. The status of the wound bed will dictate the degree of surface inflammation. Increased surface and matrix metalloproteases oxidants and other mediators of inflammation result in a continued breakdown of new tissue and stimulate fibroplasia.

## Causes of Excess Wound Inflammation

- Chronic open wound
- Surface necrosis or desiccation
- Infection, increased bacterial burden
- Foreign body, sutures

Any noxious stimulus to the wound, as described above, will accentuate the inflammatory response [10–12].

Exaggeration of the inflammatory phase, in an open or infected wound or burn, increases the concentration of growth factors known to produce increased fibroblast numbers and excess amounts of collagen and extracellular matrix [5, 7]. These growth factors include fibrosis growth factor, transforming growth factor B, platelet-derived growth factor and, most importantly, transforming growth factor (TGF-B). This cytokine, released with inflammation, appears to trigger the cell–cell and cell–matrix interactions, leading to excessive scar [5–13].

Increased mast cells leading to increased release of histamines, known to stimulate growth of fibrous tissue as well as other vasoactive mediators, are also present in proliferative scar compared to normal healing [14, 15].

An excess and prolonged neovascularisation is also found. This process leads to granulation tissue formation, which corresponds with excess collagen in the wound bed. Fibroblasts are also found in increased numbers in granulation tissue, leading to increased collagen deposition as well as an abnormal matrix [3, 4, 16]. These fibroblasts are more sensitive to growth factors compared to normal skin. Increased and persistent levels of chondroitin sulphate are present, located in the nodular areas of excess collagen, leading to a more rigid scar [17, 18]. Chondroitin increases water content, which increases scar firmness. A decrease in interferons and cytokines, that downregulate collagen and matrix synthesis, is also noted [5, 19]. This abnormality leads to less collagenolysis and less matrix degradation with remodelling.

---

**Strategies for Controlling Wound Inflammation**

- Early wound closure
  - Definitive coverage
  - Addition of dermal elements
- Controlling environmental insults
  - Moist healing
  - Early debridement
  - Infection control
- Pharmacologic control of inflammation

---

Early removal of necrotic tissue and maintenance of a moist wound bed will significantly decrease inflammation and fibroplasia. The importance of maintaining a surface moisture layer in the healing process has been well recognised. This approach also helps to improve surface immune defences (see above).

An actual infection, defined by bacterial invasion of normal tissue, is not necessary in order to negatively impact healing [10, 22]. The term excessive bacterial burden is now used to describe the deleterious effect of surface bacteria. The bacterial content, which can cause tissue fibroplasia and impair re-epithelialisation, varies with the wound and the host. Delayed healing is often the best measure of excess wound bacteria. Topical anti-microbials are indicated in this case.

There are a number of potential pharmacological approaches which can be used to control inflammation. Non-steroidal anti-inflammatory agents have been shown to decrease fibrosis through inhibition of IL-1 and prostanoids, known to stimulate fibrosis [23].

Anti-histamines have been shown to be effective not only in controlling pruritus, but also in suppressing histamine-induced tissue proliferation [24]. Some newer anti-allergic drugs also inhibit the release of histamine and prostanoids from wound mast cells [23].

Corticosteroids are the main agents in the protein synthesis inhibitor category [25]. These agents, when injected into scar, decrease fibroblast proliferation, decrease angiogenesis and inhibit collagen synthesis and also extracellular matrix protein synthesis. Complications include pain on injection, thinning of surrounding skin, systemic absorption and recurrence of scar at a later date.

Interferons are known to reduce the production of TGF-$\beta$, the major scar forming growth factor. Both intravenous and intralesion injections of interferon have shown significant clinical benefits in reducing hypertrophic scar. Popularity to date is hampered by high cost and unfamiliarity with this approach. Agents that inhibit collagen cross-linking would decrease scar rigidity and collagen deposition. The most promising agent in this category is topical putrescine, which has been reported to decrease hypertrophic scars with no side effects.

## The Open Wound

A wound which is open for more than 3 weeks has a much greater incidence of sub sequent proliferative scarring [26, 27]. This process is particularly evident in the burn wound [26, 27]. The mechanism is clearly multifactorial. Clearly, the open wound has a greater risk of insults, which increase wound inflammation such as desiccation, increased surface bacteria and use of topical anti-microbials which are toxic to epithelial cells and fibroblasts [8, 26, 27].

Also, there is an increase in the production of granulation tissue in the exposed wound bed. Increased fibroblasts are evident at the base of the chronic wound, in creasing collagen deposition. These fibroblasts tend to organise a very tense type-III collagen matrix in granulation tissue as opposed to the preponderance of type-I collagen in normal mature scar or a rapidly re-epithelialised wound. Myofibroblasts are also in abundance. These cells are most likely involved in the wound contracture formation and dense scar [26–28].

Wound closure should occur prior to 3 weeks to decrease scar. This approach is best demonstrated for burns and cutaneous wounds, which heal by secondary intent or await closure once the wound is considered to be clean. Deep dermal burns and wounds are now preferably closed surgically early by 3 weeks rather than allowed to re-epithelialise over a more prolonged time period. Studies have established that early preservation of dermis and dermal elements prior to wound-bed fibrosis decreases scar formation [29]. In addition, the more dermis that is present on the wound bed on a skin graft, the less likely is it that excess scar will form [30, 31].

## Role of Dermal Elements

It has been well established that a dermis containing active dermal elements is critical for the orchestration of a normal healing process, and the absence of dermal elements will lead to excess scar [30, 38]. The role of the dermis can be divided into its structural component and its biological messenger component.

The scaffolding or structure of the matrix, mainly collagen type I, is made up of the collagen fibres. The collagen lattice provides contact orientation for dividing and migrating cells [30–35]. This cell-guidance system allows for a more organised, less abundant scar. Providing a collagen lattice onto the wound surface prior to scar formation allows for the ingrowth of a new matrix over time. The matrix orchestration system is composed of dermal proteins like fibronectin and growth factors, hyaluronic acid, a complex carbohydrate and the glycosaminoglycan content [35–41].

A deep partial-thickness or full-thickness wound no longer has these key dermal elements. However, there are a number of collagen-matrix products now available which are designed to restore some of the dermal-like properties when placed on a clean full-thickness wound bed [41, 42]. The addition of these dermal-like properties should allow for a more normal healing process, thereby potentially decreasing scar. Providing a dermal-like layer to a full-thickness wound especially a wound, which is closing by secondary intent, should help to control scarring in cutaneous wounds, especially if the components maintain the biological activity of normal dermal elements. Several studies have demonstrated decreased scarring using some of the more novel matrix dressings.

## Summary

The causes of proliferative scar formation in cutaneous wounds is multifactorial. Although there is much not yet known about the genetic and cell–cell signals which cause scar, a number of preventable factors have been well identified. These factors are mainly concerned with the status of the wound bed itself. They can be modified using basic principles of wound care. Tension on the wound edges has been identified for centuries as a cause of scar. The role of excess inflammation has been identified more recently. Proteases and other inflammatory agents clearly stimulate fibroplasia while delaying healing. For the most part, the stimuli which increase inflammation can be significantly attenuated, if not prevented.

The effect of an open wound on subsequent scar formation is well recognised, especially in the burn wound. Waiting for granulation tissue to form on a wound prior to definitive closure is no longer considered the ideal management. Granulation tissue is a factory for excess collagen. Closure over a granulation tissue bed is more likely to lead to hypertrophic scarring. Earlier closure of a wound in the initial phases of cell proliferation and collagen deposition will result in less scar formation.

The importance of the dermis and dermal elements in orchestrating a more architecturally correct wound closure has also now been well established.

## References

1. Su C, Aladeh K, Lee R (1998) The problem scar. Clin Plast Surg 25: 451
2. Ladin DA, Garner WL, Smith DJ Jr (1994) Excessive scarring as a consequence of healing. Wound Repair Regen 3: 6–14
3. Scott P, Ghahary A, Chambers M et al. (1994) Biological basis of hypertrophic scarring. Adv Structural Biol 3: 157–165
4. Erlich HP, Krummel TM (1995) Regulation of wound healing from a connective tissue perspective. Wound Repair Regener 4: 203–210
5. Robson M (2003) Proliferative scarring. Surg Clin N Am 83: 557–569
6. Mast B (1992) The skin. In: Cohen K, Deigelmann I (eds) Wound Healing. WB Saunders, Philadelphia, pp 344–355
7. Polo M, Ko F, Bersello F et al. (1997) Cytokine production in patients with hypertrophic burn scars. J Burn Care Rehab 18: 477–482
8. Bolton L, Fattu A (1994) Topical agents and wound healing. Clinics Derm 12: 95–120
9. Falanger V (1993) Growth factors and chronic wounds. J Derm 19: 711–718
10. Brown-Etris M, Punchello M, Shields D (2000) Final report on a pilot study to evaluate porcine small intestinal submucosa as a covering for partial thickness wounds. Wound Ostomy Continence Nurses Society, June 2000 (poster)
11. Yager D, Chen S, Ward B et al. (1997) Ability of chronic wound fluids to degrade peptide growth factors is associated with increased levels of elastase activity and diminished levels of proteinase inhibitors. Wound Repair Regen 5: 23–32
12. Baxter C (1994) Immunologic reactions in chronic wounds. Am J Surg 167: 12–15
13. Border W, Ruoslahti E (1992) Transforming growth factor β: the dark side of tissue repair. J Clin Invest 90: 1–7
14. Heleda P, Collins M, Tharp M (1993) Mast cell and myofibroblast in wound healing. Dermatol Clin 11: 685–691
15. Linareo H, Kischer C, Doberkofsky M et al. (1972) The histiotypic organization of the hypertrophic scar in humans. J Invest Dermatol 59: 323–331
16. Li J (2003) Angiogenesis in wound repair: angiogenesis growth factors and the extracellular matrix. Micros Res Tech 60: 107–114
17. Linaris H, Larson D (1976) Elastic tissue and hypertrophic scars. Burns 3: 407–412
18. Weitzhandler M, Bernfield M (1992) Proteoglycan glycoconjugates. In: Cohen K, Deigelmann I (eds) Wound Healing. WB Saunders, Philadelphia, pp 195–208
19. Granstein R, Flotte T, Armento E (1990) Interferons and collagen production. J Invest Dermatol 95: 75–80
20. Treld C, Kerstein M (1994) Overview of wound healing in a moist environment. Am J Surg 167: 2–10
21. Winter G (1962) Formation of the scab and rate of epithelialization of superficial wound in the skin. Nature 193: 293–297
22. Robson M, Heggers J (1970) Delayed wound closure based on bacterial counts. J Surg Oncol 2: 379–383
23. Peacock E (1981) Pharmacologic control of surface scarring in human beings. Ann Surg 193: 592–597
24. Vitale M, Fields-Blacke C, Luterman A (1991) Severe itching in the patients with burns. J Burn Care Rehabil 12: 230–233
25. Cohen C, Dergelmonn R (1973) The biology of keloid and hypertrophic scar and the influence of corticosteroids. Clin Plast Surg 9: 297–299
26. Granstein R, Flotte T, Armento E (1990) Interferons and collagen production. J Invest Dermatol 75: 75–80
27. Deitch E, Wheelan T, Rose M et al. (1983) Hypertrophic burn scars: analysis of variables. J Trauma 23: 895–898
28. Rudolph R, Vande Berg J, Ehrlich P (1992) Wound contraction and scar contracture. Cohen K, Deigelmann I (eds) Wound Healing. WB Saunders, Philadelphia, p 92
29. Robson M, Sterbert B, Heggers J (1990) Wound healing alterations caused by infection. Clin Plast Surg 17: 485–492
30. Corps B (1969) The effect of graft thickness: donor site and graft thickness in the hooded rat. Br J Plast Surg 22: 12
31. Nakagawa S (1989) Extracellular matrix organization modulates fibroblast growth and growth factor responsiveness. Exp Cell Res 182: 572–582
32. El-Ghalbzouri A (2002) Effects of fibroblasts on epidermal regeneration. Br J Dermatol 142: 230–243

33. Badylak SF (2002) The extracellular matrix as a scaffold for tissue reconstruction. Cell Develop Biol 13: 377–383

34. Donaldson D, Mahan J (1983) Fibrinogen and fibronectin as substrates for epidermal cell migration during wound closure. J Cell Science 62: 117–127

35. Verani J, Nickoloff B, Riser B, Mitra R, Dixit V (1988) Regulation of keratinocyte motility and proliferation by extracellular matrix components and cytokines. FASEB 2: 1821

36. Raghow R (1994) The role of extracellular matrix in post inflammatory wound healing and fibrosis. FASEB J 8: 823–831

37. Weigel P, Fuller G, LeBoeuf R (1986) A model for the role of hyaluronic acid and fibrin in the early events during the inflammatory response and wound healing. J Theor Biol 119: 219–234

38. Makatsuki T (2003) Reciprocal interactions between cells and extracellular matrix during remodeling of tissue constructs. Biophys Chem 100: 593–605

39. Yates R, Nanney L, Gates R, King L (1991) Epidermal growth factors and related growth factors. Inter J Derm 30: 687–694

40. Krejii N, Houng A, Hansbrough J (1999) Fibroblast sheets enable epithelialization of wounds that do not support keratinocyte migration. Tiss Eng 5: 555–562

41. Saariatho-Kere U, Kovacs S, Pentland A, Olerud J, Welgus H, Parks W (1993) Cell-matrix interactions modulate interstitial collagenase expression by human keratinocytes actively involved in wound healing. J Clin Invest 92: 2858–2864

42. Jones I, Currie L, Martin R (2002) A guide to biologic skin substitutes. Br J Plast Surg 55: 185–193

# The Non-Surgical Management of Hypertrophic Scars and Keloids

M. GOLD

## Introduction

The management and treatment of hypertrophic scars and keloids remains one of the most challenging therapeutic dilemmas facing physicians today. A variety of both medical and surgical approaches have been used over the past 20 years in an attempt to successfully manage these lesions. At the time of this writing, the non-surgical approach to treating hypertrophic scars and keloids usually employs the use of intralesional corticosteroids, topical silicone gel sheeting and the non-invasive vascular lasers and intense pulsed light sources. This chapter will primarily focus on these therapeutic modalities but as well will review some of the other non-surgical approaches to these lesions. In order to fully appreciate the modalities to be reviewed, the chapter will also highlight the epidemiology of these lesions, their aetiology, clinical manifestations, and their pathological considerations, all of which aid in understanding the difficulties we all have when confronting these lesions.

## Epidemiology and Aetiology

Hypertrophic scars and keloids have been found to occur in all races with keloids being more common in dark-skinned individuals. Cohorts have shown that between 6 and 16% of dark-skinned individuals are susceptible to the development of keloids. Hypertrophic scars are more common in light-skinned individuals, although keloids have been described in this group as well. Hypertrophic scars and keloids occur with equal frequency in both males and females. They most commonly form in patients between the ages of 10 and 30 years. A case of congenital keloids has been described and it has been noted that these lesions are rarely found in prepubescent adolescents and in the elderly population.

Hypertrophic scars and keloids are both formed through the excess proliferation of fibrous tissue. Hypertrophic scars are most commonly formed as a physiological response to an injury pattern. The most common injury patterns seen for these lesions to develop include surgical procedures and/or infections in a wound itself. If hypertrophic scars are formed following a surgical procedure, one can usually find that the wound was poorly designed and/or there was too much tension applied to the closed wound. Hypertrophic scars undergo a rapid growth phase during the first 6 months following the injury pattern; then they will show a regression phase which can last for the following 6 months. They usually form on areas of the body which have the thickest skin, such as the back. Most importantly, pathological examination shows that these lesions will remain within the original border of the wound itself.

The most common aetiological factor for the development of keloids is trauma. Keloids can develop within 1 year of the traumatic insult – most are noted to occur within 2–4 weeks of the injury pattern. Keloids result from an inherited alteration in the development of collagen. Traumas which have been associated with keloid formation include: following a surgical procedure, laceration injuries, bite injuries, burns, vaccinations and tattoo placement, to name a few. The formation of keloids depends upon the skin tension and motion of the wound, the wound's orientation to the normal skin tension lines and factors associated with the wound-healing cascade. Most importantly, pathological examination of keloids shows that these lesions grow beyond the peripheral borders of the wound. Keloids are most commonly found on the back, shoulders, chest and earlobes.

Family history is also very important in the development of keloids. Both autosomal dominant and autosomal recessive inheritance patterns have been described. Multiple keloids in the same individual are usually associated with more symptoms and morbidities than those with a single lesion. A variety of dermatological diseases have been reported to be associated with the development of keloids. These include acne vulgaris, acne conglobata, dissecting folliculitis of the scalp, hidradenitis supporativa, pilonidal cysts, foreign body reactions, some connective tissue disorders and infections. Connective tissue disorders associated with the development of keloids include Ehlors–Danlos syndrome, Rubenstein–Taybi syndrome, pachydermoperiostosis and scleroderma. Infections associated with keloid development have included folliculitis, pyodermas, vaccinia, and varicella.

Clinically, both hypertrophic scars and keloids present as raised lesions which occur at the site of trauma in the majority of individuals. Keloids are generally more firm than hypertrophic scars, more pruritic, tender and nodular. If pruritus is seen as a symptom in these lesions, it may be severe and associated with an active growth phase component of the lesion. Both hypertrophic scars and keloids may have multiple shapes, sizes and colours seen; remember hypertrophic scars remain within the border of the wound, whereas keloids grow beyond the border of the wound.

Histologically, both hypertrophic scars and keloids exhibit a similar appearance. Both begin with an early inflammatory phase. Fibroplasia is seen with an increase in vascularity and an associated perivascular mononuclear cellular infiltrate. During this time there is an increase in the production of proteoglycans, the beginning of collagen fibre formation and bundling of these fibres, and an increase in the number of mast cells. In hypertrophic scars, the fibroplasia and vascular proliferation decreases by the end of the fifth week following the injury. The collagen fibres are seen to become more parallel at this time and compression of normal structures under the skin occurs. This phenomenon gives these lesions their typically described histological appearance of whorls of hyalinised collagen which will proceed to the border of the wound itself. Keloids, as already noted, will continue to grow beyond the wound border. In addition, keloids are more cellular than normal tissue, have more extracellular material as compared to normal skin and are more fibrous than normal skin. They have been shown to have an increase in DNA, mast cells and proteoglycans component compared to normal skin. Propyl-hydoxylase activity, associated with the synthesis of collagen is increased. The increased proteoglycans component stops collagenase digestion which allows continued growth of these lesions.

## Management of Hypertrophic Scars

The most important and perhaps simplest approach to management is prevention itself. Properly planned surgical procedures following the normal tension lines of the skin will help minimise the risk of hypertrophic scars and keloids. Proper wound closure with appropriate tension on the closed wounds will minimise the chance of development of these lesions. Early intervention as soon as the formation of a hypertrophic scar or keloid is noticed will allow the clinician to use tools available to minimise the final outcome of the scar. It is also important to keep in mind that most physicians will use a combination of therapies when treating hypertrophic scars and keloids, although we are going to evaluate these therapeutic modalities on an in-dividual basis. Also, the literature is deficient in the reporting of randomised, controlled clinical trials for many of the non-surgical approaches to hypertrophic scar and keloid management – this is important in determining whether reproducibility from small prospective trials and case reports seen in the literature is truly viable.

The non-surgical approach to hypertrophic scars and keloids consists of numerous choices. These include, among others: intralesional corticosteroids, topical silicone gel sheeting, laser and pressure therapy, radiotherapy, cryotherapy, adhesive microporous paper tape therapy and several others including the emerging therapies of interferon injections, intralesional 5-fluorouracil and bleomycin injections. A full list of therapeutic options is listed below. Of all the therapies listed, only intralesional corticosteroids and topical silicone gel sheeting have shown efficacy data in controlled randomised clinical trials. Despite our best intentions, recurrence rates for hypertrophic scars and keloids remain high, no matter which of the modalities is used. Recurrence rates as high as 40–55% have been reported – that is why combination therapies may be the best approach to these lesions.

Intralesional corticosteroids remain the most widely used and recognised therapy available for hypertrophic scars and keloids. The exact mechanism of action for their use in hypertrophic scars and keloids remains unknown. They may affect the collagenase pathway, stopping continued growth of these lesions. They may be used alone or in combination with other therapies, where their efficacy seems to be

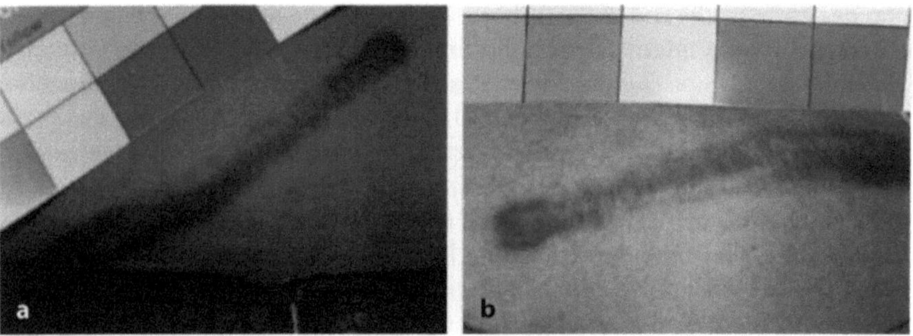

**Fig. 1. a** Prior to intralesional corticosteroids. **b** Post-intralesional corticosteroids

enhanced, especially with a surgical procedure, cryotherapy and laser therapy. Most lesions will flatten with intralesional corticosteroid therapy; complete resolution of the scar is not very common (Fig. 1). Response rates for intralesional corticosteroids have been reported to vary from 50–100%, with recurrence rates noted to be from 9–50%.

### Non-Surgical Options for Hypertrophic Scars and Keloids

- **Commonly reported**
  - Intralesional corticosteroids
  - Topical silicone gel sheeting
  - Laser therapy
  - Pressure therapy
  - Cryotherapy
  - Radiotherapy
  - Interferons ($\alpha, \beta, \gamma$)
  - Intralesional 5-fluorouracil
  - Intralesional bleomycin
- **Other therapies reported**
  - Intramuscular and oral methotrexate
  - Topical tretinoin cream
  - Electron beam radiation
  - Interstitial radiotherapy
  - Oral antihistamines
  - Oral colchicine
  - Oral pentoxyphilline
  - Oral penicillamine

There is no one injection technique or delivery system known to be superior to another. The most common medicine used for the injection is triamcinolone acetonide, in concentrations from 3 mg/ml to 40 mg/ml. Dermatologists tend to use less dilute triamcinolone acetonide than plastic surgeons; the physician must be comfortable with the dose and amount of medicine given. Intralesional injections may be given at 2- to 4-week intervals – the higher concentrations given less often than the more dilute medicine. Several delivery systems are available to administer the intralesional corticosteroids. These include the basic needle/syringe method, Leur-Lok devices, and mechanical injectors – physicians should use whichever system they are most comfortable using. Injections should be given with 30-gauge needles (on occasion 25-gauge) and at 1-mm intervals directly into the scar being treated.

The biggest drawback to the use of intralesional corticosteroids is the associated adverse effects often seen with this approach. Injection pain is seen in virtually all patients, even when physicians have tried to use lidocaine in combination with the triamcinolone. Up to 63% of patients will develop other adverse reactions to intralesional corticosteroids, including skin atrophy, depigmentation at the injection site and associated telangiectasia formation. Frank skin ulceration and skin necrosis have also been reported following aggressive intralesional corticosteroid injections.

Topical silicone gel sheeting has been used for over 20 years in treating hypertrophic scars and keloids. The first reports of its effectiveness were its use in treating hypertrophic scars from burn injuries.

Several reports followed the original descriptions documenting the effectiveness of topical silicone gel sheeting in reducing thermal injury scars. In 1985, Quinn reported that there were no effects with regard to pressure, scar temperature or oxygen tension within the scar to explain how topical silicone gel sheeting was effective in these lesions. The hydration of the skin was altered with an evaporative water loss 1/2 that of the normal skin and the stratum corneum provided a reservoir for fluid. Davey, in 1986, stated that the topical silicone gel sheet is impermeable, acts as the stratum corneum in reducing haemostasis, decreasing hyperaemia and fibrosis, and thus alteration of the final scar result. By 1989, non-burn keloids were being evaluated using topical silicone gel sheeting with improvements noted in 86% at 2 months. This author performed the first dermatological trials with topical silicone gel sheeting, published in 1993. The open-labelled trial showed over 80% improvement in scar thickness at 3 months and 75% improvement in scar colour back towards normal skin colour at 3 months. The first controlled clinical trial in dermatology followed in 1994 by the author. One half of the hypertrophic scar or keloids were treated with the topical silicone gel sheeting; the other half served as the control. The results showed between 75–90% improvement in scar thickness and scar colour returning towards normal at 3 months. In addition, several patients were treated with carbon dioxide laser surgery and either used topical silicone gel sheeting following the procedure or not – there was a significant difference in preventing recurrences in patients who used the topical silicone gel sheeting compared to those who did not in this small group. Finally, thermal injury patients with hypertrophic scars or keloids were included in the trial. One hundred percent responded in scar thickness, 80% in scar colour towards normal. A number of other investigators reported similar findings over the next several years. In all, 8 randomised controlled studies and a mega-study of 27 trials demonstrate that topical silicone gel sheeting is safe and effective for the management of hypertrophic scars and keloids. In 2000, this author published a report on the possible prevention of hypertrophic scars and keloids using topical silicone gel sheeting in susceptible individuals by using the material as prophylaxis following a surgical procedure. The results of this controlled clinical trial also supported its safety and efficacy. Examples of topical silicone gel sheeting are shown in Fig. 2.

Topical silicone gel sheeting works through occlusion and hydration for its effect. Other totally occlusive dressings such as the polyethylene films, or the semi-occlusive dressings such as polyurethane films, have not shown evidence of efficacy, and evidence of other materials, including glycerine and other non-silicone-based materials, is mixed, at best. Some formulations of silicone oil have been effective in treating hypertrophic scars, although their scope was limited. A variety of topical silicone gel sheeting products is available; the clinical trials were carried out using industry leaders containing pure adherent medical grade silicone.

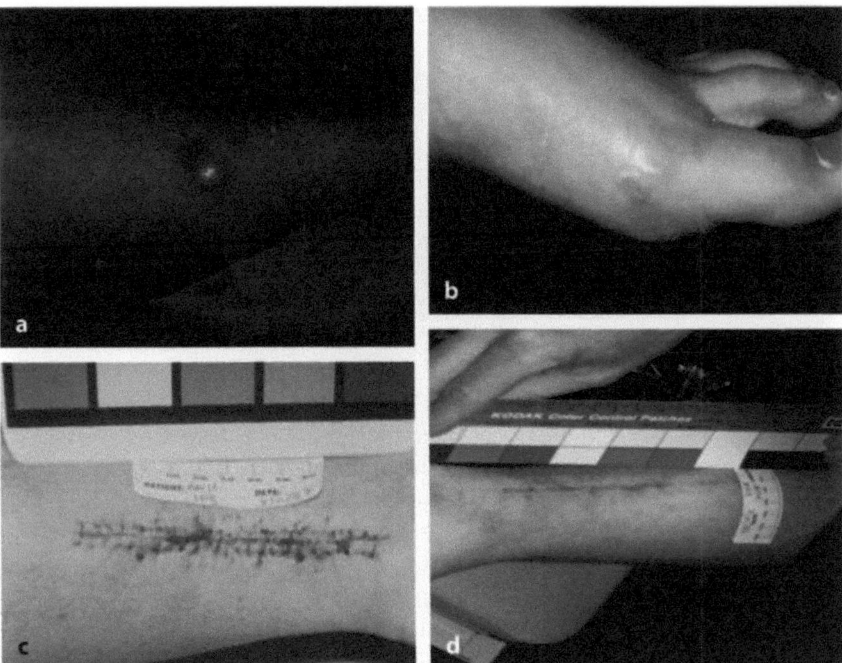

Fig. 2. **a** Prior to topical silicone gel sheeting therapy. **b** Post-topical silicone gel sheeting therapy. **c** Immediate post-operative wound in high-risk scar former. **d** Six-month follow-up of topical silicone gel sheeting used as prophylaxis

A variety of laser systems have been used to treat hypertrophic scars and keloids over the years. The primary laser system studied early on was the carbon-dioxide laser system. Carbon-dioxide lasers cause non-specific thermal destruction of the target through its natural absorption of water. Early reports suggesting good results with less scarring soon gave way to high recurrence rates when these devices were used alone. This author has reported on the successful use of the carbon-dioxide laser and topical silicone gel sheeting as prophylaxis in the treatment of hypertrophic scars and keloids.

Other laser systems have also been used for management of these lesions. The argon lasers, popular in the 1970s, failed to show long-term improvement and had high recurrence rates. More specific systems, such as the yttrium-aluminium garnet (Nd:YAG) laser, the flashlamp-pulsed dye laser and the non-laser intense-pulsed light source, have been used to target the blood vessels in the hypertrophic scar or keloid. Up to 60% of patients have had their lesions flattened with the Nd:YAG laser with long-term follow-up and several reports have demonstrated the efficacy of the pulsed dye laser and intense pulsed light device (Fig. 3), with improvements noted in 57–83% of cases treated. A recent investigation with the pulsed dye laser has shown very rapid resolution of scar stiffness and erythema as well as improvement in the quality of the final scar result when the laser therapy is performed within 2 weeks of a surgical procedure. Most laser surgeons would agree that treating the

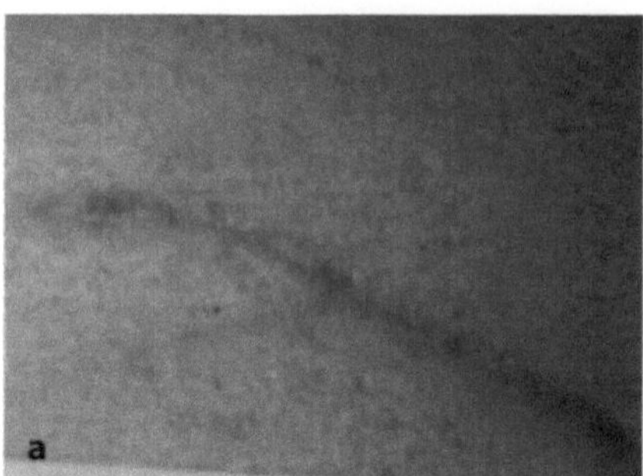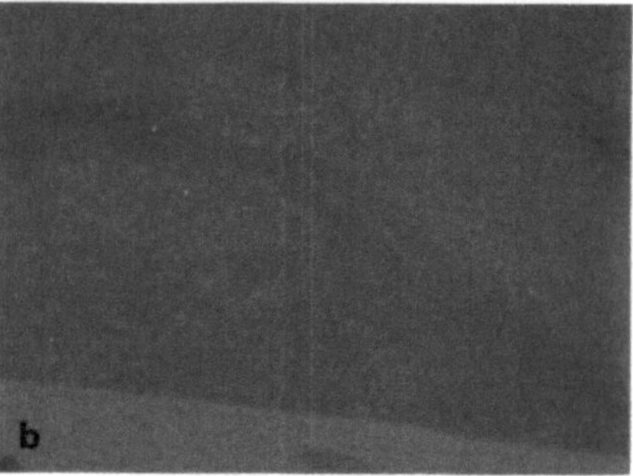

**Fig. 3. a** Prior to intense-pulsed light therapy. **b** Post intense-pulsed light therapy

associated erythema with the vascular specific light sources is a useful therapeutic option for hypertrophic scars and keloids. Combination therapy with intralesional corticosteroids may be very useful for resistant lesions.

Pressure therapy has been a standard therapeutic modality in burn centres for many years in treating hypertrophic scars and keloids. In order for pressure therapy to be effective, pressure must be maintained between 24 and 30 mmHg, which exceeds the inherent capillary pressure seen in these lesions. Up to 12 months of therapy is required, and an overall efficacy remains questionable as seen in a large prospective randomised trial of 122 patients who did not show enhanced scar maturation or diminished hospital stays by wearing pressure garments.

Radiotherapy has been used as monotherapy and in combination with surgical procedures to treat resistant and recalcitrant hypertrophic scars and keloids. Used solely, radiotherapy remains controversial, due to several reports in the literature of cancer formation following this monotherapy. Response rates of 10–94% have been reported, with recurrence rates noted to be between 50 and 100%. Results with combination therapies have been mixed, with reports showing 25–100% improvement. Randomised, prospective clinical trials with radiotherapy are lacking.

Cryotherapy has been reported to be successful in treating newly formed hypertrophic scars and keloids. Flattening of lesions has been reported in 51–74% of cases treated with this modality. Adverse effects, including pain and post-treatment hypopigmentation, limit this therapy to very skilled cryosurgeons.

Some physicians feel that the use of adhesive microporous hypoallergenic paper tape to fresh surgical incisions may be helpful in preventing hypertrophic scars and keloids. Several uncontrolled clinical trials have reported on its use; specifically on its preventative capabilities. It may work through mechanical and occlusive means.

Several other non-surgical treatment options warrant mention at this time. They include the use of interferons, intralesional 5-fluorouracil and bleomycin injections. Interferons ($\alpha$, $\beta$ and $\gamma$) have demonstrated an ability to increase collagen breakdown. Improvements in hypertrophic scars have been seen, and they may be more beneficial than triamcinolone acetonide in preventing recurrences following surgical procedures. The injections are painful and expensive. Intralesional 5-fluorouracil has been used as monotherapy and in combination with triamcinolone acetonide to treat hypertrophic scars and keloids. Preliminary data look promising and adverse effects appear to be low. Bleomycin intralesional injections have been shown to be useful in treating hypertrophic scars and keloids resistant to triamcinolone acetonide injections. More defined research with prospective clinical trials is warranted for these emerging therapies.

## Summary

The treatment of hypertrophic scars and keloids remains a difficult task for the physician faced with these lesions. The evidence-based literature for the non-surgical approach to hypertrophic scars and keloids is lacking in its scope. Intralesional corticosteroids and topical silicone gel sheeting have shown efficacy in prospective, controlled clinical trials. Other modalities for treating these lesions have also been reported to be useful, although controlled clinical trials are not very widespread. Physicians should utilise the medical literature and their training/experience in guiding them in deciding which therapies will be best for their patients who present for treatment of hypertrophic scars and keloids.

# Surgery of Scars: Hypertrophic, Keloid and Aesthetic Sequellae

T.A. MUSTOE

## Introduction

In order to develop a coherent decision tree for the surgical treatment of hypertrophic scars and keloids, it is important to understand some of the basic factors that influence the resolution of wound healing and the development of scar, and by implication how to prevent hypertrophic scars in patients that are at high risk.

## The Process of Wound Healing

The injury from a surgical incision is quickly repaired by an influx of inflammatory cells which release growth factors and cytokines that drive cell proliferation and matrix synthesis. Although there are still many gaps in the understanding of this tightly orchestrated process, even less is understood about the resolution phase of wound healing, which lasts for many months to even years. The quality of the scar is dependent on the rapid resolution of inflammation and resulting excess matrix synthesis while achieving sufficient scar strength through matrix remodelling and collagen cross-linking to prevent scar widening.

In optimal healing after incisional wounding which occurs with a minimal fine scar (the outcome in essentially all animal wounds), at 1 week post-injury, histological analysis reveals an intensely proliferative wound with a predominantly macrophage cellular infiltrate. By 2 weeks, the inflammatory cells and many of the fibroblasts are disappearing through the process of apoptosis [1], and collagen accumulation has peaked. Over the next several months collagen remodelling and increased cross-linking results in continued gains in tensile strength, and the resulting scar is a fine line. In wounds that become hypertrophic, (limited almost entirely to human wounds), the inflammatory phase is prolonged, with persistence of cellular proliferation, continued collagen accumulation, with a gradual stabili-sation in collagen accumulation over many weeks or months and eventual gradual partial resolution. The signals that result in resolution of wound healing are unknown, and therefore strategies to reduce scarring have been relatively non-specific: reduction of inflammation with agents like steroids, interference with cell proliferation (radiation and intralesion chemotherapeutic agents) and interference with collagen synthesis either directly or indirectly by interfering with the TGF-B pathway [2].

In keloids, which represent a unique situation very different from hypertrophic scars, a proliferative process ensues months to years after the initial injury, with a self-perpetuating process without a clear resolution phase. The signals that result in keloids are unclear, but have a clear genetic predisposition, and have cellular abnormalities such as altered p53 expression or altered response to stimulation by TGF-B that persist in cells cultured ex vivo [3, 4]. However, in patients with a genetic predisposition often a persistent inflammatory stimulus such as a pierced ears with irritation from earrings or ingrown hairs can be the cofactor that results in a frank keloid.

## Controllable Factors that Lead to Hypertrophic Scarring

One particularly important observation regarding the inflammatory process that occurs in normal wound healing is the dramatic effect that re-epithelisation has on inducing apoptosis in the underlying granulation tissue and the suppression of inflammation [5, 6]. Scars resulting from second-degree burns or partial-thickness injury from laser or dermabrasion virtually never become hypertrophic if epithelisation is complete within 7–10 days, and in younger patients with a more vigorous inflammatory and proliferative response, hypertrophic scars occur in essentially every patient in whom epithelisation is delayed beyond 18 days (Fig. 1). These obser-vations have very large implications for the surgical treatment and prevention of hypertrophic scars: to close incisions in a way that optimises rapid epithelisation and minimises irritation from sutures, to mimic the effects of a keratinised epithelium with the use of semi-occlusive taping or silicone gel sheeting and pay meticulous attention to achieving complete skin graft take when covering an open wound [7].

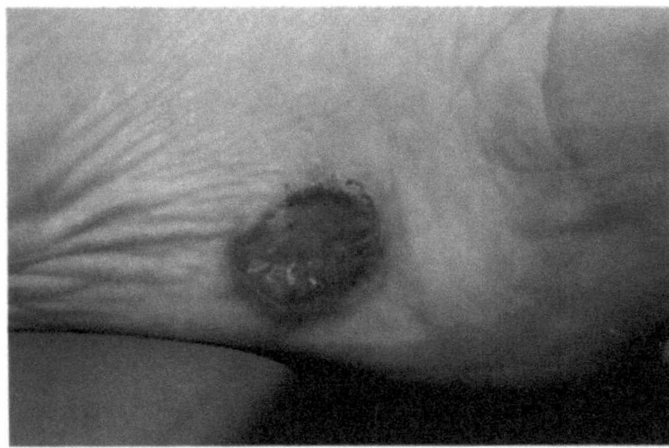

Fig. 1. This patient had a skin graft after excision of scar tissue on the sole of the foot. Note that there is a rim of hypertrophic scar at the edge of the graft where epithelisation was delayed. This is a typical location where epithelisation is delayed

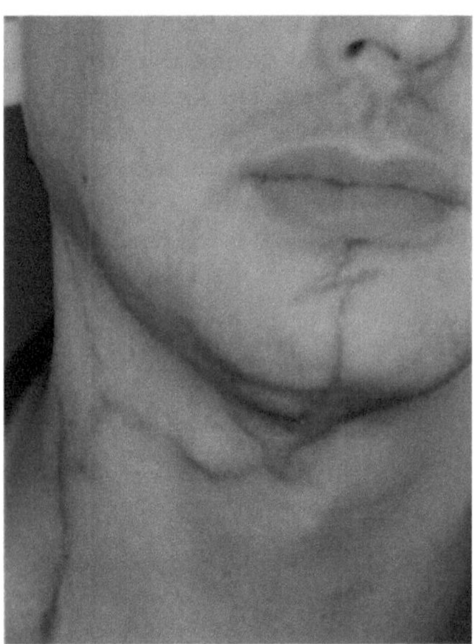

**Fig. 2.** This young adult patient with an increased predisposition to form hypertrophic scars had the entire length of his surgical incision closed with an identical meticulous technique. In areas of motion (and tension) the scar segment became hypertrophic

Another critical factor regarding the difference between a wound that heals with a fine scar and one resulting in significant collagen accumulation (scar hypertrophy) is the degree of tension at the wound site. One reason that all animals heal without hypertrophic scar formation is their loose non-adherent skin (compared to human skin), which can contract without induced mechanical tension in the dermis. There is a great body of evidence at the cellular level of the signal transduction effects on mechanical stress with induced cell migration, alignment, and – more importantly – cell proliferation and collagen synthesis [8]. In human wounds, areas of tension such as the shoulder (due to motion) and sternum (due to skin tightness) and upper breast (due to weight of breast) frequently result in hypertrophic scars, due to the mechanical stresses at the cellular level and the resulting signal transduction. Wounds closed after excision resulting in tension (such as abdominoplasty) frequently result in hypertrophic scars, unless suturing techniques are utilised which effectively splint the wound for the months it requires for the scar to regain tensile strength approximating normal skin (Fig. 2).

## Techniques to Prevent Hypertrophic Scarring in Surgical Wounds

All patients benefit from surgical techniques that minimise and optimise scarring. The key issues, aside from good surgical principles, are to minimise trauma to the dermal edges. Heavily traumatised tissue will result in inflammation that can result in hyperpigmentation and increased scarring. Sometimes excessive traction on tissues with retractors can produce an ischemia reperfusion injury which may be sufficient to result in marginal necrosis. Even a fraction of 1 mm of necrosis at the skin edge is sufficient to result in delayed epithelisation and prolonged inflammation at the skin margin as the non-viable cells need to be phagocytosed and carried off. If a small incision necessitates extensive traction for appropriate visualisation, it is often better to simply excise the damaged skin edge and accept a marginally longer incision than suture heavily injured tissue. However, skin can be gently grasped with toothed forceps to optimise suture placement, without skin injury.

### Suture Techniques

In general, no more sutures should be used than necessary to achieve an optimal closure. Intradermal sutures can later extrude (spit), causing scarring at the point of extrusion. Cutaneous sutures or surgical clips will leave suture marks if left in more than a week, and so the most widely applicable technique for suture closure is a layer of interrupted deep dermal sutures followed by a continuous superficial intradermal closure. However, multiple studies have demonstrated that surgical metal clips will give a quality of scars equivalent to sutures if properly used with careful skin approximation. Nevertheless, very precise skin closure is more achievable with fine sutures placed meticulously in areas like the face. An excellent alternative to sutures for epithelial approximation once the dermis has been closed is cyanoacrylate adhesive, which has been available in the USA since 1998. The quality of the scars is equivalent to suturing. If the closure is under no tension and the skin does not tend to gape, then absorbable sutures, or cyanoacrylate adhesive or a cuticular suture, removed soon enough to avoid suture marks will give an excellent closure.

If even mild tension is present, careful thought as to suture choice is in order. In the USA, the most widely used absorbable sutures are monocryl (Ethicon), polygalactate (Vicryl, Ethicon) and a very similar polymer, lactomer (Polysorb, United States Surgical/Davis and Geck) and polyglycone (Maxon, Davis and Geck). They all lose half their tensile strength within 3 weeks. At that time the surgical incision has gained only about 10% of its eventual strength, and if the skin is under tension, 3 weeks of dermal splinting by the sutures is insufficient to prevent scar widening and hypertrophy. In an excellent study by Elliot and Mahaffey [9], a group of patients had one half of a two layer surgical closure done with intradermal absorbable sutures, followed by a cutaneous closure with sutures that were removed in 1 week. In the other half of the incision, a single cutaneous closure was used, without intradermal sutures. After 6 months there was no difference in the width or appearance of the incisions. On the other hand, a polyprolene intradermal suture left in for 6 months had a major beneficial effect on scar width. Given the time course in gain of tensile strength based on classical animal studies, this clinical observation is expected. What is still unknown is whether sutures can be left in for less than 6 months.

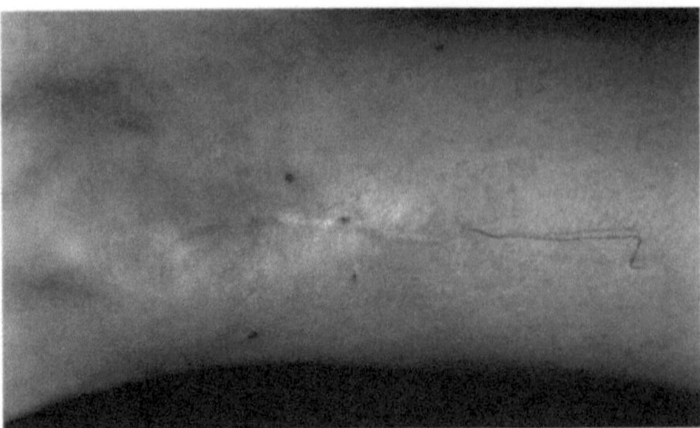

**Fig. 3.** This patient had a melanoma widely excised, with closure of the tight lower leg skin under significant tension. With placement of a prolene suture (typically left in for 6 months or greater, after cutting the end off to prevent irritation), there is no widening of the scar after 2 months, when this photograph was taken

There are some absorbable sutures available that will keep 50% of their tensile strength for up to 6 weeks (i.e. polydioxanone, PDS, Ethicon). For many surgical closures this may provide sufficient dermal splinting to give optimal scar outcomes. However, for incisions closed under significant tension such as abdominoplasties, the author has observed a significantly better outcome if sutures are left in for longer than 3 months versus removal in 6 weeks. Scars that stretch subject to tension will double their width between 3 weeks to 3 months, and will increase another 50% between 3 and 6 months. Our standard closure for incisions under tension on the torso or lower extremity has become 3–0 polygalactate or lactomer deep dermal suture, followed by a superficial continuous polypropylene intradermal stitch, which we leave in for 6 months (or indefinitely) in incisions closed under significant tension (Fig. 3). This technique has been used for many years and has a number of advantages: relatively quick closure, predictability and a complete absence of knots (the stitch is locked at either end rather than use knots). Occasionally, the polyproprolene suture will partially extrude after a few months, but the inflammatory reaction is generally minimal, and because the polyproprolene is so slippery, it can be removed with relative ease. Another alternative is to use intradermal clear 5–0 nylon sutures placed in the deep dermis with buried knots and a cutaneous closure of choice. This option can be used in areas like the face where the dermis is relatively thin.

A key issue is the effectiveness of the suture in splinting the wound. This requires large dermal bites, and a requirement that the suture be anchored so that it will not slide through the tissue, releasing tension. Polypropylene has the advantage that it is slippery, and thus is relatively easy to remove, but for shorter incisions nylon which is stickier, will more effectively resist sliding through the tissue. An alternative approach is to knot the suture at each end, but the knot may extrude before 6 months and have to be cut, releasing tension so that the suture no longer effectively splints the wound. Another very slippery stitch which is effective for evening tension in a purse string stitch (for a periareolar closure) is polytetraflourethylene (Goretex, Gore). However, even with the best techniques, if the dermis is thin or weak or the tension is great, the sutures will cut through the dermis and not effectively splint the dermis, so that scar-widening or hypertrophy can still result.

## Choice of Incisions

A key issue in achieving optimal scars is the choice of the direction of the excision. Whenever possible, the incision should fall along a relaxed skin tension line, which in general follows parallel to the direction of wrinkles in a given area of the face, or parallel to a flexion crease on an extremity. Asking a patient to contort their facial muscles is a good way to determine the direction if it is in question, but usually it is obvious, such as a horizontal incision in the forehead to follow the skin creases rather than a vertical scar.

Another important factor to consider is the tendency for linear incisions to contract such that an incision over a convex surface will tend to produce an indentation, while incisions will tend to produce a web over a concave surface. In addition, very short scars have a tendency not to be visible, because the eye is trained to notice motion or long lines. Therefore, breaking up a linear scar with a short step or zigzag will both prevent indentations or webbing over non-flat surfaces, and will also make the line difficult for the eye to follow, and therefore be less visible. For this reason w-plasty (a running w) has often been advocated for revision of a linear scar. Unfortunately, it is not always successful. The potential advantages of a running w can be more than offset by the tendency of small triangular flaps to pucker as they contract, and for minor delays in healing at the ends of the triangles. Any delay in epithelisation will prolong inflammation, and lead to enough localised scar hypertrophy to offset the theoretical benefits of a w-plasty. In the absence of pre-existing scar contracture, we have found it generally better to revise a scar by careful excision and re-approximation, using the supportive measures discussed below to prevent scar contracture and optimise healing in the post-operative period. However, if there is indeed significant contracture, serial z-plasties, which can be as short as 4–5 mm in length if necessary, can be quite effective in correcting the contracture and, with appropriate post-operative care and meticulous suturing, the trap-door deformities from the triangular flaps can be minimised.

## Post-Operative Care

As discussed above, when an open wound is epitheliased, epithelial-mesenchymal cell signalling occurs with a down-regulation of inflammation. If the wound has been open less than 2 weeks, the inflammatory process inherent with an open wound is transient enough that there is rarely hypertrophic scar formation. A well-coapted surgical incision will epitheliase within 48 h and form a water barrier. However, the epidermis over the incision will not form a mature keratin layer for a much longer period of time. This may be the reason for the observation that semi-occlusive taping (which in effect mimics the keratin layer as a water barrier) when placed on a fresh incision has a very beneficial effect in minimising incisional erythema (a marker of inflammation), and leads to improved outcome. Although this observation has not been proven with prospective randomised studies, there is a supportive study [10], and an international group of experts reached a consensus that it was beneficial [7].

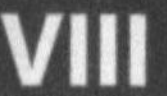



Our routine is to place two layers of paper tape (or steristrips) over the incision (parallel rather than perpendicular) with the help of an additional adhesive, and leave them in place for up to 2 weeks. If the skin is traumatised, or it is believed that there will be significant exudates resulting from oedema, inflammation and breaks in the epithelial barrier, then an alternative is to place a semi-occlusive ointment on the incision to keep the epidermis well hydrated.

In patients who are at increased risk for hypertrophic scarring, including patients under the age of 40, patients with a personal or family history of hypertrophic scarring or patients from ethnic and racial groups with increased risk for hypertrophic scarring, in addition to careful attention to appropriate choice of suturing technique as discussed above and early management of the incision with taping, consideration should be given to the use of silicone-gel sheeting which is started after removal of the surgical tapes 1 to 2 weeks post-operative, or as soon as the wound is epitheliased. There are multiple randomised studies demonstrating its efficacy in both the prevention and treatment of hypertrophic scars, as outlined in a recent review and multiple previous papers [7, 11, 12]. These points will be discussed in other chapters in more detail. For patients who are showing signs of development of scar hypertrophy marked by increasing erythema, early scar elevation and pruritis, early treatment with insoluble steroids such as triamcinolone can be very useful.

## Surgical Treatment of Established Hypertrophic Scars

The surgical treatment of established hypertrophic scars can be very challenging and frustrating. The underlying genetic predisposition to hypertrophic scarring can overwhelm the best surgical care. Once a hypertrophic scar is well established, with a widened as well as elevated appearance, non-surgical methods can only ameliorate a bad problem, but result in a narrow fine scar. In general, if the cause of the hypertrophic scar was prolonged inflammation due either to infection, poor wound closure, delayed epithelisation or failure to effectively splint an incision under tension (with sutures that maintain their tensile strength for months, or by external splints), then there is reason for optimism in the outcome. The scar can be excised, and then closed using the principles discussed above, but with particular attention to permanent sutures to splint the dermis (either clear nylon or pull-out polypropylene), early scar occlusion and later application of silicone-gel sheeting. Another extremely useful adjunct is the use of insoluble steroids (i.e. triamcinolone) which can be layered into the wound at the time of closure. The steroids will delay development of wound strength, but effective suture can overcome this problem. However, it is a mistake to inject the steroids into the tissues adjacent to the open wound: the result is a profound delay in healing that can frequently lead to secondary wound dehiscence. Running z-plasty or w-plasty should in general be avoided. The increased length of the incision and inevitable delays in epithelisation at the tip of the flaps usually more than offset any gains in disguising the scar. However, selective use of z-plasty can be used to relieve skin tension; also lengthening scars where there is contraction can be quite effective.

Hypertrophic scars in hair-bearing areas present specific challenges. The hair follicles can get caught up in the scar with resulting ingrown hairs and increased inflammation, and revising the scars may be particularly frustrating. Close follow-up, with judicious use of local steroid injections, can be useful, but often the results in these areas are disappointing. Minimising the use of absorbable sutures can be helpful.

## Surgical Treatment of Keloids

Keloids are the most challenging problems to treat. Although there is always a genetic predisposition, like hypertrophic scars, keloids often occur in the setting of recurrent or prolonged inflammation. The most common location of keloids is from pierced earrings, in which the trauma of placement of the earring, combined with irritation from foreign bodies, is an ongoing source of inflammation. Another frequent location is in hair-bearing areas where ingrown hairs are a source of ongoing inflammation, and a third area shows high sebaceous activity such as the central chest, where the combination of tension due to the relative tightness of the skin, and inflammation from blocked glands can cause a scar to develop into a keloid and then relentlessly spread as the production of scar blocks more glands, resulting in more inflammation and an ongoing stimulus. Simple surgical excision and closure without additional measures may result in a recurrence rate as high as 90%. Steroid injections will work in perhaps 50% of cases, applied at the time of surgery, layered into the wound and then used aggressively post-operatively, with any sign of recurrence almost always manifested by pruritis before hypertrophy is significant.

The more severe keloids need more aggressive treatment. Although the use of post-operative radiation is considered controversial by some authors, with appropriate shielding and use of high-energy machines, precise dosimetry is possible, virtually eliminating risks to any area other than the scar for future development of radiation-induced malignancies. Although that risk is not zero, many practitioners consider the risk acceptably low when considering the morbidity of an unsuccessfully treated keloid [13]. We have found that radiation will not have a significant deleterious effect on the take of a skin graft. For the treatment of a deforming recurrent ear keloid, we have found that partial excision of the keloid, in effect carving the remaining tissue into the shape of the ear lobule so there is no net loss of ear shape, and using the epithelium (with a thin layer of underlying dermis) taken from the excised keloid as a skin graft to cover the raw surface, and then immediately radiation (from 1200 to 2000 rads in five divided doses) is an effective way to treat the problem (Fig. 4). Even with radiation, keloids can occasionally recur, but they are amenable to re-excision and a second dose of radiation.

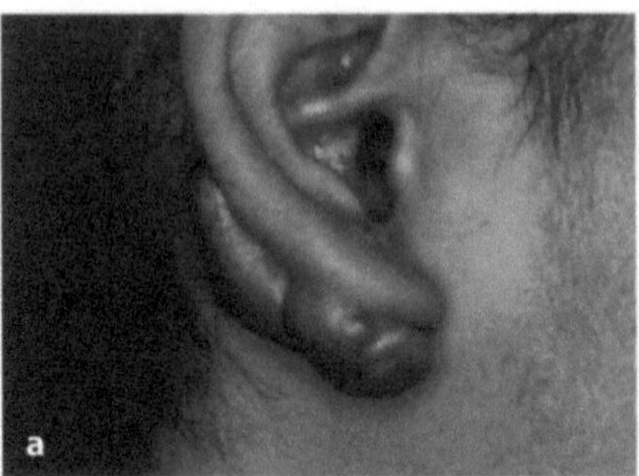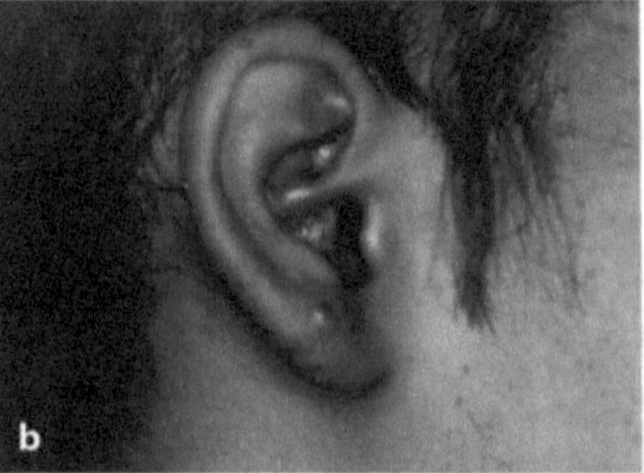

**Fig. 4.** This patient with an ear keloid that had recurred after excision and steroid injections, was treated with excision of the keloid, to preserve the natural shape of the ear lobule, and grafting of raw surface with a skin graft taken from the excised keloid and then radiated with 1200 rads over five divided doses beginning the day of surgery. **a** Prior to treatment. **b** Following excision, grafting and radiation

In summary, consideration and understanding of the general principles underlying optimal wound healing and early resolution of inflammation, and use of suturing techniques to successfully splint scars healing under tension for prolonged periods of time, will lead in a high proportion of cases to fine surgical scars that patients find acceptable.

## References


1. Desmouliere A, Redard M, Darby I, Gabbiani G (1995) Apoptosis mediates the decrease in cellularity during the transition between granulation tissue and scar. Am J Pathol 146: 56–66
2. Shah M, Foreman DM, Ferguson MW (1995) Neutralization of TGF-β1 and TGF-β2 or exogenous addition of TGF-β3 to cutaneous rat wounds reduces scarring. J Cell Sci 108: 985–1002.
3. Khouri RK, Mustoe TA (1992) Trends in the treatment of hypertrophic scars. In: Habal MB (ed) Advances in plastic and reconstructive surgery, vol 8. Mosby Year Book, St. Louis
4. Niessen FB, Spauwen PH, Schalkwijk J, Kon M (1999) On the nature of hypertrophic scars and keloids: a review. Plast Reconstr Surg 104: 1435–1458
5. Marcus JR, Tyrone JW, Bonomo S, Xia Y, Mustoe TA (2000) Cellular mechanisms for diminished scarring with aging. Plast Reconstr Surg 105: 1591–1599
6. Brown DL, Kao WW, Greenhalgh DG (1997) Apoptosis down-regulates inflammation under the advancing epithelial wound edge: delayed patterns in diabetes and improvement with topical growth factors. Surgery 121: 372–380
7. Mustoe TA, Cooter R, Gold M, Hobbs R, Ramelet AA, Shakespeare P, Stella M, Teot L, Wood F, Ziegler U (2002) International clinical guidelines for scar management. Plast Reconstr Surg 110: 560
8. Carlson, Longaker, M. J Surg Res 2002 zzz???
9. Elliot D, Mahaffey PJ (1989) The stretched scar: the benefit of prolonged dermal support. Br Journal Plastic Surg 42: 74–78
10. Reiffel RS (1995) Prevention of hypertrophic scars by long-term paper tape application. Plast Reconstr Surg 96: 1715–1718
11. Ahn ST, Monafo W, Mustoe TA (1989) Topical silicone gel: A new treatment for hypertrophic scars. Surgery 106: 781–787
12. Ahn ST, Monafo W, Mustoe TA (1991) Topical silicone gel for the prevention and treatment of hypertrophic scar. Arch Surg 126: 499–504
13. Botwood N, Lewanski C, Lowdell C (1999) The risks of treating keloids with radiotherapy. Brit J Radiol 72: 1222–1224

L. Téot

## Introduction

Problems of skin maturation can have important consequences in terms of quality of life and socio-cultural issues. More easily accepted than the price to pay after a surgical procedure, a problematic scar becomes difficult to live with in the long-term evolution of an early operated congenital malformation or a burn scar in an adolescent. Guidelines have been developed recently, based on a large international consensus, after a large review of EBM proofs obtained in the literature. Silicone and corticosteroid injection gave a good level of proofs, compressive garments are extensively used in burn scars and alternative procedures are still under evaluation. Prevention is usually proposed early in the evolution, and the clinical evaluation must be done early enough to determine the right moment when preventive management must be initiated. The management of hypertrophic scars and keloids is characterised by a wide variety of techniques. Many have been proven through extensive use over the past two decades, but few have been supported by prospective studies with adequate control groups, and in some cases even safety data are lacking. Many new therapies showed early promise in small-scale trials, but these results have not been repeated in larger trials with long-term follow up. Judgement of efficacy has further been limited by the difficulty in quantifying change in scar appearance and the natural tendency for scars to improve over time. Thus, cutaneous scar management has relied heavily on the experience of practitioners rather than the results of large-scale randomised controlled trials and evidence-based techniques.

## Prevention or Treatment

It is much more efficient to prevent hypertrophic scars rather than treat them. Prevention implies using a therapy with the aim of reducing the risk of the problem scar evolving. The transition to a treatment regimen takes place when a true hypertrophic scar or keloid, and not an immature scar, is diagnosed. Conceptually and practically, treatment and prevention regimens can be similar and the following section presents the clinical data for both. Early diagnosis of a problematic scar can considerably impact the outcome. The consensus of the authors is that the most successful treatment of a hypertrophic scar or keloid is achieved when the scar is immature but the overlying epithelium is intact, although this is not, as yet, confirmed in current literature.

## Clinical Assessment Strategy

The Vancouver scale was proposed in 1990 to rate the burn scar. Pigmentation, vascularity, pliability and scar height were assessed independently, with an increasing score being assigned to the greater pathological condition. This scale has proven to be useful for burns scars, and has been validated in this indication. The main difficulty remains to determine as early as possible if a scar will become the source of pathological problems and will require an adapted treatment.

A regular assessment, from month to month, seems useful during the first 3 months, the initial clinical evaluation being realised at the end of the first month after complete healing.

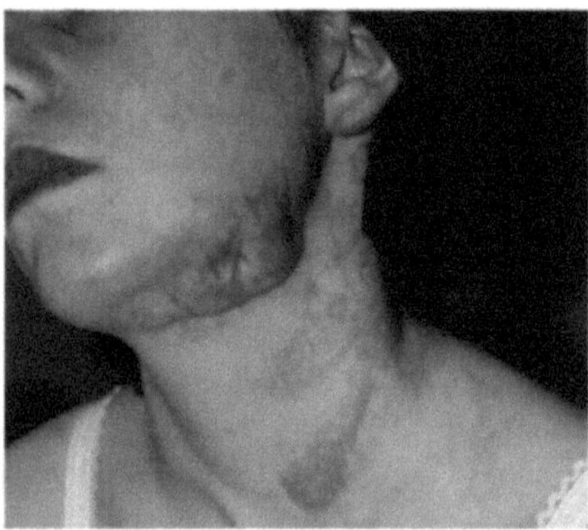

Fig. 1. Linear massive post-burn hypertrophic scar of the mandibular angle

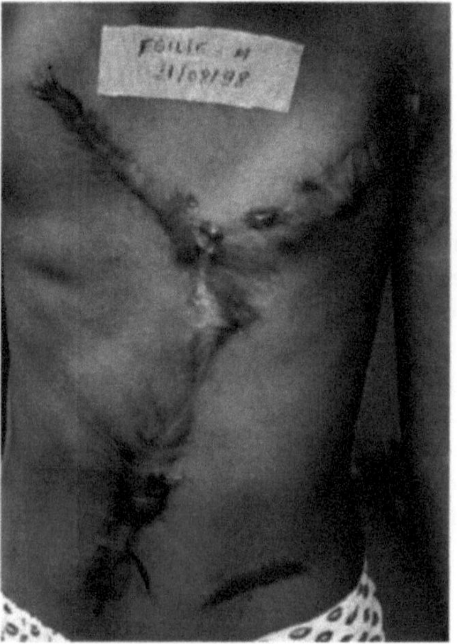

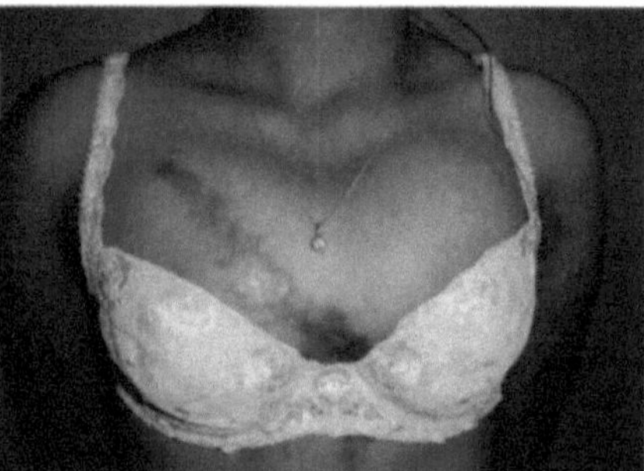

Fig. 2a,b. Large thoracic post-burn scar treated after adolescence using a bilateral mammary prosthesis

### First-Month Evaluation

Clinical assessment will determine the scar's general features, focusing on colour and elevation. At this stage, colour and vascularity seem to be the most important parameters to evaluate correctly. If a scar is red and hypervascular, risks of hypertrophic evolution are important (Fig. 1). Preventive measures such as silicone gel sheets will be useful.

Laser Doppler evaluation can be proposed as a complementary technique to assess hyper-vascularisation.

### Second-Month Evaluation

Clinically, changes in width, height and colour are more easily observed. At this stage, redness is frequently accompanied by a moderate hypertrophy. A purple aspect will reflect an intense hyper-vascularisation. Redness can change in intensity, depending on the anatomical location (more intense on limbs, close to the extremities), the muscular activity (more pronounced after movements) and the outside temperature (Fig. 2).

Itching is often present at this stage, with a maximum intensity when the patient is active and the scar red. Pain is variable, reaching an acme on lower leg scars during movement, generally appearing when standing up. Pain can considerably limit movement in post-burn scars largely extending along the lower limbs. Local treatments can be indicated in the presence of hypertrophy, redness and increase in width. Laser Doppler evaluation can confirm the scar hyper-vascularisation.

### Third-Month Evaluation

The signs are generally evident. Hypertrophy is visible, troubles in pliability and texture are patent (Fig. 3 and 4).

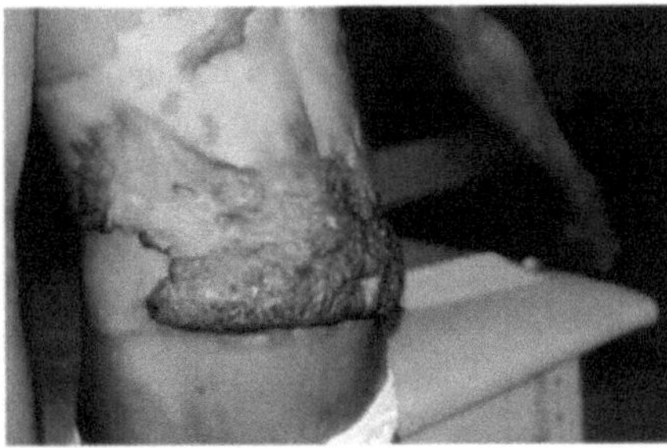

**Fig. 3.** Hypertrophy, troubles in pliability and texture

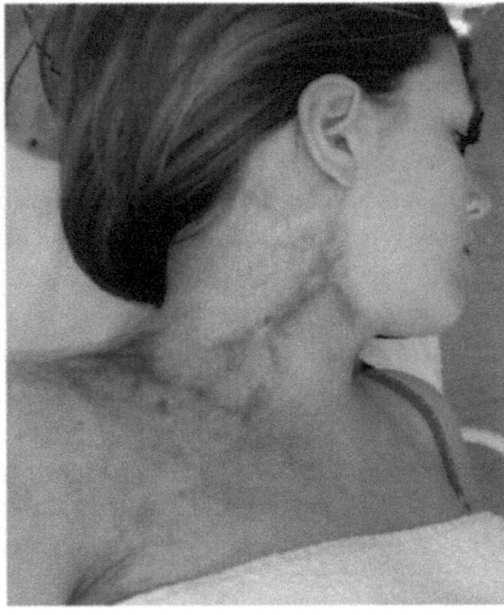

**Fig. 4.** Redness and mild hypertrophy on a post-burn scar of the neck ▸

## Prevention

The clinical evaluation of scars at regular intervals is still one of the main preventive measures. A simple distinguishing of problematic from normal scarring could be beneficial for the patients. Painful, hypertrophic or retractile scars observed after several months of evolution might be easier to manage if seen at an early stage.

An early clinical assessment strategy can be considered as a good preventive measure to control any pathological evolution of scars, whatever the origin of the scar and the intensity of the pathological process may be. The absence of validated tools concerning assessment and clinical measurement of scars must lead to clinical researches, in order to quantify the different pathological aspects, focusing on redness and elevation. Profiles of evolution are more important than one single assessment. In the opinion of many specialists, two successive evaluations realised after the first month and after the second month after complete healing are necessary to prevent transformation into problematic hypertrophy. Early determination of a keloid profile can be determinant to propose and undertake appropriate therapeutic measures.

Proofs of efficiency of silicone gel sheeting and of corticosteroid injections are statistically established. An early management of very active scars will be beneficial to the patient. Every effort must be made to prevent the development of hypertrophic scars or keloids after surgery or trauma. Excellent surgical technique and efforts to prevent post-surgical infection are of prime importance. Special attention should be given to high-risk patients, i.e. those who have previously suffered abnormal scarring, or are undergoing a procedure with a high incidence of scarring, such as breast and thoracic surgery. To our knowledge there has been no large-scale assessment of scar outcomes and risk factors.

Recommended preventive techniques include:

- Hypoallergenic microporous tape with elastic properties to minimise the risk from shearing. Use of taping for a few weeks following surgery is standard practice for the majority of the authors. Although there are no prospective controlled studies documenting its efficacy, the authors' consensus is that it is beneficial.
- Silicone gel sheeting which should be considered as first-line prophylaxis. Use of silicone gel sheeting should begin soon after surgical closure, when the incision has fully epithelialised, and be continued for at least 1 month. Silicone gel sheets should be worn for a minimum of 12 h daily, and if possible for 24 h a day, with daily washing twice. Use of silicone ointments may be appropriate on the face and neck regions, although their efficacy in preventing scarring is unsupported by controlled trials.
- Intralesional corticosteroid injections as second line prophylaxis for more severe cases.

The effectiveness of alternative therapies is limited to anecdotal evidence. Patients at low risk of scarring should maintain normal hygiene procedures, and be provided with counselling and advice if concerned about their scar.

## Surgery

Surgical excision of hypertrophic scars or keloids is a common management option when used in combination with steroids and/or silicone gel sheeting. However, excision alone of keloids results in a high rate of recurrence (45–100%).

Combining surgery with steroid injections reduces the recurrence rate of keloids to less than 50%, with the combination of surgery and peri-operative radiation therapy reducing recurrence to 10%. However, this combination approach is usually reserved for abnormal scars resistant to other treatments.

Hypertrophic scarring resulting from excessive tension or wound complications, such as infection or delay in healing, can be treated effectively with surgical excision combined with surgical taping and silicone gel sheeting. Scars that are subject to tension require substantial physical support.

The authors agreed that the most effective way of splinting scars is by surgical closure with intradermal sutures for at least 6 weeks, and when tension is substantial for up to 6 months. Surgical techniques, the use of dermal substitutes and procedures such as w-plasty and z-plasty, improve the appearance and mobility of contracted burn scars but are not appropriate for immature hypertrophic scars (Fig. 5).

## Conclusion

Scar management and prevention are becoming more and more subtle as progress in controlling the occurrence of scars develops. In most cases, prevention is much better than treatment. A standard post-operative scar must be checked until the third month, a post-burn scar must be observed each month during the first 3 months, and the preventive measures must be extensive. Silicone, corticosteroid injections and compressive garments represent the most evaluated tools.

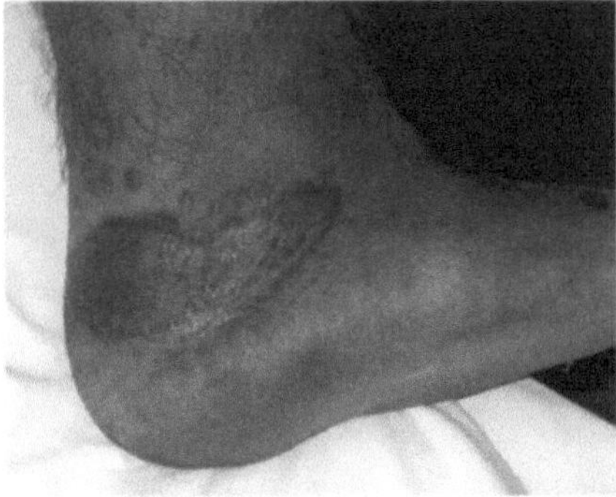

**Fig. 5.** The use of dermal substitute under a skin graft can improve the function but also the aesthetic aspect

## References


1. Baryza MJ, Baryza GA (1995) The Vancouver Scar Scale. An administration tool and its interrater reliability. J Burn Care Rehabil 16: 535–538
2. Boyce ST, Supp AP, Wickett RR, Hoat SB, Warden GD (2000) Assessment with the dermal torque meter of skin pliability after treatment of burns with cultured skin substitutes. J Burn Care Rehabil 21: 55–63
3. Dressler J, Busuttil A, Koch R, Harrison DJ (2001) Sequence of melanocyte migration into human scar tissue. Int J Legal Med 115: 61–63
4. Matsumura H, Engrav LH, Gibran NS et al (2001) Cones of skin occur where hypertrophic scar occurs. Wound Repair Regen 9: 269–277
5. Mustoe TA, Cooter RD, Gold MH et al. (2002) International clinical recommendations on scar management. Plast Reconstr Surg 110: 560–571
6. Siana JE, Rex S, Gottrup F (1992) Comparison of self-reported and observed length, width and colour of scar tissue. Scand J Plast Reconstr Surg Hand Surg 26: 229–231
7. Sullivan T, Smith J, Kermode J, McIever E, Courtemanche DJ (1990) Rating the burn scar. J Burn Care Rehab 11: 256–261
8. Téot L (2002) Clinical evaluation of scars. Wound Repair Regen 10: 93–97

# Psychological Consequences of Facial Scarring

P. PRICE, N. TEBBLE

## Introduction

Currently, dermal scarring is an inevitable consequence of surgical incision. Patients undergoing surgery have a range of issues to address in anticipating their surgical procedure, including expectations of clinical outcome, impact on quality of life and their perceptions of the severity of scarring. For many, the scars will heal well and the final outcome will be a flat, hairless, shiny area of skin; for those unfortunate enough to suffer from hyertrophic or keloid scars, the outcome will be overgrown, raised, red scars. The individual will go through periods when the scar is tight, tender and itchy, and periods of limitations on function due to the contractions that can occur. From a psychological perspective the location of scarring can be of particular importance, especially in visible locations such as the face and neck, back of the hands and lower arms – although for many, especially females, scars in areas associated with intimate contact with others can also be problematic.

It has been estimated that there are up to 400 000 people in the UK with minor disfiguring conditions [1]. However, the effect of facial injury on body image is an area that is largely neglected in the scientific literature [2], with much information coming from general literature, folklore and personal accounts [3]. Although there is growing interest in the topic, it is limited to medical journals which focus on a particular condition or to the social psychology literature [4]. One explanation for the paucity of empirical research on this topic is the basic premise that underlies such research – appearance plays an important role in the perception of an individual by society [5]; a view which many may not wish to support.

This chapter outlines some of the key issues related to the psychological consequences of scarring, including body image, societal responses to disfigurement and factors that can impact on the level of psychological reaction to scarring, as well the concerns that patients have in dealing with scars on a daily basis within a society that places great importance on "looking good".

## Body Image

Lacey and Cumming [6], Birchnell [7], Brown et al. [8] and Newell [2] have all argued that one of the main problems in the literature associated with body image, particularly outside the area of eating disorders, is that the construct has been used in a loose and ill-defined way; without a clear definition the construct is difficult to measure. As the term is not operationalised consistently, the literature has become confused in some areas.

Body image was described first in the 1920s by Head [56], but this was from a neurological perspective; he defined body image as the unity in the sensory cortex developed from past and current body sensations. There is little attempt in his definition to go beyond the location of these sensations within the brain. It is not until the work of Schilder that the construct goes beyond the purely physical. Schilder (1935 cited in [9]) defined body image as "the picture of our own body which we form in our own mind, that is to say, the way in which the body appears to ourselves". Here, body image was described in an inclusive way incorporating somatic, psychological and social aspects of self. However, Goin and Goin [10] defined body image incorporating the emotional significance that we attach to various physical parts of our bodies.

The definition of body image by Price [11] is the one most familiar to nurses: "Body image is the totality of how one feels and thinks about one's own body and its appearance". This definition brings together much of the earlier work, but also adds to the concept as for the first time three elements of body image are incorporated: body reality, body ideal and body presentation. Much of Price's work has focused on how these three elements relate to one another; Price sees the elements existing in a state of tension or balance which together make up a satisfactory body image which humans strive to maintain. The model is important as it is one of the few that goes beyond a mere description of the construct; it has gained a high profile amongst British nurses, not least because it is closely tied to clinical practice. However, many of the assumptions behind the model have not been tested empirically and, as a result, writers such as Gournay et al. [12] state that the model is purely speculative.

The list of factors affecting the development of body image are numerous, but include genetics, socialisation, fashion, peer groups, cultural influences and messages delivered through health education. We enter adulthood with a relatively static perception of our own body and its image. However, whilst age may not be associated with negative aspects [13], there can be little doubt that any significant alteration to our bodies or the image we have of ourselves outside the usual aging process will lead to a range of psychological reactions: this is known as altered body image. The work in relation to altered body image has focused on the impact of trauma, acute wounds and disfigurement, a review of which can be found in Magnan [14]. The work of Papadopoulos and Bor [15] has outlined the potential impact of poor body image on behaviour in patients with chronic skin conditions (see below).

---

### Responses of Those with Poor Body Image

- Edit out social experiences to reinforce existing negative perceptions of self
- View their bodies only as aesthetic objects
- Minimise other positive aspects of their appearance
- They have a heightened sense of body awareness
- They comply with narrow social standards in terms of what is attractive

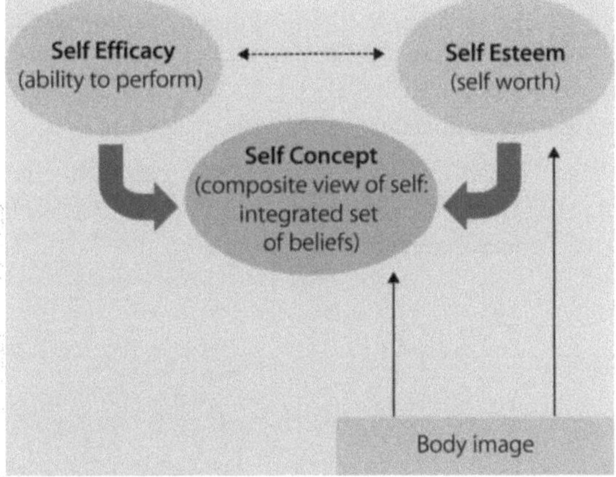


**Fig. 1.** Self and body image

With regard to self-esteem, writers such as Bandura [16] and Neil and Barrell [17] have argued that there is a lack of clarity between the concepts of "self-efficacy", "self-esteem" and "self-concept", whereby researchers and clinicians use the terms interchangeably even though they are not the same. Figure 1 defines these concepts and whilst it is clear that both self-efficacy and self-esteem relate very closely to self-concept, the relationship between the ability to perform tasks and the self-worth associated with those tasks results in a variable, and as yet unquantifiable, relationship between self-efficacy and self-esteem.

The relationship between these aspects of self is complex. The work of Bandura and colleagues has identified a set of circumstances in which the likelihood of feeling a sense of worthlessness may be exacerbated: individuals who have limited competencies in those aspects of life that they hold important, plus, they have exacting standards in terms of self-evaluation, plus, they belong to a socially or culturally disparage group or minority, are much more likely to experience poor self-esteem.

In order to maintain a high sense of self-esteem, individuals must not internalise the negative reactions of others and must remain confident about their ability to cope; this can be exceedingly difficult for patients with significant scarring. Papadopoulos and Bor [15] have shown that those who are able to maintain high self-esteem, whilst experiencing severe dermatological conditions, believe that the negative reaction of others says more about those "others" than about themselves.

Many of the writers already cited in this chapter would argue that body image is closely related both to self-concept and self-esteem. Certainly, self-concept and body image are both influenced by how positively or negatively others appraise us in both our social and cultural environment. Rogers [18] defined self-esteem as the extent to which our real self measures up to our ideal self, and the way we are perceived by others; a definition not dissimilar to that proposed by Price [11] for body image. When discussing body image, Papadopoulos and Bor have argued that

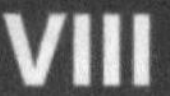



dissatisfaction with a particular aspect of self has been found to cause an overall reduction in self-esteem; this is particularly likely in situations where scarring is visible to others.

Self-esteem is a personal resource that may moderate the effects of disfigurement, incapacitating illness and injury or threatening life events. We know that an altered body image can lead to negative self-esteem in patients who experience acute wounds following trauma, those with dermatological conditions and those that live with long-term disfigurement, including scarring.

## Anxiety

It has been suggested previously that anxiety is a problem for people with facial disfigurement [19]. Sen et al. [20] found that over 30% of patients with maxillofacial trauma (mostly fractures) were anxious or depressed (using the Hospital Anxiety and Depression Scale [21]). Anxiety can have an effect on how people react to situations [22] by leading to the employment of less functional coping mechanisms [23]. Work with cancer patients has suggested that once cancer is cured and worries about physical problems and/or mortality have been removed or alleviated, the focus then shifts to psychological issues [24, 25]. For some patients with scarring as a consequence of the nature of their injuries/condition, their focus would not be concern about survival or any major functional difficulties, leaving the focus of attention on psychological issues such as anxiety.

## The Social Impact of Disfigurement

Social interaction is an area of life where many people experience difficulties – this is particularly the case for those with visible scarring [3, 5, 26, 27]. Disfigurement to the face may be particularly problematic for the patient because of the unique importance of various functions of the face [28, 29]. The face is exposed, the centre of communication, and is central in others' perceptions of us [30]: the face has been found to be the main part of the body to which we attach physical and mental importance [31].

Newell and Marks [32] suggest that the social difficulties experienced by those with facial disfigurements may be due to phobic anxiety specific to social situations. In comparing 112 facially disfigured people with 66 people with agoraphobia and 68 patients with social phobia, the authors found that those with facial disfigurements resembled people with social phobia on social phobia, anxiety and depression subscales of the Fear Questionnaire [33]. The authors refer to a fear-avoidance model that proposes that the difficulties experienced are primarily because of a fear of the response of others in a social situation [34]. The subsequent avoidance of social interactions then perpetuates the problem.

Social skills training can help to improve this situation by enabling a facially disfigured person to cope with potentially difficult situations [4, 35, 36]. However, it could be argued that cognitive behavioural approaches have a greater effect on social situations. These approaches focus on exposure and the interpretation of events [15, 32, 37–39]. In particular, Newell and Clarke [40] found that a leaflet outlining cognitive-behavioural tactics improved anxiety and depression scores (measured by Hospital Anxiety and Depression Scale [21]) as well as scores on the social leisure scale of the Social Adjustment Questionnaire [41].

## Can Minor Injuries Have Psychological Consequences?

Literature in the area has suggested that an injury does not have to be major in order to have a psychological impact on a patient [15, 42–44]. Price's model of body image emphasises the importance of recognising the potential for altered body image in all patients [45], which is an important clinical reminder to us all. It is not so much the change in appearance itself that is of importance, but how an individual reacts to it. A minor injury can still act as a powerful trigger for psychological symptoms [42] and there is no proven relationship between the severity of an injury and the psychological distress experienced [43, 46]. Smith [44] reports that research and experience at *Changing Faces* has shown that a "small mark" can present as many obstacles as a more major disfigurement. Similarly, McGrouther [47] suggests that the impact of an injury on a patient is not directly proportional to the severity of the disfigurement but that other psychological factors are involved. Indeed, current research has suggested, perhaps surprisingly, that adjustment to a major disfigurement may be more straightforward than adjusting to a relatively minor facial disfigurement [48], as minor injuries can leave the individual more uncertain about reactions of others.

These results indicate that far more research is needed in this area, as data are often contradictory. However, from a clinical perspective, we must be careful not to assume that because a wound has healed without significant medical problems and/or is of a size that would be considered medically of little consequence, that the patient is not affected by the outcome. There are many individuals who are struggling to readjust to changes in their appearance, based on physically minor scars.

## Factors that May Influence Psychological Outcomes

Previous research has suggested a number of factors that may influence the psychological outcome of disfiguring injury and scarring. People have different social influences at different ages [13] and it has been suggested that women are more sensitive than men in terms of psychological difficulty following disfigurement [25, 49]. The general health literature suggests that those in a lower socio-economic state are more affected by their health status [50] and it has also been found that the unemployed are at greater risk of developing psychological distress following acute injury [51]. Social support can have an important "buffering effect" on responses to difficult situations [52]; much of this social support is provided by family members and health-care professionals. The impact of social support can be profound: for example, social support was found to positively impact on head and neck cancer survivors' rehabilitation outcomes at 6 months [48], whilst burn survivors who were poorly adjusted were found to have less social support from friends and family [53].

In terms of location, Partridge [54] found that disfigurements located within the communication triangle of the face (between the eyes and mouth) provoked more negative reactions than disfigurements on more peripheral location on the face. In terms of aetiology of injuries, although accidents have been shown to have associated psychological sequel [43], assault has been found to have a greater psychological impact [42].

Several of these factors were tested in a longitudinal study on minor facial scars conducted in an outpatient setting. Tebble et al. [55] followed 63 patients for 6 months and demonstrated that a larger scar size (>4 cm), living alone and aetiology of injury were significantly related to higher levels of self-consciousness and anxiety: those involved in an accident were more likely than those assaulted or involved in a sports injury to have higher scores on both self-consciousness and anxiety. Initially and 6 months later, gender, age, socio-economic group, location of scar, satisfaction with appearance and number of scars were not deemed significant factors. General self-consciousness improved at 6 months but social self-consciousness and anxiety remained the same, indicating that many patients were still concerned about their appearance in social situations and felt anxious about life long after medical help ceased to be available to them. Such studies indicate the desperate need for further research in this area to investigate interventions that may assist people in coping with their scars.

## Summary

In the 21st century the western world is dominated by cultural views that reinforce the idea that "looking good" is important; literature, the media, advertising and the emphasis on celebrity status all contribute to the idea that in order to be considered important or worthwhile, or to "get on" in life, then being "beautiful" or "good-looking" is paramount. Many feel that they cannot compete in such an arena and are often left with poor self-esteem and a level of self-consciousness that can lead to depression and anger. Whilst a change in cultural and societal perspectives towards those who look different has been advocated for some time [54], such a change is likely to take some considerable time.

Those individuals with congenital conditions that lead to disfiguring consequences and those who undergo surgery for whatever reason know that each surgical intervention will result in a further scar. Scarless healing is still, at this time, on the wish-list for the future. Whilst the aim of most surgery is to save lives, and most patients accept that as the priority, once the medical emergency is over, the patient is often left with the rest of his life to deal with the psychological consequences of a new "self": for such patients, scarless healing cannot come quickly enough.

## References


1. Lansdown R, Rumsey N, Bradbury N, Bradbury E, Carr T , Partridge J (1997) Visibly different: coping with disfigurement. Butterworth-Heinemann, Oxford
2. Newell RJ (1999) Altered body-image: a fear-avoidance model of psycho-social difficulties following disfigurement. J Advanced Nursing 30: 1230–1238
3. Houston V, Bull R (1994) Do people avoid sitting next to someone who is facially disfigured? Eur J Soc Psychol 24: 279–284
4. Clarke A (1999) Psychosocial aspects of facial disfigurement: problems, management and the role of a lay-led organization. Psychol Health Med 4: 127–142
5. Bull R, Rumsey N (1988) The social psychology of facial appearance. Springer Vale, New York
6. Lacey JH, Cumming WJK (1988) The neurobiology of the body schema. Br J Psych 153 [Supp 2] 7–11
7. Birchnell SA (1986) Body-image and its disturbances. J Psychosom Res 30: 623–631
8. Brown TA, Cash TF, Milulka PJ (1990) Attitudinal body-image assessment: factor-analysis of the body-self relations questionnaire. J Pers Assess 55: 135–144
9. Dewing J (1989) Altered body-image. Surg Nurse 2: 7–20
10. Goin J, Goin M (1981) Changing the body: psychological effects of plastic surgery. Williams and Wilkins, Baltimore
11. Price B (1990) Body-image: nursing concepts and care. Prentice Hall, New York
12. Gourney K, Veale D, Walburn J (1997) Body dysmorphic disorder: pilot randomised controlled trial of treatment; implications for nurse therapy and practice. Clin Effect Nurs 1: 38–43
13. Janelli LM (1986) The realities of body image. J Gerontol Nurs 12: 23–27
14. Magnan MA (1996) Psychological considerations for patients with acute wounds. Critical Care Nurs Clin North Am 8): 183–193
15. Papadopoulos L, Bor R (1999) Psychological approaches to dermatology. BPS publications, Leicester
16. Bandura A (1997) Self-efficacy: The exercise of control. Stanford University, New York
17. Neil JA, Barrell M (1998) Transition theory and its relevance to patients with chronic wounds. Rehabil Nurs 23: 295–299
18. Rogers CR (1959) A theory of therapy, personality and interpersonal relationships, as developed in the client-centered framework. In: Koch S (ed) Psychology: A study of a science, vol 3: Formultations of the person and the social context. McGraw-Hill, New York
19. Macgregor DA (1997) Facial disfigurement: problems and management of social interaction and implications for mental health. Aesthetic Plastic Surgery 14: 249–257
20. Sen P, Ross N, Rogers S (2001) Recovering maxillofacial trauma patients: the hidden problems. J Wound Care 10: 53
21. Zigmond AS, Snaith RP (1983) The Hospital Anxiety and Depresssion Scale. Acta Psychiatr Scand 67: 361–70
22. Lazarus RS, Folkman S (1984) Stress, appraisal and coping. Springer, New York
23. Dropkin MJ (2001) Coping strategies and coping behaviours in patients undergoing head and neck cancer surgery. Cancer Nurs 24: 143
24. Gamba A, Romano M, Grosso IM, Tamburini M, Cantu G, Molinari R, Ventafridda V (1992) Psychological adjustment of patients surgically treated for head and neck cancer. Head and 14: 218–223
25. Newell R (2000) Psychological difficulties amongst plastic surgery ex-patients following surgery to the face: a survey. Brit J Plast Surg 53: 386–392
26. Malt U, Ugland O (1989) A long-term psychological follow-up study of burned adults. Acta Psychiatr Scand 355 : 94–102
27. Macgregor FC (1990) Facial disfigurement: problems and management of social interaction and implications for mental health. Aesthetic Plast Surg 14: 249–257

28. Ekman P (1978) Facial signs; facts, fantasies and possibilities. In: Sight sound and sense Indiana University Press, Bloomington
29. Shaw W (1981) Folklore surrounding facial deformity and the origins of facial prejudice. Br J Plast Surg 34: 237–246
30. Fawzy NW, Secher L, Evans S (1994) The positive appearance center. Cancer Practice 5: 345–349
31. Kreuger D (1984) Emotional rehabilitation of physical trauma and disability. SP Medical and Scientific Books, New York
32. Newell R, Marks I (2000) Phobic nature of social difficulty in facially disfigured people. Br J Psychiatr 176: 177–181
33. Marks IM, Matthews AM (1979) Brief standard self-rating for phobics. Behav Res Ther 17: 236–267
34. Newell R (1991) Body image disturbance: cognitive behavioural formulation and intervention. J Adv Nurs 16: 1400–1405
35. Robinson E, Rumsey N, Partridge J (1996) An evaluation of the impact of social interaction skills training for facially disfigured people. Br J Plast Surg 49: 281–289
36. Feigenbaum W (1981) A social training program for clients with facial disfigurations: a contribution to the rehabilitation of cancer patients. Rehabil Res 4: 501–509
37. Freedman R (1990) Cognitive Behavioural perspectives on body image change. In: Pruzinsky T (ed) Body images. Development, deviance and change. Guilford Press, London
38. Rosen JC, Retier J, Orasan P (1995) Cognitive-behavioural body image therapy for body dysmorphic disorder. J Consult Clin Psychol 63: 263–269
39. Veale D, Gournay K, Dryden W, Boocock A, Shah F, Wilson R, Walburn J (1996) Body dysmorphic disorder: a cognitive behavioural model and pilot randomised controlled trial. Behav Res Ther 34: 717–729
40. Newell N, Clarke M (2000) Evaluation of a self-help leaflet in treatment of social difficulties following facial disfigurement. Int J Nurs Stud 37: 381–388
41. Marks IM, Hallam RS, Connolly J, Philpott R (1977) Nursing in behavioural psychotherapy. Royal College of Nursing, London
42. Shepherd JP, Qureshi R, Preston MS, Levers BGH (1990) Psychological distress after assaults and accidents. Br Med J 301: 849–851
43. Bisson JI, Shepherd JP (1997) Psychological sequale of facial trauma. J Trauma 43: 496–500
44. Smith H (2000) Challenging disfigurement. Community Practitioner 73: 637
45. MacGinley KJ (1993) Nursing care of the patient with altered body image. Br J Nurs 2: 1098–1102
46. Bryant RA, Harvey AG (1996) Initial post-traumatic stress responses following motor-vehicle accidents. J Trauma Stress 9: 223–234
47. McGrouther DA (1997) Facial disfigurement. The last bastion of discrimination. Br Med J 314: 991
48. Baker CA (1992) Factors associated with rehabilitation in head and neck cancer. Cancer Nurs 15: 395–400
49. Anderson RC, Maksud DP (1994) Psychological adjustments to reconstructive surgery. Nurs Clin North Am 29: 711–724
50. Marmot MG, Stansfield D, Patel C, North F, Head J, White I, Brunner E, Feeney A (1991) Health inequalities among British civil servants. The Whitehall Study. Lancet 337: 1387–1392
51. Joy D, Probert R, Bisson JI, Shepherd JP (2000) Post-traumatic stress reactions after injury. J Trauma Inj Infect Crit Care 48: 490–494
52. Cohen S, Wills T (1985) Stress, social support and the buffering hypothesis. Psychological Bulletin 98: 310–357
53. Browne G, Byrne C, Brown B (1985) Psychological adjustment of burn survivors. Burns 12: 28–35
54. Partridge J (1997) The psychological effects of facial disfigurement. J Wound Care 2: 168–171
55. Tebble NJ, Price PE, Thomas DW (2004) Anxiety and self-consciousness in patients with facial lacerations. J Adv Nurs (in press)
56. Head H (1920) Studies in neurology, vol 2. Oxford University Press, Oxford

# IX Future Perspectives in Wound Management



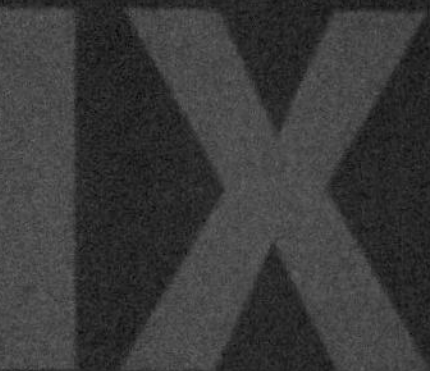

E. ERIKSSON, R. GHEERARDYN

## Introduction

Over the past 30 years our knowledge about skin cells, the extracellular matrix and their interaction through different signalling pathways has grown exponentially.

It started with Howard Green and collaborators developing methods for the in-vitro culture of keratinocytes [1]. This discovery not only allowed the study and manipulation of these cells, but also permitted long-term conservation or expansion in order to provide resurfacing of, for instance, burn wounds.

Bell et al. studied the extracellular skin matrix and developed methods to produce new matrices [2, 3]. They achieved this through modification of allogenic or xenogenic transplants, synthesis of scaffold-induced matrices, or via completely in-vitro-synthesised products. Integra and Apligraf are examples of such engineered products that are being used in clinical practice nowadays.

Cohen received the Nobel Prize for his description of the epidermal growth factor and its effect on various cell types [4]. Subsequently, a large number of growth factors, their antibodies and their receptors have been described. A large amount of research has also been done determining the potential clinical utility of these proteins. For example, PDGF-BB (Regranex) is being used in the treatment of diabetic ulcers and VEGF inhibitors have found a use in cancer treatment [5, 6]. With a large focus in this area, it is likely that more clinical therapies will evolve from this research topic.

Gene transfer, often referred to as gene therapy, is a process involving introduction of DNA or RNA molecules into cells. Its intended result is the production of small signalling proteins that act in either an autocrine, paracrine and endocrine fashion. In animals and plants, gene transfer to germ cells has been done for a few decades in order to add or delete certain characteristics in the genotype. Concerns about safety, ethics, religion and legal issues, will delay germ cell gene transfer in humans.

However, the possibility of eliminating certain birth defects, cancer or diabetes through germ cell modifications offers significant promise to patients at risk, as well as to physicians, politicians and planners dealing with public health issues.

Clinically, prefabrication or prelamination of human tissue has been carried out for at least decades. Millard prelaminated parts of a reconstructed nose in the forehead [7]. Pribaz and collaborators did similar prelamination prior to the transfer of free flaps for reconstruction of the nose and other parts of the face [8]. In addition, skin grafts, grafts of bone, cartilage and blood vessels expand the diversity and the use of these prefabricated flaps to an unexpected level.

## Tissue Engineering

There has been a rapid evolution in what Bell refers to as "the engineering triad", which includes scaffolds, cells and signalling proteins [9].

In the typical tissue-engineering experiment, an absorbable or non-absorbable scaffold is engineered. This structure is then implanted into an animal, in order to allow ingrowth of cells and deposition of the extracellular matrix. Some of these matrices have been seeded with cells prior to implantation [10, 11]. Techniques have also been designed using the matrix as a gene-transfer vehicle [12].

There has been a virtual explosion in the development of cell-culture techniques, especially in skin cells. Overall, culture systems have become more effective and less complicated. For instance, when Howard Green first cultured keratinocytes, he had to use a feeder layer of irradiated fibroblasts. Later, by modifying the keratinocyte growth medium, this layer could be eliminated.

With increased knowledge of the influence of certain factors in the medium, such as calcium ions, one can selectively promote certain cell types in the culture at the expense of other cells. It has also become possible to develop cell lines stably expressing transgenes, which allow further possibilities for research.

Most tissue-engineering experiments have consisted of growing allogenic cells in a synthetic matrix in vitro. It was subsequently transplanted to an animal, which was usually immune-incompetent or immuno-depressed. These experiments have provided proof of principle of the methodology, but two problems still remain to be solved: one is that of providing vascularisation when dealing with a large construct, and the other is overcoming the immune reaction to allogenic cells. Work in both these areas is in progress [13, 14].

## Prefabrication

Prefabrication – perhaps the term prelamination is more correct – is an innovative methodology developed to increase and refine the utility of various flaps. It is based on the idea of creating a pre-shaped flap that will be later transferred to partially or completely replace an anatomic structure. Millard used this technique for the first time to prepare composite forehead flaps, adding skin graft and cartilage in order to provide contour to the nasal alae and tip [7]. Similar principles were used later by Baudet and Pribaz for reconstruction of nasal and facial defects [15, 16].

The term prefabrication is probably best used when a completely new flap is created by the introduction of a vascular pedicle into an area of skin with desirable qualities in terms of availability, thickness, colour and texture. For this purpose, the ideal vascular pedicle might be the omental vessels. In fact, they connect an artery with concomitant veins and they can be harvested with a minimal amount of surrounding tissue. However, it requires a laparotomy and an additional microsurgical procedure for their implantation in the area of prefabrication. Other superficial vascular pedicles that provide blood supply to the skin or to superficial muscles are therefore preferentially used. Sometimes, a section of fascia or muscle is included in order to supply a more extended vascular tree. Finally, it is, of course, possible to combine both principles of prefabrication and prelamination in order to increase the utility of these flaps [16, 17].

In the future, it would be exciting to combine flap prefabrication and tissue engineering. This would not only allow the ingrowth of nutritive vessels into the tissue-engineered part, but also provide a vascular pedicle, which would be easier to use for the microvascular implantation at the recipient site.

## Growth Factors

Growth factors are signalling proteins that bind to receptors on the target cell in order to initiate, enhance or repress certain cell functions. A large number of growth factors have been described to date. A few of the common growth factors involved in wound healing are listed in Table 1.

In 1973, Stanley Cohen published his first report on epidermal growth factor [4]. This started an era of very intensive research into the identification, sequencing and production of these proteins.

However, the initial enthusiasm has been somewhat dampened by the fact that all the studies done on this topic resulted in few formulations useful in clinical practice.

This appears to be mainly due to three reasons. First, the precise molecular and cellular functions of many of the factors are still not completely elucidated. Second, although it is easy to deliver precise amounts of growth factors in vitro, we lack the appropriate tools to reach an efficient expression in vivo in most cases. Third, many pathophysiologic processes such as wound healing have a great redundancy of growth factors influencing the same molecular mechanisms. Their expression is most often overlapping and influencing each other. As a result, a single deletion or over-expression of one factor has not yet had a great impact. However, in studies of pressure sores and diabetic ulcers, PDGF BB (Regranex) was found to have significant clinical benefits [5]. Most recently, certain statins that block the effect of vascular endothelial growth factors (VEGF) in tumours have been shown to have beneficial effects on neoplastic development [6, 18].

## Gene Therapy

Somatic gene therapy, which is the introduction of DNA or RNA molecules into eukaryotic cells for the purpose of expression of a protein, is very common laboratory practice. There are also approximately 600 clinical protocols being conducted under the outlines of the FDA and the RAC related to this technique (www.wiley.co.uk/genetherapy/clinical). No treatment has yet reached a level of approval for standard clinical practice. The most notable early successes have been achieved in the case of single gene defects, such as severe congenital immune deficiency and haemophilia. The second area of early success is vaccination with gene-transfer techniques. In a European study, congenital immune deficiency could be corrected through a retroviral gene transfer protocol [19, 20]. A complicating factor has been the early development of leukaemia, which may be related to the gene-transfer process because of the non-specific integration of the retrovirus into the host genome. In the clinical treatment of haemophiliacs, factor VIII has been delivered with gene transfer [21]. Patients have been improved and the number of bleeding episodes has been greatly reduced, avoiding the need for transfusion.

A large number of gene-transfer studies have been reported in the area of wound healing, starting with a study by Andre et al. [22]. For in-vitro gene transfer, almost any described vector system can be used. For direct in-vivo gene transfer, naked DNA (delivered by particle bombardment, single injection or microseeding) has been successfully used [23–25]. Viral transfection methods using adenovirus, adeno-associated virus, lentivirus and Herpes simplex I have also been described [26]. Electroporation and liposomal gene transfer have also been utilised, both in vitro and in vivo [27, 28]. With these methods, it is possible to achieve protein expression of physiological magnitudes and above. Even more, with the addition of systems for regulation of expression, it has become possible to determine the timing of onset of expression as well as the level of expression via different mechanisms of regulation. For example, the amount of systemic or local tetracycline administered precisely controls the expression of the proteins transferred within the virus [29]. This also makes the system much safer.

## Future Avenues

Tissue engineering is a very exciting field that is likely to be of great importance in the future. It would probably benefit from combining with the areas of wound repair, gene therapy and even flap prefabrication. In the broad sense, the work in these fields aims at engineering cells and tissues. Great strides have been made, particularly in the field of in-vitro tissue engineering; but increasingly, the focus is moving toward in-vivo tissue engineering, which is creating new methodologies and potential therapies. In this context, signalling molecules, particularly the growth factors, have crucial importance. The initiation and control of their enhanced or decreased expression with gene-therapy techniques is, therefore, a promising road to further progress.

## References

1. Green H, Rheinwald JG, Sun TT (1977) Properties of an epithelial cell type in culture: the epidermal keratinocyte and its dependence on products of the fibroblast. Prog Clin Biol Res 17: 493–500.
2. Bell E (1991) Tissue engineering: a perspective. J Cell Biochem 45: 239–241
3. Bell E, Ivarsson B, Merrill C (1979) Production of a tissue-like structure by contraction of collagen lattices by human fibroblasts of different proliferative potential in vitro. Proc Natl Acad Sci USA 76: 1274–1278
4. Cohen S (1972) Epidermal growth factor. J Invest Dermatology 59: 13–16
5. Robson MC et al. (1992) Platelet-derived growth factor BB for the treatment of chronic pressure ulcers. Lancet 339: 23–25
6. Thompson WD, Li WW, Maragoudakis M (1999) The clinical manipulation of angiogenesis: pathology, side-effects, surprises, and opportunities with novel human therapies. J Pathol 187: 503–510
7. Millard DR Jr, McLaughlin CA (1979) Abbe flap on mucosal pedicle. Ann Plast Surg 3: 544–548
8. Pribaz JJ, Fine NA (1994) Prelamination: defining the prefabricated flap – a case report and review. Microsurgery 15: 618–623
9. Bell E (2000) The tissue engineering triad. In: Lanza R, Langer R, Vacanti J (eds) Principles of tissue engineering, 2nd edn. Academic Press, Orlando, USA, pp XXV–XXVI.
10. Teebken OE et al. (2000) Tissue engineering of vascular grafts: human cell seeding of decellularised porcine matrix. Eur J Vasc Endovasc Surg 19: 381–386
11. Teebken OE, Pichlmaier AM, Haverich A (2001) Cell seeded decellularised allogeneic matrix grafts and biodegradable polydioxanone-prostheses compared with arterial autografts in a porcine model. Eur J Vasc Endovasc Surg 22: 139–145
12. Bonadio J (2000) Tissue engineering via local gene delivery. J Mol Med 78: 303–311
13. Niklason LE, Langer R (2001) Prospects for organ and tissue replacement. JAMA 285: 573–576
14. Fischbeck JA et al. (2001) Genetic modification of alphaGal expression in xenogeneic endothelial cells yields a complex immunological response. Tissue Eng 7: 743–756
15. Baudet J, Pelissier P, Casoli V (1995) 1984–1994: Ten years of skin flaps. Prefabricated flaps. Ann Chir Plast Esthet 40: 597–605
16. Pribaz JJ, Fine N, Orgill DP (1999) Flap prefabrication in the head and neck: a 10-year experience. Plast Reconstr Surg 103: 808–820
17. Garfein ES, Orgill DP, Pribaz JJ (2003) Clinical applications of tissue engineered constructs. Clin Plast Surg 30: 485–498
18. Kaushal V et al. (2003) Potential anticancer effects of statins: fact or fiction? Endothelium 10: 49–58
19. Bordignon C et al. (1995) Gene therapy in peripheral blood lymphocytes and bone marrow for ADA-immunodeficient patients. Science 270: 470–475
20. Gordon EM, Anderson WF (1994) Gene therapy using retroviral vectors. Curr Opin Biotechnol 5: 611–616
21. Powell JS et al. (2003) Phase 1 trial of FVIII gene transfer for severe hemophilia A using a retroviral construct administered by peripheral intravenous infusion. Blood 102: 2038–2045
22. Andree C et al. (1994) In vivo transfer and expression of a human epidermal growth factor gene accelerates wound repair. Proc Natl Acad Sci USA 91: 12188–12192
23. Eriksson E et al. (1998) In vivo gene transfer to skin and wound by microseeding. J Surg Res 78: 85–91
24. Hoeller D et al. (2002) Gene therapy in soft tissue reconstruction. Cells Tissues Organs 172: 118–125
25. Jeschke MG et al. (2001) Possibilities of non-viral gene transfer to improve cutaneous wound healing. Curr Gene Ther 1: 267–278
26. Galeano M et al. (2003) Adeno-associated viral vector-mediated human vascular endothelial growth factor gene transfer stimulates angiogenesis and wound healing in the genetically diabetic mouse. Diabetologia 46: 546–555
27. Cupp CL, Bloom DC (2002) Gene therapy, electroporation, and the future of wound-healing therapies. Facial Plast Surg 18: 53–57
28. Jeschke MG et al. (2001) Therapeutic success and efficacy of nonviral liposomal cDNA gene transfer to the skin in vivo is dose dependent. Gene Ther 8: 1777–1784
29. Yao F, Eriksson E (1999) A novel tetracycline-inducible viral replication switch. Hum Gene Ther 10: 419–427
30. Vranckx JJ (2004) Gene transfer of growth factors for wound repair. In: Rovee DT, Maibach HI (eds) The epidermis in wound healing. CRC Press, Boca Raton, USA, p 267

# X Conclusions



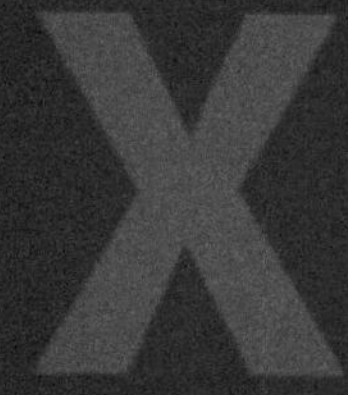

# Changing Philosophies in Reconstructive Surgery

L. Téot, P. Banwell, U. Ziegler

## Introduction

Over the past three decades, reconstructive surgery has flourished with the help of pioneering anatomical works. Isolation of a composite block of tissue on its blood supply has allowed the use of local, regional, distant and free flaps. This surgical approach has heralded tremendous advances and over recent times we have also seen the introduction of pre-fabricated and perforator-based flaps, thus adding to the sophistication of our surgical armamentarium.

However, our perspective on the interface between reconstructive surgery and the endeavours of clinically relevant wound-healing biology has shifted. Utilising these ideas, a philosophy of a staged reconstruction has now been proposed as an alternative to a one-stop-reconstructive approach. Tissues are rebuilt from the depth to the surface. The advantages of this attitude are progressively demonstrated in terms of aesthetic and functional results. Unfortunately, it has been argued in some quarters that reconstructive surgeons may utilise flap techniques too readily in the surgery for both acute and chronic wounds. Should this be the case? We therefore propose some pathways which may help the reader choose when *not* to operate using a radical procedure.

## Staged Reconstruction: Enlightenment or Controversy?

The use of flaps in reconstructive surgery is now routine throughout the world. Indeed, such techniques form the cornerstone of advanced procedures within the reconstructive ladder. Transfer of vascularised tissue to close a defect provides an instant and reliable solution to an often difficult problem. However, these advanced reconstructive procedures have purely been in the domain of plastic surgeons working with allied specialties, who have championed improvements in resuscitation, intensive therapy care and infection control.

In parallel, many surgeons have introduced topical negative-pressure (TNP) therapy into their practice. In particular, orthopaedic and traumatology departments have found this technique revolutionary in that many complex wounds may be covered with prolific granulation-tissue formation following application. In turn, this has down-staged the wound and avoided the need for flap reconstruction. Is it therefore time to change our practice and adopt a similar philosophy?

## Staged Reconstruction

### Debridement

The natural evolution of a wound allowed to heal is based upon four successive stages: debridement, granulation-tissue formation, keratinisation and maturation. At the end of this process, a scar will form, and its quality and suppleness will determine final outcome and patient satisfaction. In the future, we anticipate that patients will become increasingly aware of their scars after surgery. In particular, plastic surgeons and dermatologists will commonly see the psychological sequelae concerning their scars.

For many years, sharp surgical debridement has demonstrated its efficiency in the wound-healing process, but many other techniques, initially developed for chronic wounds, have demonstrated an important role. Surgeons have to be trained to practice elective debridements using the scalpel, but alternative techniques like powerful hydrojets and bio-surgery are becoming progressively available in some units.

### Granulation Tissue

Over the past decade, topical negative-pressure therapy has modified the management of wounds in many ways and has penetrated many surgical disciplines. Looking at published reports on efficiency of the technique, it is obvious that colleagues involved in different disciplines have successfully tested the technique.

In the arena of trauma, results have surpassed the expected thus changing practices at a level which is close to revolution. Previously, the number of reconstructive surgical flap procedures performed was significant, often leading to large blood loss and potential complications during the post-operative period, especially when using the micro-surgically revascularised flaps. However, the introduction of topical negative-pressure therapy to downgrade surgical procedures has been met with considerable success. Simplification of the global procedure is one of the most striking points of this technique. Versatility and adaptation to the different anatomical situations and to the aetiologies (burns, degloving trauma, amputations, partial loss of substances) has made the therapy a standard of care in many trauma units. The simple principles of the therapy also relate to the dressing procedure itself, and nursing staff are easily trained to control and manage the dressing changes, with or without the presence of a surgeon.

However, most of the plastic surgeons, trained in flap surgery, have been more cautious in integrating this therapy into their practices; in contrast, trauma surgeons, thoracic surgeons and most of the medical disciplines have readily adopted its use. The ideal situation should be a good collaboration between plastic surgeons trained in TNP therapy working together with other disciplines. In fact, TNP therapy can be considered as the first step towards reconstructive process, even if in some situations the TNP can end in a rapid complete closure of the wound. When integrated in the staging reconstruction process, TNP obtains a granulation tissue covering the entire surface of the wound.

The granulation tissue observed in chronic wounds or acute wounds becoming chronic (over than 6 weeks of evolution) has always been considered in the past as a potential source of infection. This heterogeneous tissue was always considered as tenuous and skin grafting sometimes unsuccessful. Since the demonstration of a minimal bio-burden resulting from treatment with TNP, a new era has commenced. This granulation tissue can now be covered with skin grafts, but also by skin substitutes, highly susceptible products whose sensibility to micro-organisms is well known. It is likely that TNP has an important role in augmenting skin substitute take rates.

## Dermal Reconstruction

Artificial dermis is now used all over the world and the results can be considered as promising. In acute wounds, post-cancer resections, as well as in burns and in resurfacing procedures, the use of artificial dermis is now accepted by most surgeons around the world. Based on bovine collagen, this structure does not induce immunological problems, and can be considered as a transient scaffold progressively revascularised, issuing to a dermis covered secondarily with a thin skin graft bringing a souple aspect, with a real dissociation between the skin graft covering it and the underlying aponeurosis.

Artificial dermis has been progressively adopted as a secure technique, leading, in trained hands, to a scar whose volume is very different from the one obtained with skin grafts alone. The obtained skin is flat, supple and following the movement, due to the lack of adherence to the underlying aponeurosis. Colour of the recipient site can more or less be chosen when harvesting the skin graft close to the recipient area.

Integra, and other dermal substitutes do not contain any cells susceptible to cause immunological problems or to transmit diseases. They are now also being used in various clinical situations such as after skin-tumour excisions, in acute burns, in trauma and in scar resurfacing.

## Epidermal Formation

Cultured epithelial autografts have now been used for over a quarter of a century with take rates approaching in excess of 75%. Many factors influence this take, and particularly the ability of the cells to promote angiogenesis. Some attempts of "boosting" the cells using gene therapy are under progress. Covering a wound using such techniques is still exceptional, but new alternatives have emerged. Skin substitutes, including living dermal and epidermal cells, are now available and have demonstrated their potential role in large randomised control trials in chronic wounds.

## Infection

Young surgeons, confronted with these methods, may feel somewhat daunted with the prospect of deciding appropriate usage. In particular, new technologies are developing very quickly and we are now faced with solutions we did not expect some years ago.

In the area of local infection, new dressings and silver-based anti-infectious agents can now help the surgeon in correcting the local disorders imposed by the bio-burden. The use of general antibiotics is progressively regressing, due to a better understanding of local mechanisms in bacteriology.

## Discussion

The staged reconstruction concept is not very different from what was called the spontaneous healing process previously, except that the spontaneity is encouraged by solutions adapted to the cell behaviour and respecting them. A flap will in most of the cases be considered as a foreign body when analysing the dynamics of the anatomical area of the recipient site. Results obtained after staged reconstruction look promising, essentially because results observed at distance of surgery are more close to a natural healing.

## Conclusion

Much fundamental and clinical research is still required in the field of tissue reconstruction. Whilst flap surgery has demonstrated its usefulness in saving limbs, covering vital structures and bringing new functions to denervated and devascularised areas, it is now possible to utilise alternative solutions to map the surface and depth of the wound defect and approach clinical wound healing from a staged perspective.

# XI  Appendix



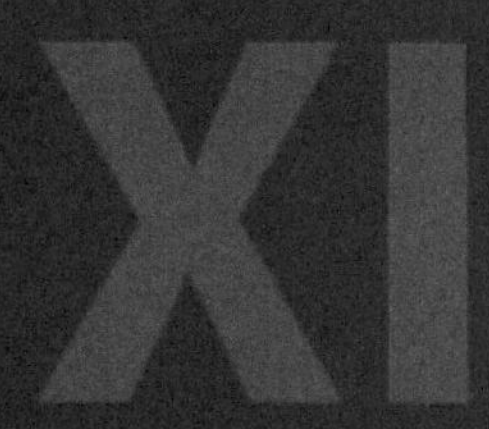

# Index